Fifth Edition

HEALTH IN THE LATER YEARS

Rebecca L. Ferrini, MD, MPH
Medical Director
Edgemoor DP SNF
County of San Diego Health and Human Services Agency

Armeda F. Ferrini, PhD
Professor Emerita
Department of Health and Human Services
California State University, Chico

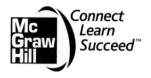

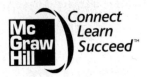
HEALTH IN THE LATER YEARS, FIFTH EDITION

Published by McGraw-Hill, a business unit of The McGraw-Hill Companies, Inc., 1221 Avenue of the Americas, New York, NY 10020. Copyright © 2013 by The McGraw-Hill Companies, Inc. All rights reserved. Printed in the United States of America. Previous editions © 2008. No part of this publication may be reproduced or distributed in any form or by any means, or stored in a database or retrieval system, without the prior written consent of The McGraw-Hill Companies, Inc., including, but not limited to, in any network or other electronic storage or transmission, or broadcast for distance learning.

1 2 3 4 5 6 7 8 9 0 DOC/DOC 1 0 9 8 7 6 5 4 3 2

ISBN 978-0-07-802849-6
MHID 0-07-802849-3

Vice President and Editor-in-Chief: *Michael Ryan*
Vice President & Director Specialized Publishing: *Janice M. Roerig-Blong*
Publisher: *David Patterson*
Executive Editor: *Christopher Johnson*
Developmental Editor: *Darlene M. Schueller*
Marketing Coordinator: *Colleen P. Havens*
Senior Project Manager: *Joyce Watters*
Design Coordinator: *Margarite Reynolds*
Cover Designer: *Studio Montage, St. Louis, Missouri*
Cover Image Credit: *Marianna Gontarz York*
Buyer: *Laura Fuller*
Media Project Manager: *Sridevi Palani*
Compositor: *Cenveo Publisher Services*
Typeface: *10/12 Times Roman*
Printer: *R. R. Donnelley*

Library of Congress Cataloging-in-Publication Data

Ferrini, Rebecca L.
  Health in the later years / Rebecca L. Ferrini, Armeda F. Ferrini. — 5th ed.
    p. cm.
  Armeda F. Ferrini's name appears first on the earlier editions.
  Includes bibliographical references and index.
  ISBN 978-0-07-802849-6 (alk. paper)
  1. Older people—Health and hygiene. 2. Health. I. Ferrini, Armeda F. II. Title.

RA777.6.F46 2013
613'.0438—dc23   2011048959

The Internet addresses listed in the text were accurate at the time of publication. The inclusion of a Web site does not indicate an endorsement by the authors or McGraw-Hill, and McGraw-Hill does not guarantee the accuracy of the information presented at these sites.

www.mhhe.com

BRIEF CONTENTS

CONTENTS

PREFACE

The population of older people in the United States is growing at a rate that is unprecedented in American history. The continued growth in the number and proportion of older people in the United States impacts us all—socially, politically, and financially. Extensive federal and state resources are consumed paying for the healthcare needs of an aging population.

Health status is an important variable in determining the length and quality of life. And, as we grow older, health status is no longer taken for granted. Older people commonly assert that, "when you have your health, you have everything." Most people do not consider themselves as old until their health begins to fail and it becomes harder to do the things they are accustomed to do.

Learning about health in the later years will help you to prepare yourself to age healthfully and to better understand and care for your aging family members. If you are planning a career in health and human services, this information is key to providing effective care to your future patients and clients.

AUDIENCE

This text is designed for use in college-level courses in health and aging. Students enrolled in these courses usually come from diverse fields, such as biology, medicine, dietetics, social work, psychology, nursing, sociology, recreation, public health, and allied health professions. Some students are preparing to work with older people, while others may just wish to know how to help themselves and their loved ones age successfully. Graduate students and professionals who want to continue their education in health and aging will find this text useful. Students often share this text with their older family members as a starting point for discussions about the many and varied issues surrounding aging.

NEW TO THIS EDITION

This text includes chapters that address the major influences on the health of older persons. It is amply referenced to enable advanced students to study health issues in more depth. In this edition, we have given more attention to helping readers better understand the nature of research to enable them to read, interpret, and evaluate current research in professional journals, in the news and on the internet.

For the fifth edition, the majority of the text has been revised to reflect the rapid expansion of knowledge about health and aging:

- Demographics have been updated and new information from current research is presented.

- Tips for communicating with those with visual, hearing, and cognitive problems are included.
- The theories of aging have been consolidated to summarize the major lines of thinking to explain how we age. The "Blue Zones" are discussed, including strategies to increase the chance of living longer.
- New material includes the metabolic syndrome.
- Expanded section on infections, dehydration, and the cascade to delirium.
- New material discusses how elders fare in a major disaster and how to better plan to meet their needs.
- The section on psychoactive medications has been expanded to include uses, side effects, and risks. New material discusses common behaviors in dementia and practical methods to cope with them.
- The text includes an extensive discussion of Medicare changes, including Medicare Part D. Expanded the section on the issues and advances of medical care including health literacy, patient safety, the doctor–patient relationship, electronic medical records, and the patient-centered medical home. Other new additions include a discussion of health care reform and its impact on elders, and sections outlining the impact of new technology and how it can improve health care for elders.
- Nursing home updates regarding new federal regulations and assessments, five-star rating systems, the Advancing Excellence campaign, and expanded sections on "hot button topics" such as staffing, hospital readmissions, physical and chemical restraints, and person-centered care.
- The chapter on death and dying is expanded to include new initiatives in end-of-life planning, consent, and surrogate decision making.
- The physical activity and nutrition chapters incorporate the latest recommendations for elders with focus on the role of exercise and nutrition in the prevention and treatment of disease and disability and discussion of community-based programs to improve the eating and exercise habits of older Americans.

These include the National Physical Activity Plan and Physical Activity Guidelines for Americans as well as the new "My Plate" initiative.

- Preventive health care for elders addresses primary, secondary, and tertiary prevention and updated recommendations of the U.S. Preventive Task Force as well as Healthy People 2020.
- This edition provides reputable Web-associated resources to supplement the written material in the text, allowing for more in-depth study of many topics.
- Interactive exercises, such as "What Is Your Opinion?" and end-of-chapter activities provide students with an opportunity to apply their knowledge to real-life experiences.
- New case studies, most from Rebecca's personal experience as a physician, illustrate the complexity of care involved in working with elders.
- Instructor resources are available at **www.mhhe.com/ferrini5e**

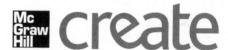

McGraw-Hill Create™

Craft your teaching resources to match the way you teach! With McGraw-Hill Create, you can easily rearrange chapters, combine material from other content sources, and quickly upload content you have written like your course syllabus or teaching notes. Find the content you need in Create by searching through thousands of leading McGraw-Hill textbooks. Arrange your book to fit your teaching style. Create even allows you to personalize your book's appearance by selecting the cover and adding your name, school, and course information. Order a Create book and you'll receive a complimentary print review copy in 3–5 business days or a complimentary electronic review copy (eComp) via email in minutes. Go to www.mcgrawhillcreate.com today and register to experience how McGraw-Hill Create empowers you to teach your students your way.

ELECTRONIC TEXTBOOK OPTION

This text is offered through CourseSmart for both instructors and students. CourseSmart is an online resource where students can purchase the complete text online at almost half the cost of a traditional text. Purchasing the eTextbook allows students to take advantage of CourseSmart's web tools for learning, which include full text search, notes and highlighting, and email tools for sharing notes between classmates. To learn more about CourseSmart options, contact your sales representative or visit www.CourseSmart.com.

ACKNOWLEDGMENTS

It has been a quarter of a century since we began to write the first edition of this text. During the majority of those years, Armeda was professor and chair of the Department of Health and Community Services and coordinated the Gerontology Program. She taught countless students about health and aging at California State University, Chico, and is now retired. Her interest in aging has moved from the theoretical to the experiential as she approaches 70 years of age.

Over the last 25 years, Rebecca has married, birthed five children, and worked in preventive medicine, hospice care, nursing home medicine and administration. She currently works as Medical Director for Edgemoor, a county-run long-term care facility in Santee, California. In 2009, she was honored by the American Medical Directors Association as Medical Director of the Year.

In continuing the intergenerational development of this project, Rebecca's daughter, Allison, now a student at University of California, Davis, assisted with editing the revision, and provided a student's perspective on the material and presentation.

We would like to dedicate this edition to Albert Ferrini, father and grandfather, who died in 2005 after a brief illness at the age of 93. He was so proud that his daughter and granddaughter wrote a book that he had all the editions on his end table for years. He served as a good role model for healthy aging as he ate well and exercised vigorously until the last month of his life.

We are thankful for the various forms of assistance we have received from many individuals. We are proud to share the photographs of Marianne Gontarz York, who is both a photographer and social worker. This is the first edition in which all photographs, including the cover, are from her portfolio. We are sure you will agree that they capture a vibrant, sensitive, and realistic portrait of older people. We would also like to thank those instructors who reviewed the previous edition and provided us with critical feedback to use in preparation of this edition: Lois Steichen, Forsyth Technical Community College; Lorilla Leckie Hawkins, Brigham Young University; Betty Boyle, West Chester University; Mark Kelley, University of Wisconsin-La Crosse; Mary Helen McSweeney, University of Scranton; and Debra Sheets, California State University-Northridge.

We would also like to acknowledge the assistance of the book team: Tricia Louvar, Van Brien & Associates, developmental editor; Joyce Watters, senior project manager; and Margarite Reynolds designer.

Rebecca L. Ferrini
Armeda F. Ferrini

The Study of Health and Aging

Old and young, we are all on our last cruise.

Robert Louis Stevenson

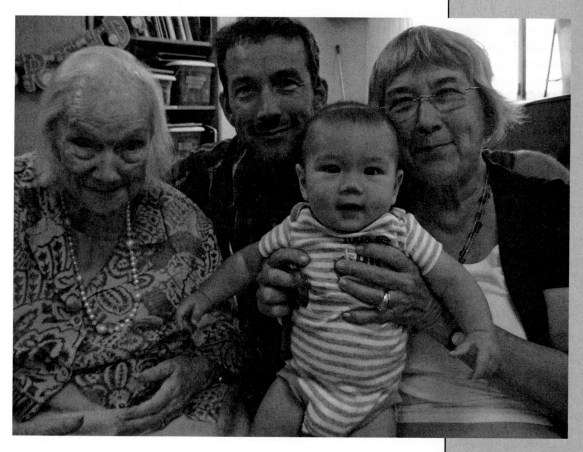

HOW OLD IS OLD?

Although death is inevitable, living to be old is not. It is only in the last century that a significant number of people have lived long enough to be classified as old.

The definition of *old* varies over time, culture, and situation. Today, we consider age 65 or so to be old; 200 years ago, age 50 might have been considered old. The age at which one is considered old may depend on the age of the person defining the word. A child may consider someone over 20 to be old, a teenager may think 40 is over the hill, and a 60-year-old may consider 70 as elderly. In essence, old is generally thought of as an age beyond one's own. Most elders do not consider themselves old until they become sick or dependent on others.

Aging is a complex, continuous process that begins at maturity and continues until death. Although we commonly think of stages of life (childhood, young adulthood, middle age, elderly), it is difficult to pinpoint exactly when one stage begins and another ends. The simplest way to classify age stages is by chronological age. In the United States, age 65 defines the beginning of old age because this used to be the age of full retirement benefits from Social Security. Researchers often use age 65 as a cutoff point to define old age, many

businesses use this age to begin "senior citizen discounts," and even elders themselves look at this age as the beginning of their later years.

Some gerontologists make distinctions between the young-old (65 to 74) and the old-old (75 and above) because there are significant differences between these groups. Generally, the young-old are more vigorous, have higher incomes, are more likely to be married, and have fewer health problems than the old-old. But even these divisions are not absolute.

Use of chronological age to determine old age is limiting in obvious ways. First, it is apparent that no abrupt change occurring on the eve of one's 65th birthday automatically transforms a person from "middle-aged" to "elderly." Second, profound differences between individuals of the same age make generalizations problematic. Some elders are in extremely good health well into old age, while some individuals in midlife exhibit many disabilities and illnesses that are generally associated with older people. For this reason, many gerontologists distinguish chronological (numerical) age from functional age, the physiological capacity of the body. Thus, a marathon runner may have a chronological age of 80 but physiologically function as well as an average 40-year-old. Some individuals psychologically

---

Terms Used to Describe Individuals 65 and Older

History has shown us that the language we use to define a particular group reflects our attitude and behavior toward that group. Although most of us do not intend it, inadvertently some of the terms we use to describe the older population create negative images of being old. Consequently, it becomes easy to disregard their contributions and needs.

Many terms have been used to describe older people: senior citizens, seniors, golden agers, retired persons, mature adults, elderly, aged, and old people.

Among older people there is no clear preference for any of these terms. Some grimace at being called a senior citizen, while others like the term. Many gerontologists, and the authors of this text, choose to use "elder" and "older person" to refer to individuals who are 65 and older. The term "elder" emphasizes the accumulated experience, knowledge, and wisdom associated with aging. The term "older person" emphasizes that aging is a continuum, with older people at one end and younger people at the other.

and socially grow old before their time. For example, there are individuals who use their age as an excuse for inactivity, dependence, and disengagement from society. In a sense, these individuals have died before their bodies. Without a doubt, sociological and psychological age is also an important part of aging.

Despite these caveats, the definition of *old* that we use in this text is the chronological age of 65 and older because most data are available in this form. When available, information on age subgroups is included.

THE STUDY OF AGING

Gerontology is the term used to describe the study of aging. Gerontology is a multidisciplinary field with a major focus on the biological, behavioral, and social sciences. However, gerontology may be applied to such diverse areas as interior design, history, literature, and marketing.

The term *geriatrics* refers to the medical care of older people. In contrast to gerontology, geriatrics is primarily concerned with changes that occur with age as a result of disease. Geriatricians and geriatric nurses are medical professionals who specialize in meeting the medical needs of elders.

As the number of elders grows, the study of gerontology and geriatrics will become increasingly important. These experts provide guidance regarding social and public policy changes, medical care innovations, and the future direction of medical services to respond to this increasing consumer pool.

Why study health and aging? One of the most powerful incentives to study health as it relates to aging is a personal one. Information about the many variables affecting health status in the later years can help people make better-informed health choices to increase the quality of their later life.

Whether old age is to be endured in an unhealthy, debilitated state or with energy and vigor is largely up to individual responsibility and the value placed on healthy behavior. One common response of an individual who is practicing an unhealthy behavior (e.g., smoking cigarettes, overeating) is, "I'm going to die anyway, might as well be from this." However, this reasoning is flawed. The chance of growing old with disabilities due to poor health behaviors is much greater than the chance of dying quickly from them. It is ironic that many of the diseases and disabilities formerly believed to be inevitable are now known to be due to our own thoughtless behaviors. Thus, the short-term enjoyment of unhealthful activities exacts a long-term cost on health. Whereas health may not seem of great concern when we are young, when we become old, health becomes a crucial concern. Perhaps the most important reason to discuss health in later years is to get a perspective on the direction in which our own health behaviors may be leading us.

Aside from the impact on our personal lives, the study of health and aging will assist us to better manage the aging process of those close to us—our friends and families. It is more likely now than it was 50 years ago that our parents, grandparents, and other kin will live to old age. Also, it is more likely that family members will spend some of their lives dealing with impaired spouses or relatives. Accurate knowledge about health and disease, appropriate measures to minimize health problems, and available medical and social services and means to finance them will be valuable in meeting that challenge.

The study of aging and health may enhance our professional careers. With the demographic shifts in the next few decades, the number of careers for those who choose to work directly with elders will increase dramatically. Researchers, teachers, social workers, physicians, nurses, nutritionists, counselors, psychologists, pharmacists, physical therapists, and many others with special knowledge of the needs of elders will be in demand. Those entering other careers, such as advertising, fashion design, tourism, and mass communications, will do well to understand the needs and desires of elders as

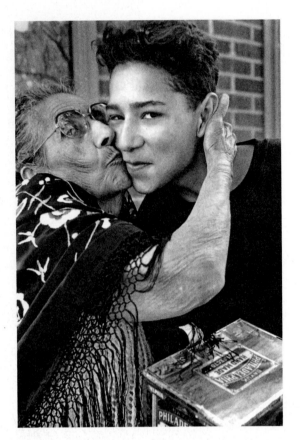

older consumers become an increasing proportion of the total population.

Finally, as enlightened citizens and voters, it is our duty to be knowledgeable about issues regarding health and aging. Health care provision for all the nation's people is a critical economic, political, and moral issue. Health care expenditures currently account for 18 percent of the U.S. gross domestic product, costing more than two and a half trillion dollars annually, and this number is expected to increase as health care costs rise and the population ages. The medical expenses of elders account for about a third of that expenditure. Even though Medicare pays a substantial portion of these increasing costs, elders are paying more from their own pockets than they did before Medicare was enacted. With the expected population shifts, important issues will have to be faced: Who should pay for health care, and what should it include? How can health care policy be modified to better meet the needs of elders? Barring early death, sooner or later we all will join the ranks of elders and will be either helped or harmed by these policy decisions. Answers to questions such as these are crucial for our nation and for our own future.

CHAPTER I

Our Nation's Elders

The Facts

By the year 2030, one of five people in the United States will be aged 65 and over. How old will you be?

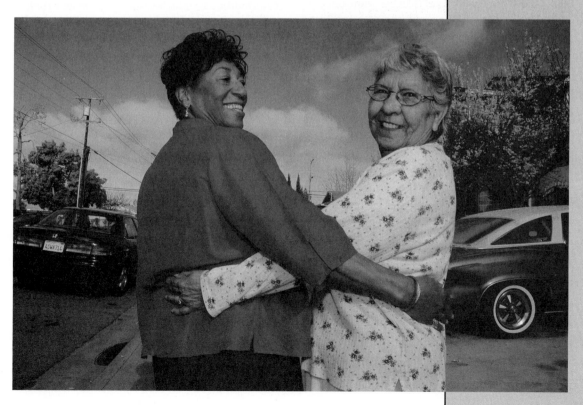

One of the first tasks in the study of health and aging is to understand the characteristics of the 65 and older age group in the United States. Who are elders? Are they rich or poor, white or nonwhite, sick or well, educated or not? To answer these questions, we need to gather information from many sources to form a portrait of what it means to be an elder in the United States. Looking at the facts and figures is necessary, for life expectancy, marital status, living arrangements, income and poverty levels, educational level, and racial and ethnic composition tell us a lot about health status and medical care needs, no matter what age group is studied.

In the twenty-first century, our country is experiencing the largest elder growth spurt in history as the baby boomer generation turns 65. This population shift will have profound effects on our politics, economy, values, and culture and will affect every American. Further, for the first time in U.S. history, racial and ethnic groups who are aged 65 and older will expand faster than the white population. By the year 2030, about one of four elders will be a member of a minority group. The four largest minority groups are black Americans, Hispanic Americans, Asian and Pacific Islanders, and Native Americans. All individuals, particularly those who work in the health and social service fields, need to become aware of the varied backgrounds, needs, and concerns of elders in order to better serve them.

AGEISM

Each of us has perceptions of elders and of growing old. Those perceptions are influenced by our interactions with family members, neighbors, and friends who are old. Further, our current age affects our attitudes toward aging: The closer we are to becoming an elder, the more realistic we become about growing old. Our cultural beliefs and attitudes about older people also influence our perception of older people. The media—including movies, books, television, greeting cards, magazines and the Internet—play a very large part in shaping our view of elders and aging.

Robert Butler, a prominent gerontologist, coined the term "ageism" to describe prejudice and discrimination against the old. These generalizations, whether negative or positive, are usually based on limited experience with older people. Although commonly held beliefs about aging may be true for some older people, ageism is the practice of applying these stereotypes to all elders.

The best way to learn about individuals' beliefs and attitudes toward growing old is to ask them. In 2000, a study conducted by the National Council on the Aging explored the public's attitudes toward aging.[1] As part of that study, 25-minute phone interviews were conducted with a nationally representative sample of over 1,000 individuals who were 65 and older to better understand elders' perception of growing older. The results of that study were compared to the results of a similar study conducted in 1974, over a quarter of a century earlier. In the more recent study, elders reported a more positive experience with aging: A significantly lower proportion of individuals 65 and older reported poor health (42 percent), fear of crime (36 percent), insufficient money to live on (36 percent), and loneliness (21 percent) as serious personal problems.

It is interesting to note that even though most elder respondents did not report that they experienced those problems, about 80 percent believed that those problems were serious for "most people over 65 these days." This response exemplifies the impact of society's portrayal of elders on individual elders' views of their age group. In essence, many older people also exhibit ageism, seeing their peers as unhealthy, lonely, fearful, and poor, but seeing themselves as the exception.

The study also revealed that older persons' views of themselves were generally optimistic. Almost half the individuals 65 years of age and older and one-third of those 75 years of age and older saw themselves as young or middle-aged. The survey also asked the elder respondents what was the best indicator of old age. The two most commonly mentioned were decline in physical ability (44 percent of respondents) and in mental functioning (35 percent). Further, most elders in this study had positive views about their aging process and wanted to live longer. About 90 percent agreed with the statement "As I look back on my life I am fairly well satisfied," and 70 percent agreed that "As I grow older things seem better than I thought they would be." More than 60 percent would like to live at least 10 more years, and almost half agreed with the statement "These are the best years of my life." These answers bode well for our future selves.

WHO ARE OUR NATION'S ELDERS?

We define elders as aged 65 and over, but the group is very heterogeneous. Some older people are at their peak of personal and political power (e.g., physicians, judges, CEOs, politicians, artists), while others have debilitating physical and mental illness and are living out their final days in a skilled nursing facility. Our health status, marital status, living arrangements, education, income, degree of social support, and cultural background strongly influence who we are, no matter what our age. The following cases exemplify the diversity among elders and the complex interactions among the physiological, socioeconomic, and environmental factors that influence health in the later years.

- A 75-year-old woman is partially blind and walks with a cane because of osteoporosis. She is unable to drive and lives in a rural area, but her friends provide transportation to church and take her to visit members of the historical society of which she is the chairperson. She is mentally alert, reads well with glasses, and has a positive attitude about life. She has some college education and lives alone.
- A 65-year-old black man with a history of congestive heart failure lives in a three-story walk-up because he does not have enough money to move. His children live nearby and help him with housecleaning and meal preparation. He has refused their offer to stay with them. He has been prescribed medication for his heart trouble but takes it only when he experiences pain because he cannot afford to take the medication daily.

- An 83-year-old Asian woman has recently returned from the hospital to her apartment in the city after hip surgery and is temporarily disabled. She needs physical therapy but cannot get there because she fears she will be attacked in the city neighborhood as she waits for the bus. Her neighbors help her fix meals, but she is very hesitant to ask for any other type of help because she does not want to burden others.
- A 72-year-old white woman is a retired dancer and continues to dance daily in a local studio. She is highly motivated to exercise and eat well to maintain her health. She lives with her husband in a house behind her adult daughter's family and helps her with babysitting and light housework.

Even though everyone is an individual with a story, generalizations help us understand the population, its needs, and how to meet them. This section provides an overview of the demographic factors that directly or indirectly affect the health of older people. *Demography* is the study of the size, geographical distribution, and vital statistics of a particular group. Demographic data may be collected in various ways, but the most common way is through surveys. Survey research commonly uses personal interviews, written questionnaires, or phone interviews to collect data on the incidence, distribution, and interrelationships of psychological and social variables. By selecting random samples of people, researchers hope that survey data can be used to make generalizations about a group of people or the population as a whole.

Unless noted otherwise, the facts and figures cited in this chapter were gathered from *A Profile of Older Americans: 2010*,[2] compiled of data from the U.S. Census Bureau, the National Center for Health Statistics, and the Bureau of Labor Statistics. A yearly update can be found on the Administration on Aging Web site: www.aoa.gov under Aging Statistics. When interpreting the statistics, remember that the data are displayed as averages and do not reveal the tremendous variability among individuals. Thus, it is important not to use these general data to make predictions about the situation of a particular older person.

Number and Growth of the Older Population

The number of people who are 65 and older continues to grow rapidly and will accelerate over the next three decades. At the beginning of the twentieth century, fewer than one in twenty-five people in the United States was 65 or over (4.1 percent). By 2009, the percentage had tripled: One person in eight (13 percent) was 65 or over—almost 40 million people. It is estimated that between 2000 and 2030 the number of elders will almost double, growing to one in five (20 percent) of the nation's total population. Individuals who are 85 and older are increasing the fastest.

Why is the older population growing so rapidly? More people are surviving to old age, and the birthrate is relatively constant. Up until 2010, the rate of increase was slower because few babies were born during the Great Depression of the 1930s. However, starting about 2010 through 2030, an unprecedented increase in the proportion of individuals reaching age 65 is expected because the baby boomers have started to "come of age."

Historically, ethnic minorities have been underrepresented in the elder population because of their shorter life expectancy. As the life expectancy and birthrates of ethnic populations increase, however, they will comprise a greater

The National Census

Probably the best-known example of a survey is the population census conducted by the U.S. Census Bureau. Although the national census was originally designed to count the number of individuals in each state to determine how many representatives each state could send to the federal House of Representatives, the data are now used by researchers, policy makers, and local, state, and federal governments in a variety of ways. Census data help the policy makers understand trends, set priorities, and monitor progress. The data are also used in financial decisions about allocating money to various groups and in determining funding, political representation, and societal trends. The information gathered from the national census, called *vital statistics,* is the major source of data about the U.S. population.

Every 10 years, the Census Bureau mails a questionnaire to each household in the United States with an address. Most households receive a short questionnaire asking for name, gender, age, relationships within the household, race and ethnicity, and whether the respondent rents or owns the house. About one in six U.S. residents receives a long form that includes questions regarding disability, economic status, and monthly expenses, and detailed questions regarding the respondent's living space. If the questionnaire is not returned, a census taker visits the addressee to collect the information. In the 2000 census, about two-thirds of those sent the questionnaire (281,421,906 individuals) were counted. The table showing the number and percentage of elders according to race and Hispanic origin is an example of the type of information gathered.

Census 2000 Data on the Aging Population

Total 65+	Numbers	Percent
Non-Hispanic		
Black	2,787,427	8.0%
American Indian/ Alaska Native	124,797	0.4%
Native Hawaiian/ Pacific Islander	19,085	0.1%
Asian	796,008	2.3%
Two or more races	264,588	0.8%
Other race	21,397	0.1%
Hispanic (any race)	1,733,591	5.0%
White	29,244,860	83.6%
Total 65+	34,991,753	100.0%

Source: www.census.gov/mso/www/c2000basics/00Basics.pdf

proportion of the elder population. In 2009, almost 20 percent of all elders were minorities. About 8 percent were black, 7 percent were of Hispanic origin, more than 3 percent were Asians or Pacific Islanders, less than 1 percent were American Indians or Native Alaskans, and 1 percent identified themselves as of two or more races. It is estimated that by the year 2020, almost one in four older adults will be from a minority group. It is projected that Hispanics will increase the fastest—doubling their current elder population.

The increased number and proportion of elders in the United States will have profound consequences on our society, especially on the demand for medical care. Higher numbers of elders, especially those over 75, increase the need for medical services, long-term care facilities, and home health services. Furthermore, government insurance programs that serve elders, such as Medicare and Medicaid, will have to carry a heavier burden.

Life Expectancy

Life expectancy for both men and women in the United States continues to increase. Those born today can expect to live about 30 years longer than those born in 1900. In 2009, the average life expectancy at birth was 78.2 years.

Gender has the largest influence on life expectancy, although the difference is narrowing somewhat. No matter what ethnicity or race, generally women live longer than men. Women outnumber men in every age group. In 2009, there were almost 23 million older women and almost 17 million older men, making a sex ratio close to 140 women for every 100 men. This sex ratio increases with age; from 65–69, the ratio of women to men was 114 women to 100 men, but by ages 85 and older the ratio was 216 to 100—more than twice as many women as men in the 85+ age group.

Ethnicity also has a strong influence on life expectancy. In 2009, blacks on the average died more than four years earlier than whites. Native Americans have the shortest life expectancies of all minority groups, estimated to be six years less than the general population. The reduced life expectancy among ethnic and racial groups is thought to be due primarily to poverty, increased rate of some chronic illnesses, and reduced access to health care.

Regardless of gender, ethnicity, or race, life expectancy increased rapidly in the last century largely because of reduced deaths of infants and children, primarily through control of infectious diseases. A greater proportion of the population is now living to be old, even very old. In 2009, about 64,000 centenarians (people aged 100 or over) were living in the United States. It is estimated that there are more people over the age of 100 alive today than all those who ever lived to be 100 prior to the twentieth century.[3]

Housing and Geographic Distribution

In 2009, four of five older persons owned their own homes, with a median value of $150,000. Almost two-thirds of them had paid off their mortgages. In general, their homes were older than those of younger age groups. Many lived in the same homes in which they had raised a family. As expected, the median income of those who rented their homes was lower ($15,774) than the median income of those who owned their homes ($30,400). Elders are less likely to change residences than younger groups. Even when older people do move, most stay in the same county.

More than four of five elders in the United States live in metropolitan areas, either in the city or in the suburbs. About one in five elders lives in rural areas, primarily small towns. In 2009, the states with the greatest number of older people were California (4.1 million), Florida (3.2 million), New York (2.6 million), and Texas (2.5 million). The states with the highest proportion of older people were Florida (17 percent) and West Virginia (almost 16 percent).

Marital Status and Living Arrangements

Marriage is generally very beneficial for both partners in later life. It can provide companionship, help with daily living activities, and personal care when a partner needs assistance. In addition, married people generally have a higher household income than single people. Those who are married are less likely to need home health services and institutional care. Most elders are married during the early part of their later years. However, with advancing age and the failing health of their partners, many become widowed. Because women live longer than men and have a tendency to marry men older than themselves, there are more than four times as many widows (8.9 million women) as widowers (2.1 million men). Older men are much more likely to be married as older women. In 2009, 72 percent of older men and 42 percent of older women reported being married. The proportion of older women who are widowed (41 percent) equals the number who are married (41 percent).

The number of elders who are divorced is increasing. The proportion of divorced (and not remarried) or separated older persons represented almost 12 percent of all older persons in 2009. This figure has more than doubled since 1980. It is estimated that the proportion of elders who have been divorced may climb significantly by 2020.

Two-thirds of the nation's older people who are not institutionalized live in a family setting. "Family setting" means that they live with at least one other person, most commonly a spouse. Living arrangements generally reflect marital status; those who are married are more likely to live as part of a family. However, the number of elders living with family members decreases with advancing age. And older women are less likely to live with their families than older men because the majority of older men are married and the majority of older women are widowed.

The proportion of elders living alone is increasing. In 2009, about 30 percent of older people lived alone. The proportion of older women living alone was more than twice that of older men (39 percent vs. 19 percent). The likelihood of living alone increases with advancing age. Among women 75 and older, half lived alone. Most elders choose to live alone and prefer that lifestyle to

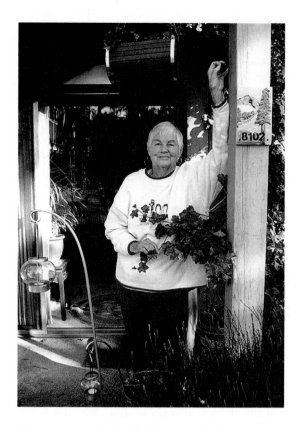

living with adult children. However, living alone can be a liability because these elders are more likely to have lower incomes and are at greater risk of institutionalization than those who live with families.

Contrary to what we may think, a very small proportion of elders reside in nursing homes. In 2009, only about 4 percent of elders resided in a nursing facility. However, the chance of living in a nursing home increases with advancing age. Less than 1 percent of those 65 to 74 resided in a nursing home, but 14 percent of those 85 or older lived there.

Marital status, living arrangements, and the availability of children play a major role in determining whether an older person resides in a nursing home. When a spouse or child is not present, elders are more likely to be institutionalized. Most older people have children, but not all live nearby or are willing to provide care. A few older people have no children.

Some elders have to provide care for their disabled children or care for grandchildren. In 2009, about 475,000 elders had primary responsibility for their grandchildren who lived with them. Current trends, such as the increasing divorce rate, tendency to have fewer children, and more women in the workforce, will likely affect the living arrangements of future elders.

Education

As a group, older people have completed fewer years of schooling than younger adults. However, this gap continues to narrow: From 1970 to 2009, the percentage of those aged 65 and older who had completed high school more than doubled, from 28 percent to 78 percent. In 2009, almost 22 percent of those 65 years and older had a bachelor's degree or higher. Educational attainment differs by race and ethnic origin: 83 percent of whites, 72 percent of Asians and Pacific Islanders, 64 percent of blacks, and 46 percent of Hispanic Americans completed high school. Since the baby boomers are the most educated cohort in history, it is expected that the elders of the future will be more educated than those of today. Nonetheless, it is likely there will still be significant disparities in educational level among elder subgroups, particularly minority immigrants.

Although older adults may have completed fewer years of formal education than those younger than 65, many elders are lifelong learners, enrolling in educational programs in their later years. Some elders choose to enroll in community classes, and others are enrolled in courses at community colleges and universities that offer reduced-tuition programs to attract older people. As the educational level of the elder population increases, it is expected that many retirees will return to education to enhance their quality of life, develop their interests, and acquire new skills.

Income

There have been dramatic changes in the income level of elders over the past few decades. With the onset of Medicare and Social Security, they are no longer the most financially vulnerable age group. With increased protection from high medical bills and a guaranteed income, elders have more financial security than ever before. Nevertheless, as a group, elders in the United States have a lower annual income than other adult groups (children have the highest poverty level). For all older persons reporting income in 2009, the median yearly income was $19,167 ($25,877 for males, $15,282 for females); but 20 percent of older persons reported incomes of $10,000 or less, and close to 40 percent reported $25,000 or more.

Elders living in a family setting fare better than those living alone. In families headed by elders in 2009, the annual household income averaged $43,702 ($45,400 for non-Hispanic whites, $35,049 for blacks, $32,820 for Hispanic Americans, and $47,319 for Asian Americans), accounting for about 60 percent of the median income of the 25–64 age group. In 2009, 6 percent of families headed by elders had incomes below $15,000, and about 60 percent had incomes of $35,000 or more.

About 9 percent of the older population was classified as poor or near poor in 2009. That year, the federal poverty threshold for those 65 and over was $10,289 per year for individuals and $12,968 for two individuals living together. Close to 9 percent of elders lived below the poverty level in 2009. Another 5 percent of elderly were classified as near poor with incomes up to 25 percent above the poverty level. Almost 14 percent are considered either poor or near poor. The current poverty rate among elders is lower than in 1970, when 25 percent of elders had incomes below the poverty level, or in 1959, when 33 percent of elders were poor. Even though a lower percentage of elders are subsisting below the poverty line, a disproportionately high number are still living on marginal incomes.

There are significant gender, racial, and ethnic disparities among elder groups. Women aged 65 and older have much higher rates of poverty than men aged 65 and older (11 percent vs. 7 percent in 2009). And those living alone in 2009 were three times more likely to be poor than those living with their kin (16 percent vs. 5 percent). There is a great disparity in income level with race and ethnicity. In 2009, one of fifteen white elders was poor or near poor, but one in five blacks and Hispanic Americans was poor or near poor. Being female, being an ethnic minority, and living alone increase the risk of poverty. For example, in 2009, over one-third of older black women who lived alone and close to half of older Hispanic women who lived alone were classified as poor. Those who are over 85 generally have the lowest income of all.

While many young and middle-aged adults rely on income from work and may even have health insurance funded by their employers, the majority of older people are no longer employed. As a consequence, their income is lower than that of other adult groups. There have been dramatic changes in the income level of elders over the past few decades, primarily due to an important government retirement program: Social Security. Aside from Social Security, other major sources of income for older people are private and government pensions, assets (e.g., savings and home equity), and earnings. In addition, the Supplemental Security Income program is available to augment the income of those at or below the poverty level who qualify. In this section we describe the major sources of income for older people.

Social Security

The Social Security Act of 1935 guaranteed a monthly income to individuals 65 years of age and older who paid into the program during their working years. At its inception, the Social Security Act provided minimal income to the worker. Four years later, new benefits were added: payments to the spouse and minor children of a retired worker (dependent's benefits), survivor's benefits paid to the family in the event of the premature death of the worker, and benefits to workers who become disabled. This change transformed Social Security from a retirement program for individuals into a family-based economic security program. Over the years, Social Security benefits were augmented further. Disabled individuals of any age and children of disabled workers became beneficiaries of Social Security. Other benefits added were automatic cost of living increases and the ability to retire at age 62 with slightly reduced benefits. In 2000, legislation was passed to enable individuals who began to collect their retirement benefits at 62 years of age and were still working to retain their retirement benefits if they earned less than $15,000 a year. Further, individuals who continue to be employed at age 65 and older can earn as much as they want while collecting their full retirement benefits. These relaxed earning restrictions enable hundreds of thousands of working elders to augment their incomes while collecting Social Security. Those who work must pay Social Security taxes on their earnings. The age of retirement to collect full Social Security benefits for individuals born before 1938 is 65 years. Retirement age gradually increases after that until those born in 1960 or later will not receive full retirement benefits until age 67. See www.socialsecurity.gov for more information about the Social Security program and for a retirement table for those born between 1938 and 1960.

Social Security is financed by taxes on the salaries of working adults. The employer withholds a portion of the amount earned by employees, matches that amount, sends those taxes to the Internal Revenue Service (IRS), and reports the employees' earnings to the federal government. People who are self-employed pay Social Security taxes when they file their tax returns, and IRS reports their earnings to Social Security. Workers who pay Social Security taxes earn "credits" that count toward eligibility for future Social Security benefits. An employee must earn at least $1,120 per quarter to receive one quarter of coverage

(1 credit).[3] A maximum of four credits can be earned each year. Most people need 40 credits (10 years of work) to qualify for benefits. In general, the longer a person works, and the higher the salary a person earns, the higher will be the Social Security benefit upon retirement. Younger people need fewer credits to qualify for disability or survivor's benefits.

Social Security is now viewed as an essential part of life in the later years, and the number of people receiving benefits from the program has grown. About 98 percent of all workers are in jobs covered by Social Security. When Social Security was instituted more than 70 years ago, only 222,000 individuals received benefits and many for only a short time. Now, close to 38 million retired workers enjoy them. In 2011, according to the Social Security Administration, the average monthly benefit was $1,177 (refer to www.ssa.gov for updated facts).

Social Security provides a lifeline to the majority of older Americans. In 2009, close to 90 percent of of all elders received Social Security. It provided about 40 percent of all income of elder Americans. And, for more than one-third of the elder population, Social Security provided 90 percent or more of their total income. It is particularly helpful to those who are unmarried. In 2009, 22 percent of married elders and 43 percent of unmarried elders relied on Social Security for 90 percent or more of their income. Social Security benefits provide income security not only for the elderly but also for the nearly one in three beneficiaries who are younger disabled individuals and children of disabled parents. In addition, due to advances in life expectancy and earlier ages of retirement, people collect benefits for many more years, and some collect more than they contributed. Social Security, pensions, other financial assets, and earnings have enabled millions of retirees to enjoy a financially secure retirement. Although poverty is still a significant problem among adults of all ages, Social Security provides a safety net for elders that other age groups do not enjoy.

Minority elders are less likely to collect retirement benefits because they are more likely to die before they are eligible because of their reduced life expectancy. Ninety percent of elder whites earned Social Security, but only 81 percent of blacks, 74 percent of Hispanics, and 66 percent of Asians earned Social Security.

Since the Social Security fund is primarily supported by taxes paid by workers, the retirement of the baby boomer generation will require that adjustments be made to continue the fund's viability for future retirees. Several solutions have been proposed: increasing the percentage of taxes on earnings, starting to tax incomes earned above the current maximum, increasing retirement age, decreasing benefits, privatizing the fund, and others.

Supplemental Security Income (SSI)

Social Security provides the lion's share of retirement income for the elderly. However, if Social Security benefits are insufficient to cover living expenses, public assistance is available from the Supplemental Security Income program (SSI). The SSI program was established in 1974 to assist all aged, blind, and permanently disabled people who had inadequate income and little to no assets. Unlike Social Security benefits, SSI eligibility is not tied to participation in the workforce. The program is financed by the federal government through general taxes with contributions and management by the states. The size of monthly payments varies from state to state. In 2011, the SSI program provided needed income support for more than 8 million needy people, 2 million of whom were 65 and older. Although the size of monthly payments varies from state to state, the average monthly payment was about $400.[3]

Other Income Sources

Many older people have income sources beside Social Security: personal assets, private or public pensions, and earnings. Personal assets include savings, proceeds from businesses, and home equity. Except for home equity, ownership of these assets is concentrated among a few, relatively affluent retirees. A little more than half the elder population reported private assets in 2008. However, they are generally not adequate to supplement Social Security. For example, the median income from financial assets is less than $1,000 a year for elder women.[3]

Pensions are monies set aside by employers during the employee's working years to be paid to the retired employee monthly after retirement. The government has established tax incentives to employers to offer pensions. In 2008, 28 percent of the 65+ age group reported private pensions and 14 percent reported public pensions. Unmarried women were the least likely to receive any type of pension. Pensions, like Social Security, serve to provide a steady income, and some even provide health coverage to supplement Medicare; but they have their drawbacks. Employers may not adequately fund their pension plans or may offer pensions to only some classes of workers. Although today's elders may have had pension plans, these plans are becoming less common. Further, pension benefits are skewed toward more affluent households who are more likely to be saving adequately for retirement even without pensions. Generally, pension benefits are meager among lower- and middle-income households. Pension rules are often complex and favor the employer over the employee. And pensions are not guaranteed: Employers have been known to steal employees' pension funds, and when companies file for bankruptcy, workers and retirees may lose some or all of their pensions.

Instead of traditional pensions, which guarantee employees a level of benefit, the trend is for employers to offer *Individual Retirement Accounts (IRAs)*, in which individuals contribute a portion of their paycheck to an investment fund, usually consisting of various combinations of stocks and bonds. The employer may also contribute to the employee's IRA. There are several types of IRAs. Some contributions are not taxed until the fund is used (usually after retirement, when the individual has a lower tax rate). Other contributions are taxed before being placed into the investment fund, but any interest earned over the years is not taxed when the money is withdrawn. Depending on the markets and investment choices of the individual or broker, this money is expected to grow over many years so that, by the time a person retires, the fund has increased significantly in value and the money is available to use on an as-needed basis.

Retirement accounts are more risky than pensions. The major drawbacks of savings through retirement accounts is that the money is not in a bank—investments are not guaranteed to grow and may even lose money. The rules for withdrawing money from Individual Retirement Accounts are very complicated.

Some individuals who are 65 years of age and older continue to work. They may begin a second career after retirement, they may continue to work for personal satisfaction, and many continue to work for financial reasons. Seventeen percent of the elder population was in the workforce (employed or actively seeking a job) in 2009.

Health Status and Health Care

In 2009, a national survey reported that almost 42 percent of older persons living in the community classified their health as excellent or very good (two-thirds of those in the 18–64 age group reported their health as excellent or very good).[4] Elder men and women differed little on their evaluation of their health, although minority groups were less likely than elder whites to report excellent or good health.

Morbidity (or illness) rates provide information about the incidence of disease and disability. Elders have the highest morbidity rates of all age groups because of their high prevalence of chronic illness. Most elders have at least one chronic condition. In 2006–2008, the most common conditions reported by those 65 and older were hypertension (38 percent), arthritis (50 percent), heart disease (32 percent), cancer (22 percent), and diabetes (18 percent). As expected, the number and severity of chronic illnesses increase with advancing age. Elders are less likely to report that they suffer from psychological disorders than younger groups, but rates of cognitive impairment (such as dementia) increase with age. Alzheimer's disease is the leading cause of cognitive impairment in the elder population.

Limitations in activity due to chronic conditions increase with age. Some limitations are so severe that the individual is unable to perform a major daily activity (including bathing, dressing, eating, and getting around the house). A large study of elders in 2007 reports that about one-fourth have problems completing one or more activities of daily living, and among those living in institutions, more than four fifths had those problems.

Because elders have a higher prevalence of chronic illness than the rest of the population, they have longer hospital stays, visit physicians more often, and are prescribed more drugs than younger groups. Also, older people are the prime users of long-term care institutions. In 2009, the average out-of-pocket health expenses (paid by elders themselves) averaged $4,241, close to 13 percent of their total income.

The Older Foreign-Born Population

In 2004, there were 3.7 million foreign-born individuals aged 65 and older living in the United States. About 40 percent were from Europe, 31 percent from Latin America, 22 percent from Asia, and 8 percent from other parts of the world. Almost two-thirds of the foreign-born have lived in the country for more than 30 years and one-third lived in the western states. Their living arrangements differ from those who are natives in that the foreign-born are more likely to live with families and more likely to be poor. They are also more likely to be uneducated and unable to speak English.

RACIAL AND ETHNIC DIVERSITY

Today's elderly are a highly diverse group, and an important aspect of this diversity is race and ethnicity. The status and resources of several racial and ethnic elder groups are reflective of the continued social and economic discrimination experienced throughout their lives. Many minorities also face cultural and language barriers. In general, minority elders are more likely to face the hurdles of fewer years of education, substandard housing, higher poverty, and poorer health than white elders.

Although the minority groups are incredibly diverse, they have two characteristics in common—high poverty level and racial discrimination. Differences in language, education, appearance, and customs keep many minorities out of well-paying jobs, positions of authority, and consequent financial security. These disparities generally begin during their working years, consequently leaving most with no resources for their later years. Despite the negative impact of discrimination throughout their lives, these elders possess some unique resources. Identification with an ethnic group and cultural traditions are a source of support in the later years. In addition, ethnic groups tend to maintain strong extended social networks, within both the family and the local community. However, acculturation is changing this practice among some groups.

Those working with elders need to be sensitive to cultural differences. Culture is a unified set of values, beliefs, and standards of behavior shared by a group of people. Our culture influences the way we accept, order, interpret, and understand experiences throughout our lives. Many cultures are represented in the United States today. This diversity broadens our perspective. It is important to learn about cultural differences within the specific population groups so that we can be better able to meet their needs. Keep in mind, however, that describing cultural differences can be like stereotyping—be certain to understand that there is within a culture that will impact a person's response to any situation.

An important distinction among cultures is the difference between individualism and collectivism. Whether one believes in individualism or collectivism has an impact upon determining how someone sees the world and his or her health and illness.

Individualism is the belief that people are independent of each other. Those with individualistic beliefs are concerned with personal autonomy and self-fulfillment. The United States is an individualistic culture with a focus on individual achievement, responsibility, and fulfillment. In contrast, those from Latin or Asian cultures often have more collectivistic beliefs. These cultures focus less on the role and value of individuals for their own gain and more on how an individual fits into a web of family or community. Collectivist cultures focus on interdependency.

Even within each ethnic group, there is much variation in education level, financial status, cultural background, length of time in the United States, family structure, geographical distribution, and degree of adherence to cultural practices. The Native American and the Asian and Pacific Islander groups in particular include many subpopulations, each with its own cultural heritage and language. Statistics necessarily focus on generalities, but the reader should be aware of the diversity within these ethnic and racial groups, for it strongly influences their health and medical care needs and their response to the medical care system.

In this section, we consider the health of the four largest groups of minority elders: black Americans, Hispanic Americans, Native Americans, and Asians and Pacific Islanders. These four minority groups comprise about 20 percent of the total elder population, but their numbers are increasing due to higher fertility rates and gains in life expectancy over the past few years. Currently, the growth of the minority elderly population is outpacing the growth of the white population. As mentioned earlier, the fastest-growing groups are Hispanic Americans, Asian Americans, and Pacific Islanders.

In order to effectively work with the many ethnic groups, it is important to learn about their historical background and their beliefs about health, illness, and health care. The reader is directed to the Ethnogeriatric Curriculum Modules edited by Gwen Yeo in which experts on each of 12 elder ethnic populations present an extensive training module for the professional.[5] The modules can be accessed on the Web at www.stanford.edu/group/ethnoger Much of the material presented below is based on that source.

Black American Elders

The black American (also called African American) population is the largest group of minority elders in the United States, comprising about 8 percent of the total elder population. These figures include those who have moved here from the Caribbean, Central and South America, and Africa. Because the category of black Americans is extremely varied, there is a great diversity in their cultures, income, education, and living arrangements.

Just as in other elder populations, black women outnumber black men, most men are married, and most women are widowed. However, black older men are less likely to be married and are more likely to live alone than white older men. Even though the life expectancy of blacks is increasing, whites live longer on average than blacks. In 2009, the life expectancy of black women was 77.4 years, over three years less than that of white women, and the life expectancy of black men was 70.9 years, almost six years less than that of white men.

A high proportion of elderly blacks are living in poverty. Figures from 2009 indicate that older blacks were almost three times as likely to be poor as their white cohorts (blacks, 20 percent; whites, 7 percent). Older black women who live alone are the most likely to be poor. Like other ethnic minorities, elder blacks are generally less educated, have had lower-paying jobs, and have less financial security than their white cohorts. Because of their job record, they have not contributed as much to Social Security. Thus, in their later years, they continue to be poor. Because they are also less likely to have pensions and assets than their white counterparts, they are more likely to depend on Social Security as the mainstay of their income. However, all elder blacks are not poor. Those with a college education and

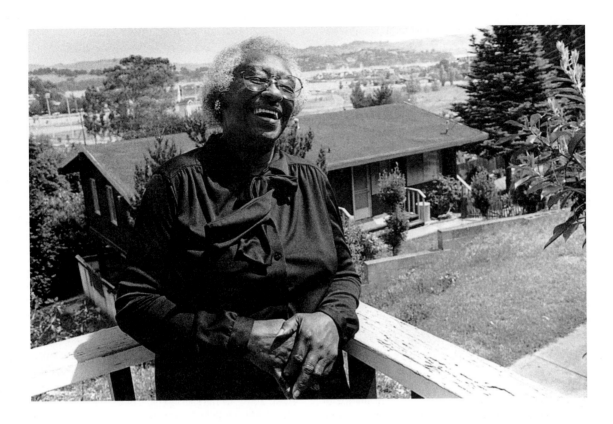

professional careers in their working years have income levels similar to those of white elders.

As a group, black elders are more likely to suffer from chronic health problems than their white counterparts. Although heart disease, cancer, and stroke are the three major causes of death in both blacks and whites, these diseases are more prevalent in the black population. Black elders also have a significantly higher prevalence of glaucoma, diabetes, and prostate cancer than do white elders.

The incidence of lung cancer and deaths from other lung diseases is dramatically increasing among older black men and women, and hypertension mortality rates are increasing among older black women. When compared with whites their age, black elders have more restricted activity, disability, and lost workdays per year. Blacks visit physicians less often, are more likely to postpone seeking medical attention until health problems become severe, and stay longer in the hospital. They are less likely to use home health services and nursing homes than white elders.

It is hypothesized that health professionals' prejudicial attitudes toward blacks may, in some cases, restrict needed access to health and social services, or result in services of inadequate quality. A classic example is the 40-year Tuskegee Experiment (1932–1972), in which government researchers recruited black men who had syphilis to be part of a research project to determine at autopsy the effects of the disease on the human body. Even after penicillin was discovered, the black men were not treated, and some transmitted the disease to their wives, many of whom died or suffered permanent disability.

Unfortunately, even as racism seems less prominent in the United States, there are still widespread differences in health care treatments offered and outcomes achieved when blacks are compared with whites. It is understandable that blacks are suspicious of health care personnel. Many view their interactions with health professionals—with physicians and other medical personnel—as degrading. The long waits, the medical jargon, and feelings of racism, alienation, and powerlessness at clinics are not uncommon.[6] It is important that those in the health and social services who work with elder blacks treat them with respect, take time to establish rapport, and put them at ease.[7]

Hispanic American/Latino Elders

Hispanic American elders are the fastest-growing ethnic minority in the United States. In 2009, they represented 7 percent of the elder population. It is predicted that the number of Hispanic elders will surpass the number of elder blacks by 2028.

The word *Hispanic* does not define a race; most Hispanics are Caucasian. It is an umbrella term for a number of different, varied ethnic groups hailing from countries in Latin America (Latino/Latina), Cuba, Puerto Rico, or Spain (the origin of the term *Hispanic*). Subgroups within the Hispanic population are highly diverse. The largest group originates from Mexico, a significant number comes from Cuba and Puerto Rico, and fewer originate in other Central and South American countries. The largest concentrations of elder Hispanics live in California, Texas, New York, and Florida. Mexican

Mrs. H.: A Black Woman[7]

Mrs. H. is an 83-year-old black woman with type II diabetes and severe vision loss from diabetes. She is widowed and lives alone in a small house she bought with income from 45 years of working as a domestic. She is very proud of her home but cannot see well enough to keep it up. She has two surviving children, but both live several hundred miles away, and she doesn't see them often. Until two years ago she was active in the local senior center, where she participated in crafts programs. She was also active in her church. Now, however, unless someone comes by to pick her up, she can't participate in either because she can't see well enough to walk or take the bus.

Her physician recently retired and referred her to a new doctor. She called the senior transport service for a reservation for the day of her appointment and was told they would have to pick her up three hours before her appointment because the day was so busy. When she arrived at the clinic, the receptionist asked Mrs. H. lots of questions and asked her to fill out many pages of forms. Finally after two hours of waiting, the nurse came to the waiting room and called, "Ruby, the doctor is ready to see you." The doctor seemed rushed and preoccupied. During their conversation he told her about a new research project she was eligible for that would provide a new treatment for her diabetes, low vision assistive devices, and homemaker services. She said she would think about it. When the nurse called two days later to enroll her in the project, Mrs. H. said she didn't want anything to do with the experiment and didn't want anyone coming to her house.

DISCUSSION QUESTIONS

What factors contributed to Mrs. H.'s difficulties with her new health care provider? What could the physician's office have done to improve the initial visit?

Why do you think Mrs. H. refused the assistance offered to her, even though she might have benefited from it? How might you convince her to accept this assistance?

What might be done differently by the senior transport dispatcher, clinic receptionist, physician, and nurse to better serve Mrs. H.?

Americans tend to reside in the Southwest, those from Central and South America often settle in New Mexico, most of the Cuban American population resides in Florida, and the Puerto Rican American population has settled in New York and New Jersey.

The Hispanic American population is considerably younger than the white population. This age difference is due to higher fertility rates (more babies born per family), shorter life expectancies, and historical patterns of immigration and emigration. For instance, many middle-aged and elder Hispanics voluntarily return to their homelands. However, some elders arrive in the United States in their later years because their children send for them.

Demographic data on the Hispanic population are often inadequate because Hispanics may be classified as "white" or may be under-reported on the census as some of their population are in this country illegally.

Of all minority elderly, those of Hispanic background are the least educated. A little more than one-third of the elder Hispanic population completed high school. In comparison, three-fourths of the white elder population completed high school. As a group, Hispanic elders are more likely to retain their native language. Numbers vary by subgroups regarding the ability to speak English. Over half the Cuban American elder population and a quarter of Mexican Americans cannot speak English. Inability to speak English serves as a barrier to accessing health and social services.[8] Further, their lack of education and inability to speak English have forced Hispanic Americans into jobs with low pay and no pension or health insurance (e.g., employment as domestic helpers and farm workers and other "under the table" occupations). Consequently, they are less likely to collect Social Security.

Elderly Hispanics are much more likely to be poor as the white population (18 percent vs. 7 percent in 2009). As in all elder populations, poverty rates among Hispanic Americans are higher among older women than among older men, particularly among women who live alone. In 2009, 45 percent lived below the federal poverty level.

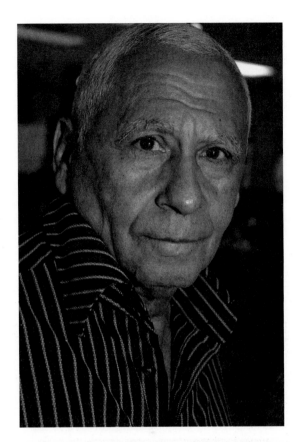

Elderly Hispanics are more likely to depend on Supplemental Security Income (the federal assistance program for the poor, blind, and disabled) than the elder white population.

Elder Hispanic Americans suffer poorer health than their white counterparts. Overall, they are less likely to die from the three top killers: heart disease, cancer, and stroke. They are more likely to suffer from diabetes and obesity. There is some evidence that Hispanic American elders are at higher risk of depression, particularly those who have not adjusted to American culture.[9] Elder Hispanics are significantly more disabled than white elders.[10] They are also more likely to visit a physician than white elders, and they are more likely to be hospitalized. However, they are less likely to be covered by Medicare or to have private insurance.

Hispanic elders rely more heavily on their families than do white elders. As a group they are more likely to live with relatives than are whites, usually with their adult children. It is not clear whether they live together because families may not have enough money for a separate household, because elders have more disabilities and cannot function independently, or because they have strong family ties and choose to help one another.

Traditionally, Hispanic American elders are highly respected by their children and are the core of the extended family network. They act as repositories of cultural traditions, values, and history. More than the younger Hispanic Americans, they have retained their native language and culture. In comparison to whites, Hispanic Americans often have more kin in town, interact more frequently with relatives, and are more likely to help family members financially. However, as adult children are quickly being integrated into American culture, the extended family network of the Spanish-speaking population is disintegrating, threatening the emotional and financial support of Hispanic American elders.[8]

Elder Hispanic Americans can be cynical and suspicious of governmental institutions and workers, but they are often extremely respectful of health care providers. With the exception of going to the doctor, they are less likely to utilize social and educational programs, mainly because many cannot speak or read English. However, their underutilization of services does not mean that the services are not needed. The term *personalismo* means displaying mutual respect and building trust. *Personalismo* is an important cultural value within the Hispanic American elder population. Simple actions by the health provider such as exchanging pleasantries before the examination begins and addressing the patients by their last names are two giant steps toward delivering culturally competent care.[11]

Native American Elders

In the 2000 census, about 125,000 Native American elders (includes American Indians and Alaska Natives) were counted, comprising one-half of 1 percent of the U.S. elder population.

Mrs. G.: A Mexican American Woman

Mrs. G., a 67-year-old Mexican American woman with diabetes, high blood pressure, and obesity, required amputation of part of her foot because of poor circulation and an ulcer that would not heal. A home health nurse visited her at home. The nurse found the house quite crowded. The woman was living with a daughter, grandchildren, and a niece in a two-bedroom apartment. Her daughters all worked and were unable to change the dressings on the wound. Mrs. G. took her medications sporadically, based on her own assessment of how she felt and whether she needed them. Her family would go across the border to Mexico and bring back medications—some of them were homeopathic, and others were versions of U.S. prescription drugs. She would medicate herself with these as needed. She expected her daughters to care for her and was upset to discover that the doctor had talked to them about placing her in a nursing home.

DISCUSSION QUESTIONS

Identify at least five issues that might concern you as a health or social service provider to Mrs. G. and her family. Which issues are the highest priority and why?

How might you initiate a discussion regarding one of these issues with Mrs. G. and her family? Role-play the discussion with a peer.

With whom would you talk first regarding nursing home admission: Mrs. G. or her daughters?

About one-quarter of Native American elders live on American Indian reservations or in Alaskan Native villages. Over half of the Native American population is located in five states: California, Oklahoma, Arizona, Texas, and New Mexico.

It is important to underscore the diversity within the Native American group: More than 560 tribes exist, and over 100 tribal languages are spoken.[12] Native Americans have significantly higher death rates than the general population. The Indian Health Service reports that American Indians and Alaska Natives have a life expectancy that is about five years less than the general elder population.

In addition to having the shortest life expectancy, Native Americans are the poorest minority group in the United States. Because of the high unemployment rate among Native Americans (50 percent), most elders are ineligible for Social Security benefits and must depend on government support as their sole source of income. Some experts believe they should be eligible for Social Security benefits earlier than the rest of the population because many Native Americans do not live long enough to collect their benefits.

Although the majority of younger Native Americans have moved from reservations to urban areas, their elders for the most part still live on reservations or in rural areas. On the average, the quality of their housing is very poor. As a group, elder Native Americans are less educated than other elders in the United States.

Many Native Americans have an extended family network with a strong commitment to their elders. Due to a high rate of unemployment among the younger population, the family often stays together because the elder in the family may be the only one with a steady income. Elders may provide a significant proportion of the family income through their government subsidies. This provision of support may indirectly preserve the status of elders within the family. However, traditional family support is ineffective in families with no resources, and many Native American elders are left impoverished on the reservation when their children leave to seek a better life.

Native Americans have the unenviable reputation of having the poorest health status in the United States. They have a higher death rate than other groups for alcoholism (more than six times

Mrs. T.: A Native American Woman

Mrs. T. is a 65-year-old Native American woman living on a reservation in Wyoming. She lives in an old recreational vehicle with a generator to provide power. She does not have running water inside her home but does have access to a well nearby. She does not consider herself poor because she lives similarly to others. A mobile physician sees her every three months; she calls her a "daughter." Mrs. T. has diabetes, she is overweight, and she has arthritis and high cholesterol. She had tuberculosis last year and spent some time in a hospital and does not want to go back. She is very respectful of the nurse who visits, but the nurse suspects she does not follow her advice. Mrs. T. seems unconcerned about her medical problems and prefers to discuss her life with the doctor only. When the nurse arranged for a social service worker to visit and provide her with a new refrigerator for her insulin and the delivery of fresh food, Mrs. T. gave them away to a young mother who lives nearby.

DISCUSSION QUESTIONS

How might a health care worker build rapport with this client and convince her to follow his or her advice?

If you were the health care worker, what would be your goal in this case, and how might you best achieve it? From whom might you elicit help?

more), fatal accidents (more than double), homocide (almost double), suicide (almost double), and tuberculosis (six times more). They are almost three times as likely to have diabetes. On the other hand, their rates of the four top killers are similar to the rest of the elder population (heart disease, cancer, stroke, and lung disease). The major health problems of Native American elders include pneumonia and diabetes; women have more than double the diabetes rate of the general elder population.[13,14]

Despite the high prevalence of illness among elder Native Americans, this group has a low level of use of health and social services.[15] One reason is lack of access to health care. The Indian Health Service is responsible for the health care of those who live on reservations. However, the Indian Health Service is often a long distance away from the reservation. Lack of transportation and inability to communicate with health personnel further reduce access to needed health care. Those who do not live on the reservation or do not belong to a registered tribe must seek care outside the Indian Health Service.

Because the Indian Health Service does not provide long-term care services, individual tribes are responsible for providing any long-term services that do exist. Currently there are only 12 tribal-run nursing homes, and many people who need them must be placed far from their family and their land.[15] Consequently, most sick elders are cared for in the home by family members. Because many of the young and middle-aged Native Americans have moved from the reservation to urban areas for economic reasons, the availability of family caregivers is reduced. Elder Native Americans may not utilize health care because of the lack of sensitivity of the staff to the Native American culture and the lack of respect for the patients. Furthermore, older Native Americans are more likely to have a different view of disease and healing and are more likely to rely on ritual folk healing than on visits to a physician.

Even though health care expenditures have increased consistently for the rest of the population,

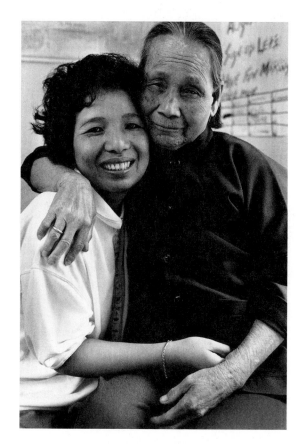

per capita health care expenditures for Native Americans have not. Because the U.S. Congress and the Bureau of Indian Affairs, not the individual states, are responsible for developing and implementing programs to meet the health and social service needs of Native Americans, older Native Americans may not have access to government assistance programs available to the rest of the population. As a result, they are at higher risk for substandard housing, poverty, and poor health.

In sum, the poor state of health of elder Native Americans is worsened by their low income and educational level, their serious health problems, and their lack of access to and stringent governmental controls on health and social service programs for Native Americans.

Levanne R. Hendrix suggests that the cultural values of American Indians have an impact on service delivery to that group: listening over talking; calmness and humility over speed and self-assertion; and the high value placed on silence. She suggests that the provider slow down when communicating with American Indian elder clients and not interrupt them. Other adaptations mentioned were allowing elder American Indian clients more personal space, not looking them in the eye, and not touching them without their permission.[12]

Asian and Pacific Islander Elders

Asian and Pacific Islander elders represent less than 4 percent of all people aged 65 and older in the United States. This population includes 60 ethnic

---

Mr. W. and Mr. L.: Asian American Men

Mr. W. is a 75-year-old Chinese American male who presents with vague and multiple physical complaints that he reports he has had for several weeks. Prior to this he was in good health and would come in only for periodic physical exams. His son tells you he has been complaining of "heart pain," indigestion, and weakness. He was seeing the herbalist but has continued to complain to his son. The patient does not speak much English, and his son interprets for him. During the interview you find out that Mrs. W., his wife of 50 years, died last year. His son is busy and sees him about once a month and will be moving to a job in another state. Your exam and laboratory and diagnostic tests are normal. On a return visit, you bring up the possibility that Mr. W. may be depressed. The son and the patient get very upset and vehemently deny any depression. The patient states that he is sick, not crazy.[17]

Mr. L., an elderly Korean American man with liver cancer, sits placidly in his hospital bed during various tests and visits from specialists. Because he does not speak English, little communication is directed toward him, although he is always smiling and allows any examination. Chemotherapy is administered, based on the assumption that this is what he wants. His granddaughter, who is working full-time, takes calls at work and acts as a translator. She mentions that he feels nauseated and has pain, but she is not able to follow up on whether those symptoms are treated. She does not tell Mr. L. that his illness is terminal. When he begins to get weaker, a large number of family members come and sit at his bedside,

spilling over into other areas of the hospital and bringing pungent foods to tempt his appetite. They crowd into his room, which he shares with two other patients, and someone is present at all times. Visits by medical personnel and updates about the patient's medical status are communicated through the granddaughter, who is expected to relay the information to her relatives. When the patient dies, the granddaughter calls and asks for his body to remain in the bed for hours, which is a Buddhist tradition. The hospital denies her request, informing her that they need the bed immediately.

DISCUSSION QUESTIONS

What common threads run through both cases? How might cultural factors influence diagnosis and treatment?

What cultural factors might contribute to Mr. W.'s and his family's reaction? How might you bring up issues of mental distress? Why do you think the son reacted to the diagnosis in the way he did? Why did the father?

What are some problems that may occur with using members of Mr. L.'s family as translators? How can these problems be reduced?

Does the patient have a right to know his diagnosis and prognosis? What is your responsibility to the patient? What if the patient's family forbids the health care team to tell the patient the truth about his health?

groups originating from 20 different countries. The largest three elder subgroups are Chinese, Japanese, and Filipino. The Asian and Pacific Islander population also includes people originating from Korea, the East Indies, Cambodia, Guam, Hawaii, Samoa, Vietnam, Thailand, Laos, Malaysia, and elsewhere. Those of Asian descent make up more than 95 percent, and Pacific Islanders comprise 4 percent.[16] It is estimated that between 2010 and 2030, the number of Asian and Pacific Islander elders will increase by 150 percent (as compared to the elder white population, which is projected to increase by 60 percent).

The vast majority of Asian American elders live in metropolitan areas, and half live in the West. The length of residence in the United States is also variable. Some have lived here for several generations; others, such as the Vietnamese, Hmong, and Laotians, migrated in the 1970s.

The diversity in language and cultural background within this population is immense. However, the common cultural influence is Confucianism. The philosophy originated in China but was later brought to Japan and many other Asian countries. One of the foundations of Confucian thought is filial piety. Children are expected to obey and respect their parents, to bring honor to their parents by being successful, and to care for their parents when they become old. For Asian Americans, however, filial piety has begun to take a backseat to such traditional American values as independence and self-reliance. Still, older Asian Americans tend to retain their old ways, living in small, close-knit groups with others who share their language and culture. However, such strong social support tends to isolate these populations from the rest of society.

Although Asian American elders have a higher median income and lower poverty rates than elder whites, many elder Asian Americans suffer the same poverty, discrimination, and language difficulties as other ethnic minorities. Many receive no Social Security benefits because they were employed as seasonal farmworkers or self-employed.

The health status of Asian and Pacific Islander Americans as a group is similar to that of white elders. However, generalizations ignore the tremendous diversity among populations: Some are in better health than whites, and others are in poorer health. Health status relates somewhat to *acculturation* (adapting to a new environment). Acculturation has both positive effects (e.g., increased reliance on preventive care, better communication with medical providers) and negative effects (e.g., change from traditional low-fat Asian diets to high-fat American diets). Asian American elders have a higher incidence of some types of cancers, hypertension, and infectious diseases such as hepatitis and tuberculosis than white elders. As a group, elder Asian Americans have a higher incidence of suicide—three times that of their white counterparts.

Like other minorities, elder Asian Americans are less likely to utilize medical care services than white elders, probably because of language barriers and unfamiliarity with Western medicine. They may be recent immigrants and may not have access to Medicare or Medicaid services. Many do not have private health insurance.[16]

For more information on Asian American elder subgroups (Asian Indian, Chinese, Filipino, Japanese, Korean, Native Hawaiian, Pakistani, Vietnamese, Cambodian, Hmong, and Laotian), refer to the ethnographic modules edited by Yeo[17] on the Web, at www.stanford.edu/group/ethnoger/efiles.html

WORKING WITH MINORITY ELDERS: OBSTACLES AND OPPORTUNITIES

The elder population in the United States is incredibly diverse. Health and social services professionals are in a good position to appreciate the challenges posed by working with individuals of differing economic, educational, and cultural backgrounds.

The cases presented in this chapter illustrate the barriers to effective health care that elders of different racial and ethnic groups face. Among these barriers are cultural beliefs and practices regarding illness and health; inability to speak or understand English; feelings of confusion, anxiety, and isolation; and the clash between traditional beliefs about illness and treatment and the Western technological medical model. Ignorance on the part of the health worker regarding the patient's culture and traditional health beliefs and behavior leads to miscommunication among the patient, family, and provider and ultimately results in inferior care.

Researchers have identified disparities in health and health care across racial, ethnic, gender, and socioecomomic groups, even among individuals with the same insurance status. A study by the Johns Hopkins Center for Health Disparities Solutions calculated the direct and indirect costs of racial and ethnic disparities in health care in the United States. The estimated cost for the period 2003 through 2006 was $229.6 billion.[16] What accounts for these disparities? A number of factors have been postulated. The main reason is socioeconomic and geographical. Many minority populations are poor, with less access to healthy food, high quality education, safe communities, and high quality insurance and medical care. Minority populations may face increased stress—from overcrowding, financial insecurity, poor employment, lack of control, and discrimination. Even with Medicare funding at 65, minority groups continue to fare worse than their white Non-Hispanic counterparts: Minority groups spend longer in the hospital for the same problem, have more complications, are subject to more medical errors and longer wait times, and receive less "evidence-based" and preventive care.

Since it is projected that one of four elders will be a member of a minority population by 2030, momentum has been building in the field of health and human services to train professionals to work effectively with diverse groups. It is clear that race and ethnicity are related to health disparities (inequalities) in life expectancy, morbidity (illness rates), and mortality (death rates), especially among the four subgroups discussed here.

The variations are believed to be due in part to the inaccessibility and underutilization of needed health and social services. In other words, the staff or the programs themselves may not be "culturally sensitive."

A body of literature is developing to increase understanding of the problems and to find ways to decrease the disparities between white and ethnic/racial subgroups. One of the thrusts is to better train health and human service professionals and to develop or modify health and social services organizations and programs to reflect culturally competent care. What is cultural competence? A culturally competent professional is someone who is knowledgeable about cultural differences and their impact on attitudes and behaviors; is sensitive, understanding, nonjudgmental, and respectful in dealing with people whose culture is different from his or her own; and is flexible and skillful in responding and adapting to different cultural contexts and circumstances.[18] A culturally competent service is one that is culturally appropriate, culturally accessible, and culturally accepted by the group it is intended to serve.

Achieving culturally competent health care includes:

- Evaluating the clients you are serving and their needs and preferences and setting up your systems to address them.
- Hiring staff who are bilingual and bicultural and soliciting their input into your systems of care.
- Viewing your care from the perspective of a client/patient.
- Having translation services available as well as written materials and methods to enhance and verify client understanding.
- Training staff in understanding, appreciating, and being able to communicate with members of other cultures.
- Setting up the service to appeal to those of various cultures (e.g., location, decorations, the way clients move through the offices).

Obstacles to Effective Health Care Delivery to Minority Elders

ECONOMIC AND EDUCATIONAL
- They may not be eligible for Medicare.
- They are more likely to have a low income level.
- They are less likely to be able to pay for services.
- They are more likely to have a low educational level.
- They are not likely to understand medical and bureaucratic jargon.

CULTURAL
- They are less likely to be able to speak and understand English.
- They are less likely to know about available services, eligibility standards, and application procedures.
- They are more likely to have many health care needs.
- They are more likely to distrust the health system.
- They may have had prior negative experiences.
- They may not be legal U.S. residents.
- Their loved ones may not be in this country.
- They may have strong values about healing and may be using other types of healing therapies at the same time (herbs, traditional healer).
- They may have particular beliefs about shots, pills, taking blood, and X-rays.
- They may not communicate, and their silence may be misinterpreted.
- They may be there because of family pressure, not because they want to be.
- They are more likely to use a kin network for emotional support.
- Their values and worldview affect their health and illness beliefs and practices.
- They are more likely to have traditional views of health beliefs and illness behavior.

GEOGRAPHICAL
- Fewer services are available in remote areas, so the elders must travel long distances.
- Public or private transportation may not be available.
- In urban areas, crime may deter elders from leaving home to seek services.
- Family and friends may not be nearby to accompany them.

INSTITUTIONAL
- The service provider may be biased that minority groups take care of their own elders.
- Services may be fragmented with different qualifications for care.
- The care facility may require excessive paperwork, making it confusing for the illiterate.
- The facility may not have personnel who can speak their language.
- There may be a shortage of outreach personnel.
- Educational materials targeting common health problems of specific populations are not common.
- Community support for long-term care for minority groups is inadequate.
- Unavailability or reduced availability of services is a problem.
- Discrimination by providers resulting in no care or poor care is common.
- There may be a cultural insensitivity toward the minority consumer.
- Minorities have little, if any, input on program planning.

Note that the definition of a culturally competent professional implies more than knowledge. It also implies an attitudinal shift at recognizing and honoring differences in approaches, attitudes, beliefs, and values and finding common ground with the client. An individual cannot be culturally competent unless he or she has compassion and respect for people who are culturally different. Further, the individual must be aware of personal biases and *ethnocentricity* (believing one's own way of thinking and behaving is the best way). Resources to learn more about culturally competent care are at the Office of Minority Health at www.minorityhealth.hhs.gov

Although working with ethnic elders can be challenging, most health and social service professionals find working with these populations gratifying. Because of lower educational attainment, some elders may benefit tremendously from relatively simple educational efforts. These individuals appreciate services and respect the expertise of health care professionals. In many cases,

their larger extended families mean that more loved ones are available to provide help in the home, reducing the need for institutionalization. Regardless of age, race, or ethnicity, religious and educational background, or cultural values, it is important that those who choose to work in the field of health and social services treat all clients with honesty, compassion, and respect. Further, awareness of one's own prejudices and willingness to learn and change in order to become a more effective professional are crucial to meeting the needs of individuals in any population group.

SUMMARY

Familiarity with demographic data is crucial to understanding elders and the multiple factors that affect their health status. Information concerning the living situation, financial status, health care utilization, morbidity, and geographical distribution of older people allows a realistic appraisal of their characteristics and needs. Statistical data may lead one to the erroneous conclusion that elders are a homogeneous population rather than a widely varied group. Nevertheless, statistical information is invaluable in giving us accurate information to effectively meet the future demands of that group. Finally, since the elder group is one we all eventually will join, the information can assist us to be more realistic about our own later life.

ACTIVITIES

1. Visit your local Area Agency on Aging or the document section of your library or use Web sites to find the demographic characteristics of elders in your community. Find the proportion of older people, the proportion of ethnic group elders, levels of income, and other pertinent material. Compare with national figures.

2. From the material you gathered for activity 1, what health needs can you predict for your community? Interview a public health official, social worker, or planner at the local Area Agency on Aging to get other perspectives on the status and needs of elders in your community.

3. Analyze current television programming, newscasts, and television commercials to determine whether the media's view of older people is consistent with the demographic picture presented in this chapter.

4. Discuss beliefs you have held about older people. What did you learn from this chapter to change those beliefs? What information reinforced your beliefs?

5. Do the statistics outlined in this chapter accurately define the elders you know? How do your friends or relatives differ? Discuss some of these facts and figures about elders with your friends and family. Which ones were surprising?

6. The median yearly income in 2009 for an older woman was $15,282. Use this figure to develop a monthly budget. What expenses could not be covered in your budget? List the ways low income might interfere with the quality of this woman's life.

7. Interview an elder, and write a brief case history. How do demographic characteristics (e.g., marital status, income, family support) contribute to his or her health status? How does this elder report personal health in comparison with others his or her age?

8. Given the expected increase in the proportion of elders in 2030, discuss how society will have to change to better meet the future health care needs of its older population.

BIBLIOGRAPHY

1. Cutler, N.E., Whitelaw, N.A., and Beattie, B.L. 2002. *American perceptions of aging in the 21st century*. Washington, DC: National Council on the Aging.

2. Administration on Aging. 2011. *A profile of older Americans: 2010*. Washington, DC: Administration on Aging, Department of Health and Human Services.

3. Social Security Online. *Monthly statistical snapshot,* May 2011. www.ssa.gov/policy/docs/quickfacts/stat_snapshot/
   Social Security Online. *Research statistics and policy analysis: Income of the population 55 or older, 2008.* www.ssa.gov/policy/docs/statcomps/income_pop55/index.html
   Beard, B.B. 1990. Centenarians: The new generation. In Wilson, N.K., and Wilson, A.J.E. (Eds.), *Centenarians*. New York: Greenwood Press.

4. National Center for Health Statistics. 2010. *Summary health statistics for U.S. adults: Health Interview Survey, 2009.* www.cdc.gov/nchs/data/series/sr_10/sr10_249.pdf

5. Yeo, G. (Ed.). 2001. *Curriculum in ethnogeriatrics.* Stanford Geriatric Education Center, Stanford University, www.stanford.edu/group/ethnoger/

6. Spector, R.E. 2000. *Cultural diversity in health and illness*. Upper Saddle River, NJ: Prentice-Hall Health.

7. Scott, V., and Module Committee. 2001. Health and health care of African American elders. In Yeo, G. (Ed.), *Curriculum in ethnogeriatrics*. Stanford Geriatric Education Center, Stanford University, www.stanford.edu/group/ethnoger/ebooks/african_american.pdf

8. Talamantes, M., Lindeman, R., and Mouton, C. 2001. Health and health care of Hispanic/Latino American elders. In Yeo, G. (Ed.), *Curriculum in ethnogeriatrics*. Stanford Geriatric Education Center, Stanford University, www.stanford.edu/group/ethnoger/ebooks/hispanic-latino_american.pdf

9. Gonzales, H.M., Haan, M.N., and Hinton, L. 2001. Acculturation and the prevalence of depression in older Mexican Americans: Baseline results of the Sacramento area Latino study on aging. *Journal of the American Geriatrics Society* 49: 948–953.

10. Ostchega, Y., Harris, T.B., Hirsch, R., Parsons, V.L., and Kington, R. 2000. The prevalence of functional limitations and disability in older persons in the United States: Data from the national health and examination survey III. *Journal of the American Geriatrics Society* 48:1132–1135.

11. Warda, M.R. 2000. Mexican American perceptions of cultural competent care. *Western Journal of Nursing Research* 22(2):203–224.

12. Hendrix, L.R. 2001. Health and health care of American Indian and Alaska Native elders. In Yeo, G. (Ed.), *Curriculum in ethnogeriatrics*. Stanford Geriatric Education Center, Stanford University, www.stanford.edu/group/ethnoger/ebooks/american_indian_alaskanatív.pdf

13. Indian Health Service. 2011, January. *IHS fact sheets: Indian health disparities.* U.S. Department of Health and Human Services.

14. Indian Health Service. 2002, September. *Facts on Indian health disparities*. Office of the Director, Public Affairs Staff.

15. John, R. 1999. Aging among American Indians: Income security, health, and social support networks. In Miles, T.P. (Ed.), *Full color aging: Facts, goals, and recommendations for America's diverse elders* (pp. 65–91). Washington, DC: Gerontology Society of America.

16. *The economic burden of health inequalities in the United States.* Johns Hopkins Center for Health Disparities Solutions, Sept. 2009. Web, Dec. 2009. Blanchette, P.L. 2001. Health and health care for Asian and Pacific Islander American elders. In Yeo, G. (Ed.), *Curriculum in ethnogeriatrics.* Stanford Geriatric Education Center, Stanford University, www.stanford.edu/group/ethnoger/ebooks/asian_pacific_islander.pdf

17. Tom, L. 2001. Health and health care for Chinese American elders. 2001. In Yeo, G. (Ed.), *Curriculum in ethnogeriatrics.* Stanford Geriatric Education Center, Stanford University, www.stanford.edu/group/ethnoger/ebooks/chinese_americans.pdf

18. Administration on Aging. 2001. *Achieving cultural competence: A guidebook for providers of services to older Americans and their families.* Washington, DC: Administration on Aging, Department of Health and Human Services.

Biologic Aging Theories and Longevity

Young man,
Seize every minute
Of your time.
The days fly by;
Ere long you too
Will grow old.

Tsu Yeh

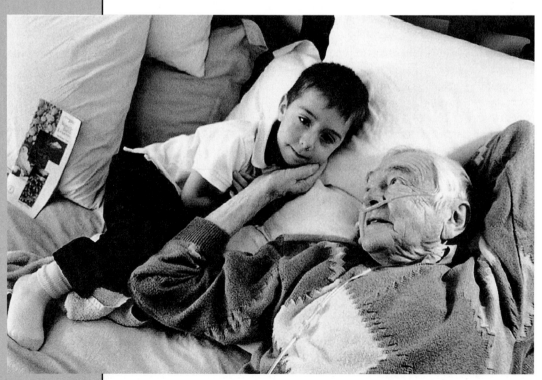

Why do we age and die? What factors influence the rate of aging and determine how long we live? What can we do to increase our chances of a long life? These questions are spurring researchers all over the world as they search for behavioral, cultural, psychological, physiological, and biochemical factors associated with longevity. Currently, researchers are interested in understanding the genetic and cellular basis of aging. Despite extensive scientific inquiry, how and why we age remains a mystery. In fact, each new discovery raises more questions than answers.

This chapter begins by describing the many factors that affect how long we live. Some of these are under our control, while others are not. Next, we discuss what is known about why our bodies age. Finally, we explore efforts to counteract the effects of aging, including anti-aging medicine.

LIVING LONG AND WELL

Life span is a term used to define the theoretical limit on the length of life, given ideal conditions. Life span does not vary by culture or nation—it is fixed for the human species. For humans, the life span is generally assumed to be around 115 to 120 years and has not changed for centuries. In contrast, *life expectancy* is the number of years an individual can expect to live and is highly variable. Life expectancy in humans depends on many factors—year of birth, age, gender, race, and culture—and is affected by some health behaviors, such as smoking.

Life expectancy can be calculated for any age. In general, life expectancy is calculated from birth. For example, the National Center on Health Statistics reports that the life expectancy from birth for an infant born in the United States in 2007 was 77.9 years. However, in 2007, the life expectancy for a person aged 65 years was close to 19 years—that is, the average 65-year-old in 2007 will live almost 19 more years. Although it seems paradoxical that someone born 65 years ago will live longer than someone born in 2007, those who lived long enough to reach 65 are "survivors," and the "average" is calculated on a smaller population—those who already have shown that they have the genes and health habits and lack of disease to live to at least age 65.

Life expectancy has dramatically increased over the last century, particularly in developed countries. This increase is largely due to improvements in public health, including sanitation and vaccination, antibiotics, and increased survival of infants, young children, and birthing women. For instance, life expectancy at birth in the United States in 1901 was 49 years. At the end of the twentieth century it was 77 years, an increase of greater than 50 percent. More people are living to the age of 60, 70, 80, or even 90, but only a few surpass the theoretical life span of 115–120 years of age. A French woman, Jeanne-Louise Calment, holds the world record for longevity. She was 122 years old when she died in 1997.

There are great variations in life expectancy, both within and among different countries, and there are variations between groups within single countries. For example, in the United States in the early twentieth century there were even larger differences in life expectancy between people of different ethnicities than there are now. In almost all countries, women have a longer life expectancy than men.

How long do you want to live? Nobody wants a long life if it includes being debilitated, demented, or dependent. If a long life could be guaranteed to be a healthy one, most people would want to live long.

It is generally agreed that the best way to age is to live a healthy, vigorous life for as long as possible, then die quickly and painlessly, preferably during sleep. Although nobody escapes mortality (death), each of us hopes to escape morbidity (illness) and disability. Morbidity is the period of reduced function, disability, and illness that occurs in a population. Morbidity becomes more prevalent in the later years, especially before death.

James Fries has conducted extensive research on a concept he calls the "compression of morbidity." Fries asserts that the ideal aging process is to keep disease and disability at bay until close to the end of life, then to die quickly.[1] With his model, older people would have a longer period of vigor and a shorter period of chronic illness, disability, and frailty, enabling a highly functional old age. Each of us probably knows one or more older individuals who exemplify Fries's model.

Over the years, several studies have documented that the "compression of morbidity" does occur, particularly among those who have a low health risk. For example, the health risk level and extent of disability of more than 1,700 university alumni were first recorded in 1962 when they were about 43 years old, and then assessed yearly from 1986 to 1994. Their level of health risk was defined by smoking, body mass, and exercise patterns; disability was determined by a health assessment questionnaire. Individuals who had a high health risk score had twice the disability of those with a low health risk score. Further, the onset of disability was delayed by more than five years in the low-risk group when compared with individuals in the high-risk group. The researchers concluded that the individuals in their study who smoked the least, were not overweight, and exercised lived longer, and the disability they experienced was compressed into fewer years at the end of life.

STUDYING LONGEVITY

How can we find out what characteristics and behaviors are associated with long life? Several types of research can answer this question. One common way is to study actuarial data. Actuaries calculate the life expectancy of people from various states, ages, races, and educational levels, with several health habits. They determine the precise effect of particular characteristics and behaviors on life expectancy. For instance, smoking is associated with a reduced length of life, but by how many years? Actuarial studies use statistics based on groups of people and averages. They do not tell us why women live longer than men, or why nonsmoking is associated with fewer driving accidents; they just describe the patterns they see by looking at a great deal of data about people collected over time. Actuarial studies can give you the "statistical probability" of your life expectancy that depends on the data you

enter: age, gender, height, weight, blood pressure, family history, smoking history, and health habits. A popular one is the "Living to 100 Life Expectancy" calculator at www.livingto100.com

Animal studies are conducted to determine the factors affecting longevity because it is not feasible to use human subjects in such studies. Animals can be bred to be genetically identical to one another except for one or two genes that the scientist has decided should differ. This allows the scientist to see the effect of one gene upon longevity. Further, experimenters can place animals in tightly controlled environments so that only one variable can be manipulated at a time. For example, some mice can be placed in a smoke-filled atmosphere and some in a smoke-free atmosphere to determine the difference in average life expectancy. Finally, animals have a shorter life span than humans, and results can be gathered much more quickly.

Animal studies can yield extremely powerful and interesting data. But there is always one critical difference: Humans, though they are mammals, behave differently from laboratory animals, and it is not always clear whether the results obtained from animal studies will apply to humans.

One of the most intuitive ways to determine how to live longer is to look at people who live to be very old and try to identify why. We can ask those who have lived more than 100 years what their secret is for living so long. Usually the answers are not scientific. For example, the answers may range from "a lot of sex" to "love" to "a shot of whiskey every day." We may ask them whether they smoked or how much they drank or what they ate, but it is difficult to compare their responses to those of elders who did not make it to 100, for they are already dead! Researchers involved in the New England Centenarian Study are examining individuals who live to be more than 100, their siblings, and their children to try to understand what factors are associated with extreme aging. Although this study is necessarily imperfect, it provides some glimpses into possible reasons why they live longer, healthier lives than most people.

When we study the factors that influence longevity, we must realize the tremendous variability

Studying People over 100 Years Old

The New England Centenarian Study is based on the hypothesis than centenarians as a group age more slowly and either delay or escape diseases normally associated with aging (heart disease, cancer, stroke, Alzheimer's disease). The study began in 1994 with centenarians from the Boston area and has expanded to include an international sample of more than 1,500 centenarians, their siblings and children, and a group of younger controls. To date, the researchers report that their hypothesis is supported: The centenarians they studied have lower rates of major diseases and later ages of onset of illness and disability than the general population.

Many of them are still independent and living alone into their 90s (90 percent at age 92 and 75 percent at age 95). In addition, few are obese or have a history of smoking, and longevity runs in their families (at least half have a close relative who reached extreme old age). The researchers concluded that, for centenarians, older doesn't mean sicker; instead, centenarians show us that "the older you get, the healthier you have been." For details on this interesting study, the findings, and profiles of several centenarians in the study, go to http://www.bumc.bu.edu/centenarian/

among individuals. Although there are a few individuals with poor health habits who live long lives and, conversely, some with good health habits who die prematurely, on the average, choosing a healthy lifestyle increases our chance of living long and well. Although certain factors are associated with longevity, there is no simple formula or collection of traits that guarantees any one of us a long life.

Longitudinal studies provide important information but are lengthy and expensive. Ideally, the researcher would begin the longitudinal study with a sample of pregnant women and follow their intrauterine environment, then, after the children are born, monitor the children's diet, their activities, family environment, psychological state, and so on until their deaths. But this study would take more than 75 years, and keeping track of these data for all these people would be intrusive, and very expensive. If you started the study later—say, with a group of 65-year-olds—you could get some useful information, but even this study would be lengthy and expensive. In addition, you have to be certain you measure the variables that are important at the beginning of the study, even though you are not sure what they are or what will be discovered

in the future. How many of the older studies measured details on diet, or the specifics of intensity, frequency, and duration of physical exercise, or reaction to stressful life events—all factors we now associate with health and longevity?

Factors Influencing Longevity

Gerontologists generally consider 115 to 120 years to be the maximum limit of human life, yet most people live less than two-thirds of that. Why do so few reach this upper limit? In an attempt to answer this question, scientists have identified a number of genetic and environmental factors that are associated with longevity. Some believe heredity to be the primary determinant, while others assert that psychosocial and lifestyle factors are more significant. Regardless of which determinants are most important, most agree that several factors influence our length of life. Some are beyond our control (e.g., genetics, gender), and others are modifiable lifestyle choices (e.g., smoking, weight control, and physical activity). Since none of us can change our genetic makeup, we can choose a healthy lifestyle, making the best of what we have. As Robert Louis Stevenson said: "Life is not a matter of getting good cards, but of playing a poor hand well."

Heredity

Experts agree than longevity has a genetic component. Animal studies support the role of genetics in longevity. Among humans, twin studies provide evidence that genetics play a role in determining length of life. For example, both life expectancy and cause of death are more similar in identical twins than in fraternal twins. Parental longevity is significantly correlated with longevity of the offspring—an observation that is likely related to both genes and parenting style. Parents probably influence the longevity of their children in the way they raise them—by their diet, their activity level, their ways of managing stress, and whether they have harmful habits (such as being a couch potato or a smokestack). Further support for the theory that genes are the basis of longevity is the wealth of research conducted to better understand the relationship of genes and disease. The Human Genome Project, an awe-inspiring attempt to understand the entire human genetic code, is making many exciting discoveries.

Genetic studies of centenarians and their relatives have revealed that living to extreme old age has a genetic component. The large-scale New England Centenarian Study found that at least half of the centenarians have first-degree relatives or grandparents who also achieve very old age. Many centenarians have exceptionally old siblings. Brothers and sisters of centenarians maintain half the death rate of other people born in the same time period, from age 20 until extreme old age. The cumulative effect of this year-to-year survival advantage is that the brothers of the centenarians have a 17 times greater chance of living to age 100 and the sisters have an 8 times greater chance.[2]

Information from the human genome has provided new tools to researchers who study longevity. A study utilizing a gene scan of over 300 centenarians and their siblings shows a group of genes on chromosome 4 that occurs more commonly than would be expected by chance. That region likely contains one or more genes that exert an influence on aging or susceptibility to disease. This finding gives researchers hope that there is a gene or group of genes that influences the ability to live to an

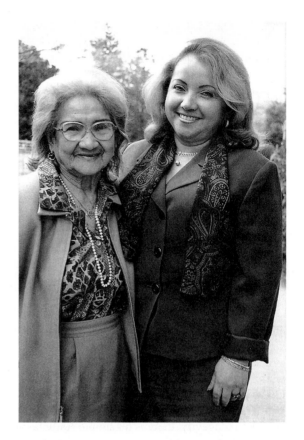

extremely old age.[3] Identifying genes that influence the length of life can eventually provide information about how people age differently and what genetic factors influence susceptibility to various diseases associated with growing old.

Gender

There is a strong relationship between gender and longevity. In almost every country and among all racial groups, females live longer than males. This differential holds in all age groups, even in the prenatal period. In those few countries where men live longer than women, researchers have attributed this differential to a high rate of maternal death during childbirth and, in some cases, to the neglect or infanticide of girls. In the United States, men have a higher death rate for the top 15 causes of death, except for Alzheimer's disease. The average life expectancy in the United States for males born in 2007 was 75.4 years; for females it was 80.4 years. The difference in longevity between men and women is thought to be due to a combination of environmental, behavioral, and biological factors.

Males are at higher risk for accidents, homicide, and suicide and are more likely to smoke and drink excessively than females. Further, men are less likely to visit doctors and practice positive health behaviors than women.

Since females of almost all animal species have a longer life expectancy, scientists hypothesize that females have a genetic advantage that enables them to live longer than males. The physiological basis for this advantage is the subject of ongoing research. The X chromosome (females have two, males have one) carries important genes for immune system functioning and possibly genes that repair damage within the cell. This might make females more resistant to infectious diseases and cell damage. Females may also produce more antioxidant chemicals that inactivate harmful free radicals, reducing damage to genetic material. The X chromosome also directs the production of sex hormones, namely estrogens, which affect cholesterol levels or other factors. It is known that women become more susceptible to heart disease after menopause, when their levels of naturally occurring estrogens drop. Women also have lower metabolic rates than men, which may partly explain their increased longevity.

In the past, it was believed that testosterone, produced in greater quantity by men than by women, was responsible for the differences in life expectancies. Testosterone is produced in the male testes and in the adrenal glands in both sexes. Before laws to protect people who participated in research were in effect, one study of mentally retarded adults found that castration (removal of the testes) increased life expectancy; castrated men lived an average of 13.5 years longer than their virile counterparts and 6.7 years longer than women.[4] However, current research suggests that the picture is much more complicated. Men with lower levels of testosterone and other androgens (male hormones) actually have higher mortality than those with higher levels, and the range of "normal" is very broad. It is clear that too little is known about hormones to fully explain the gender differences in longevity.

Although gender differences in life expectancy are pronounced, the gap is narrowing. Over the last 25 years, men have continued to make larger gains in life expectancy than have women. In 2007, the difference was smaller than previously recorded: only five years. Can you think of reasons for this trend?

Race and Ethnicity

Race and ethnicity strongly influence life expectancy. Blacks on the average die almost five years earlier than whites. Native Americans have the shortest life expectancies of all minority groups, dying about six years earlier than the general population.

What accounts for these differences? Many studies have attempted to answer this question; and although we have some ideas, it is still not clear why there are such marked differences. Some studies suggest there are genetic differences in populations that impact longevity. It is difficult to determine this, for many individuals who are ethnic minorities in the United States are from developing countries with lower life expectancy rates. It may also be possible that immigrants to the United States differ in some important ways from persons who remained behind—being either more healthy or less healthy, for example. It is clear that different minority groups have different rates of disease and that many develop diseases earlier (such as high blood pressure, heart disease, or diabetes) and suffer more severe consequences of the disease compared to their white counterparts. For instance, Native American rates of disease and disability from smoking, alcoholism, accidents, diabetes, obesity, and heart disease are much higher than rates within the white population.

It is clear, however, that even if genetic differences explained some of the longevity differential, they do not explain it all. Many researchers hypothesize that socioeconomic factors are very important. As a group, ethnic minorities have lower incomes, reduced access to health care and to health insurance, and lower educational attainment. These factors relate to what you do, what kind of jobs you hold, whether you smoke, drink, or use drugs, or live in areas with a high rate of violence. They affect the type of car you drive and whether it has safety features such as airbags, the kind of air you breathe, and the amount of close contact with others who may have infections.

Stress level is also important. It cannot be said that rich people do not have stress, but their stress is different from fear of personal injury, fear of being unable to make ends meet, fear of crime, fear of discrimination and of being singled out.

A growing number of studies have documented the deleterious health consequences of the experience of racial discrimination among black Americans. Interestingly, those minorities who reach old age live as long as, or even longer than, their white counterparts.

Cigarette Smoking

Gender and race cannot be changed, but cigarette smoking can. Inhaling smoke from tobacco plants is the most detrimental health habit among Americans. It results in a significant and pronounced reduction in life expectancy. The leading cause of preventable death in the United States is cigarette smoking. About 440,000 deaths in the United States each year are attributed to cigarette smoking. It is estimated that men who smoke cut their lives short by 13.2 years and women who smoke lose 14.5 years of life.[5] Further, an estimated 8.6 million persons in our country have serious illnesses attributed to smoking.[6]

Experts agree that the single most important action an individual can take to increase life expectancy is to not smoke cigarettes. The link between tobacco use, serious health problems, and decreased life expectancy is well documented. People who smoke cigarettes die significantly earlier than those who do not, mainly from lung cancer, heart disease, and emphysema. The risk of illness and death is directly related to the degree of cigarette smoke exposure: number of cigarettes smoked per day, total years of smoking,

and degree of inhalation. The latest report from the Surgeon General regarding the health consequences of smoking revealed important new information for the public regarding older people: Smoking reduces bone density among postmenopausal women, increases risk of hip fractures in men and women, doubles to triples the risk of cataracts (a leading cause of blindness and vision loss), and increases the risk of chronic obstructive pulmonary disease.[5]

The good news is that the rate of disease and premature death decreases in proportion to the number of years since quitting. Healthy 35-year-olds who quit smoking can extend their life expectancy by six to seven years. Even 65-year-olds can gain two additional years of life (men) to four additional years (women).[7] Insurance companies are well aware of the higher mortality rates of smokers and offer reduced premiums for nonsmokers.

Genetic and Acquired Disease

Although it may appear obvious, one of the most important determinants of length of life is the presence or absence of disease. While it is true that some people die suddenly without disease (for example, in an automobile accident), the overwhelming majority of deaths in the United States are among people who are ill. The more diseases an individual has and the number of body systems affected, the more likely the person is to die. Many inherited genetic diseases (e.g., hemophilia, sickle-cell anemia, Down syndrome, and juvenile diabetes) and acquired health problems (heart disease, cancer, diabetes, obesity, and Alzheimer's disease) decrease life expectancy.

Body Weight and Height

Overweight people are more likely to have a chronic illness that reduces their life expectancy. Obesity has been correlated with an increased risk of premature death and disability and an increased likelihood of diseases that increase mortality rate: diabetes, coronary heart disease, and hypertension. It is hypothesized that overeating and increased body size have promoted an epidemic of chronic disease. It is not known whether obesity itself causes a decreased life expectancy or whether obesity accompanies other more important risk factors, such as sedentary lifestyle or high-fat diet, which cause premature death.

Several researchers have reported that shorter people have lower death rates and fewer diet-related chronic diseases than taller people. Shorter people also live longer than those who are taller. Animal studies also show that smaller animals within the same species generally live longer.[8]

Physical Activity

Most experts agree that a high level of physical activity retards many age-associated changes, reduces the incidence of some diseases, and increases longevity. The physiological benefits of physical activity that influence longevity are well documented: Exercise strengthens the heart, decreases the likelihood of obesity, increases the good cholesterol in the blood, and reduces blood clot formation. These benefits are more fully discussed in Chapter 9, "Physical Activity." A higher level of physical activity also is associated with a lower death rate, not only from heart disease but from all causes of mortality. The higher the degree of fitness, the lower is the risk of death.

It is difficult to tease out the effect of physical activity on longevity, however, because of confounding factors. For example, individuals who are physically active may be that way because they are healthier in the first place, and those who are unable to be physically active are often ill or disabled and so may face a higher mortality. No study has conclusively documented the effect of physical activity or the type, frequency, or duration of activities that promote long life.

Alcohol Use

Light consumption of alcohol appears to be associated with cardiovascular benefits. Light to moderate use is defined as one drink a day for women and two drinks a day for men. Suggested biological

mechanisms for the benefits of alcohol are that alcohol increases the production of certain beneficial types of blood cholesterol (HDLs) and that alcohol may decrease the clotting tendencies of the blood.

It is still not clear whether the association of alcohol consumption with longer life is due to the alcohol consumption itself. For example, it may be that moderate drinkers as a group have other lifestyle characteristics in common that predispose them to living longer. As a group, teetotalers have a lower socioeconomic status than moderate drinkers. They may also have more rigid personalities that make them more susceptible to stress. On the other hand, it may be that those who do not drink have health problems that prohibit them from drinking, including alcoholism.

Heavy drinking (drinking three or more alcoholic drinks a day) is associated with reduced life expectancy and a higher risk for a number of physical and mental health disorders, such as liver damage, nutritional deficiencies, cardiovascular problems, nervous system conditions, suicide, accidents, and certain cancers. Heavy drinkers also are at significantly higher risk of early death.

Marital Status

Being married is associated with longer life expectancy. People who are married at the time of their death live significantly longer than those who were widowed, divorced, or never married. In 2007, the never married group had the highest death rate (more than two times those who are married) followed by those who were divorced, and widowed at the time of their deaths.[9]

Exactly how might marriage promote longevity? Some suggest that marriage provides an individual with a friend—someone who cares about the individual—thereby reducing stress. Studies consistently show that people with few social relationships have more illnesses and die earlier from a variety of causes than those who have a good social support network.

The advantage of being married, however, is not just a matter of togetherness. Marriage also promotes healthful habits. Excessive rates of smoking

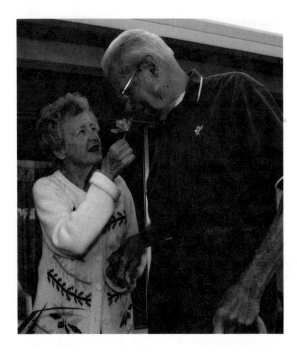

and drinking are more common among the single, divorced, and widowed than among married men. Another reason may be that a proportion of those who remain single or get divorced may have mental or physical illnesses or disabilities that predispose them to an earlier death. Married people have better financial status and are more likely to remain at home when ill as the spouse can give care.

Since societal mores regard married life as the ideal, being single may induce stress. The stress of losing a spouse of many decades during old age may also contribute to the shortened life expectancy observed among those not currently married when death occurs. Some studies suggest the health benefits for men in marriage are greater than those for women. It is not yet known exactly which aspect of marriage confers benefits and whether these same benefits may be realized in other ways, for example, by living with a friend or sibling.

Psychological Factors

Mounting evidence supports the hypothesis that some people are resilient to the effects of stress and disease while others are vulnerable and disease-prone. It is hypothesized that negativity in daily interactions, or a repressed/depressed personality style may be associated with a high risk of illness and premature death, comparable to having high blood pressure or high cholesterol. Personality traits such as bitterness, hostility, and a suspicious, frustrated nature are associated with increased cardiovascular disease and premature death.[10] Conversely, individuals able to handle stress constructively may live longer. Such personality traits may influence longevity by affecting hormones, immune function, cholesterol level, or other biochemical processes within the body. Further, negative personality characteristics may predispose some individuals to select life-shortening behavioral patterns (such as smoking cigarettes and drinking alcohol).

Social Class: Education, Income, and Occupation

Because income level, education, occupation, and social class are so closely interrelated, it is difficult to isolate which are the most important determinants of longevity. High educational and occupational levels are correlated with higher income and standard of living. People in the middle and upper classes live considerably longer than those in the lower classes. It is clear that higher educational attainments and social class, more prestigious occupations, and above-average income levels contribute to greater longevity. It may be that those with more education have more healthful habits and so have lower risk of smoking and obesity. An important consideration is that those with more money can spend more on health care and wellness, are more likely to have health care, have more dietary variation, and may live in less polluted, crowded, or toxic environments. These social factors are likely to play a role in explaining racial and ethnic differences in longevity.

Interesting demographic studies have been conducted in various urban areas showing the impact of zip codes on life expectancy. Those who live in zip codes of wealthier areas live years longer and have fewer chronic diseases than those who live in poorer zip codes. This "zip code effect" shows the impact of socioeconomic status on health.

Cultural Factors

It is well documented that life expectancy varies widely from one country to the next. In general, people from developed countries have a longer life expectancy than those from less-developed countries. However, much of the influence on life expectancy in less-developed countries is explained by their increased rates of infant and maternal mortality; many individuals die very young, but others can live to be very old. Multiple factors affect rates of longevity, such as sanitation and prevalence of infectious diseases, dietary factors, and access to health care. In addition, life expectancy in other developed nations (such as Canada) is increasing faster than in the United States, even among whites. It is hypothesized that a greater disparity of income between the richest and poorest members of a society contributes to decreased life expectancy statistics.

The Physical Environment

A number of factors in the external environment may affect longevity. Radiation and air and water pollution have been associated with variations in life expectancy.

Humans are exposed to low levels of radiation every day. This low-level radiation can impair cell function by causing mutations in the genetic code. Higher levels of radiation can shorten life by accelerating the aging process. Radiation is thought to damage the immune system, making the body less resistant to infection. Leukemia and tumor development are more prevalent after irradiation.

Air pollution is inversely related to life expectancy. Death rates in areas with dense air pollution are higher than those in pollution-free communities. Studies consistently show that air pollution is associated with increased rates of illness, hospitalization, and death among people of all ages, but the elderly are particularly vulnerable. Air pollution weakens the cardiac and pulmonary

systems, leaving elders more susceptible to illness, pneumonia, heart attacks, and death.

Expanding populations and increased consumerism combined with the unpopularity of constraints on industry make it unlikely that groundwater pollution, acid rain, increased pesticide and herbicide use, and increased air pollution will be reduced in the near future. It is more likely that the effects of pollution on human health and longevity will increase.

OVERVIEW OF CELL REPRODUCTION AND REPAIR

To understand how our bodies age, we must understand how cells work and how they age as cells are the basic building block of all life. Cells join together to make tissues, tissues to make organs, and organs to make organ systems. Cells carry on functions inside themselves, cells communicate with each other, and cells can make chemical messengers to send to other cells or organs or tissues elsewhere in the body.

Each cell is at least somewhat self-contained and self-maintaining: It can take in nutrients, convert these nutrients into energy, carry out specialized functions, eliminate waste, and reproduce as necessary. Cells take in amino acids, sugars, fats, vitamins and minerals and use these to make various proteins and other molecules. Some of these proteins and molecules are used within the cell. Proteins may build and repair cell parts, are used for energy, or create enzymes which facilitate chemical reactions. Other proteins and molecules made by cells are used outside the cells—hormones or neurotransmitters, for example, help one cell communicate with another. A typical cell contains 10,000 different proteins. Cells may all have the same genetic material, but they become specialized to do different jobs—some cells become nerve cells, others muscle cells and others are liver cells. Individual cells respond to the environment by making different proteins, making more of a certain kind of molecule, or speeding or slowing production. Cells take in nutrition and release waste products into the blood.

The body is composed of millions of cells. Each cell is specialized for a particular function. For instance, some cells (neurons) conduct electrical messages from one part of the body to another, some (blood cells) serve to carry oxygen to body tissues, and some (somatic cells) combine with other cells to form tissues and body organs. More than 200 types of cells make up the structure of the body.

How does a cell know what to do? Every cell in the body contains instructions, or genes, housed in a library of chromosomes in the cell nucleus. Humans have 23 chromosome pairs, one member of each pair contributed by each parent. Chromosomes are often referred to as *DNA* because they are composed of deoxyribonucleic acid. Chromosomes carry genetic messages, which direct the cell's assembly of amino acid building blocks into proteins that are ultimately used in the cell for growth, maintenance, and repair. The directions are in a chemical code composed of four types of nucleotides, identified by the letters A, C, T, and G, each of which stands for a different chemical. These four nucleotides are arranged on the chromosome in precise three-letter word combinations, called *codons,* that are interpreted by a compound called ribonucleic acid or *RNA.* The RNA molecule reads a group, or sentence, of these codons within the cell nucleus. Then the RNA travels out of the nucleus to other parts of the cell where it directs the production of proteins. The DNA is like the master computer working in a large but private part of a company. The RNA compounds are the messengers who read the code, then exit to the factory to direct the production of proteins, enzymes, or other cellular components.

Almost every cell in the body has an identical and complete set of genetic information. Thus, a nerve cell in the brain and a cell in the kidney are identical genetically, even though they have very different functions. Although every cell contains all the information for development and maintenance of the body that is stored in chromosomes within the cell nucleus, only the section of the information that is applicable to a particular cell is used; the rest of the genetic information is ignored. All chromosomes have a type of cap at each end, called a *telomere.* Similar to the tips that cover the ends of shoelaces, the telomeres keep the DNA from unraveling and assure that the cell divides correctly.

A *mutation* is any alteration in the genetic code. Mutations may be random errors that occur in the daily life of a cell, or by outside influences such as radiation and chemical exposure. Mutations may be insignificant if they affect a part of the genetic code that is not used by that particular cell or if the cell can repair the damage. However, mutations can be lethal to a cell if they affect a gene that is crucial to cell function.

Most cells in the body can reproduce by dividing in two, a process called *mitosis.* After growth and development are completed, mitosis is the usual way the body replaces damaged cells. Mitosis results in two cells that look identical to the parent cell. If one cell dies, another can divide and make a new one just like it. Cells that can divide are called *mitotic cells.* Skin cells and cells in the intestines are mitotic. However, some cells in the body (*postmitotic cells*) cannot divide after the individual reaches maturity. This is true of some neurons and muscle cells. Once these cells die, they are never replaced.

When damage occurs in DNA, genes are able to direct cells to repair damage by making various enzymes that recognize and correct abnormalities. Cells make new proteins and destroy the old ones. Cells are constantly checking for damage to the DNA and have complex repair methods. Extremely abnormal cells are destroyed. These processes of damage and repair are complex, and when they no longer work, they have a significant impact on cellular aging.

BIOLOGIC THEORIES OF AGING

There is probably no area of scientific inquiry that abounds with as many untested or untestable theories as does the biology of aging.

—Leonard Hayflick

We know that cells age, organs age, and the body eventually weakens and dies. But what causes the body to age? Can anything be done to stall or eliminate the process? While the younger body can respond well to stress and damage and has low rates of disease, as we age, our bodies become less able to handle stress (not just emotional stress, but the stress of heat, cold, prolonged physical activity), it becomes more difficult to repair damage, and we are at increased risk of disease. Could aging really be a type of disease that is treatable or even curable? Many scientists spend their lives trying to answer this question.

Today, there are two major schools of thought, or theories, on the causes of aging: *random* and *programmed*. Those who follow the random theories assert that aging is the result of accumulation of errors, wastes, damage, and misrepair that slowly reduce the ability of the cell to function. Random events occur throughout our lifetime, both from the environment and within the body, that weaken and eventually destroy the genetic material (DNA) that keeps the cells functioning properly, causing cell death. Another school of thought is that the aging process is programmed in our genes. These theorists assert that aging is not random but is predetermined by characteristics of our genetic material or cells. It is likely that the aging process incorporates some aspects of both theories.

The following sections provide overviews of the major theories that attempt to answer why and how we age.

Random Aging: The Accumulation of Errors

Those who support theories of random aging assert that a variety of circumstances causes the cell to malfunction and eventually to die. The most important part of that decline seems to happen in the nucleus with the DNA. What can happen? Some people think the main problem is too much waste, which can accumulate and clog up the functions of the cells (called waste accumulation theories). Others postulate that the DNA gets damaged by viruses, radiation from the environment, pollution, chemicals, free radicals and so on. This "wear and tear" reduces the efficiency of the cell (called wear and tear theories). Perhaps the DNA gets "cross-linked" and doesn't match up correctly— this makes it hard for the cell to read the mangled instructions and thus makes poor-quality proteins (cross-linkage theory). Scientists also postulate that time results in the buildup of errors in the DNA (error accumulation theory), or cells take shortcuts in repair that diminish their efficiency of DNA (DNA misrepair theory). The cell repairs the DNA quickly just to get it back into production, but the repairs are not perfect, and with time the DNA becomes too damaged to work. Mutations are changes that occur in our genetic instructions and can occur through "copying" errors or from the environment (diet, pollution, chemicals, solar radiation). If too many mutations build up and are not repaired correctly, the cell cannot function well.

The *free radical* theory of aging suggests that damage from highly reactive molecules within the cell causes aging. Free radicals are one of the toxic by-products of normal cell metabolism. For instance, free radicals are produced when a cell metabolizes oxygen to make energy to maintain itself. Free radicals also can be created through diet or environmental exposures (tobacco smoke, pollution, sunlight, radiation, nitrites used as preservatives for meats). Free radicals are parts of molecules that have either an extra or a missing electron that makes them highly charged and likely to combine with and destroy important parts of the cell.

Fortunately, the body produces enzymes to inactivate free radicals before they wreak damage and to repair damage after it occurs. Melatonin produced in the pineal gland also has been found to be a strong antioxidant. Further, some vitamins and minerals, such as vitamin E, vitamin C, vitamin A, and selenium, help to inactivate free radicals. Although enzymes made by the cells "mop up" much of the damage caused by free radicals, their efficiency wanes with age. The destruction accumulates over time, likely contributing to cell malfunction and eventual cell death.

Free radicals can damage genetic material, especially DNA, preventing it from making important enzymes needed for cell metabolism or from dividing correctly. They also can cause damage to other cell components, such as the mitochondria (site of oxygen metabolism), other cell membranes, or connective tissue. For example, free radical damage to the inner wall of blood vessels can cause abnormal blood clotting and the formation of atherosclerotic plaques, increasing the risk of heart disease and stroke. Damage to connective tissue can cause increased stiffening of the blood vessels and lungs and skin wrinkling.

The effect of free radical damage on the cell's DNA, in combination with the decreased efficiency of the cell to repair such mistakes, can lead to an accumulation of errors in the genetic material, altering its ability to function properly. This can lead to abnormal cell growth or cancerous tumors.

Programmed Aging: Born to Die

Some scientists argue that random events are not enough to account for all that is observed in human aging. They believe that aging is much more a matter of destiny, that cell growth, maturity, and decline are programmed as part of the DNA within the genes for each cell or by the gradual, but expected, decline in how our cells, organs, and bodies function.

Perhaps all animals have a *biological clock* that is programmed to shut down at a specific time. An example of a biological clock phenomenon is the menopause, when hormonal changes around midlife result in the cessation of the ovary's production of eggs on a monthly cycle and a loss of fertility. Proponents of the biological clock theory (also called the *pacemaker* theory) suggest that the nervous system, the hormonal or endocrine system, or the immune system gradually shut down and the organism weakens and eventually dies.

Evidence to suggest that there are hormonal declines that lead to aging and death come from studies of the hypothalamus. The hypothalamus is a part of the brain that links the nervous system and the endocrine system by sending chemical messages to the pituitary gland. The pituitary gland, in turn, sends chemical messages to other endocrine glands of the body. The hypothalamus regulates the hormones of the ovaries, testes, adrenal glands, and thyroid glands. As we age, this system becomes less functional, and this decline

can lead to high blood pressure, impaired sugar metabolism, and sleep abnormalities. When laboratory mice had the hypothalamus removed and were given all the hormones that the researchers felt the body needed, these mice lived longer than those who had aging hypothalamus glands. It is unclear whether changes in hormone levels with age would cause aging, or perhaps the pituitary secretes an additional hormone that we have not yet discovered. This hormone may promote longevity (and less is secreted with age), or it may cause decline and death, with higher levels being secreted with advancing age.

The immune system is often thought to play a key role in the aging process of cells and eventual cell death. Components of the immune system are able to differentiate "foreign" from "self." Not only do parts of the immune system combat foreign invaders, such as bacteria and viruses, but also infected, abnormal, or cancerous cells are recognized and destroyed.

Like hormones, some parts of the immune system decline as we age. The body is more likely to produce immune cells that make mistakes, inadvertently attacking normal cells or tissues or failing to attack abnormal ones. Perhaps the decline in immune function is what makes us more susceptible to cancers and other abnormalities in our own bodies. It may be that the decline in immune function is somehow programmed, perhaps to ensure that our tissues do not destroy themselves. However, an effect of this reduced specificity is that the immune system is less likely to destroy abnormal cells, such as cancer cells. A combination of more abnormal cells, and a reduced immune system to keep them in check, may result in an increased rate of cancer, inefficiency, and cell death.

Proponents of the genetic theory of aging believe that life span is determined by the genes we inherit. Researchers note that life span is consistent across species and that females live longer than males in almost every species. As discussed earlier in the chapter, it is clear there are genes that influence the rate at which we age.

Some research suggests that cells have a finite life span, a type of biological clock that programs their death. The biological clock may reside in the DNA of the cell. Human cells cannot grow and divide forever; instead, they have a finite life span. For instance, human embryo cells may divide no more than 40 to 60 times before death. Leonard Hayflick, a preeminent researcher in longevity and aging, reported that cells have the capacity to remember their maximum life span: The older the cell donor, the fewer times the cell divides before it dies.[11] Even if a cell has divided 20 times, is frozen, and then is thawed, it continues to reproduce about 30 more times before death. Interestingly, most people die long before they reach the limit of their cells. Hayflick hypothesizes that as the cells gradually grow older, a number of biochemical decrements occur that decrease cell function and reproductive capacity.[12]

Scientists believe that aging may be related to a tiny cap on the tips of the chromosomes called *telomeres.* It is known that some cells can divide throughout their life, while others lose their ability to divide. If you look at the cells of the skin and sperm cells, which are cells that continue to divide throughout their life span, you note a difference. These "immortal cells" have longer telomeres.

Telomeres are like protective caps adhered to the ends of DNA strands. They have been compared to those little plastic caps that tip your shoelaces, which make it easier to lace up your shoes. Every time a cell divides, these telomeres shorten slightly. Once the telomeres reach a certain critical length, the cell can no longer divide, and some cells weaken and die. You can think of this as shoelace damage that keeps shortening the shoelace until it is too short to lace up anymore.

However, something different happens in cells that are immortal. It seems these cells have more of an enzyme called telomerase, and this keeps the telomeres long, even though the cell is dividing. In the lab, if scientists can activate the telomerase in previously "mortal" cells, these cells can go on dividing forever and become immortal too. However, there is a downside to telomerase. Telomerase is commonly found in cancer cells, which often have a mutation in the telomerase gene and make too much telomerase. The telomerase appears to help

cancer spread by "helping" these cells become immortal, allowing them to divide and grow out of control. Perhaps there is a reason that our cells are not supposed to keep growing forever. Some fear that if we tried to activate the telomerase in each cell, then we might have increased cancer or other abnormalities in our bodies.

Are telomeres our biological clock, and when they reach a critical length, is it the end? The evidence to support this idea is that telomeres shorten in humans and animals with advancing age. According to one study, individuals with shorter telomeres in their blood cells died four to five years earlier than those with longer telomeres, and they are also at higher risk of dying of heart disease or an infectious disease.[13] We also know that individuals with *progeria,* a disease of accelerated aging, have shorter telomeres than the general population. If telomerase enzyme is added to cells, they grow and divide endlessly.

Other evidence argues against the central role of telomeres in the aging process. Many important cells, particularly in the heart and brain, never divide after maturity and survive for years or decades, so the role of telomeres in these cells is less clear. Further, shortened telomeres may be the result of other detrimental processes to the DNA, likely free radical damage, and not the cause of the decline. In addition, some species have much longer telomeres than humans yet have a shorter life span.

The importance of telomeres and their role in the aging process and cancer are still not well understood, and this is a fruitful area of research. For more detailed and current information on research on telomeres, go to the Telomeres Information Center at the American Federation for Aging Research Web site: (www.infoaging.org) and type telomeres in the search option.

Is Aging Random, Programmed, or Both?

Recognizing the interplay between our genes and the external conditions to which we subject them should lead to a deeper understanding of the process of aging. Today, most experts in the biology of the aging process believe that a combination of

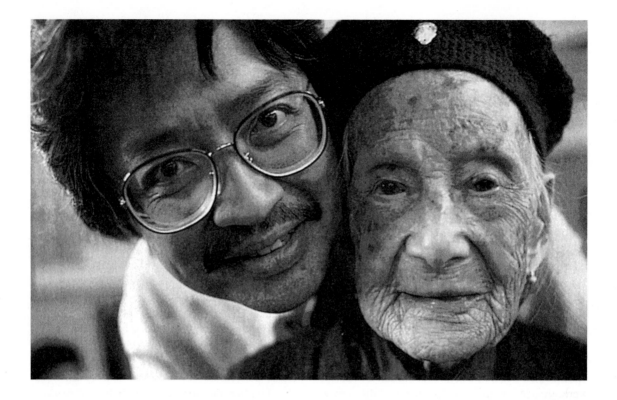

genetic and random events is responsible for aging. Any single limited theory of aging is certain to be insufficient. Much more remains to be learned about this physiological yet very mystical process of growing old.

One of the greatest difficulties researchers encounter is determining which changes are the underlying causes of aging and which are only manifestations of a process that originated elsewhere. Most likely, a combination of these events and some yet undiscovered contributes to the complex and intriguing process of aging.

ATTEMPTS TO EXTEND THE LENGTH OF LIFE

Although immortality continues to be beyond our grasp, scientists throughout the world still seek ways to deter aging and extend life. Researchers

have not yet discovered the mythical fountain of youth, but their attempts continue to provide a better understanding of why and how we age.

Anti-aging medicine has received much attention in the gerontological literature in the last couple of years. The term refers to any intervention that delays the development of age-associated diseases and other adverse age-related changes. At this time, no convincing evidence exists for any of the substances touted to slow the aging process, reduce the onset of disease, or extend life in humans. Claims that foods or supplements will extend your life have been made for centuries, and the public often clamors to buy the latest "scientific," natural, or 100 percent guaranteed product. Although the claims may appear scientific and convincing, the fact is that no compound has been tested and found effective at extending life in humans. Not that wheat grass, olive oil, garlic, red yeast, soy, blueberries, acacia berries, or almonds are not great foods and part of a healthful diet, there is just no evidence that they extend your life. These compounds may have been found in some animals to extend life (generally working in one species but not another), or they may be shown in correlational studies to be associated with longevity, or perhaps they are shown in a laboratory to "reverse free radical damage" or "prevent cross-linking."

If you want to live longer, the best strategy would be to eat less. The only intervention proven to extend life expectancy, prevent and reduce many age-related diseases, and maintain physiological function in animals is to restrict calories, but not nutrients. Early rat studies showed that if you underfed baby rats, they lived longer—the underfeeding gave the rats fewer calories, but still all the nutrients they need. Now the underfed rats were smaller and grew slower, but they did live longer and seemed less prone to disease. A study was done on monkeys, which showed similar results. The study covered 25 years and 117 rhesus monkeys. Those that were allowed to eat as much as they wanted had a 2.6-fold greater risk of death than the monkeys that were restricted in their caloric intake. The average life expectancy of the monkeys allowed to eat as much as they wanted was 25 years; those that were calorically restricted lived an average of 32 years. The calorically restricted group also had lower diabetes risk and fewer age-related diseases, although the study was criticized.[14]

How caloric restriction extends life in those animals is not clear. Maybe the lower metabolic rate reduces the number of free radicals that damage cells, or the cells might be better able to repair the damage. On the other hand, maybe eating all the food the animals wanted led to overfeeding, which reduced the life expectancy of those with a restricted diet.

At this time, no human studies have shown that caloric restriction increases longevity. Even if caloric restriction is shown to be beneficial, it is unlikely that many people would significantly alter their diets to take advantage of its benefits. The dietary regimens imposed on laboratory animals are far too severe for human subjects who might be less willing to trade stunted growth, delayed maturity, or hunger pangs for the possibility of a longer life. For more information, visit the American Center for Federation for Aging Research (www.infoaging.org) and type "caloric restriction" in the search option.

The free radical theory of aging suggests that antioxidants like selenium, vitamin C, vitamin E, beta carotene, coenzyme Q-10, lipoic acid, and others might extend human life. However, not only have studies failed to show life expectancy improvements from using supplements, but some studies actually show an increased mortality rate for those taking beta carotene and vitamin E. For more scientific information on antioxidant supplements, refer to the Web site of the National Center for Complementary and Alternative Medicine at www.nccam.nih.gov/health/antioxidants

Because some hormone levels decline with age, there is a suggestion that hormone replacement may increase longevity. Hormone therapies have been suggested to extend life and improve feelings of well-being and youthful vigor. Examples include estrogens in various forms, progesterones, testosterone, and DHEA, which is a testosterone-like hormone as well as a growth hormone. Once again, there is no scientific evidence of benefits and significant risks, but this doesn't keep people from experimenting.

Futuristic ideas for life extension include nanotechnology, the development of tiny, targeted molecules, which may be able to enter the body and repair cells or organs; stem cells, which theoretically provide an unlimited supply of new cells; and cloning, which might permit the growth of new body parts. For those with a lot of money, cryopreservation (freezing the body at a very low temperature) may extend life—those who do it hope that the future may bring new technologies that can repair and rejuvenate the body (including repair damage caused by death and freezing). However, this process is quite costly and the freezing must occur immediately after death, accompanied by cardiopulmonary support. Genetic engineering is a process of sending artificial genes inside the body that enter the cell nucleus and the DNA to replace defective ones. This might allow us to restart youthful genetic processes, repair damage, or turn on or off specific genes.

A look at even the most reputable methods of extending life reveals that few have shown to be effective with large scale placebo-controlled trials on human subjects. Treatments that either promote longer life or postpone the diseases and symptoms of old age will continue to make headlines. As consumers, we need to make rational decisions about new longevity treatments that do nothing more than give false hopes and take our money.

Some gerontologists believe that the quest to extend life in the laboratory is misplaced. They assert that the goal should not be to extend the length of life but to enhance the quality of life in the later years by modifying the factors that we already know to affect the rate of aging and onset of disease (e.g. cigarette smoking). In this way, the individual follows the compression of morbidity model: remaining healthy and vital until the very last days of life, then dying quickly. Good health habits, a rewarding social situation, and a positive mental attitude are more likely to extend life than the treatments discussed above.

Man's subconscious quest for a measure of immortality continues unabated; yet paradoxically, he jeopardizes his small share in the immortality of his species by his actions.

—Leonard Schuman

The Blue Zones

When looking at a longevity map of the entire world, scientists and researchers led by Dan Buettner found something curious. In some areas of the world, there were pockets of people who lived a lot longer than others—even others in the same country. In these "Blue Zones" they found that people reach age 100 at rates 10 times greater than in the United States, and, what's more, they have fewer illnesses and live out their years in health and vitality. Buettner and his team began an odyssey to try to find out why these people lived so long. What were the characteristics of the people, their lifestyle, and their community that might contribute to a long life? Buettner and his team identified factors that were common across all the Blue Zones and identified nine habits that are shared by the world's longest-living people. These Power 9™ habits should be familiar as they also happen to reflect the best evidence we have about what habits are associated with the longest and healthiest life. These lessons emphasize not only personal choices but making changes to your environment that will influence your habits.

1. Just Move.   The world's longest-lived people don't pump iron, run marathons, or join gyms.

Instead, they live in environments that constantly nudge them into moving without thinking about it. They live in places where they can walk to the store, to their friends' houses, or their place of worship. Their houses have stairs; they sleep on the floor; they have gardens in their yards.

Consider making things a little inconvenient. Make that extra trip up or down the stairs instead of loading things at the top or bottom to take up later. Walk to your airport gate instead of taking the moving walkway. Park far from the entrance, walk a dog, do your own yard and house work, get rid of some of the time-saving electronics and power equipment that have "simplified" your life.

2. Purpose Now.   Knowing your sense of purpose is worth up to seven years of extra life expectancy. The Okinawans call it ikigai and the Nicoyans call it plan de vida; for both it translates to "why I wake up in the morning." Do an internal inventory. Be able to articulate your values, passions, gifts, and talents. What are the things you like to do and the things you don't? Then incorporate ways to put your skills into action.

Continued

The Blue Zones

3. Downshift.   Even people in the Blue Zones experience stress. Stress leads to chronic inflammation, which is associated with every major age-related disease. What the world's longest-lived people have that we don't are routines to shed that stress. Okinawans take a few moments each day to remember their ancestors, Adventists pray, Ikarians take a nap, and Sardinians do happy hour. Find a stress-shedding strategy that works for you and make it routine.

4. 80 Percent Rule.   Marketers tell us we can eat our way to health. America is eating its way well beyond health. Our strategy focuses on taking things out—instead of putting more things in—our diet. "*Hara hachi bu*"—the Okinawan 2,500-year-old Confucian mantra said before meals reminds them to stop eating when their stomach is 80 percent full. The 20 percent gap between not being hungry and feeling full could be the difference between losing weight or gaining it. Serve food at the counter rather than at the table and choose smaller portions, store leftovers, then sit down to enjoy the meal. Replace your big dishes with 10-inch plates. Remove TVs from the eating area. People in the Blue Zones eat their smallest meal in the late afternoon or early evening, and then they don't eat any more the rest of the day.

5. Eat Mostly Plants.   Go ahead and eat meat if you want. But consider it a condiment and try the leanest, finest meat you can afford. Try to limit it to a portion the size of a deck of cards and only twice per week. Beans, including fava, black, and soy, and lentils are the cornerstone of most centenarian diets. Snacking on nuts—about a handful a day—has been associated with an extra two to three years of life expectancy.

6. Wine at 5.   Moderate drinkers outlive nondrinkers. The trick is to drink 1–2 drinks per day (preferably wine), with friends and/or with food. And no, you can't save up all week and have 14 drinks on Saturday.

7. Belong.   All but five of the 263 centenarians interviewed belonged to some faith-based community. It doesn't matter if you're Christian, Buddhist, Muslim, Jewish, or some other religion that meets as a community. Research shows that attending faith-based services four times per month will add 4–14 years of life expectancy.

8. Put Loved Ones First.   Successful centenarians in the Blue Zones put their families first. This means keeping your aging parents and grandparents nearby or in your home. (It lowers the disease and mortality rates of children in the home too.) Work on being in a positive, committed relationship (which can add up to three years of life expectancy), and invest in your children with time and love. (They'll be more likely to care for you when the time comes.)

9. Hang with the Right Tribe.   The world's longest-lived people chose—or were born into—social circles that support health behaviors. Okinawans created moais—groups of five friends that committed to each other for life. Research from the Framingham Studies show that smoking, obesity, happiness, and even loneliness is contagious. Assessing who you spend time with, and then proactively surrounding yourself with the right friends, will do more to add years to your life than just about anything else.

Not only did the group identify factors associated with longevity, they developed methods to assess life expectancy and to improve it and put their tools into practice. Teaming with AARP and the University of Minnesota, the group participated in a community health experiment in a Minnesota town called Albert Lea to see if they might be able to "build" a Blue Zone. The City of Albert Lea adopted 28 evidence-based ways to change its environment to live longer and better. These included developing walking paths and walking groups, improving food offerings, and changing public policies. In less than a year, the community raised expected life expectancy by three years, got residents active, reduced weight collectively by 12,000 pounds, and dropped the health care costs of city workers about 40 percent. For more information on the Blue Zones, visit www.bluezones.com

Used with permission from Dan Buettner, Blue Zones.

SUMMARY

One of life's enduring questions is "Why do we age, and how might aging be prevented or at least postponed?" We now know there are many and varied factors that influence the length of life. Genetic determinants such as gender, ethnicity, and race, familial history, and predisposition to genetic diseases play a role. In addition, a number of factors associated with a longer life are under our control: eating healthfully, abstaining from cigarette smoking, participating in regular physical activity, and learning how to cope with stress. Changing our destructive habits may not guarantee a longer life, but it will at least increase our chance for a healthier old age.

A number of gerontologists are conducting research to support hypotheses on why and how we age at the cellular level. To better understand why the body deteriorates, even in the absence of disease, researchers are trying to understand the genetic basis of aging and how the endocrine and immune systems fit into the aging puzzle. They have already documented the importance of the finite life span of our body cells and the accumulation of damage to cells, predominantly from free radicals.

Based on epidemiological associations and biological theories of aging, researchers are studying many ways to prolong life. Perhaps the best is dietary restriction, whereby laboratory animals maintain better health and longer lives if fed a well-balanced diet that is low in calories. Other methods show promise but have not been subject to rigorous scientific scrutiny in humans. Some methods may affect life expectancy, the amount of time an individual can expect to live, but few affect life span, the maximum time a human can live, which is 115 to 120 years. Thus far, no "magic bullet" has been discovered that ensures a longer life. Although more difficult than mindlessly swallowing a pill, the tried-and-true way to improve the quality of remaining life, and perhaps its length, is to begin a program to change negative health behaviors (such as stopping smoking, increasing physical activity, losing weight, or altering diet). In the long haul, it will show more results than the "quick fix" of unproven anti-aging medicines.

ACTIVITIES

1. What is the single most important thing you could do to prolong your life? What is the most difficult? How long do you want to live? Ask these questions to people of different ages—your parents, grandparents, children. How do their answers differ? Why?

2. The Living to 100 Healthspan Calculator was developed by Thomas Perls, a geriatrician at the Boston Medical Center. The Healthspan Calculator is a good tool for quickly assessing positive and negative health behaviors that will have an impact on your length of life and identifying your greatest health risks. Complete the quiz at www .agingresearch.org/calculator/ Discuss the positive health behaviors that will lengthen your life and the negative ones that will likely shorten it. Critique the quiz. What did you learn by participating?

3. Collect and analyze five advertisements from magazines or newspapers that boast about one or more products' ability to lengthen the life span or reduce the rate of aging. How could you determine if the claims are fraudulent?

4. Devise an experiment or a set of experiments in which you attempt to isolate one of the factors that influence longevity. Would your experiment show a causal relationship or merely a correlation between the factor and longevity? Can you see the difficulty in isolating one factor?

5. If everyone lived to be 120 years old, what would be the effect on our society—politically, socially, economically, medically, and psychologically? What might some of the consequences be, and how might we surmount them?

6. How long do you want to live? Why? Would you want to live longer if you could be guaranteed good health? Do you think it would be a good idea to extend the life span? Why or why not?

7. Read the Executive Summary of the Surgeon General's report on the health consequences of smoking, at www.surgeongeneral.gov/ library/smokingconsequences/ Write a report on its major findings. What is most surprising? What facts would you particularly

want to tell a friend who smokes? Do the same for the Surgeon General's report on the health consequences of involuntary exposure to tobacco smoke at www.surgeongeneral.gov/library/secondhandsmoke/

8. Debate the topic: Life extension studies should be supported by the U.S. government.

9. Imagine that you are given an opportunity to take an anti-aging drug guaranteed to double your life span. Would you take it? Why or why not?

10. Interview a long-lived individual. What personal characteristics enabled her or him to live so long? Can you see additional positive characteristics? Write up the material in the form of a biography.

11. Design an informational pamphlet for elders on a topic of your choice, targeting the design of your brochure for those with visual problems.

BIBLIOGRAPHY

1. Fries, J. 1980. Aging, natural death, and the compression of morbidity. *New England Journal of Medicine* 303:130–135.

2. Perls, T.T., Wilmoth, J., Levenson, R., et al. 2002. Life-long sustained mortality advantage of siblings of centenarians. *Proceedings of the National Academy of Science USA* 99:8442–8447.

3. Puca, A.A., Daly, M.J., Brewster, S.J., et al. 2001. A genome-wide scan for linkage to human exceptional longevity identifies a locus on chromosome 4. *Proceedings of the National Academy of Science USA* 98(18):10505–10508.

4. Hamilton, J.B. 1948. The role of testicular secretions as indicated by the effects of castration in men and by studies of pathological condition and the short life span associated with maleness. *Recent Progress in Hormone Research* 3:357–362.

5. U.S. Department of Health and Human Services. 2004. *The health consequences of smoking: A report of the Surgeon General.* Washington, DC: U.S. Department of Health and Human Services, Centers for Disease Control and Prevention, National Center for Chronic Disease Prevention and Health Promotion, Office on Smoking and Health.

6. Centers for Disease Control and Prevention. 2003. Cigarette smoking-attributable morbidity—United States, 2000. *Morbidity and Mortality Weekly Report* 52(35):842–844.

7. Taylor, D.H., Hasselblad, V., Henley, J., Thun, M., and Sloan, F.A. 2002. Benefits of smoking cessation for longevity. *American Journal of Public Health* 92(6):990–996.

8. Samaras, T.T., Elrick, H., and Storms, L.H. 2003. Is height related to longevity? *Life Sciences* 72(16):1781–1802.

9. Xu, J., Kochanek, K.D., Murphy, S.L., and Tejada-Vera, B. 2010. Deaths: Final data for 2007. *National Vital Statistics Reports* 58(19):1–136. Hyattsville, MD: National Center for Health Statistics.

10. Friedman, H.S., Hawley, P.H., and Tucker, J.S. 1994. Personality, health and longevity. *Current Directions of Psychological Science* 3:37–41.

11. Hayflick, L. 1961. The limited in vitro lifetime of human diploid cell strains. *Experimental Cell Research* 37:614–636.

12. Hayflick, L. 1975. Current theories of biological aging. *Federation Proceedings* 34:9–13.

13. Cawthon, R.M., Smith, K.R., O'Brien, E., Sivatchenko, A., and Kerber, R.A. 2003. Association between telomere length in blood and mortality in people aged 60 years or older. *Lancet* 361:393–395.

14. Bodkin, N.L., Alexander, T.M., Ortmeyer, H.K., Johnson, E., and Hansen, B.C. 2003. Mortality and morbidity in laboratory-maintained Rhesus monkeys and effects of long-term dietary restriction. *Journals of Gerontology: Biological Sciences and Medical Sciences* 58A(3):212–219.

CHAPTER 3

Changes in the Body with Age

Everyone wants to live a long life but no one wants to look old.

Albert Klingman

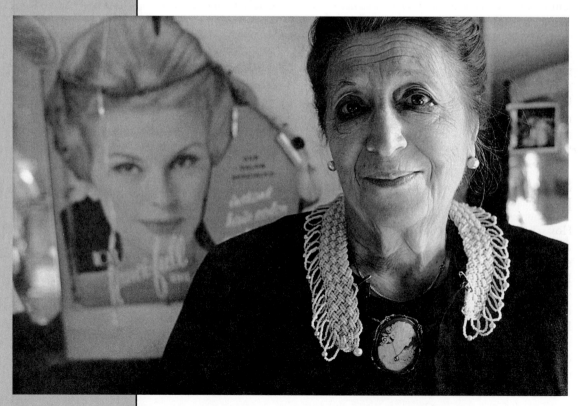

If you were asked to list the ways in which the human body changes with age, you would probably start with wrinkled skin and graying hair. As obvious as those external signs of aging are to the casual observer, they do not affect physical function. Other changes associated with aging are less noticeable but are more likely to affect the quality of later life, such as the decline of vision and hearing. In general, the aging process is associated with a decreased efficiency of body organs, but these decrements vary widely among individuals. Further, it is difficult to determine how much of the decline is due to aging itself and how much is due to environmental influences, such as disease, poor diet, lack of exercise, and cigarette smoking.

This chapter begins with an overview of the ways that researchers gather accurate information regarding the physiological process of aging. The pros and cons of each type of study are also addressed. In the remainder of the chapter, we describe the structure and function of each body system and its major age-associated changes. The term "age-associated" is used throughout the text to describe changes that commonly occur with age. Even though many of these changes are inevitable, it must be stressed that the rate of decline is highly variable. Many older adults maintain the level of function that rivals those of others who are many years younger. We have all seen extraordinarily "young" 80-year-olds and inordinately "old" 40-year-olds.

STUDYING THE PHYSIOLOGICAL PROCESS OF AGING

How do we know which changes are due to age and which are due to other factors? Researchers seek to answer these questions in a variety of ways. In a *cross-sectional approach,* researchers gather a sample of individuals from different age groups and collect data on the presence of a certain trait. For instance, to find out whether bones become thinner with age, the bone density of young people (aged 20 to 39), middle-aged people (40 to 59), and older people (60 to 79) might be measured. Then statistical methods would be used to compare the

three groups. If the researchers found that the youngest group had the highest bone density, the middle group had less, and the eldest group had the lowest bone density, they might conclude that bone mass decreases with age. Using another example to find out if height is lost with advanced age, researchers might collect height data on various age groups and compare the averages to determine if inches in stature are lost with increasing age.

Even though cross-sectional studies are relatively inexpensive and quick to conduct, they have their limitations. An alternative conclusion from the bone mass study described above is that the older individuals in the study became less active over the years, with a consequent reduction of bone mass. Thus, insufficient exercise, rather than age, may be the cause of reduced bone mass.

In a cross-sectional analysis, the groups to be compared must be similar. For example, the groups should have the same proportion of men and women, the same educational level, the same number of smokers or persons with chronic illnesses, and the same ethnicity. Suppose researchers select a group of 20- to 30-year-old college students and compare them to a group of 60-year-old college students. They might find fewer differences in memory than if they compared the same college students to 60-year-olds who have not completed high school. The researchers can "match" subjects by education, race, gender, or other factors or use statistical methods to control, or compensate, for these differences.

Cohort effects also influence the results of a study. A *cohort effect* is evident when the groups to be studied are different from one another in ways that might affect the results. Each "generation" of people may be different in some way from "generations" coming before or after. In the previously mentioned loss-of-height study, the conclusion that older people lose stature with age may be erroneous because the researchers did not take into account the fact that average heights have increased with every decade in the United States. Thus, older people may not have significantly shrunk in stature with advancing age but may have been shorter to begin with.

The results of some studies may be due to a *survivor effect*. If a researcher compared a group of younger people with older people and found more overweight people in the younger group, he or she might mistakenly conclude that weight is lost with age, when, in fact, the heavy people died and those who had average or below-average weight are still living.

Some of the difficulties of cross-sectional research can be overcome by conducting longitudinal studies. In a *longitudinal study,* a series of measurements are taken on the same group of individuals over an extended period, generally for at least seven years. For instance, mental function may be measured in a group of 50-year-olds, and then the same individuals may be retested at age 60, 70, and 80. Because the same individuals are tested over an extended period of time, it is more likely that any changes uncovered are due to age rather than to generational differences.

Even longitudinal studies cannot perfectly tease out what changes are due to age, which might be genetic, and which are affected by lifestyle. For example, a study may reveal a decline in cardiovascular capacity. However, some of the individuals may be inactive because they had a heart attack, some have become less active because of lack of motivation, some are less able to be active because of age changes, and a few actually had an improvement in status, but their numbers are dwarfed by the average. Longitudinal studies, by definition, require a long-term commitment by the individuals in the study. It is difficult and costly to keep track and maintain sufficient participants to gather needed information. Finally, individuals may become familiar with the testing situation or interviewer with time, possibly influencing the study results.

Clinical trials are better able to sort out the various factors influencing aging. In *clinical trials,* researchers are able to change some single or specific aspect of behavior in a group and monitor what happens. These are also called controlled trials because the researchers have a lot of control over the experiment. For example, a clinical trial to study the effect of exercise on bone mass of 70- to 90-year-old women may enroll 100 women. The researchers would assess bone mass and cardiovascular capacity of the full sample at the beginning of the study, then place half of the women on a weight-bearing exercise program for three days a week while the other half attends nutrition lectures. At the end of 12 weeks, all 100 individuals would have another assessment of bone mass and cardiovascular capacity, and the results would be compared. If the study finds that bone mass increases in the group on the exercise program, it may be concluded that a decrease in bone mass is at least partially caused by physical inactivity.

When subjects are randomly selected by the researcher either to have or not have an intervention, this is a *randomized trial.* When the researcher who measures the outcome (e.g., bone density) does not know which group the person was in (exercise or nutrition group), then this is called a *blinded trial.* If the subjects do not know which group they are in, it is a *double-blind trial.* Double-blind trials are used to determine medication effectiveness: Individuals in one group take the medication, and those in another group take a placebo (a pill made of sugar or other inert ingredients made to look like the real pill). Neither the researcher nor the participants knows who is taking the real pill or the sugar pill.

A *randomized controlled trial* is considered the "gold standard" type of research. However, even the gold standard is not perfect. For instance, what about people who drop out of a study? What if people in the bone mass study who watch a nutrition video also engage in a five-day-a-week exercise program without the researcher's knowledge? Another inherent problem is to correctly identify individual and subgroup differences when trying to match the two groups. Exercise may increase the bone mass of some white women with bone density more than 50 percent below the average but not do much for black women with bone density at average levels.

A problem inherent in any research methodology is sampling. It is obvious that all older people cannot participate in every study, so researchers attempt to choose a sample that is representative of the entire population (in terms of income, education, living situation, and other variables). The results of the study can be generalized to the entire population. Since studies often rely on voluntary participation, the results may be biased. Those who volunteer for experiments may be healthier, more outgoing, intelligent, and independent than those who do not volunteer. If researchers gather their volunteers from hospitals and nursing homes, the presence of medication, chronic illness, and inactivity may affect the results.

Studies are limited by funding—researchers study what is paid for. Who pays for studies? Companies will support studies that have the potential for profit, such as a new drug or a new piece of equipment, a new food or supplement. Studies may be funded by organizations (like the American Heart Association or the Huntington's Disease Society of America) to address their particular needs. Studies may be funded by universities or governments based on projects approved by representatives or boards. Studies are said to "follow the money," meaning researchers study what they can get paid for.

Another difficulty with studies is that we tend to study what is easily measured. We might want to answer a big question like "What can I do to live a long and healthy life?" However, we can only study what we can define and measure. How do I define what is happy or healthy? How do I measure happiness? Does my definition work for other people? How do I keep track of all the factors that might be important?

It is clear that no piece of research is perfect; every type of study has its strengths and limitations. Seeing the whole picture involves a review of several different types of studies, each looking at the same problem from different angles. Each study builds on ideas or associations or trends or findings reported by previous studies and tries to further clarify an issue or answer a question. There are often hundreds of studies on even the smallest topic. New evidence is constantly being discovered. What was "fact" 10 years ago, or even six months ago, may be called into question at any time. It is important when reading about the results

of a study that you put on your critical thinking cap and ask questions: Why might this association be true or false? What are the strengths and weaknesses of this study? What other conclusions could have been drawn? What other studies support these findings? What further studies may be done to clarify this issue? You and your peers will likely play a pivotal role in the future to clarify issues that are unclear today. There is so much left to discover!

DEFINING AGE CHANGES

In order for a physical change to be the consequence of advancing age, it should meet the following five requirements: (1) The decline must be universal—that is, it occurs in all members of the species to a certain degree. (2) The decline must be intrinsic (e.g., caused by age or genetics) and not due to environmental influences. (3) The onset of the decline must be progressive—a gradual process rather than a specific event. (4) Changes due to age have to be irreversible, although it may be possible to slow the process. (5) The change must be deleterious—that is, it must lead to a loss of function.[1]

Although these requirements seem clear-cut, it remains very difficult to distinguish which physical decrements result from the aging process alone and which are influenced by other factors. Cross-cultural studies of physiological changes accompanying age are sparse, so the requirement of universality remains unfulfilled. In addition, separating out environmental influences, diseases, diet, changes in other systems, physical activity, and mental attitude from aging can be problematic. Furthermore, when the "average" decline is reported in research studies, it includes some individuals who maintain or even improve in function and others who are totally debilitated.

Growing old is inevitable, but the rate of aging is highly individual. Chronological age is not a good indicator of biologic age after midlife. Without a doubt, genetic, environmental, and lifestyle differences play a critical role in the rate of aging. Furthermore, the degree at which each organ declines varies within an individual. For instance, a 70-year-old woman may have excellent vision and hearing but poor lung capacity. The ability to adapt to such changes also varies among individuals. Some elders adapt easily to heavy losses and are minimally affected in their daily routine, while others have minimal losses but adapt so poorly that they require major lifestyle changes. Whether an elder is debilitated or challenged by a loss of body function depends on the person's physiology, emotional state, and presence of social support.

Why study body changes with age? We need to learn to differentiate changes that are associated with aging from changes that are caused by disease. Because elders often have chronic illnesses, it is often difficult for health professionals and elders themselves to determine if a complaint is a symptom of disease or of "old age." If physicians erroneously attribute symptoms of a disease to old age, they may miss a treatable condition. And when elders themselves attribute their symptoms to old age, they may not seek treatment. For example, an elderly man with severe joint pain that limits his mobility may not bring his problem to the attention of his physician because he believes aches and pains are just part of growing old. In reality, his pain may be due to any of several treatable conditions.

Knowledge of the physiological aging process gives us a realistic view of aging. Professionals and laypersons alike need to know that people do not suddenly become frail at age 65. Even though each of us experiences some changes that are attributed to aging, they do not significantly affect everyday functioning. Further, some individuals exhibit "usual" aging (what is average for the population), and others experience "successful" aging (achieving the maximal functional capability in the later years).

Although this chapter focuses on age-related decline, it is important to realize that none of these decrements is life threatening. The deterioration caused by disease has a much more significant effect on health and lifestyle. The intent here is not to categorize older people as different but to emphasize that everyone experiences gradual changes with advancing age. Many changes are occurring in your body even as you read this page—some cells are no longer functioning as effectively, and others

are gradually dying. Eventually those changes will be interpreted as signs of aging as they become more visible to you and to those around you.

THE INTEGUMENTARY SYSTEM

The skin and its accessory organs comprise the *integument*, the largest and most visible body system. The skin has many functions. It protects underlying tissues from harmful environmental influences and minimizes water loss. The large surface of the skin and its capacity to sweat and shiver are important in the regulation of body temperature. The skin also eliminates salts and other waste products through sweating. Sensory receptors in the skin permit us to respond to environmental changes such as heat, cold, pain, or light touch. Upon exposure to ultraviolet light, the skin synthesizes vitamin D from a hormone in the skin. Vitamin D plays a vital role in building bone. Subcutaneous fat cushions the body from injury and forms a large part of energy reserves. Because the skin is able to absorb certain drugs, dermal patches are becoming a common method to administer medication.

The skin has three layers: the epidermis (tough protective outer layer), the dermis (below the epidermis), and subcutaneous tissue. The surface of the epidermis is covered by a layer of dead cells that is constantly being worn away as new cells form beneath. Skin cells thicken and harden as they are pushed toward the surface. The epidermis produces a pigment, called melanin, to protect the skin from sunlight by absorbing light. Skin and hair color are determined by the amount of melanin in the epidermal cells. Individuals with dark complexions have more melanin in their skin cells than those with fair complexions.

The dermis consists of nerve cells, capillaries (the smallest blood vessels), sweat glands and sebaceous glands, and connective tissue. The capillaries direct nutrients to all skin cells and also regulate body temperature. When we are too hot, the capillaries dilate and the skin feels warm as heat leaves the body. When we are cold, the capillaries constrict, directing blood away from the skin toward the body core. Also, specialized nerve endings that are receptive to heat, cold, touch, pressure, and pain are found in the dermis. Sebaceous glands secrete an oily substance that keeps skin and hair lubricated. Subcutaneous tissue lies below the dermis and connects the skin to the organs beneath it. It contains more blood vessels, nerves, connective tissue and fat. The fat serves as a shock absorber and insulator to protect internal organs and control body heat.

Hair and nails are another type of skin. Hair follicles occur in almost every part of the skin except the soles of the feet, palms of the hand, eyelids and lips. Hair serves to keep us warm and protects the sensitive areas of the body. The hair cycle within the hair follicle has two phases—a growth phase (2 to 6 years) and a resting phase (2 to 3 months), after which the hair falls out. A new hair then starts growing from the follicle. It is estimated that the average human scalp has 100,000 hairs and on the average, 50–100 scalp hairs are lost each day. Nails protect the sensitive parts of fingers and toes from injury.

Age-Associated Changes in the Integumentary System

No one dies of old skin.

—Leonard Hayflick

Although most people consider wrinkled, loose, leathery skin a necessary accompaniment to old age, much of the wrinkling, roughening, and mottling of skin is due to sun damage. This is easy to document: Compare the skin on an area of your body that is not often exposed to the sun with the skin on your face and arms.

When the skin is exposed to the sun, a chemical action is initiated that creates *free radicals,* destructive molecules that can damage the ability of the skin cells to function and reproduce. Even though the body produces substances that can neutralize free radicals, those substances are not sufficient. In fact, the thickening and darkening of the skin that follows sun exposure—a suntan—is a signal of skin damage. When exposed to the sun's ultraviolet radiation, the skin produces melanin to protect itself from UV damage. As a result, photoaging (aging caused by sunlight) occurs that is manifested as wrinkled, mottled, and sagging skin.

Because the face and neck are more likely to be exposed to sun and wind than the rest of the body, they are most likely to show sun damage, especially wrinkles, sags, and pigment changes. The degree of skin degeneration is directly related to the amount of sun exposure. And the damage accumulates with time, resulting in what most of us think of as aged skin. Genetics also plays a role: Naturally dark skin contains a greater degree of melanin so it resists sun damage, ages more slowly, and deteriorates much later in life than white skin. People with freckled or fair complexions, red or blond hair, and blue eyes are most susceptible to sunlight damage to their skin. Sunlight also stimulates the development of age spots and premalignant and malignant (cancerous) skin lesions. Solar (actinic) keratoses, or roughened patches, commonly appear on the face and other sun-exposed areas in old age. These may develop into skin cancers and should be monitored by a physician.

Cigarette smoking can profoundly alter the texture of the skin, creating tiny vertical wrinkles around the lips and increased wrinkling in the area around the eyes. This explains why cigarette smokers look older than those who do not smoke.

Only a few facial furrows are believed to be a consequence of aging. These natural wrinkles include "laugh lines" around the eyes and between the nose and upper lip, and other furrows created by habitual facial expressions. The elastin fibers that keep the skin taut loosen over time, allowing the skin to sag. The skin is stretched when facial muscles move in characteristic expressions. Over time, the skin is less likely to return to its original shape so that by age 40 most of us have creases that reflect our habitual facial expressions.

Physiologically, the skin becomes more fragile and translucent with age due to the thinning of the dermis and epidermis. The connections between the epidermis and the dermis flatten out, making the two layers more easily separable and increasing the propensity of the skin to tear. The skin may feel rough because the cells in the outermost

What Is Your Opinion?
Reversing Wrinkles

Although wrinkling and age spots have little effect on longevity, they may profoundly affect feelings of self-worth, especially for people who strive to look youthful. Society places more pressure on women than on men to maintain a youthful appearance. Thus, women are a receptive market for a lucrative cosmetic industry that offers formulas to delay wrinkling, age spots, and loosening of skin. Cosmetics and lotions, however, do little more than lubricate the superficial layers of the skin, causing it to appear less roughened and dry. The best way to reduce wrinkles is prevention: Reduce sun exposure and don't smoke!

Wrinkles come to all of us to a greater or lesser degree. Many techniques are available to counteract the imprint of the sun on the skin. To a great extent, the choices depend on the pocketbook. Tiny wrinkles can be reduced by dermabrasion—mild abrasion that uses a spinning wheel or brush to remove the outer skin layer—or by a chemical peel that does the same but with acid. Laser resurfacing is a newer technique to remove the sun-damaged outer skin layer. It destroys the outer skin layer by using a focused light beam to vaporize the water in the skin cells. No matter how the top layer of skin is removed, the success of the technique depends on the regeneration of smoother skin during the healing process.

Perhaps the most effective cream documented to reduce skin wrinkles and some precancerous skin conditions is tretenoin or Retin-A, derived from vitamin A. This drug seems to work by increasing the thickness of the epidermis, skin circulation, cell turnover, and connective tissue synthesis. However, it can be irritating to some individuals, and increases sensitivity to the sun. Currently, it is sold only by prescription in the United States.

Another method of reducing wrinkles is to inject collagen (taken from elsewhere in the body or from cows) into them, thereby reducing the shadows and skin folds that wrinkles cause. The effect of collagen injections is temporary, lasting up to two years. Silicone implants and injections have received much negative publicity and are no longer recommended.

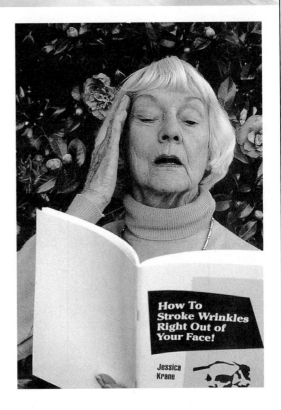

How To Stroke Wrinkles Right Out of Your Face!

Jessica Krane

Cosmetic surgery is the most expensive way to look younger and is more effective than the nonsurgical approaches. Common procedures are face-lifts, eye-lid lifts, and neck tightening.

Botox injections are currently the fastest-growing cosmetic procedure to reduce wrinkles. Botox is made from the bacterial toxin responsible for botulism, a form of serious food poisoning. The toxin causes muscle paralysis. When Botox is injected into wrinkles, underlying muscles become temporarily paralyzed and can no longer contract to form frowns. The results last from four to six months. Although the FDA approved the drug only for frown lines between the eyebrows, Botox is commonly injected at other sites on the face.

Continued

What Is Your Opinion?
Reversing Wrinkles

DISCUSSION QUESTIONS

What is your opinion about trying to look as young as possible?

What procedures are you willing to undergo to reduce the effects of aging on your skin?

Should the medical procedures mentioned above be covered by health insurance? Why or why not?

Do you believe that wrinkles should be treated?

If someone were willing to pay for a Botox injection for you, would you get one? What about a face-lift?

layer of the epidermis are not replaced as quickly. Fewer functioning sebaceous glands are available to lubricate the skin. The collagen and elastin connective tissues become less uniform and are replaced with inelastic fibrous tissue, reducing the resilience of the skin. The effect is greatest on skin exposed to sun, and least on unexposed areas.

The number of active sweat ducts in the skin diminishes with age. Although the decline reduces the potential for body odor, it decreases the ability to perspire and to regulate body temperature. Blood circulation in the skin is reduced with age. Most elders feel cold more than do younger people. The smallest blood vessels (capillaries) that feed the surrounding skin cells become fragile and more susceptible to rupture with even a slight injury: Older people bruise more easily, and their wounds heal more slowly. Sunlight accelerates the loss of elasticity in the capillary walls that are seen as fine blue lines, commonly called spider veins. The sun also damages the walls of the small blood vessels, increasing the likelihood of bruising.

Older people cannot produce as much vitamin D in their skin as younger ones. Thus, they need to eat more foods with vitamin D in them, take supplements, or increase the time they spend in the sun (without burning!).

Both the aging process and sun exposure combine to reduce the number of melanocytes (cells that produce the pigment melanin) and, in turn, melanin production itself. Further, reduced melanin increases susceptibility to sun damage. The melanin that remains may clump, causing pigmented

blotches on the skin that are commonly called liver spots. These can be removed by cryosurgery (freezing with liquid nitrogen), electrocautery (burning with low-dose electricity), or laser surgery (vaporizing with a focused light beam). Tretenoin (Retin-A) has been documented to fade age spots.

Subcutaneous fat smoothes out body contours. With advancing age, subcutaneous fat is generally reduced in the face, hands, shins, and feet and increased in the midsection of men and women and the thighs of women. Less subcutaneous fat, combined with diminished skin elasticity and gravity, causes the skin to sag and fold. These changes make underlying bones, tendons, and blood vessels more prominent. A reduction in muscle mass further contributes to the loosening of the skin.

With advanced age, nails grow more slowly and appear thinner and duller. The crescent at the bottom of the nail may disappear, and the nail may develop longitudinal ridges. Also, the nail may become thickened and hard to cut. Some elders, especially those with deteriorating vision, poor coordination, obesity, or arthritis, may be unable to cut their own toenails. They may need to see a podiatrist to prevent foot discomfort, infections, and mobility problems.

Graying hair in the middle years, widely recognized as an age change, is caused by a reduction of hair pigment. Almost everyone experiences a change in the texture and thickness of hair with advancing age. The number of hairs on the scalp, pubic area, and underarms is reduced. In males, some hairs become coarser, particularly on the ear ridges and eyebrows and in the ears and nostrils. In women,

Minimizing Sun Damage

Even though most people acknowledge that sunlight ages the skin, individuals of all ages, especially the young, too rarely protect themselves from the sun. Further, the thinning of the ozone layer is causing increased ultraviolet light exposure. In addition, with migration and travel, fair-skinned people, who traditionally lived in latitudes far from the equator, now live in sunny climates all over the world. It is difficult to stay out of the sun. Sunlight feels pleasurable and relaxing, and many leisure activities are conducted outdoors in sunny weather. Additionally, in our culture, a person with a suntan is considered to look healthful, attractive, and sexually appealing.

The sun is the single most important cause of the wrinkling, sagging, and thickening of the skin, also called *photoaging*. (The only other known factor that ages the skin is cigarette smoke.) To maintain healthy skin, it is critical to protect skin from the harmful effects of ultraviolet (UV) radiation. Sunlight contains two types of ultraviolet rays: UVA and UVB. UVB rays are most intense in the summer and at high altitudes. In contrast, the intensity of UVA radiation does not vary with the time of day, the seasons, or the altitude. Although UVA rays are not as powerful as UVB, they penetrate more deeply into the skin. It used to be thought that UVB rays were the main cause of sunburns, skin damage, and basal and squamous skin cancers, but we now know that both types of UV rays are responsible. There is increasing evidence that UVA is related to the deadly skin cancer melanoma.[2] Tanning booths, especially those that use UVA radiation, should be avoided as they also cause photoaging.

The best way to prevent skin cancer is to reduce exposure by spending less time in the sun, especially during the hours when the sun is the brightest. Outdoors, photoaging and skin cancer risk are reduced by the use of protective clothing (hat with brim, long-sleeve shirt). A third option is to use sunscreen and sun-block products. Sunscreens work in a chemical reaction with molecules in the skin to chemically absorb ultraviolet light. In contrast, sun blocks are opaque (like zinc oxide) and physically block the sun's rays. The strength of a sunscreen is denoted by its sun protection factor (SPF), a measure of the length of time the product protects against UVB (but not UVA). New sunscreen rules were enacted in 2011 that limit the claims manufacturers can make about these products. For instance, products labeled "broad spectrum" must protect against both UVA and UVB rays; no product can call itself waterproof; if the SPF is less than 15, the product must carry a warning that it does not prevent skin cancer; and no product can claim an SPF above 50.

Individuals should apply sunscreens about a half hour before going into the sun and reapply it every two hours. Experts recommend that SPF 30 be used if sunlight exposure will last more than an hour. A common mistake is using an insufficient amount of lotion and not reapplying it as needed for the full protection. Because many medications cause photosensitivity of the skin, which markedly increases the risk of sunburn, it is especially important for individuals using such drugs to use sun protection.

There is some controversy about the use of sunscreens. It is clear that they reduce sunburn and some types of skin cancer (actinic keratosis related to sun exposure), but it is not known whether use of sunscreen protects against melanoma, the most deadly type of skin cancer. Some experts feel that individuals may have a false sense of security with sunscreens and stay out in the sun longer with sunscreen without burning but still expose themselves to harmful rays. Others fear that some of the chemicals in sunscreens may be harmful or that sunscreens may cause vitamin D deficiency if used every time an individual is outdoors. Experts do agree that physical sun protection, such as hats and long sleeves, provides the safest way to enjoy the sun.

hairs may coarsen on the upper lip and chin because of changes in the balance of sex hormones.

Perhaps the most dramatic alteration in hair distribution is baldness among men. About half of the male population can expect some degree of baldness, which may begin as early as the late teens or not until the late 40s. In male-pattern baldness, the hair follicle gets progressively smaller, resulting in a shorter, finer hair, until finally there is no hair. The inability of the follicle to grow a new hair is associated with a genetic predisposition and the presence of dihydrotestosterone (DHT), which is converted from testosterone. The pattern of male baldness starts with a gradually receding hairline. Eventually hair on the top of the head is lost until there is only a fringe of hair above the ears and around the back of the head. Females with the genetic trait do not exhibit baldness, although their hair may become thin.

There is no cure for baldness, but some medications can increase hair growth and some individuals opt for cosmetic surgery. Minoxidil (Rogaine), a drug for high blood pressure, reduces hair loss in men and women who rub the medication into their scalp twice daily. This over-the-counter drug is costly, and it takes at least four months to a year to see any benefit. The individual must have had recent hair loss, and the loss must be on the crown of the head, not at the hairline. The drug is better at slowing the loss of hair than it is at making new hair grow and must be used continuously to be effective. Another drug, finasteride (brand name Propecia), was first approved to treat prostate enlargement but was found to encourage hair growth.

Because many people perceive baldness as a sign of old age, much money is spent to counteract hair loss. Wearing a hairpiece is probably the least expensive option. Surgery is the only way to permanently restore hair. The most common surgical approach is hair grafting. Hair follicles are removed from an area of the scalp with hair and are transplanted to a bald area, one follicle at a time, using microsurgical techniques. Another surgery involves moving a flap of hair-bearing scalp to the top of the head. A third surgery is scalp reduction, removing a bald spot by bringing the hair-bearing scalp closer together.

THE MUSCULOSKELETAL SYSTEM

Muscles and bones work together to protect and support the organs of the body; preserve body structure, posture, and stability; and enable body movement. The skeleton consists of over 200 bones; cartilage and ligaments bind bones together at the joints. Bone is a specialized type of connective tissue composed of calcium, salts, and some other minerals. Although bones look inactive, live bone tissue is constantly remodeled as salts in the bone and calcium in the blood are continuously interchanged. The bone stores calcium and other minerals and releases them into the bloodstream when calcium is needed in other parts of the body. The bone also produces red and white blood cells in the bone marrow.

The strength and thickness of bone depends on gender (men have stronger bones than women), health status (many illnesses and medications are associated with bony weakness), genetics, and physical activity. Race influences bone mass. For instance, Africans have thicker bones than northern Europeans. Physical exercise increases bone mass by causing stress on the bones as the muscles and ligaments pull against bones. Without physical activity, bones become weaker and thinner. People who have physically taxing jobs or are athletes have thicker and heavier bones than those who are sedentary. Bones lose calcium with inactivity, thus reducing bone mass and bone strength.

Muscles support the skeleton and account for almost half of the body's weight. Active muscles release a large amount of heat that is conducted to other body tissues by the blood to maintain body temperature. Muscles can be divided into three categories based on their structure: skeletal (or striated), smooth, and cardiac. *Skeletal muscles* are primarily attached to the skeleton and act on the bones to produce voluntary actions such as those needed for posture, facial expressions, and locomotion. In contrast, *smooth muscles* line the walls of the digestive tract, windpipe, bladder, and blood vessels. The movement of smooth muscles is slow and sustained, often wavelike. *Cardiac muscle* is composed of a network of fibers that contract as a unit. These muscles initiate their own contractions and are responsible for the continual pumping action of the heart.

Just as bones are strengthened with physical activity, skeletal muscles also become strengthened with use. A muscle that is not used becomes significantly reduced in size and strength, called atrophy. Muscles can atrophy rapidly, as one can tell by observing how much thinner an arm or leg looks when immobilized by a cast. Muscle atrophy occurs gradually among those who are sedentary.

Age-Associated Changes in the Musculoskeletal System

Sarcopenia, the age-related decline of skeletal muscle mass, is common among people over 65. The ability to climb stairs, get out of a chair, do housework, and walk is dependent on lean muscle mass. Loss of muscle mass predisposes elders to falls, decreased bone density, diabetes, and decreased tolerance to heat and cold.

To study the extent of sarcopenia among older adults, one research project sampled the skeletal muscle mass of over 300 healthy individuals between the ages of 65 and 92 and compared the figures with a group of young individuals from other studies. In general, the older group had 25 percent less muscle mass than the younger group. Differences in loss of muscle mass were more pronounced among those over 80—particularly among the men. Women over 80 had an average muscle mass that was one-third that of younger women while men over 80 averaged about half the muscle mass of the younger men.[3]

We know that muscle mass decreases with age, but it is still not clear how much of the loss is due to aging and how much is due to the decreased activity and increased disease common among older people. Men lose a higher proportion of muscle mass over their life span than do women. Among men, level of physical activity, testosterone level, and the presence of disease are associated with reduced muscle mass.

A decrease in muscle mass is associated with a decrease in muscular strength and seems to be associated with age. One longitudinal study measured the strength of knee and elbow flexor and extensor muscles of 120 individuals between the ages of 46 and 78 over a 10-year period. The rate of decline in strength averaged about 15 percent per decade, with the older participants declining at a faster rate than the younger ones. However, the changes were not inevitable; some individuals increased muscle strength by increasing their muscle mass with exercise. Interestingly, other individuals declined in strength even though they maintained the same amount of muscle mass.[4]

The loss of muscle mass and strength can be reduced by weight-bearing exercises, even among the very old. Longitudinal studies report that elders who maintain higher levels of activity have less deterioration of muscle mass and strength than those with lower activity levels. In contrast, those who are immobile show very high rates of muscular atrophy. Even when an exercise regimen is initiated late in life, studies commonly report that deterioration can be significantly slowed or reversed. For more information on increasing muscle mass and strength among elders with exercise, refer to Chapter 9, "Physical Activity."

One consequence of the loss of muscle mass with age is an alteration in the *basal metabolic rate,* the number of calories the body burns at rest. Because muscle tissue needs more oxygen than other tissues, when muscle mass declines, fewer calories are needed to fuel the body. The basal metabolic rate begins to decline in young adulthood and continues throughout the life span. With each decade, individuals must eat less and exercise more or they will gain weight. It is estimated that the body needs about 12 fewer calories a day for each year of age after age 30. For example, a 60-year-old person would need 360 fewer calories per day than a 30-year-old.

As adults lose muscle mass, their percentage of body fat increases. The average 25-year-old woman is composed of about 25 percent fat, whereas the average elder woman has more than 40 percent fat. Also, fat distribution changes in middle age. For men, fat becomes more prominent in the middle torso; for women, fat is deposited in the middle torso, hips, buttocks, and thighs. Body weight generally increases until age 55; then it begins to fall, mostly due to loss of muscle, bone, and water.

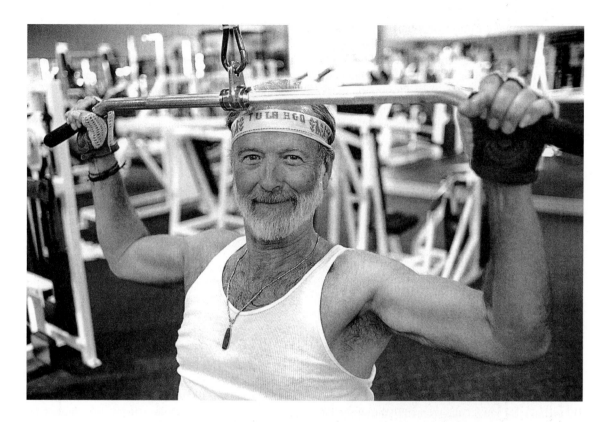

Joints become less flexible with age, creating minor stiffness and limited movement. Although joint degeneration is associated with old age, the aging of the joints begins even before skeletal maturity. Thus, joint problems may occur in adults of any age and increase in frequency as aging progresses. Calcification, fraying, or cracking in the cartilage and ligaments contributes to joint movement difficulties. Cartilage may become eroded in heavily used joints (especially the knee and hand) causing bone pain, stiffness, and loss of flexibility. In joint pain of the knee, obesity plays a significant role. Limitations in limb and neck joints may cause moderate alterations in posture, gait, and balance. Although extremely common, joint problems are not inevitable in old age. Like muscles, joint problems can be reduced with regular exercise and, in some cases, weight loss.

Reduced bone strength and mass are also associated with advancing age. The bones lose mineral content and become more porous and susceptible to

fractures. Experts believe this occurs because the rate of bone rebuilding does not keep pace with the rate of bone breakdown. Although bone loss is inevitable with age, the degree and rate are highly variable. A strong determinant of bone mass in the later years is the amount of bone mass built up before the third decade.

Gender plays a significant role in bone loss. Women commonly lose up to 30 percent of their bone mass over their lifetime; men lose about half that amount. For women, the most rapid bone loss occurs within five to ten years after menopause. Since women start with a lower bone mass than men, such loss can be significant. Because of this difference, it is important that women build up bone mass before maturity. Building sufficient bone mass when young reduces the risk of low bone density and consequent fractures in the later years.

Building strong bones is important throughout the life span. Before the age of 30, bone mass is increased by exercise and a diet rich in calcium and vitamin D; among middle-aged and older adults, these same practices slow the rate of bone loss. In contrast, a diet low in calcium and vitamin D and high in phosphorus (found in meat and sodas containing phosphates) is correlated with reduced bone mass. Estrogen also plays a role in bone strengthening. At this writing, the effect of hormone replacement therapy on bone mass is in question. Many large-scale studies are in progress to address this critical issue.

Reduced bone mass affects elders by increasing minor aches and pains and fractures. Furthermore, when older bones break, they take longer to heal. Ironically, the immobility necessary to heal them can worsen bone loss. Finally, brittle bones may further reduce physical activity because elders become overly cautious, inadvertently promoting further decline.

Both men and women become shorter with advancing age. The ongoing longitudinal Baltimore Study on Aging reported that, starting at about age 30, both men and women lose stature and the loss in height accelerates with increasing age. Women lose more height between ages 30 and 70 than men (women lose 2 inches; men lose 1.2 inches). By age 80, the women in the study had lost an average of 3.2 inches, the men 2 inches.[5] A gradual reduction of height is due to the cumulative effects of gravity on the spine, particularly the disks. Osteoporosis, poor posture, and musculoskeletal changes are likely contributors.

Why is it rare to see an older person with the erect posture of a young person? Changes in muscles and bones produce alterations in posture with advanced age. Spending too much time sitting hunched over a computer or phone, and too little time exercising and strengthening the core muscles in the abdomen and spine leads to an epidemic of poor posture. Further, bad posture in youth is accentuated with advancing age. Some elders may assume a stooped posture: head and neck held forward, bent or stooped shoulders, forward thrust of the hips, and slightly bent knees. These changes may be caused by compression of the vertebral disks in the spinal column, a decrease in elasticity of joints and ligaments, a loss of strength and shortening of tendons or muscles, or degenerative changes in the central nervous system. Poor posture affects a number of body functions. It interferes with stability and balance, increases back problems, and may also impede movement. Curvatures of the back may reduce lung capacity or compress internal organs. Also, poor posture detracts from general appearance, contributing to a decreased sense of self-worth. It is important to note that good posture can be maintained with exercise and is not inevitable in old age. Chronic conditions such as osteoporosis, spinal deformity or injury, foot problems, and obesity have a greater effect on posture than does the normal aging process.

THE CARDIOVASCULAR SYSTEM

The major function of the cardiovascular system is to transport nutrients to and wastes from all cells in the body. The cardiovascular system includes the heart, blood vessels (arteries, capillaries, and veins), and the blood.

The *heart* is a muscular pump that rhythmically moves blood and dissolved substances through the blood vessels to every cell in the body. The blood brings oxygen from the lungs, nutrients from the digestive system, hormones from the endocrine glands, and antibodies from the immune system to all cells throughout the body, and it returns waste products from the cells to the lungs and kidneys for removal through the blood. Blood also maintains body temperature by transferring the heat generated by the skeletal muscles to the rest of the body.

The heart consists of four chambers, two upper (atria) and two lower (ventricles). The atria and the ventricles are separated by valves that control the timing and amount of blood flow into each of the chambers and between the large arteries and the ventricles. The right side of the heart receives deoxygenated blood from the veins and pumps it to the lungs to be oxygenated. Oxygen-laden blood returns to the left side of the heart to be pumped to the rest of the body via the arterial system. Special arteries, called *coronary arteries,* supply the heart muscle with blood. The heart beats about 72 times a minute and pumps about 170 gallons of blood in an hour.

Unlike other types of muscle, the muscle fibers in the heart wall initiate contractions that spread through specialized fibers to all parts of the heart. Heart fibers called *pacemaker cells* initiate a rhythm of contraction that signals the other heart muscle fibers to contract. Heart rate can be altered by hormones or by nerve signals from the brain.

The heart pumps blood into the *arteries* to be transported to all parts of the body. Because the arteries are under pressure, the blood is able to travel uphill from the heart to the head and from the feet to the heart. Arteries provide more blood to organs as they need it. For instance, during exercise, the arteries to the muscles relax and widen, and more blood is routed to exercising muscles. After eating, blood vessels widen to send more blood to the stomach. Arteries contain elastic fibers that allow them to expand under pressure and spring back with decreasing pressure with each heartbeat over a lifetime. Arterioles branch from the arteries, carrying blood from the heart to the smallest blood vessels, the capillaries. In the capillaries, oxygen and nutrients move from the blood to the cells, and waste products from the cells move into the blood. Blood that is depleted of nutrients and oxygen moves into the veins to return to the heart and lungs for replenishing.

In contrast to arteries, the *veins* have fewer elastic fibers and rely on one-way valves within the veins and on adjacent muscles to return the blood against gravity to the heart and prevent backflow. Physical activity contracts the muscles that push blood upward from the veins in the legs back to the heart and lungs. Veins are under less pressure and expand much more than arteries.

Age-Associated Changes in the Cardiovascular System

With age, the cardiovascular system gradually loses efficiency. Although the system usually works well into advanced age, the maximal capacity of the system lessens over time. For example, it becomes more difficult to sustain high levels of exercise over a long period of time, and it is harder to achieve maximal exercise tolerance. Both longitudinal and cross-sectional studies have documented a decrease in maximum heart rate (the number of

beats per minute achieved with exercise) with advancing age. The decline in heart rate is constant, starting at birth. Maximum heart rate can be estimated by subtracting one's age from 220. For example, if you are 25, the average maximum heart rate for your age is 195. However, this number is highly variable among individuals of the same age and is not related to health problems.

Most age-related alterations in cardiac efficiency affect only peak levels of performance and do not affect the ability to carry out daily activities. In addition, cardiovascular performance in elders is highly correlated with level of physical fitness: Those who exercise regularly maintain a higher level of cardiovascular function when compared to their inactive cohorts.

Certain structural changes in the aging heart may contribute to decreased maximal efficiency and increased risk of cardiovascular disease. The walls thicken and the heart increases in weight with age. These changes increase the pumping force of the heart and may compensate for the slightly increased blood pressure that usually occurs with age. The heart valves become stiffer. The coronary arteries supplying the heart muscle with blood become twisted, and the aorta, the major vessel carrying blood out of the heart, becomes larger. There is also a reduction of pacemaker cells, which slows the heart rate.[6,7]

Changes in the arteries throughout the body may contribute to the reduced cardiovascular efficiency in elders. Arterial walls become thicker and progressively less elastic with age due to calcification, resulting in a smaller artery diameter and a hardening of connective tissue. "Hardening of the arteries" occurs whether or not vascular disease is present: It is an age-related condition and is not associated with lifestyle. Over time, these changes contribute to a gradual increase in *systolic* blood pressure (the top number in blood pressure readings, referring to the pressure of the blood on the walls of the arteries when the heart is beating), but the *diastolic* blood pressure (the bottom number, denoting the pressure of the blood on the walls of the arteries at rest) does not change. Hardening of the arteries also places more pressure on the heart.

In contrast, atherosclerosis, the buildup of cholesterol within the walls of the arteries, is a disease that is caused by a combination of genetic and behavioral influences. Atherosclerosis progresses with age and, in the United States, even appears among children.

Effects of age on the venous system have not been studied as extensively as age effects on the arterial system. Researchers do know that the veins become thicker and more twisted, and some of the larger veins increase in capacity due to decreased elasticity of the walls. Deterioration of the venous valves creates increased venous pressure and pooling of blood in some areas. Stretched and distorted veins caused by blood pooling in the legs are called *varicose veins*. When the veins in the legs do not effectively move the blood to the heart and lungs, swelling of the legs and feet may occur. When distorted veins appear in the anal canal, they are called *hemorrhoids*.

Blood flow to the internal organs diminishes with age. Since many body organs lose mass with age, the decrease may be in response to a reduced need for oxygen and nutrients by each organ.

THE LYMPHATIC AND IMMUNE SYSTEMS

The lymphatic system has two major functions. The first is to collect excess fluid from around cells and return it to the bloodstream. The second function is protective. *Lymph nodes,* located throughout the body, contain immune cells that inactivate bacteria and viruses and filter foreign matter from body fluids. These lymph nodes enlarge when a person has an infection or is invaded by cancerous cells. The nodes are located in the neck, under the arms, inside the chest and abdomen, in the groin, and around joints such as the elbow. Two other organs of the lymphatic system are related to the lymph nodes: the thymus and the spleen.

The *spleen,* the largest lymphatic organ, is located in the upper left part of the abdomen. Its function is to store blood and to fight infections. When the body needs blood because of exercise or hemorrhage, the blood stored in the spleen is expelled into circulation. Also, the spleen filters blood as do the lymph nodes. Some of its cells

(phagocytes) destroy damaged red blood cells, and other cells (lymphocytes) help to defend the body against infection.

The immune system includes the complex system of cells and chemicals in the blood that identify and destroy foreign invaders. The system fights infections from bacteria, viruses, and yeasts. The system also searches and destroys our own abnormal cells. On the negative side, the immune system is capable of rejecting transplanted tissues and organs and destroying healthy cells. It is also responsible for allergic reactions to foods, plants, some environmental toxins, and medications.

Our bodies are engaged in a constant battle with foreign invaders and use many mechanisms to defend themselves. The skin provides a strong barrier against invasion by microorganisms, stomach acid deactivates organisms that we may swallow, and enzymes in the mucous membranes (mouth, nose, vagina) inactivate invaders. The body also has many internal lines of defense. The liver, spleen, and lymph nodes filter the blood and contain many antibodies and immune cells to attack invaders. When there is an infection, these organs become more important and may enlarge. *White blood cells,* specialized cells that seek out and destroy foreign bodies, are perhaps the most important mechanism of the immune system. White blood cells may do their work while circulating in the blood or body fluids, or in the spleen or lymph nodes.

Every day, studies are identifying many and varied chemicals and reactions that play a role in immunity. The actions of the immune system are predominantly mediated through white blood cells and associated chemical pathways that are complex and not fully understood. There are many types of white blood cells. The most well known are B-cells, T-cells, and macrophages.

B-cells "remember" infections fought in the past and create antibodies to fight infections in the bloodstream. In the presence of infection, B-cells make specialized proteins called *antibodies,* which bind to the surfaces of bacteria or viruses and target them for destruction. The body makes several different kinds of antibodies to combat a single microorganism. These antibodies also protect us against future infection from the same type of bacteria or virus. For instance, if you have had measles, you will carry antibodies that are specifically directed against measles for the rest of your life.

T-cells search and identify cells that are "foreign" to the body, and they initiate a cascade of reactions to destroy them. T-cells work directly to inactivate invaders and indirectly to begin a complex series of chemical reactions that cause inflammation, fever, swelling, itching, rash, and other symptoms of infection or allergy. T-cells have multiple functions, depending on their type: T-helper cells aid B-cell function, T-killer cells attack bacteria or foreign cells, and T-suppressor cells protect the body's own cells from attack by the immune system.

Macrophages also serve an important immune function. There are many types of macrophages, each type protecting a particular tissue. They are attracted to injured tissue, and when they contact bacteria or viruses, they secrete a chemical that activates T-helper cells. In addition, they engulf injured cells and foreign invaders, then digest them. Many macrophages die during the process as do the cells of the injured tissues. The accumulation of dead macrophages and tissue debris forms the whitish fluid called pus. Pus continues to form until the infection or tissue damage is brought under control.

Age-Associated Changes in the Lymphatic and Immune Systems

It is generally agreed that immune function declines with age, placing elders at a higher risk of infectious diseases than the rest of the population. It appears that the number of functioning lymphocytes is reduced with advancing age. The general consensus is that there is a slight decrease in T-helper cells and possibly increased activity of T-suppressor cells. Neutrophils, a type of white blood cell that specifically fights bacteria, are less efficient with advanced age. With advancing age, T-cells are less likely to proliferate in response to an infection, and the immune response is blunted. Thus, elders may not develop a fever or inflammation as younger adults would with the same infection.

The antibodies produced by older persons do not respond as vigorously to foreign antigens as do younger adults' antibodies. Cancer becomes more common in the middle years. This may be because body cells have had longer to be exposed to damaging toxins or radiation in the environment and are more likely to be injured or mutated. In addition, there may be a change with age in the body's ability to distinguish normal cells from abnormal cells and to repair abnormal cells.

With advancing age and peaking around age 70, the body seems to make an increased number of antibodies in response to slightly changed proteins in its own tissues. Researchers thought that such an increase in autoantibodies might cause autoimmune disorders, a host of diseases (e.g., rheumatoid arthritis) that occur in people of all ages. However, even though these antibodies increase with age, there is no evidence that autoimmune diseases are more common in the later years. In fact, they are more likely to occur in the middle years.

THE RESPIRATORY SYSTEM

All body cells require oxygen to survive. Since cells and tissues are unable to store oxygen, a new supply must be delivered continuously from the mouth and nose to the lungs and into the bloodstream; otherwise, the cells will die. The waste product of oxygen metabolism, carbon dioxide, is excreted from the body cells into the circulatory system and back through the lung. The major function of the respiratory system is to transfer oxygen from the air into the bloodstream and to remove carbon dioxide from the bloodstream into the environment.

Air enters the nostrils and is filtered, warmed, and moistened in the nasal cavity. Air then passes through the *pharynx* (a flexible tube that also carries food to the esophagus), then through the larynx (voice box) to the trachea (windpipe). The *trachea* divides into two tubes (bronchi), and these continue to divide and subdivide into smaller and smaller cartilage-ringed branches that reach deep into both lungs. The *bronchial tubes* are lined with cells that secrete mucus. Protruding cells with hairlike projections (cilia) trap foreign particles that are inhaled and moved upward to the pharynx. Once in the pharynx, mucus and foreign material pass through the esophagus and into the stomach.

Each of the smallest tubes, *bronchioles,* ends in an air-filled sac called an *alveolus.* Nearly a billion microscopic balloon-like alveoli are housed in the lungs, giving the lungs a spongy appearance. The walls of the alveoli are one cell thick and covered with capillaries. They are the site for oxygen and carbon dioxide exchange. The inhaled oxygen passes through the alveolar walls, diffuses through the capillaries, and binds to hemoglobin molecules inside red blood cells in the bloodstream. At the same time, the blood from the veins containing carbon dioxide—the waste product of oxygenation—dissolves in the blood, then moves through the alveoli walls to be exhaled. For a diagram of the respiratory system and details about how the lungs work, go to www.lungusa.org; then click on "Your Lungs."

The mechanism of breathing is very complex. With each inspiration, the *diaphragm* (a sheet of muscles separating the chest from the abdomen) contracts. The contraction causes the diaphragm to lower. This lowering decreases pressure inside the lungs and causes air to enter the respiratory passages. During exhalation, the diaphragm muscle relaxes, bowing upward again. This movement constricts the lungs and forces the air out. Movement of the intercostal muscles (between the ribs) increases the depth of inhalation or expiration by lifting the chest. When extra respiratory effort is needed (such as during intensive exercise or in cases of chronic lung disease), muscles in the neck, shoulders, and abdomen become involved.

The rate and depth of breathing are regulated by a respiratory control center in the brain. Either high levels of carbon dioxide or low levels of oxygen in the blood can trigger an increase in breathing rate or depth by altering the muscle contractions.

Age-Associated Changes in the Respiratory System

The respiratory system is constantly exposed to environmental pollutants. Because of this exposure, it is extremely difficult to differentiate the extent of respiratory deterioration due to age from that caused by accumulated damage from pollutants. Although noticeable respiratory decrements are associated with age, the degree and rate of loss also depend on the state of the other body systems, exposure to pollutants, and extent of physical activity.

The main effect of age on the respiratory system is the reduced amount of oxygen taken up by the blood. With age, air tends to distribute less evenly within the lung, which lowers the efficiency of gas exchange. Lung tissue becomes less elastic with age, decreasing the amount of time the airways in the lungs are kept open. This decrease in elasticity affects the amount of air that can fill the alveoli, especially in the lower portion of the lung. Respiration becomes less efficient because blood still flows through the areas that are poorly ventilated.

Gas exchange is also limited by other age-related factors. The alveolar walls break down and flatten, reducing the area for gas exchange. The chest wall muscles and skeleton become more rigid, increasing the effort of breathing and reducing the ability of the lungs to expand during inspiration and compress during exhalation. Because of these changes, maximum breathing rate decreases with age.

The most consistent change in breathing capacity with age is a decrease in *vital capacity,* which is the amount of air that is moved in and out of the lungs when a person is inhaling and exhaling as hard as possible. Also, the amount of air left in the lungs after maximal exhalation is noted, called *residual lung volume.* When air in the lungs is not replaced with each breath, less oxygen is brought to the bloodstream and more carbon dioxide builds up in the lungs.

Despite the many changes due to aging in the respiratory systerm, the lungs maintain an adequate gas exchange for daily functioning. However, changes become obvious when an individual needs to perform at maximum exertion levels in an emergency or when reserves are needed during an acute event. Depending on their physical condition, older people may need more rest periods during heavy physical exertion than the young because they tire more easily and take longer to recover. Generally, older people are less able to cope with environmental pollutants and are more susceptible to pulmonary distress or death during periods of high pollution than younger people.

As in other age changes, tremendous variation exists among elders regarding these measures of pulmonary efficiency. A regular exercise program can help many elders to minimize most of these decrements. Smoking cigarettes and inhaling polluted air exacerbate them.

THE DIGESTIVE SYSTEM

The digestive system is a modified, muscular tube that extends from the mouth to the anus. Portions of this tube are specialized for different functions. Each portion plays a role in the breakdown of food into usable nutrients, absorbing them into the blood and temporarily storing the waste products until elimination. Accessory structures, such as the pancreas and gallbladder, release chemicals into the alimentary canal to facilitate digestion and absorption. A diagram of the digestive system can be found at www.nlm.nih.gov/medlineplus/digestivesystem.html

Other body systems also affect the workings of the digestive system. The nervous system regulates contractions of the muscles in the wall of the alimentary canal and the blood flow to these organs. Digestion also involves the secretion of enzymes and hormones by the endocrine system. The cardiovascular system transports food molecules from the digestive system to body cells.

Digestion begins in the mouth, where *teeth* (a complete set numbers from 28 to 32) mechanically break down food particles. *Saliva,* secreted by three major pairs of salivary glands, moistens the food and contains an enzyme that breaks down complex carbohydrates into simple sugar molecules. Salivary secretions also help taste-bud functioning and keep the oral cavity clean. The *tongue* mixes food with saliva and also moves food from the mouth into the passageway of the esophagus.

When food is swallowed, rhythmic muscular contractions of the *esophagus* push food toward the stomach. When the esophagus contracts, a valve opens at the entrance to the stomach. As the sphincter closes, the muscular stomach wall churns to break down the food. Although the *stomach's* major function is storage, some digestion occurs there. An enzyme (pepsin) and hydrochloric acid initiate the digestion of proteins. Gastric juice also contains other enzymes, one of which aids in the absorption of vitamin B_{12}. This mixture of partially digested food and secretions then passes from the stomach into the *duodenum,* the first part of the small intestine.

Both the liver and the pancreas are essential to normal functioning of the small intestine. The *liver* is located on the upper right side of the abdominal cavity under the rib cage. The liver regulates the metabolism of carbohydrates and fats, synthesizes proteins, removes wastes, and stores vitamins. The main digestive function of the liver is to produce bile, which is stored in the *gallbladder.* Bile from the gallbladder subsequently travels through the bile duct to the small intestine to break up fat globules so the small intestine can absorb fat and cholesterol. Some of the ingredients in bile travel back to the liver through the bloodstream to be used again. Bile also contains waste products from the liver that are eventually excreted in feces. The *pancreas* is a soft spongy organ located behind the stomach and is attached to the small intestine. The pancreas produces juices that flow into the pancreatic duct to the small intestine. The pancreas opens into the small intestine, secreting bicarbonate to neutralize the strong stomach acid and enzymes to break down carbohydrates, fats, and proteins.

The *small intestine,* almost 10 feet in length, is the main site for the absorption of nutrients, water, and salts. Its lining also secretes a number of different enzymes that further break down proteins, complex starches, sugars, and fats. As food moves through the small intestine, fingerlike outgrowths (villi) with hairlike projections (microvilli) absorb the water, salts, and small molecules of the meal into the bloodstream. After four to six hours in the small intestine, the unabsorbed contents empty into the large intestine through another valve.

The *large intestine* consists of the *colon,* the *rectum,* and the *anal canal.* The *appendix* is a tubular pocket that extends from the entrance of the large intestine. It has no digestive function; it contains lymphatic tissue that may resist infection in the area. The large intestine has little significance in absorbing nutrients; it absorbs water and salts, forming and storing solid feces. When the muscular terminal portion of the colon (the rectum) is filled, feces are eliminated through the anal sphincter. Feces usually contain 50 to 75 percent water, indigestible plant matter, dead cells, and bacteria.

Age-Associated Changes in the Digestive System

The digestive system has a high turnover of cells and a substantial reserve capacity, enabling it to withstand considerable deterioration before any effect is noted on digestive functioning. Thus, few age-associated changes in this system have been noted. Although pepsin production in the stomach is reduced in middle age, healthy older people show no additional decline. Structurally, there is a reduced blood flow through the intestinal mucosa in older people. There is some evidence that reduced absorption of calcium, iron, and vitamins B_1 and B_{12} is common in late life. However, if an older person is healthy and eats well, these changes are not problematic. No significant functional changes in the gallbladder, liver, or pancreatic secretions into the intestine have been reported.

Perhaps the most obvious change affecting digestion associated with advancing age is tooth loss. Since the 1970s, more people are keeping their teeth. The latest National Health and Nutrition Examination Surveys (1999–2004) report that black seniors, current smokers, and those with lower incomes and less education have fewer remaining teeth. Elders over age 65 have an average of 19 remaining teeth, and more than one of four elders has no remaining teeth.

Tooth loss is also associated with poor oral hygiene, gum disease, malnutrition, diabetes, and drugs that dry the mouth. With advancing age, there is generally a receding of the gums that exposes more and more tooth area, but it can be slowed with good oral hygiene. Teeth also wear down over a lifetime of use, but the extent is not significant.

Experts predict that, in the future, increasing numbers of elders will retain their original teeth. Today's children and young adults benefit from a bevy of oral care products, fluoridated water, improved dental hygiene, more frequent checkups, and dental education in the schools.

The Urinary System

Waste products are formed when each body cell breaks down oxygen and food into molecules necessary for cell growth and energy. Cells contain and are surrounded by a fluid that takes nutrients from blood and returns waste. The respiratory system eliminates one waste product, carbon dioxide, from the body. The urinary system rids the body of other waste products and toxic substances. In addition to transporting waste, the urinary system also regulates the amount and composition of body fluids.

The urinary system includes a pair of kidneys. Each kidney is attached to a muscular tube called a ureter, which transports urine from the kidney to the bladder. The bladder stores the urine until the urethra, a narrow tube connected to the bladder, carries the urine outside the body. For a diagram of the urinary system, refer to kidney.niddk.nih. gov/kudiseases/pubs/yourkidneys

The *kidneys* are located behind the digestive organs in the middle of the back, one on each side of the spine. Each kidney is about 4 inches long and is composed of millions of tubules, called nephrons, that selectively remove waste from the blood, returning almost all the fluid and nutrients back to the body. The waste products and water become urine, which passes through the kidneys into the ureters and then to the bladder. Kidneys regulate the concentration of urine. When we are dehydrated, our kidneys make more concentrated urine to conserve water; when we drink a lot of water, the kidneys make the urine more dilute. The urinary filtration system is very efficient: The entire volume of blood in the body is filtered almost 50 times a day.

The *bladder,* an expandable muscular sac, can store up to a pint of urine for several hours. It expands as it fills, and when it is filled close to capacity, nerve endings within the bladder wall transmit a message to the brain that initiates the urge to urinate. One sphincter at the neck of the bladder and another surrounding the urethra keep urine from leaking out. When the bladder is about half full, sensors in its wall signal the brain, resulting in the urge to urinate. Even when the bladder is full, it will not empty until it gets a signal from the brain, allowing time to get to the bathroom. When the time is appropriate, an individual relaxes the sphincters at the opening of the bladder and squeezes down on the bladder, emptying the urine into the urethra. From the urethra, the urine passes out of the body. In males, the urethra is about 8 inches long; in females, about 2 inches. The male urethra also carries semen.

Age-Associated Changes in the Urinary System

During middle age, the kidneys gradually become less efficient at filtering the blood. This leads to a reduced ability of the body to make concentrated urine and thus, less ability to deal with dehydration. When kidneys are less efficient, many medications stay in the body longer. Thus, older people and those with kidney problems need lower doses of many medications.

Reduced efficiency of the kidneys also results in changes in the hormones secreted by the kidneys that regulate salt-water balance. This in turn, affects the "day-night" rhythm of urination. Starting in childhood, urine is produced according to a day-night cycle (called circadian rhythm). Generally the urine produced during the day is twice that produced at night. This pattern changes at around age 60, when elders gradually shift to producing more urine at night. In the later years, the amount of urine produced at night may equal or even exceed the day rate. As a result, older people are more likely to wake up at night to urinate (a condition called nocturia).

The bladder also undergoes age-associated changes that begin around 50. Muscles in the wall of the bladder weaken, reducing bladder capacity.

The reduced capacity of the bladder to fill sends a message that the bladder is full when it is not, causing increased urinary frequency (polyuria).

Just as in other systems, some age-associated decline in kidney and bladder function can be expected, but the severity and rate of decline are highly variable. Most individuals maintain stable kidney and bladder function thoughout their lives.

THE NERVOUS SYSTEM

All body functions are monitored and controlled by a complex communication network involving the nervous and endocrine systems. In general, these systems function well into advanced age. However, age-associated changes in the neurosensory system, particularly those affecting hearing and vision, are inevitable in the later years.

The nervous system has two main components: the central and the peripheral. The *central* nervous system (brain and spinal cord) gathers input from the sensory organs, integrates it, and sends messages to the peripheral nervous system. The *peripheral* nervous system controls the work of body organs, glands, and muscles. Both the central and the peripheral nervous systems are composed of *neurons*—nerve cells, which store and conduct information. It is believed that the brain alone is composed of a billion to a trillion neurons that direct the function of the body.

Neurons transmit information to muscles, to glands, and to each other by both chemical and electrical stimulation. The shape of neurons varies and depends on their role and location. A neuron receives information from another neuron by an electricity-conducting fiber within the neuron that is able to both receive information from and send information to other neurons. The speed of information passing from neuron to neuron is up to several hundred miles an hour, enabling a neuron to transmit information hundreds of times each second. When the information reaches the ends of the nerve cell branches (axons), it triggers the release of neurotransmitters, chemical messengers that allow communication to flow between the nerves to enable the body to function.

Many types of chemicals serve as neurotransmitters, and each type has a specialized function. The importance of neurotransmitters cannot be overstated. They facilitate muscle contraction, keep the heart beating, control the secretion of hormones, and are involved in learning, memory, sleep, mood, and emotion. Much research on Alzheimer's disease, Parkinson's disease, mental illness, and pharmaceutical drugs to alter mood involves the study of the workings of neurotransmitters.

Another major component of the nervous system is the tissue that surrounds and supports the neurons, called *glial cells* (also called neuroglial cells). These cells do not transmit information but protect and nourish the neurons. Glial cells are ten times more common than neurons. There are several types of glial cells, each type having a specialized function. Glial cells may make chemicals to facilitate message transfer from one neuron to another, increase the speed of nerve transmission, make cerebrospinal fluid, or protect against infection by engulfing microorganisms.

The brain is extraordinarily complex, and many of its functions are not well understood. Each area of the brain has a different purpose. The largest portion, the *cerebrum,* is responsible for intellectual activities: speech, thought, learning, memory, and reasoning. The cerebrum also interprets messages from the sense organs and controls voluntary muscle action. The *cerebellum* coordinates voluntary muscle movements and maintains muscle tone, posture, and equilibrium. The *brain stem* connects the spinal cord and brain and is the main relay center for messages traveling to and from the brain. It controls involuntary processes: heartbeat, blood pressure, respiration, temperature, and the release of some hormones. The spinal cord is a bundle of nerves encased within the vertebral bones of the spine. Spinal cord neurons receive messages from various body parts and transmit directions to the brain or to other parts of the body.

Neurons that branch out from the spinal column and brain constitute the peripheral nervous system. Some of these peripheral nerves regulate voluntary actions (such as movement of the skeletal muscles in the arms and legs). Others regulate involuntary actions such as breathing, digestion, and hormonal release. Sensory messages are received in the skin and other organs and are transmitted to the spinal cord.

The nervous system depends on specialized sensory neurons called *receptors* to gather information about the internal and external environment. The receptors include neurons needed for vision, hearing, smell, taste, touch, equilibrium, temperature, and pain sensation. Although each sensory receptor responds to only one type of input, all convert the input into electrochemical impulses that travel along peripheral nerves to the central nervous system for processing. Sensory decrements are the most crucial physiological changes associated with the aging process because they affect an individual's perceptions and response to the world. The reader may want to download the online 74-page booklet *Brain facts: A primer on the brain and nervous system* published by the Society for Neuroscience for more detail on the structure and

---

Tips to Effectively Communicate Health Information to Elders

Aging results in normal changes in cognition: It takes longer to process information, it is easier to become distracted, and it is more difficult to remember new information. When information is presented too quickly, when there is background noise, and when the information is not repeated, understanding and recall suffers. When health information needs to be communicated to an older person, specific details need to be understood. For example, directions on when and how to take a medication is important. Another important consideration is to avoid mixing positive and negative information. Doing so may cause people to remember instructions incorrectly, especially when the

Continued

Tips to Effectively Communicate Health Information to Elders

information is new. For example, you may repeatedly remind a patient, "Do not take this pill with food." But that patient may actually remember the instruction as, "Take this pill with food." The following tips can help you to be more effective when you communicate health information to elders.

What You Can Do	Starter Tips
Repeat essential information.	Repeating information several times may help people with memory problems. When writing, be specific and repeat your points. Use pronouns such as "it," "this," and "that" sparingly because they are indefinite in meaning.
Focus on important details.	When communicating, stay focused on important details. Personalize information when possible and minimize distractions. Be sure details such as timing and the order of health-related actions are understood.
Emphasize desired actions.	Communicate directions and advice that older adults *need to follow,* not actions they *should avoid*. This helps boost memory for appropriate action and reduces confusion. Be aware that familiarity may be interpreted as truthfulness. Avoid using a "myth vs. fact" format.
Use plain language.	Writing and speaking in plain language boosts understanding for people with health literacy problems. Organize your information with the most important points first. Break information into chunks. Use simple words and active voice. If you need to use a difficult word, explain it.
Consider the effects of stress and fatigue.	Know that the stress that comes with illness and self-care can make anyone tired. Understand that mistakes in judgment, errors, and depressed mood may result more from sickness than cognitive changes. If managing technology or a medical device is important to a person's health, be sure that the person can use the technology or device when tired and stressed. Ask stressed older adults to bring family or friends with them to appointments. When possible, communicate important information during times of low stress.
Be aware of the effects of illness and recovery.	Illness, or recovery from treatments such as chemotherapy and surgery, can temporarily reduce cognitive function. A person's ability to self-manage treatment or recovery can be compromised under these conditions. Some medical conditions can result in permanent changes in executive function.
Be sensitive to individual needs.	Not every older adult is the same, and not every older adult will experience significant mental decline. Some just need help in specific areas, so look for ways to clarify those needs.
Provide adequate time for instruction.	A slower pace may be needed when working with older adults. Factor in extra time so you can adjust the pace with which you deliver instructions.

RESOURCE
PlainLanguage.gov includes a large amount of information and resources on plain language.

function of the brain and nervous system: www.sfn.org then search for Brain Facts.

Some age-associated changes in the structure of the nervous system are well documented. Brain weight starts to decline in the 20s, and up to one-tenth of brain mass is lost by very advanced age. With decreased brain size, there is a corresponding reduction in blood supply to the brain. A decline in cerebrospinal fluid is also evident with age. Structural changes occur in some neurons and glial cells although there is no evidence that they affect function. Glial cells increase in number in some parts of the brain and decrease in others with advancing age. Furthermore, neurons accumulate lipofuscin, an age-associated pigment. Despite the changes in structure, there is not a corresponding decrease in function.

Cognition and Age-Associated Changes

Cognition is the process by which one becomes aware of, perceives, or understands ideas. Studying cognition is challenging because there are so many different and interrelated components. It includes, but is not limited to the following: perception, attention, thinking, reasoning, executive function, and memory. Motivation also affects cognition.

Perception is receiving and processing input from the environment that involves the senses (e.g., light, noise, pain, heat, cold) as well as emotions (fatigue, hunger, or emotions like anger, sadness, or elation).

Attention is the ability of the person to choose what to focus on in the environment and is related to concentration (or the ability to sustain attention on one task) and to distraction (or how easy it is to get your mind off a topic). For instance, if there is a lot of noise in the restaurant, can you focus your attention on your dining partner and have your own conversation? Or, you are trying to learn how to use a new smart phone. Can you concentrate on reading the manual and not be distracted by the washer beeping, your aching back, and the list of other things you need to do today?

Knowledge refers to the accumulated data you store throughout your life about what you have experienced and what you have learned. Knowledge is related to the brain's ability to store, organize, categorize, and retrieve information.

Intelligence is the ability to acquire and use knowledge, to reason and think abstractly, to understand other's emotions and needs in a social context, to evaluate, judge, and decide, and to think original thoughts.

Thinking refers to the ability to acquire and apply knowledge accumulated throughout life, whether it be from book-learning or past experience.

Reasoning is the ability to draw conclusions and make judgments from information.

Executive function is a part of cognition that manages other cognitive processes—sometimes considered as the "adult" brain—putting off gratification and controlling impulses, facilitating problem solving, making hypotheses, learning from past mistakes, and staying organized.

Memory is the ability to store, retain, and recall information and experiences. Memory includes immediate memory (what we might use to recall a phone number for a short time), short-term memory (this includes what you did this morning or recalling what the major themes are in an article you are reading), long-term memory (recognition of people or experiences from your childhood, or remembering how to do calculations), and the deepest kind of memory, which is intuitive, subconscious knowledge.

Studying cognition in elders is challenging. For one thing, elders are less familiar with test-taking environments and more likely to be intimidated by the testing situation. Imagine you were giving a 90-year-old a test on a computer, for example, and comparing her results to those of a 30-year-old. The elder may not have much experience with tests or computers and may not perform well when compared to a younger adult who is familiar with computers and is used to taking computerized tests.

Another limitation in measuring the effects of age on personality, cognition, and memory is the measuring instruments themselves. How do we define and measure memory or cognition or personality? How do the measuring tools relate to function and abilities in day-to-day life? Most paper-and-pencil tools that measure cognition, memory, and personality include a series of questions. Although these tools have been tested to ensure they are valid and reliable, there is a lot of debate about whether they are appropriate for elders or those of different ethnicities. For example, someone may be able to recall a list of words after three minutes but may constantly lose his car keys. Does he have good memory or poor memory? Did an elder do poorly on the test because he could not see well? Because he was unable to focus on the question and too easily distracted? Alternatively, perhaps his brain is less flexible now and more "customized" to his current life and its demands. Thus, he may be able to solve a complex problem related to his job experience, but be less likely to work through problems that are irrelevant (for example, subtracting a series of numbers).

Studies consistently show a high amount of variability among individuals of all age groups. However, it is not always easy to assure that those with early dementia are excluded from the study of elders—is the cognitive decline due to age or due to early dementia? Further, cognitive skills are highly interrelated and deficiencies in one affect the other. For example, let's say testing identifies an elder with a problem with memory. This may be a problem with concentration—the elder did not focus and concentrate well enough when the information was learned and therefore did not store it correctly. Or the memory problem can be related to the inability to "find" the information and "access" it (for example, later after the test, the elder may be able to recall the information, but not quickly enough to get a high score). The tests used to measure cognitive function are not designed for elders who are more often unfamiliar or intimidated by testing situations. Memory deficits may be related to the inability to store and organize information or to difficulties accessing and finding information.

Despite their limitations, studies consistently show a decline in some cognitive functions with advancing age, beginning in midlife. The overall trend is a decline in intelligence scores, a decrease in attentiveness, and increased time to process new information. Memory, particularly short-term memory, also declines with age. The challenge of cognition research is that the complexity of cognitive function makes it difficult to distinguish which cognitive function is declining and whether or not it has an impact on everyday life.

Because we are still learning about the brain, we cannot fully identify which changes are age-related and which are related to disease or cohort effects or to differences in how the brain works with age. For instance, perhaps processing speed is reduced because there is so much more accumulated knowledge to review and sort through to find the particular piece of information desired. Further, people learn to compensate for their weak areas, making it even more difficult to study. For example, studies show that older people may learn more slowly than younger people skills such as using a cellular telephone or a computer. However, elders may compensate for slower learning times with more perseverance, a greater store of knowledge, experience, and self-motivation.

New science suggests the brain is a lot more "plastic" and can adapt throughout the life span to changing conditions and pressures. Thus, it is likely that the older brain is not necessarily worse, just different. It is difficult to measure the impact of a larger store of memories and experiences that provides elders with more data to make decisions—which laypersons called "wisdom."

Probably the most studied component of cognition and older people is the study of memory as memory loss is one of the most feared events associated with growing old. Some memory loss is a normal part of growing older; both cross-sectional and longitudinal studies confirm this. However, only certain kinds of memory seem to be affected. Older people are more likely to perform poorly on memory tests requiring speed or a high degree of focused attention.[7] In addition, compared to younger adults, elders show more decline in ability to take tests that require them to recall or to process new information. However, older subjects show less decline in the ability to access previously acquired information or skills. Vocabulary generally improves with age, and the ability to reason and solve problems does not decline. Studies seem to suggest that episodic memory, the ability to remember specific ongoing events (e.g., what I ate for dinner yesterday), is most affected by the aging process.

The type of memory least affected by aging is *reminiscing,* the ability to recall events in the personal past. Particularly for institutionalized elders, reminiscence is highly enjoyed perhaps because it is a reminder of the "good old days" when they were not sick. Many psychologists believe that encouraging reminiscence in elders is an effective way to increase self-esteem and decrease depression.

Maintaining good emotional and physical health and living in a stimulating environment reduce the risk of memory loss. Many techniques, called *mnemonics,* have been developed to improve memory. One popular way is to put what has to be remembered into small, manageable units that can be more easily remembered (e.g., dividing the grocery list into categories such as fruits and vegetables). Another technique is to visualize what needs to be remembered (e.g., envisioning what will be in the grocery bags). Probably the best technique is to write things down, whether it is a grocery list, phone number, name, or when medicine was taken last. Linking something known with what is to be remembered, such as making up a song about a name, is also helpful.

What factors influence the decline in cognition, memory, and processing speed? Dementia affects memory, learning, and executive function as well as motivation. Elders who are noted to have cognitive losses may be experiencing the symptoms of early dementia—these symptoms are rarely diagnosed until they are more serious. For others, it is likely that physical disorders, such as atherosclerosis, sleep problems, and reduced blood flow to the brain reduce cognition. High blood pressure, alcohol ingestion, surgery, lung disease, depression, and decreased cognitive exercise such as occurs in institutionalization may also impact memory. In addition, memory may be impaired due to reduced

attention and increased distractibility. Those who are not smokers, who exercise their brain with activity, exercise, and maintain good health are less likely to experience memory loss.

A body of research suggests the "use it or lose it" adage applies to cognitive function throughout the life span. Compare an older adult who volunteers in the community, works in an intellectually stimulating office, reads in various genres, uses a smart phone, and does Sudoku to one who spends the day passively watching television in a recliner chair. Generally, the mentally and physically active person will be higher functioning than one who is not. Studies show that reading, discussions, socialization, crossword puzzles, stimulating work, and seeking out opportunities to exercise the brain reduce loss and even encourage growth in cognitive function.

Personality and Age-Associated Changes

Personality is a collection of individual traits, qualities, and attributes that are consistent over time and across situations and, when considered together, describe the essence of a person. Such traits may include dependability, sociability, friendliness, willingness to try new things, irritability, tolerance, or guilt, to name a few. We may all have these traits to some extent, but we differ in how much and how often. Scientists think that more than half of our personality comes from our genes and the rest is determined by a complex interaction between genetics and environment. No matter which tests are used, multiple studies suggest that personality remains remarkably stable over time. There are some age-associated differences. There seems to be a "mellowing" of extreme personality with age, and elders are less likely to have personality disorders. There may also be a move toward androgyny with age. This means that women exhibit more traditionally masculine traits (such as assertiveness) and men exhibit more traditionally feminine traits (such as nurturing). Although some researchers assert that these are psychological changes, others suggest that the move toward androgyny may be biologically based because women have reduced estrogen production and men have reduced testosterone production.

Personality changed are so uncommon that abrupt changes occurring at any age should be investigated. Personality changes can indicate a brain tumor stroke, or dementia. More information can be found in the book *Changes in Cognitive Function in Human Aging.*[8]

Reaction Time and Age-Associated Changes

Reaction time is the time interval between a nerve being stimulated and the body's response to it. The average human reaction time depends upon the type of nerve stimulated and can be as little as one-seventh of a second. Response to visual images takes longer, close to a half-second. A number of studies have demonstrated that reaction time lengthens with age. Visual and auditory reflexes and time to complete a physical or mental task decline 20 percent or more from youth to old age. This decline may be due to physiological alterations in the neural pathway, alterations in vision or hearing, difficulty with testing situations, or increased cautiousness with age. Chronic illness and physical inactivity may also play a role. Even though there is a statistically significant lengthening of reaction time with age, in real life this translates into an increase of only hundredths of a second and does not interfere with most everyday activities. Older adults may compensate for their diminished reaction time in tasks such as driving with increased cautiousness, leaving more space between them and the car in front of them, limiting driving to less crowded times, and reducing distractions while driving.

Vision and Age-Associated Changes

Eyelashes, eyelids, tear glands, and tear ducts protect the eye from dirt, injury, or dryness. The sclera is the white, outer layer of the eyeball. The cornea is a transparent membrane that covers the front of the eyeball. The iris is the circular, colored part of the eye that lies behind the cornea and in front of the lens. The opening at the center of the iris is the pupil. When the light is dim, the pupil opening expands to allow more light to stimulate the receptors. When the light is bright, the pupil contracts to protect the receptors from damage from intense light.

The lens is a clear disk located behind the pupil and is suspended by fibrous tissue. The function of the lens is to focus light rays entering the pupil so they merge to a point on the retina located in the back of the eye. The lens focuses the image by changing its shape with the help of supporting fibers. This capacity allows for sharp vision at any distance. In some people, the shape of the eyeball or lens focuses light rays at a point beyond the retinal surface, which causes *farsightedness* (hyperopia), an inability to focus on near objects. In others, light rays come to a focus at a point in front of the retina instead of directly on it, causing *nearsightedness* (myopia), an inability to focus on distant objects. Both disorders can usually be corrected with eyeglasses, contact lenses, or laser surgery.

Vision receptors are located in the retina and consist of rods to distinguish general outlines and cones for color vision and sharp outlines. The rods and cones connect with neurons to form the optic nerve. A blind spot, the place in which the optic nerve connects to the retina, has no visual receptors. Viscous fluids (the aqueous humor in front of the lens and the vitreous humor behind it) maintain proper eye pressure and fluid balance to allow the eye to function properly. See www.nei.nih.gov/health/eyediagram/ for a diagram of the eye.

Reduced visual acuity is one of the most significant changes that accompany aging, especially the gradual changes that occur in the lens. With advancing age, the lens thickens, yellows, clouds, and becomes less elastic. The thickening of the lens reduces the amount of light that can pass through the lens. Visual clarity is further reduced by a clouding of the lens called a cataract. The term is derived from the Latin word *cataracta*, which means "waterfall," because the visual effect can be likened to looking through a sheet of water. A normal

Tips to Communicate with Elders with Visual Problems

Many older adults have problems with vision. When you create graphics, text, or other visuals, consider the needs of older audiences.

What You Can Do	Starter Tips
Make information easy to see.	Effective materials have a simple design with sharp contrast between text and background. Use a large font size, preferably 16- or 18-point. Try 1-inch margins and at least 1.5 blank spaces between lines of text. When using a table, make it simple and easy to follow.
Design Web sites that are senior friendly.	Web sites for seniors require readable text presented in a carefully organized format. Font type and size, spacing, justification, color, and backgrounds all need to be planned with older audiences in mind.
Consider using Braille and audiotaped information whenever necessary.	Braille and audiotape are necessary for some adults with low vision or blindness.
Be sensitive to individual needs.	Degrees of impairment vary, as do the ways people overcome such challenges. Ask older adults with vision problems if they want assistance with these issues and, if so, how you can help. It may help to research vision aids, such as magnifiers, so that you can understand how they help people.

RESOURCES

The following resources can help you as you design materials and Web sites to meet the needs of older adults with visual impairment.

- *Making Your Web Site Senior Friendly* is an informative checklist Web designers can use while creating online material for older adults. This checklist, published by the National Institute on Aging and the National Library of Medicine, is available at www.nlm.nih.gov/pubs/checklist.pdf
- *Making Text Legible: Designing for People with Partial Sight.* These guidelines provide good examples of effective legibility choices for anyone. It is available from Lighthouse International at www.lighthouse.org/accessibility/legible
- *Effective Color Contrast: Designing for People with Partial Sight and Color Deficiencies.* These guidelines provide specific examples of effective color contrast. It is available from Lighthouse International at www.lighthouse.org/accessibility/effective-color-contrast
- *In Other Words . . . When Vision Is an Issue . . . Communicating with Patients Who Are Visually Impaired* is a concise article that offers practical tips for designing materials for people with visual challenges. You can find it at www.healthliteracy.com/article.asp?PageID=3774
- *Making Web Sites More Accessible for Users Who Are Older and/or Have a Disability* includes background information on visual disabilities and offers strategies for improving accessibility. It is available at www.adrc-tae.org/tiki-index.php?page=TAEIssueBriefs

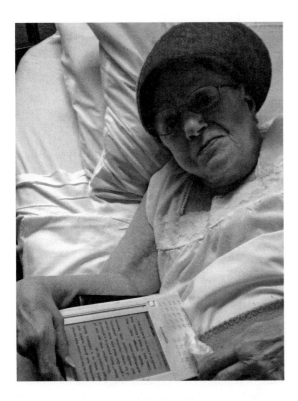

close work. Some people may need bifocals, which are glasses with lenses that incorporate one prescription for close focus on the bottom part and another prescription in the upper lens that enables the eye to focus on distant objects. Bifocal contact lenses are an alternative that may work for some. Some can wear contact lenses—one fitted for close and one for distant vision. Laser surgery for presbyopia is another alternative.

Another universal change in the eye is the yellowing of the lens with advanced age. Because of this change, more light is necessary to stimulate the light receptors in the retina, and night vision is impaired. Besides the yellowing of the lens reducing light to the retina, it also impairs the ability to differentiate blue, green, and violet. People who design visual materials for older people need to be aware of this impairment.

The amount of light entering the eye is also reduced because of age-related reductions in pupil size and thickening of the cornea. The reduction in pupil size is caused by atrophy of the muscle that dilates the pupil. As the pupil becomes less responsive, the eye loses its ability to adapt to abrupt changes from light to darkness. Also, light sensitivity is reduced because the fluids located in the eye become cloudy.

The cornea becomes thickened and less transparent with age. The thickened cornea causes light to scatter inside the retina, making glare more of a problem. To further increase visual acuity in elders, the amount of glare in the environment should be minimized. Generally, individuals who are 60 years old need three times more light to read than they needed when they were 20. Thus, great improvements in vision are possible by installing higher-wattage light bulbs in elders' living space.

Corrective lenses enable individuals of all ages to adjust to many vision problems. Those with presbyopia alone may be able to use inexpensive nonprescription magnifying eyeglasses. These, however, will not correct for other vision problems. Most experts recommend that elders have eye examinations every one to two years to detect glaucoma, cataracts, and other visual problems.

lens allows light to pass to the back of the eye; a cataract disperses and reduces the incoming light. In the early stages, elders experience a dulling of colors, difficulty with glare, and problems with night driving. Any clouding of the lens is considered to be a cataract. However, depending on the size, location, and density of the cataract, vision may or may not be impaired. Although cataracts are associated with advanced age, not all older people get cataracts. We discuss cataracts in Chapter 5, "Other Chronic Diseases and Conditions."

In middle age, almost everyone experiences problems with near vision called *presbyopia*. The lens becomes less elastic, and the fibers supporting the lens weaken, reducing the capacity of the lens to bend in order to focus on close objects. A common symptom of presbyopia is the need to hold reading material farther and farther away. Presbyopia usually starts around age 40, and by age 60, the lens is incapable of focusing at close distance.

Presbyopia responds very well to corrective lenses or to a magnifying glass for reading and

Three types of health professionals deal with eye care. An *ophthalmologist,* a physician with special training in eye diseases, can diagnose eye disease, perform eye surgery, and prescribe correction for inadequate vision. An *optometrist,* though not a physician, is trained to examine for visual defects and prescribe proper correction. If a disease is suspected or surgery is required, the client is referred to an ophthalmologist. An *optician,* following the directions of the ophthalmologist or optometrist, grinds and fits the lenses.

As of this writing, neither vision examinations nor corrective lenses are covered by Medicare, although treatment of eye diseases is reimbursed. However, for those who qualify, Medicaid (MediCal in California) may pay all or part of the expense of eye examinations and corrective lenses. In some communities, the Lions Club assists individuals with expenses related to vision problems.

Eye Care America has a program for people 65 and older in which volunteer opthalmologists across the country provide free eye exams and treatment for those who cannot afford it otherwise (www .eyecareamerica.org). The Medem Network has a physician-patient communication network for access to information and care with over 90,000 physician participants and patients (www.medem.com).

Hearing and Age-Associated Changes

The ear is composed of three distinct sections. Sound waves enter the *outer ear,* are conducted into the *middle ear,* and are translated into nerve impulses in the *inner ear.* Specialized receptor cells in the inner ear transmit sound messages to the brain for processing by way of the auditory nerve. The inner ear is also important in maintaining body equilibrium, for special fluid-filled canals signal the brain whenever they sense motion.

The most visible structure of hearing is the cartilaginous outer ear (pinna). Inside is an auditory canal lined with hair and wax-secreting glands. Earwax (cerumen) cleans and protects the ear from dirt, repels water, wards off infection, and prevents dryness. The funnel-shaped canal collects sound waves and guides them to the eardrum (tympanic membrane), which separates the outer from the middle ear.

In the middle ear, three small bones—the hammer (malleus), anvil (incus), and stirrup (stapes)—work together to transmit sound vibrations from the eardrum through the middle ear. The eustachian tube connects the throat and middle ear. This connection maintains equal pressure outside and inside the head, permitting the eardrum to vibrate normally. This explains why swallowing can relieve pressure in the ears during an airplane flight: It equalizes the pressure on both sides of the eardrum. Extreme pressure differences may cause the eardrum to rupture.

Sound waves are transformed into nerve impulses in the inner ear. The inner ear is completely filled with fluid and houses the cochlea, a snail-shaped tunnel also filled with fluid. The cochlea contains rows of hair cells that convert sound into electrical impulses that are transmitted from the auditory nerve to the brain. The hair cells respond selectively to sounds of different frequencies, depending on their location on the membrane within the cochlea. For a diagram of the ear, go to www.nlm.nih.gov/medlineplus/ and search for Ear Anatomy.

Hearing loss is very common among older adults, and the proportion with hearing difficulties increases with advancing age. Overall, about 15 percent of the adult population in the United States report hearing difficulties. More than one in four elders 65–74 years of age report hearing problems; 45 percent of those 75 and older report hearing problems.[9] Even though it looks as if the loss is due to age itself, researchers believe hearing deficits are attributable more to an accumulation of noise damage than to actual age changes, for elders in less technologically advanced countries do not exhibit hearing loss to the extent of those in our society.

Men are more likely to have a hearing loss than women, and the loss is evident earlier in life. It is not yet known whether the gender difference is due to physiological differences or to different noise exposure history. Significantly more whites report hearing difficulties than blacks, Hispanic Americans, or Asian Americans.

Over the past 40 years, a higher proportion of those aged 50 and older have become hard of hearing. It is hypothesized that the increase is due to more workplace and environmental noise and use of medications that affects hearing acuity. Many hearing authorities predict there will be even more widespread hearing difficulties because of the increasing noise in our country (e.g., city noises, rock concerts, and portable music devices). Very loud noises, such as explosions, immediately destroy the sensory cells of the inner ear; lower-level chronic noise inflames the hearing mechanism, slowly destroying the sensory cells.

There is marked variation among individuals regarding noise susceptibility and hearing loss, but generally the danger level begins at 80 to 85 decibels (e.g., garbage disposal rumbling) and increases at higher levels (e.g., rock concerts, video arcades, firearms). The louder the sound is, the less time it takes a person to suffer hearing damage. For example, one can listen to a lawn mower for eight hours without damage but can tolerate only 15 minutes of a loud rock concert or car horn. Temporary hearing loss and ringing in the ears after exposure to loud noise are warning signs in some individuals. Noise damage can be reduced with protective devices such as earplugs. Hearing loss is not only caused by excessive noise; it can also result from disease (measles, meningitis, repeated ear infections) and some medications (e.g., antibiotics and diuretics).

There are three categories of hearing loss: *conductive* (difficulty in conducting sound in the small bones of the ear), sensory (deficits in the nerves that sense sound in the cochlea), and *neural* (damage to the auditory nerves or other nerves in the brain). *Sensorineural* hearing loss refers to hearing loss caused by a combination of difficulties with sensory receptors and the nerves that transmit auditory information to the brain.

Presbycusis is the term used to describe the sensory hearing loss associated with the aging process. The word originates in the Greek roots *presby* meaning "old" and *cusis* meaning "hearing."

Almost all hearing loss in the United States is due to loss of sensory cells within the cochlea, primarily due to presbycusis and noise-induced hearing loss. The condition affects both ears. With presbycusis, elders typically do not complain of hearing difficulty but rather are unable to understand ordinary conversation in social settings because of background noise interference. Affected individuals have difficulty with high-frequency consonant sounds such as *f, g, s, z, t, sh,* and *ch.* Communication with an elder with presbycusis is optimized by speaking slowly in a quiet room.

Because hearing loss is gradual, individuals may not realize that they need a hearing aid. Further, many people believe that some hearing loss is inevitable with age, so they do not seek treatment. Correcting hearing loss, however, may correct psychological distress and social problems. The inability to hear well may limit enjoyment of social activities and the stimulation that other people and television provide. The following behaviors may indicate a hearing problem:

1. Preferring radio or television at a higher volume than others in the room
2. Complaining that others are not speaking clearly or loudly enough
3. Consistently turning one side of the head toward the speaker or cupping one ear with a hand
4. Commonly asking others to repeat phrases or words or frequently saying "What?" or "Huh?"
5. Having difficulty hearing at large gatherings with background noise, such as lectures, church sermons, and social events
6. Having difficulty in locating the origin of sounds
7. Confusing words or making silly mistakes
8. Understanding men's voices better than women's

The inability to hear in social situations may result in frustration and withdrawal, leading to social isolation. Individuals with presbycusis may also exhibit paranoid ideas and behavior, depression, suspiciousness, and lack of contact with reality. Family members and friends may withdraw from the hearing-impaired person because they are frustrated by their failed efforts to communicate. Common problems are having to continually repeat words and sentences, coping with a blaring television, and dealing with feelings of loss of a former confidant, among others. Consequently, conversation dwindles to the necessities. Furthermore, people who are hard of hearing are commonly misjudged as "senile" because they are not able to communicate easily, appear inattentive, or seem withdrawn.

In addition to presbycusis, elders may suffer hearing loss due to other age-associated changes in the ear. The wall of the outer cartilaginous portion of the auditory canal collapses inward with advancing age, narrowing the passage and making the canal less efficient in receiving and channeling sound waves to the middle ear. Furthermore, earwax (cerumen) tends to thicken and accumulate with age. It may occlude the auditory canal, contributing to hearing loss. Cotton swabs should not be used to clean the ears because they can push the earwax deeper into the ear canal. Over-the-counter wax-softening agents (e.g., Debrox) can be used at home as can warm water irrigation. However, caution is needed as older people have more sensitive skin and less coordination, and may inadvertently injure the ear canal. For a severe buildup, medical help may be needed.

Unfortunately, there is no way to increase the amount of sensory cells to restore hearing loss. Treatment almost always involves the use of sound amplification devices, usually a battery-operated hearing aid. Although hearing is not restored, it is noticeably improved. Since presbycusis usually occurs in both ears, it is recommended that a hearing aid be purchased for each ear for optimum improvement. Although hearing aids amplify sound, they cannot distinguish between speech and background noise, despite claims to the contrary.

Hearing aids are becoming more and more sophisticated. The ideal one varies based on the severity of hearing loss, lifestyle, vanity (whether you want it to show), cost, and your manual dexterity. A built-in hearing aid may be part of an eyeglass frame. Some hearing aids worn behind the ear have a clear plastic tube that transmits sound into the ear canal. Other hearing aids fit in the outer ear, and a few are custom-fit in the ear canal and are not visible to observers. Some have several channels that allow reception tailored to the environment; others are programmable, responding to changes in hearing loss.

Although various types of hearing aids are available, all use the same mechanism. A tiny microphone in the aid converts sound to electrical impulses. An amplifier boosts the signal to a speaker, which changes it into sounds. The digital technology uses a microchip to convert sound waves into digital signals, and a computer chip is programmed to suppress background noise.

Despite the available technology, most people who might benefit from one do not wear one. Why not? It may be due to the fact that most hearing aids do not restore hearing to a normal level; instead, they amplify all sounds, which can be annoying. In addition, hearing aids are often fitted incorrectly and are uncomfortable to wear. Some older people refuse to wear a hearing aid for cosmetic reasons or because they believe it to be a sign of growing old. Even when elders do wear hearing aids, the aids may not be in good repair. Furthermore, many elders cannot afford to purchase a hearing aid. Medicare covers neither the examination nor the appliance. Medicaid may pay all or part of the cost if the individual qualifies.

For moderate to severe sensorineural hearing loss, an implantable hearing aid is available that stimulates the remaining hair cells of the cochlea. The device is implanted within the middle ear (not placed in the ear canal as traditional hearing aids), and its processor (microphone and power source) are tucked behind the outer ear.

For individuals with profound sensorineural hearing loss, cochlear implants may be utilized. A cochlear implant is an electronic device that is surgically inserted inside the cochlea within the inner ear. Because those who are deaf and nearly deaf often have insufficient sensory hair cells, the electrodes bypass the sensory cells and directly stimulate the auditory nerve, which transports sound signals to the brain.

Tips for Communicating with a Hearing-Impaired Individual

1. Speak clearly, distinctly, and slowly; do not shout or exaggerate your mouth movements.
2. Face the individual when talking and look him or her in the eyes. If the person to whom you are speaking is in a wheelchair, lower yourself to eye level.
3. Be sure there is enough light for the person to see you speaking, but no glare.
4. Try to avoid noisy areas.
5. Give visual cues, such as hand movements and facial expressions, in addition to your verbal message.
6. If you are asked to repeat what you said, find other words to say the same thing.
7. In a group situation, sit in a circle so everyone can see everyone else's lip movements and expressions. Clue participants into the conversation by summarizing occasionally.
8. Be patient. Don't create the feeling that you are in a hurry.
9. Learn to read the individual's reaction to be certain she or he heard and understood what was said.
10. Keep hands, scarves, and tobacco away from your mouth. Don't chew gum, eat, or smoke while talking.
11. Get the person's attention before you start to speak.
12. Don't talk from too far away.
13. Make an attempt to discuss topics other than what is absolutely necessary, even though these are harder to communicate. Don't resort to curt, necessary exchanges.

A number of health professionals are available to assist elders with hearing problems. Physicians, either an *otologist* (ear specialist) or an *otolaryngologist* (ear, nose, and throat specialist), can diagnose the problem and determine if surgical or medical treatment is necessary or if a hearing aid is indicated. *Audiologists* are highly trained, nonmedical specialists who can evaluate hearing problems and counsel a patient on hearing aids and rehabilitation. A *hearing aid dispenser* measures hearing loss, helps to select the proper aid, custom-fits the apparatus, and explains proper use and care techniques. Hearing aid dispensers must be licensed by the state to perform these tasks, but they are not qualified to diagnose hearing problems or to prescribe medication. Selecting a hearing aid is a difficult, expensive, and time-consuming process, and the quality of work among hearing aid dispensers varies.

Other assistive devices can help the hard of hearing, including telephone and mobile phone amplifying devices, TV listening systems, auditorium-type assistive listening systems, and lipreading. Hearing ear dogs are pets trained to respond to the phone or doorbell. For more information, contact Dogs for the Deaf at www.dogsforthedeaf.org

For more information on hearing loss and hearing aids and extensive links to other sites, see the Administration on Aging site. Also see the site for the National Institute on Deafness and Other Communication Disorders, www.nidcd.nih.gov/health/hearing/older.asp To participate in a free screening test by phone in your area, call 1-800-222-EARS. Or use the Web site www.betterhearing.rg/hearing_loss/quickhearingcheck.cfm to complete a questionnaire about your perception of your hearing, and submit it online to compare yourself to others who have a hearing loss. To find an audiologist in your area, or for advice on hearing aids or protection, call the American Speech-Language Hearing Association's consumer help line (1-800-638-8255). For information on protecting yourself from hearing loss, call the National Hearing Conservation Association at 515-266-2189.

Taste and Smell and Age-Associated Changes

Taste buds, the sensory organs of taste, are located predominantly on the tongue, although a few may be found in other places in the mouth. Chemicals from food activate taste buds when they are dissolved in saliva. When the receptor is triggered, it sends a taste message to the brain. There are certain types of cells that sense different tastes—sweet, salty, bitter, sweet and savory. Each taste bud is thought to contain multiple types of taste cells and serves to synthesize taste sensations. The greater the number of taste buds, the better is the sense of taste. Taste buds constantly regenerate, having a life span of about 10 days. The sense of smell further influences taste.

Humans are able to smell by a group of receptor cells (about one-quarter inch in diameter) located high in the nose. Smell receptors turn over every 30 days. These cells are very easily fatigued; a receptor will get used to a smell and stop sending messages to the brain after only a minute of exposure. The sense of smell influences the ability to taste and enjoy food, to be aware of dangers (such as gas fumes, burning electrical wires, smoke, or spoiled or burning food), and to detect body odors and pleasant smells.

Many adults have a reduced ability to taste and smell as they age. One cross-sectional study reported that elders had a reduced bitter and salt taste acuity when compared with young adults, but their ability to perceive sweet and sour tastes was similar

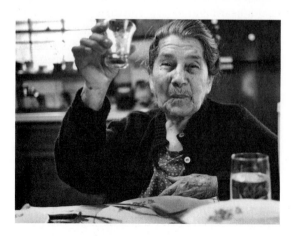

to that of the younger group. Further, in older people the sense of smell seemed to be more impaired than the sense of taste.[10] Another cross-sectional study reported that elders were less able to discriminate the quality of tastes and odors and generally had a higher threshold before they were able to taste or smell when compared with younger people.[11]

Although age plays a role, other factors influence the sense of taste and smell. Elders may have chronic illnesses, sinus or nasal problems, poor oral hygiene, nutritional deficiencies (e.g., zinc), or heartburn or other digestive disorders that impact taste and smell. They may take medications that dry the mouth, and this dryness may affect taste and smell perception. Those who smoke suffer even more decrements in taste and smell. Alzheimer's disease also reduces ability to taste and smell, likely because of cognitive deficits. Good oral hygiene may enhance taste sensitivity.

Losing the perception of taste and smell can have a significant effect on an older person's health. The loss of salt perception may make it harder for individuals with high blood pressure to restrict salt. Further, older adults are less likely to detect the bad taste of spoiled food and thus are at high risk for food poisoning. Those with a reduced sense of smell are less likely to respond to environmental dangers such as smoke, gas leaks, and other toxic fumes.

Reduced ability to taste or smell also makes eating less enjoyable, lessening the motivation to eat. This may explain why food intake declines with age and why older people frequently report a decrease in appetite. Undernutrition is a major cause of involuntary weight loss, increased susceptibility to disease, and reduced immune function among elders. A way to reduce the impact of poor taste and smell ability is to augment the natural taste of foods with seasonings, instead of relying on excessive sugar and salt.

Balance and Equilibrium and Age-Associated Changes

There are three components of balance or equilibrium: the vestibular system, the visual system, and peripheral balance receptors. These systems work together to keep our balance; if any are impaired, we are more unsteady. The vestibular system in the inner ear is responsible for sending messages to the brain about the position of the head. Located in the inner ear, the three semicircular canals are oriented in three planes and are filled with a jelly-like substance that moves against microscopic hairs connected to receptor cells. These cells send a message to the brain that the head is changing position. The brain reacts by sending motor impulses that either contract or relax particular involuntary muscles to maintain balance. The vestibular system is responsible for maintaining balance during quick moves, such as jumping off a wall, or turning your head rapidly to the side to look for oncoming traffic. The vestibular system is aided by the visual system: Our eyes tell us where we are in space.

Peripheral balance receptors are located throughout the body and may be the most crucial aspect of balance in later life. These receptors tell us how our body is positioned in space—whether we are going uphill or down, whether we are walking on an uneven surface—and generally help us maintain our balance with respect to the ground.

These three systems work together to keep our balance. As long as two of the three components (vestibular, visual, and peripheral receptors) function, balance is maintained. For instance, if you are walking into a dark movie theater, you should not lose your balance even if you cannot see. However, if two systems are inadequate (e.g., an elder has vestibular problems and is walking in a dark movie theater), the risk of an accident or fall is increased. Age is associated with decrements in vision, in vestibular balance, and in peripheral balance receptors. Up until age 65, there is increasing reliance on vision for stability, but thereafter, as vision declines, elders more often depend on the other systems.

Elders commonly experience vertigo (a sense that the surroundings are spinning) and dizziness (light-headedness and unsteadiness). These may be related to age-associated development of small stones (otoliths) in the semicircular canals or to changes in the sensory neurons. In addition, vertigo and dizziness are common side effects of many medications. Dizziness may be due to a cardiovascular condition called *postural hypotension,* a condition in which the cardiovascular system responds to a position change more slowly than usual. This slow response causes dizziness or light-headedness when a person moves quickly from lying or sitting to standing.

Somatic Receptors and Age-Associated Changes

Somatic receptors tell the brain about touch, pressure, heat, cold, pain, or body position in space. Upon stimulation, the receptors send impulses through nerve pathways to the spinal cord and brain for processing.

Touch and pressure receptors are located in the skin. The hairless portions of the skin (lips, fingertips, palms, genitals, and soles of the feet) are particularly sensitive to touch because they have a higher concentration of touch receptors. These receptors tell the brain when something is touched or felt. However, after prolonged exposure, the receptors adapt. This explains why we do not "feel" our clothing all day. Receptors that respond to heavy pressure are found deeper in the skin.

Thermoreceptors respond to either cold or heat. They sense changes in temperature, but once exposed to a certain temperature for a period of time, they adapt or cease to respond until there is another alteration in temperature.

Pain receptors are widely distributed throughout the skin and internal organs. Unlike the receptors for cold, heat, touch, and pressure, pain receptors do not adapt and stop sending messages. As long as the pain continues, the pain messages are sent to the brain.

Receptors that respond to changes in body position are located mainly around the joints. These sense changes in joint movement and relay the message to the brain.

How can age-related changes in the somatic senses be measured when the response to pain or heat or cold is so individual and subjective? This research is challenging to say the least. Nevertheless, experts believe that somatic receptors become less sensitive with age. Elders may need a greater stimulus before the nerve endings fire and send a message to the brain.

Elders may experience a decreased sensitivity to pain with advancing age. However, this may be due to less attention to pain, less reporting of pain, less brain perception of pain, or perhaps nerve changes in pain messaging. A decreased ability to feel pain may carry both positive and negative consequences. Elders may be better able to cope with common, painful chronic diseases (e.g., arthritis). On the other hand, since pain signals danger, an elder with decreased pain sensitivity may be unaware of disease symptoms or minor injuries.

Many elders exhibit a decreased perception of heat. Experts believe that reduced sensitivity to heat may contribute to the high incidence of burns among older people. Extremes in temperature are more likely to affect elders, and they recover more slowly after exposure to temperature stress.

THE ENDOCRINE SYSTEM

Body functions are regulated and coordinated through the interdependent workings of the nervous and endocrine systems. As previously described, the nervous system rapidly transmits electrochemical impulses across nerve fibers that send messages to and from the brain and spinal cord. In contrast, the endocrine system transmits its chemical messages (hormones) much more slowly through the bloodstream to tissues and organs throughout the body, and its effects last longer.

Endocrine glands, located in the brain and other parts of the body, manufacture and release chemical messengers or hormones into the blood to affect body metabolism and sexual development and function in another area of the body. Hormones affect particular cells by changing the rate of certain cell processes. Even though the hormones have the capacity to reach every cell, they attach themselves only to the receptors located on the cells (called target cells) they are designed to reach. Those hormones that do not combine with a receptor are usually inactivated by the kidneys or liver and released as waste.

Over 200 hormones have been identified. Each has a different molecular structure and function, although all hormones generally slow or speed a particular metabolic process. For instance, insulin, the hormone produced by the pancreas, increases the rate at which sugar enters into body cells. For an overview of the location and major functions of the hormones within each endocrine gland, go to www.hormone.org/endo101/glands.cfm

Age-Associated Changes in the Endocrine System

Comparatively little is known about the endocrine system, and even less is understood about the effect of aging on the function of each gland. The complicated interrelationship between the endocrine glands and the circulatory and nervous systems makes the distinction even more difficult. However, many hormones have been reported to decrease with increased age: estrogens, androgens (includes testosterone), insulin, and thyroid and growth hormones. Further, hormone receptors frequently decline in numbers or efficiency with age.

The most-studied endocrine gland is the pancreas and its associated hormone, insulin. After eating, food is broken down and absorbed, and its chemical components travel throughout the bloodstream. The liver converts some of the components into glucose, which the body cells use for energy. However, to extract the glucose from the bloodstream, the cells require insulin. With age, there is a decline in the ability of the blood to maintain normal glucose and blood sugar levels. There is also a decline of sensitivity of the cells to insulin. However, this decline is only partly attributed to advancing age and more likely is due to a combination of aging, obesity, alteration in body fat distribution, and physical inactivity.

Levels of adrenal and thyroid hormones tend to decrease in the later years. Reduced thyroid hormone levels result in a decreased metabolic rate. Although the thymus gland shrinks significantly after maturity, levels of its hormone, thymosin, remain constant throughout adulthood.

Perhaps the most well-known age change for women is *menopause,* the cessation of menstrual periods. Estrogen production is significantly reduced in the female after menopause. Menopause, however, is a gradual process, not a discrete event. In general, women in their 40s begin to experience hormonal changes that result in a gradual reduction in fertility and increasing variability in length and intensity of menstrual periods. At approximately age 50, menses and fertility cease. When a woman completes two years without a period, she has gone through menopause. The term *climacteric* refers to the duration of the period of hormonal fluctuations, which may last up to 15 years.

During the climacteric, the menstrual cycle decreases in length and regularity due to the decreased ovarian production of estradiol, one of the most potent of the estrogen hormones. After menopause, estradiol production drops even further, and cyclical variation in hormone production ceases. However, this does not mean that the body no longer produces estrogens. Androstenedione, a hormone secreted by the ovaries and the adrenal glands, is converted into estrone in fatty tissues. Estrone is a less potent form of estrogen that compensates somewhat for the decreased estradiol production.

The hormonal declines accompanying menopause initiate changes in several body systems: increased rate of bone loss, unfavorable alterations in cholesterol levels, and an increased risk of cardiovascular disease. Hot flashes and vaginal dryness are common symptoms of menopause. Many women experience no menopausal symptoms, while others notice hot flushes, vaginal dryness, sleep disorders, and changes in mood or concentration.

Some women choose to undergo hormone replacement therapy to reduce the short-term symptoms (vaginal dryness, hot flashes) and the long-term consequences of menopause (thin bones and increased risk of heart disease). Recent large-scale studies, however, have called into question the benefits and risks of long-term continuous hormone replacement therapy, causing a shift in recommendations and practices.

Women may take estrogen alone in various forms. Women who have a uterus generally take estrogen in some combination with progesterone to reduce the risk of uterine cancer that is associated with estrogen. Hormone replacement therapy varies in the type of estrogen and progesterone chosen, method of administration, dosage prescribed, and timing. When the hormones are administered cyclically, women usually experience periodic bleeding, similar to a menstrual period. In other cases, smaller doses of one or both drugs are given continuously, and bleeding does not occur. Estrogen creams, prescribed to reduce the thinning and drying of the vaginal walls, and a transdermal estrogen patch, worn on the abdomen, are other less invasive ways to deliver estrogen.

Early observational studies suggested that women who took hormone replacement therapy had a reduced risk of osteoporosis, better lipid profiles, reduced risk of cardiovascular disease, and even a lower risk of Alzheimer's disease. Hormone replacement therapy was thought to be a "fountain of youth," improving appearance (reduced wrinkling, producing a more youthful distribution of weight) and mood (assisting in depression and mood swings) and reducing the chance of suffering and dying from major killers. Many experts were recommending widespread use of the hormones for preventive reasons, and many women were taking them. However, a nagging question remained, "Were the women who chose hormone replacement different (higher education, more health-conscious) from those who did not? Might the difference explain their lower risk of some diseases?"

To address those questions, a large-scale randomized controlled trial was implemented, the Women's Health Initiative. Unexpectedly, one part of the study that followed women who were taking a continuous dosage of estrogen and progesterone (brand name Prempro) had to be terminated early because women who started taking the drug after menopause had a higher risk of breast cancer than subjects who did not use hormone replacement therapy. Later, another part of the study, in which women were taking progesterone in another form, was also terminated due to increased risks. This and other studies suggest that hormone replacement therapy may not offer protection against cardiovascular disease and osteoporosis and may have negative health consequences. Experts are still not sure whether the estrogen or the progesterone is responsible for the negative effects noted. However, there is a great deal more caution these days regarding use of hormone replacement therapy.

Many women utilize alternative treatments for menopausal symptoms, particularly hot flashes. Common treatments include soy products (phytoestrogens), the herbs dong quai and black cohosh, evening primrose oil, and acupuncture. Multiple studies have reviewed these alternative treatments for menopausal symptoms and, to date, there is insufficient data indicating that any alternative treatments reduced menopausal symptoms. Sometimes androgens are used in the postmenopausal period to stimulate women's sexual drive and energy. These can cause masculinizing effects in the short term and the long-term effects are not known.

In males, both longitudinal and cross-sectional studies have documented that the level of the male hormone, testosterone, declines at a rate of 1 percent a year after age 40. It is estimated that one of five men over 60 and half over 80 have testosterone levels below the normal range of young men.[12] The decline in testosterone is highly variable, however, with some healthy, physically fit older men maintaining levels that are higher than those of some younger men. Factors other than age are likely to contribute to changes in testosterone level. Men who have diabetes, heart disease, high blood pressure, or obesity, or are inactive exhibit decreases in testosterone levels. Testosterone is important in maintenance of muscle and bone mass and sexual desire; lower levels can result in abnormal lipid profiles, abnormal body fat distributions, muscle wasting, lack of sexual desire, and depression.

The term *andropause* is used to describe a complex of symptoms in aging men who have low testosterone levels. For those men, supplemental testosterone (androgen replacement therapy) may improve muscle mass, bone density, energy and mood, and sexual interest and ability. However, long-term consequences are not known. Studies suggest that androgens increase the risk of prostate cancer and blood clots.

THE GENITAL SYSTEM

After menopause, women lose the capacity to reproduce. Elderly men, though still capable, are rarely interested in fathering children. This section describes the male and female genital systems and age-associated physiological changes. Psychological and social aspects of aging and sexuality, changes in sexual response with age, sexual dysfunction, and therapy are discussed in Chapter 11, "Sexuality."

The Female

The hypothalamus, ovaries, and anterior pituitary glands secrete hormones that modulate the female menstrual cycle, pregnancy, and the development and maintenance of secondary sexual characteristics. A pair of ovaries, located in the lower abdomen, produce estrogens (female hormones) and eggs.

The uterus is a muscular, pear-shaped organ held in place by four ligaments. It is connected to the vagina, a muscular tube that serves as the birth

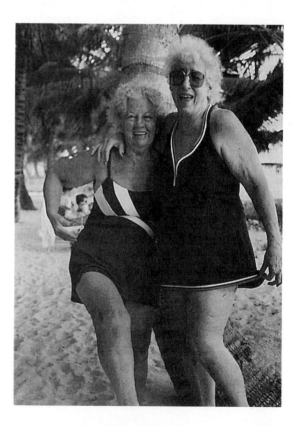

passageway and receives the erect penis during sexual intercourse. The external genital organs include the vulva, composed of the outer and inner lips (labia majora and labia minora) and the organ of sexual arousal, the clitoris.

During excitation, the labia and the clitoris become engorged with blood and are sensitive to tactile stimulation. When sexually stimulated, the veins around the vagina become filled with blood, resulting in a pressure that forces a liquid to pass from the veins through the surface cells of the vagina. The liquid provides a coating for the entire vagina. A pair of Bartholin's glands, located on either side of the vaginal opening, secrete a small amount of mucus that facilitates genital sexual activity.

Age-Associated Changes in the Female Genital System

Most of the changes in the female genital system are associated with menopause and its associated hormonal changes. The ovaries, uterus, and fallopian tubes become smaller when they cease to be stimulated to produce estrogens. The external genitalia lose subcutaneous fat, and pubic hair thins. Reduction in circulating estrogens causes the vaginal walls to be less elastic and thinner with decreased lubrication and decreased acidity. Reduced vaginal acidity and thinner walls increase the risk for yeast and bacterial infections or other irritations. These symptoms can be ameliorated with estrogen cream and lubricants. Clitoral sensation remains throughout life so that older women retain the capacity for orgasm. Changes in sexual response are discussed in Chapter 11, "Sexuality."

The Male

The male genital system consists of the penis, testes, scrotum, accessory ducts, and fluid-producing glands. Two oval-shaped testes that produce sperm and secrete testosterone (the male sex hormone) are contained within the scrotum. Under the control of the pituitary gland, androgens are secreted (within the testes) to facilitate the production of viable sperm and maintain male secondary sex characteristics. The testes release the sperm into the epididymis, where sperm cells mature and are stored.

The epididymis empties into the vas deferens. Two glands, the seminal vesicles and the prostate, empty into the vas deferens. The seminal vesicles contribute fluid to aid the movement of the sperm. The prostate gland, a chestnut-shaped structure surrounding the first inch of the urethra, deposits fluid in the urethra, which activates the sperm.

Upon ejaculation, both the sperm and the fluid from the seminal vesicles enter the ejaculatory ducts. Semen is forcibly ejaculated from the urethra through the penis, a cylindrical-shaped organ equipped to carry both urine and semen. The penis is composed of erectile tissue enabling it to enlarge with sexual excitation.

Age-Associated Changes in the Male Genital System

Like many other changes with age, most functional changes in the male genital system are highly variable and depend on the man's psychological status, presence of disease, and medication use. Older men have more difficulty achieving and maintaining erections, and exhibit a decreased ejaculatory force than younger adults. In addition, a longer time interval is required for a second erection. Changes in the sexual response cycle with age are more thoroughly discussed in Chapter 11, "Sexuality."

Males experience a universal, age-related decline in the number of viable sperm. Even though the sperm count per ejaculation remains the same, the proportion of immature sperm increases with advanced age. Nevertheless, men generally retain the ability to father a child into very old age.

Perhaps the most well-documented structural alteration with age is the enlargement of the prostate. When it enlarges, it may constrict the urethra, causing difficulty in urinating. The gland begins to enlarge in the fourth decade, and by the age of 80 almost all men have an enlarged prostate, a condition known as *benign prostatic hypertrophy*. Although sexual performance is not altered, prostate enlargement can cause symptoms of urinary frequency, urgency, decreased force of stream, and urinary retention. Benign prostatic hypertrophy is discussed further in Chapter 5, "Other Chronic Diseases and Conditions."

SUMMARY

Age-associated changes in body systems vary greatly. Some structural alterations occur in nearly every body system, many affecting maximal function far more than everyday function. Although the majority of age-associated changes do not cause significant functional impairment, some changes do require adaptation. Skin becomes more wrinkled and less elastic, and hair may thin and become gray. Elders lose muscular strength, joint flexibility, and bone strength and mass, but the losses are highly variable among individuals. The cardiovascular system becomes less efficient, especially at maximal exertion. Immune system function declines with age, making elders more susceptible to infections. Lungs become less elastic with age, decreasing the efficiency of gas exchange. Because the digestive system has high reserve capacity, age has little effect on its function. With age, the kidneys become somewhat less efficient at filtering wastes from the blood, which may increase the length of time an active drug remains in the body. Because of this, physicians should adjust the dosages of elders' prescriptions and medications.

Changes in the communication networks of the body—the sensory, neural, and endocrine systems—can affect an individual's internal equilibrium as well as the ability to respond to the environment. The most significant age-associated changes occur in vision and hearing. Structural changes in the eye create problems with near vision (presbyopia) and decreased color discrimination. Environmental noise and structural changes in the ear result in almost universal hearing loss with age, especially in the high frequencies (presbycusis). Eyeglasses and hearing aids significantly reduce the impact of changes in vision and hearing. Some structural changes occur with age in the nervous system, but the functional changes vary among individuals. Perhaps the greatest endocrine system change for women is a decline of estrogen production in the ovaries. The most obvious change in the genital system with age is women's inability to reproduce. Among men, sperm production is reduced but they can father children in late life. Reduced sexual interest and capacity with age among both men and women is highly variable and is dependent upon psychological and physical health status and medication use rather than age itself.

Changes occurring in body systems are highly variable among individuals. Some older individuals have a higher level of function than others. Some of the declines we associate with aging are due not to aging itself but to disease processes, environmental factors, or modifiable behaviors such as cigarette smoking, physical inactivity, and poor nutrition. Understanding the systems that are affected by age can help us interact more effectively with the elderly.

ACTIVITIES

1. List health behaviors you currently practice that may hasten your aging process. Which systems do these habits affect? How might these behaviors affect your functioning ten years from now? Twenty years? What practices are likely to enhance your health?

2. Make a list of physiological changes you believe are inevitable with aging. Which of these changes have you seen in all the elders you know? How are the elders you know affected by these aging processes? How do they adjust?

3. What do you think you will look like at age 80? Draw or describe your appearance and lifestyle at age 80. What physiological changes do you expect? Which changes may be minimized by different health habits?

4. Individuals of all ages often say, "I must be getting old." Explain the circumstances surrounding why you or others say this. Are they valid signs of aging, or are they due to disease or environmental factors?

5. Select a characteristic of older people that you believe is an age-related change. Using the criteria given in this chapter and recent literature, design a study that would demonstrate whether your supposition is valid.

6. Design a printed advertisement or a radio spot aimed at young people advocating sunscreen use. How will you convince them to take care of their skin before they notice damage?

7. Many companies prosper from products designed to make the public feel or look younger. Collect advertisements that promote this theme and share them with your classmates. Are claims valid? If not, write a letter to one of the companies protesting its false advertising.

8. A number of activities enable students to simulate age-related sensory and mobility decrements. Try some of the following and discuss the possible effects on daily routine and self-concept. To simulate decreased touch sensitivity, put rubber cement on your fingertips. To simulate decreased visual acuity, put Vaseline on your eyeglasses. Place cotton or plugs in your ears to simulate hearing losses. An Ace bandage wrapped around joints simulates stiffness. A scarf draped from your neck and tied to your belt simulates postural changes. Spend a whole day using a wheelchair or walker. If your college has a theater department, ask to be made up and dressed as an elder; then go shopping. Record your feelings and the reaction of others. Can you think of other simulation activities?

BIBLIOGRAPHY

1. Rowlatt, C., and Franks, L.M. 1978. Aging in tissues and cells. In Brocklehurst, J.C. (Ed.), *Geriatric medicine and gerontology*. New York: Churchill and Livingstone.

2. Wang, S.Q., Setlow, R., Berwick, M., et al. 2003. Ultraviolet A and melanoma: A review. *Journal of the American Academy of Dermatology* 48(3): 464–465.

3. Iannuzzi-Sucich, M., Prestwood, K.M., and Kenny, A.M. 2002. Prevalence of sarcopenia and predictors of skeletal muscle mass in healthy, older men and women. *Journal of Gerontology: Medical Sciences* 57A(12):772–777.

4. Hughes, V.A., Frontera, W.R., Wood, M., et al. 2001. Longitudinal muscle strength changes in older adults: Influence of muscle mass, physical activity, and health. *Journal of Gerontology: Biological Sciences* 56A(5):B209–B217.

5. Sorkin, J.D., Muller, D.C., and Andres, R. 1999. Longitudinal changes in height of men and women: Implications for interpretation of the body mass index: The Baltimore Longitudinal Study of Aging. *American Journal of Epidemiology* 150(9): 969–977.

6. Cheitlin, M.D. 2003. Cardiovascular physiology— changes with aging. *American Journal of Geriatric Cardiology* 12(1):9–13.

7. Ferrari, A.U. 2002. Modifications of the cardiovascular system with aging. *American Journal of Geriatric Cardiology* 11(1):30–33.

8. Glisky, E.L. 2007. Changes in cognitive function in human aging. In Riddle, D.R. (Ed.), *Brain aging: Models, methods, and mechanisms*. Boca Raton, FL: CRC Press; Chapter 1. Frontiers in neuroscience.

9. National Center for Health Statistics. 2010. *Summary health statistics for U.S. adults: National health interview survey, 2009*. Series 10 249. 207 pp. (PHS) 2011–1577.

10. Winkler, S., Garg, A.K., Mekayarajjananonth, T., Bakaeen, L.G., and Khan, E. 1999. Depressed taste and smell in geriatric patients. *Journal of the American Dental Association* 130(12): 1759–1765.

11. Kaneda, H., Maeshima, K., Goto, N., et al. 2000. Decline in taste and odor discrimination abilities with age, and relationship between gustation and olfaction. *Chemical Senses* 25(3):331–337.

12. Harman, S.M., Metter, E.J., Tobin, J.D., Pearson, J., and Blackman, M.R. 2001. Longitudinal effects of aging on serum total and free testosterone levels in healthy men. Baltimore Longitudinal Study of Aging. *Journal of Clinical Endocrinology Metabolism* 86:724–731.

Chronic Illnesses:

The Top Five Killers

If I'd known I was going to live so long, I'd have taken better care of myself.
Songwriter Eubie Blake, on approaching his 100th birthday

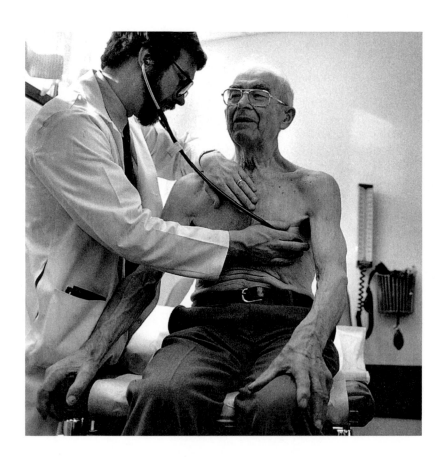

Although we would prefer to maintain the health and vigor of our young adulthood into advanced old age, our genes and our lifestyle conspire against us. For too many, the older years are associated with increased rates of death and disability. Sure, there are exceptions—some older people are healthy and vigorous into their ninth decade or beyond. But everyone dies, and most people die of something that disables them for at least a short while before taking their life.

In this chapter we discuss the nature of chronic illnesses (also called chronic diseases) and explore the five that are the major killers of older people: heart disease, cancer, stroke, lung diseases, and diabetes. Another chronic disease that is a major killer, Alzheimer's disease, is discussed in depth in Chapter 7, "Mental Health and Mental Disorders." Chronic diseases that are not as deadly but impact the quality of life in the later years are explored in Chapter 5, "Other Chronic Diseases and Conditions."

Although studying details of the many chronic diseases may seem daunting, it is important for people in the health and human service field to be familiar with these illnesses to better understand their influence on the everyday lives of older people and to work with them to minimize their impact. Further, understanding ways to prevent, treat, and manage chronic illness can help us to care for our aging relatives, and even to reduce the risk of chronic disease in our own lives.

Chronic diseases, in addition to their significant physical impact, are often accompanied by long-term social and psychological consequences. Before describing the individual diseases, we explore the nature and unique characteristics of chronic illness and its psychosocial impact on older persons.

THE NATURE OF CHRONIC ILLNESS

Being sick is generally associated with conditions from which the individual expects to recover, such as the common cold, flu, sore throat, or pneumonia. These *acute illnesses* have an abrupt onset and are generally caused by bacteria or a virus. They generally run their course or can be easily cured with medication. Some acute illnesses can even be avoided with vaccinations. With advancing age, however, the most troublesome health problems are due to arthritis, dementia, heart disease, cancer, diabetes, or other *chronic illnesses,* conditions that are generally incurable, worsen over time, and endure over many years, if not a lifetime. In general, the causes of chronic illness are multiple and are due to a combination of lifestyle or environmental agents (e.g., diet, cigarette smoking, inactivity), heredity, and other factors not yet known. Physicians usually cannot cure chronic conditions; they can only reduce the symptoms and deterioration caused by their progression (Table 4.1).

Although there are differences between chronic and acute illnesses, there is some overlap. A heart attack is an acute illness—it occurs suddenly and it needs to be treated quickly. However, acute diseases like heart attacks are often caused by a chronic disease (atherosclerosis of the blood vessels, diabetes, high blood pressure, elevated cholesterol). Acute diseases can also lead to long-term, chronic ailments. For example, if the heart attack damages the heart, heart failure (a chronic disease) can result. An individual may have an acute illness and a chronic illness (or more than one) at the same time. In fact, the presence of chronic illnesses makes it easier for older people to contract an acute illness. For example, an individual with emphysema (a chronic illness) is more likely to get pneumonia (an acute illness). Some complications of chronic illnesses are treated as acute illnesses. For example, an elder with diabetes (a chronic illness) may develop a urinary tract infection (an acute illness). Some chronic illnesses, such as a stroke or heart attack, may seem to have a rapid onset, but they likely were developing for years. Finally, with effective treatment, acute illnesses may become chronic. For example, AIDS is caused by a virus and would be terminal were it not for effective antiviral therapy. Currently, adults with AIDS are living longer and must continue to deal with a variety of symptoms, much like controlling a chronic illness. Thus, the

TABLE 4.1	Difference Between Chronic and Acute Illness	
	Chronic	**Acute or Infectious**
Length of illness	Lifetime	Brief
Cause	Often unknown, multiple, environmental	Known, often a virus or bacteria
Treatment	Treat symptoms, limit further damage	Kill microorganism, surgery
Prognosis	Generally progressive	Self-limiting, improves with treatment
Physical consequences	Irreversible	Usually reversible
Goal of care	Symptom control, maintenance, rehabilitation	Cure
Duration of care	Long, often lifetime	Brief
Cost of care	Expensive, may involve long-term drug and physician therapy and medical supervision	Often costs less because treatment is short-term

decision to call some illnesses acute and some chronic is somewhat arbitrary and changeable.

Another distinction can be drawn between illness, disease, and disability. Illness can be thought of as a poor state of health in which people feel badly or "sick." Disease is an abnormal condition affecting the body. Disability is when something—either a disease or an accident, perhaps—has caused an impairment of a body function that restricts the person from some aspect of daily living. So, for example, a disease (stroke) may cause an illness at first when a person feels poorly and needs help right away, but later develops into a disability (the person can no longer speak or walk, for example). However, the elevated cholesterol, diabetes, obesity, or high blood pressure that caused the stroke, if still present, remains a "disease." Likewise those with diabetes often do not feel "ill" and instead are accustomed to living with their condition and any disability (for example, numbness in the feet) they experience.

Chronic diseases are the major case of death in our country: Of the top 10 causes of death, most are chronic illnesses. Although chronic illnesses can occur at any age, the proportion of deaths caused by chronic disease increases with advancing age and is highest among those aged 65 and older (Table 4.2). Even older people who die of an acute illness, such

as pneumonia, likely suffered from one or more chronic illnesses that contributed to their death. Many people live with chronic illness for years. Although some chronic diseases have mild symptoms, many are responsible for extended suffering, disability, and a decreased quality of life for millions of people.

As Table 4.2 indicates, the top 10 causes of death vary by age group, but for the nation as a whole, the most common causes of death for the general population are very similar to the most common causes of death for the elderly. Why? Most people who die in the United States are older people. This has not always been the case. In the past, with higher rates of infant and maternal mortality, more childhood infections, and a lower average life expectancy, fewer people lived to old age. Children were more likely to die than adults, and infections accounted for a higher proportion of deaths. Since the discovery of penicillin and sanitation principles, infections have become less common and in their stead are chronic illnesses such as heart disease, cancer, and stroke.

Various indicators give us a snapshot of the impact of chronic disease in the lives of older people. Evidence demonstrating the burden of chronic illness in the elder population is the primary diagnosis received by individuals hospitalized

TABLE 4.2	Ten Leading Causes of Death in Specified Age Groups: United States, 2009

15–24 Years

1. Accidents
2. Homicide
3. Suicide
4. Cancers
5. Heart diseases
6. Congenital malformations
7. Influenza and pneumonia
8. Pregnancy and childbirth
9. Cerebrovascular diseases (strokes)
10. Chronic lower respiratory diseases

45–64 Years

1. Cancers
2. Heart diseases
3. Accidents
4. Chronic lower respiratory diseases
5. Chronic liver disease and cirrhosis
6. Diabetes
7. Cerebrovascular diseases (stroke)
8. Suicide
9. Influenza and pneumonia
10. Kidney diseases

25–44 Years

1. Accidents
2. Cancers
3. Heart diseases
4. Suicide
5. Homicide
6. Human immunodeficiency virus infection
7. Chronic liver disease and cirrhosis
8. Cerebrovascular diseases (stroke)
9. Diabetes
10. Influenza and pneumonia

65 Years and Over

1. Heart diseases
2. Cancers
3. Chronic lower respiratory diseases
4. Cerebrovascular diseases (stroke)
5. Alzheimer's disease
6. Diabetes
7. Influenza and pneumonia
8. Kidney diseases
9. Accidents
10. Septicemia (blood poisoning)

Note: Data from Kochanek, K.D., Xu, J., Murphy, S.L., Miniño, A.M., and Kung, H.-C. 2011. Deaths: Preliminary data for 2009. *National Vital Statistics Report* 59(4). Hyattsville, MD: National Center for Health Statistics.

in the United States each year. Most diagnoses are chronic diseases. By far, the most common diagnosis for hospitalization of individuals 65 and older is heart disease for both men and women. Analysis of similar data regarding physician visits in the United States by persons 65 years of age and older indicates that the major reason for visits to a physician each year is chronic illness.[1]

Chronic illness is associated with a reduced ability to function. Depending on what measures are used, between one-third and one-half of elders have some limitation in function, and the number who have disability and the number of limitations increases with advancing age. The Activities of Daily Living Scale (ADL) measures the limitations an individual might have in performing self-care activities in the home (bathing, dressing, using the toilet, transferring from a bed or chair, maintaining control of bladder and bowel, and eating).[2] Those with higher scores require more help. Another measure, the Instrumental Activities of Daily Living Scale (IADL), assesses the limitations of an individual in engaging in more complex activities needed to live independently: use of the telephone, driving or using public transport, shopping, meal preparation, housework, being able to take medications appropriately, and managing money.[3]

It is no surprise that chronic diseases account for the majority of health care costs in our country. Individuals with chronic diseases often take multiple drugs over a long period of time, sometimes for life. They must visit physicians regularly to manage, rather than cure, their diseases, and they often visit physicians for routine visits, even if they do not have symptoms. They often need medical equipment and supplies to deal with their conditions. And sometimes the illnesses create a crisis in which hospitalization and nursing home care, or home health care and rehabilitative services, become necessary. The cost of treating chronic illnesses is enormous. It is estimated that chronic illness care accounts for the majority of the nation's medical care expenses.

Factors that cannot be modified, such as family history, gender, and age, place some individuals at higher risk for a disease. Often, however, the type and extent of chronic diseases endured in later life are a consequence of bad health habits practiced in the early or middle years: being overweight, not exercising enough, smoking cigarettes, eating an unhealthy diet, or abusing alcohol. Those bad habits are called *risk factors* because they are known to increase the risk of particular diseases. Individuals who have two or more risk factors are considered "at risk" for chronic conditions. The "at risk" population is much more likely to be limited in their ability to participate in daily activities (bathing, dressing, eating, using the toilet, walking, getting in and out of bed) than adults with no risk factors.

Chronic diseases among older people may be difficult to diagnose. First, elders may not exhibit any symptoms. If they do, the symptoms often differ from younger groups: They may complain of multiple, nonspecific symptoms such as weakness, dizziness, or lack of appetite. Second, because elders are likely to have more than one chronic disease, the symptoms of one disease may be mistakenly attributed to an already existing disease and be ignored. Third, if elders are taking medication for one condition, the side effects of the medication may be misinterpreted as another condition. Finally, symptoms of chronic illness may be ignored because they are incorrectly attributed to normal age changes.

Management of chronic illnesses in elders can be complicated. Age changes in body systems

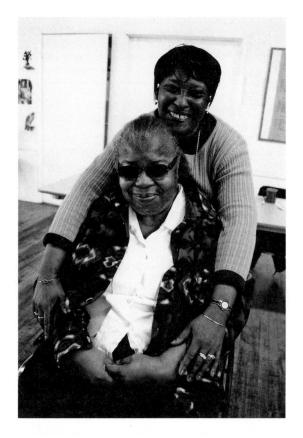

reduce the ability to respond to the stress of illness. In addition, elders often have more than one condition, often in more than one organ system, and may require multiple medications or medical interventions. Because of this, they have an increased risk of medication side effects. Some older people do not follow their physicians' directions for treatment and do not understand the cause or management of their condition. For these reasons, elders often exhibit more complications with chronic disease than do younger groups.

A discussion of the multiple chronic illnesses that affect older people is not intended to paint a portrait of debilitated, disabled old age. Although chronic disease and disabilities accumulate with age, most elders, especially the young-old, maintain reasonably good health. When a chronic disease develops, the individual can control many symptoms and reduce the progression of the disease with the help of health professionals. Despite the degree of chronic illness in the older population, close to three-fourths of a national sample report their health to be good or excellent.[1] Finally, even though a high prevalence of chronic disease is evident in the later years, it is not inevitable. Many diseases can be prevented by changes in lifestyle made as early as possible—improving diet, eliminating tobacco use, losing weight, and increasing physical activity. (Have you memorized these yet?)

Psychosocial Aspects of Chronic Illness

When and if sickness does occur, some approach it with a determination and try to overcome it with all their power. Others greet it placidly, accepting treatment but making no effort on their own. Still another small group, believing it cannot be overcome, will themselves to die and accept nothing that would delay their death.

—Eber Swope

Professionals who work with elders with chronic illnesses need to understand their medical problems and become aware of how the symptoms of disease impact their everyday life. Although chronic illnesses affect individuals differently, those who are chronically ill share many of the same problems. A. L. Strauss, a sociologist, developed a framework to look at the psychosocial problems of the chronically ill and their families.[4] Although the same framework can be used for any chronic illness, some illnesses are complex, and coping with them takes up most of the day. Other diseases have little impact on a person's daily routine. As you learn about the many problems of daily living for the chronically ill by reading Box 4.1, you might think of a particular disease and envision the day-to-day physical, social, and psychological adaptations that must be accomplished in order to live with that disease. Strauss asserts that, unless one understands how the chronically ill handle their illness on a daily basis, one cannot give effective care.

Because chronic illnesses are permanent and full recovery is not possible, elders with chronic illnesses should not be treated as if they are "sick." Concerned professionals and families may unconsciously promote dependence by allowing the chronically ill person to misuse the "sick role." Described by Talcott Parsons, a medical sociologist, the *sick role* is a phenomenon whereby a sick person is allowed to be dependent and is relieved of familial and societal responsibilities until she or he is well.[5] For example, the sick person does no household chores and is allowed to "take it easy." The ill person is not blamed for incurring the illness. However, understanding that sickness is undesirable and deviant, the sick person feels obligated to do everything possible to get well. Usually family members are supportive, and the sick person continues in the sick role until he or she is healthy enough to resume normal functioning. This model provides an excellent representation of what we do when we contract an acute illness such as influenza. Luckily, acute illnesses generally don't last long, and, as soon as we are able, we resume our normal responsibilities and interactions with significant others at home and at work.

For those who are chronically ill, the sick role must be modified because of the extended period of disability. When a chronically ill elder constantly assumes a dependent, egocentric role to cope with illness, both the chronically ill person and his or her family suffer. The inability, or reduced ability, to participate in the daily activities in the home or at work removes the person from those activities and roles that originally promoted self-esteem. Furthermore, preoccupation with the disease by both the chronically ill person and the family may encourage dependence. Instead, the ill person should attempt to do the most he or she can despite the illness and go on with life as effectively as possible.

Although the sick role is sometimes appropriate for an elder who needs special care, health professionals and families should be wary of supporting overly dependent behaviors of chronically ill elders. Often family and professional caregivers

BOX 4.1

Problems of Daily Living for the Chronically Ill

1. *Preventing medical crises and managing them when they occur.*
   Some chronic diseases are characterized by potentially fatal medical crises (e.g., diabetic coma, heart attack, epileptic seizure, and stroke). To prevent a crisis, the person's life must be organized for crisis management—that is, the signs of impending crisis must be recognized and appropriate action taken when they occur.

2. *Controlling symptoms.*
   Although the physician prescribes a regimen intended to control symptoms, the individual must rely largely on personal judgment to control symptoms. The individual needs to be aware of the present capacity of his or her body and come to terms with its reduced capability. Even minor symptoms may require a change in behavior, and major symptoms may call for redesigning daily life.

3. *Carrying out prescribed regimen and managing the problems associated with it.*
   The physician usually prescribes a treatment regimen to control the symptoms and progression of the disease, but the individual must learn the regimen and, to a greater or lesser degree, must organize the day around it. Some treatments are simple, such as ingesting a pill; others may take up a significant portion of the day. Whether or not a regimen is followed depends on a number of factors: Is the regimen easy to learn? How much time and energy does the regimen take? Is it painful? Are there side effects? Is it effective? Is it expensive? Does it lead to social isolation? When an individual has more than one chronic illness, the regimen often becomes more complicated and requires considerable juggling of time and energy.

4. *Preventing or coping with social isolation.*
   Many chronic illnesses are accompanied by lessened energy and mobility, impairment of sensory processes, visible physical disfigurement, or other deficits that may result in reduced social contact and isolation. The sick individual may withdraw from social activities, or former social contacts may withdraw. The more serious the disease, the more likely it is that isolation will occur.

5. *Adjusting to changes in the course of the disease.*
   Both the sick individual and people close to him or her need to cope with the downward course of the illness. Every downward step requires the sick person to reassess health status and make arrangements to manage symptoms, social interactions, and activities of daily living. Those close to the sick person may also need to be involved in such arrangements since dependence increases as the illness progresses. The impact of the downward course of illness on personal identity depends on the illness. If the downward course is predictable, preparation is possible in advance of each new downward phase; if it is unexpectedly quick, then adjustment is more difficult.

6. *Attempting to normalize lifestyle and interaction with others.*
   The chief task of one who is chronically ill is to live as fully as possible despite the symptoms and the disease. How normal life can be depends on the extent of symptoms, disability, and the regimen required to keep the disease under control. The task of normalization is most difficult when the disease is fatal.

7. *Financing treatments and survival.*
   As chronic illness is usually life-long, it is nearly always accompanied by financial problems. One important characteristic of chronic disease is the cost of required treatment, especially drugs, machinery, physician visits, and home-based health services. Health problems can wipe out life savings rapidly, and the chronically ill have to seek other funding sources. The problem of seeking adequate funds for treatment and survival becomes more complex when one is also dealing with physical disability.

For more information refer to Strauss, A.L. 1975. *Chronic illness and the quality of life*. St. Louis: C.V. Mosby.

inadvertently promote dependency by excessive care, which reduces coping effectiveness and encourages further decline in function. For example, a caregiver might dress and spoon-feed someone who could dress and feed herself, albeit slowly.

The term "miscarried helping" has been coined to describe a behavioral cycle of chronically ill individuals and their families. Miscarried helping occurs when well-intentioned attempts of support fail because they are excessive, untimely, or inappropriate. It may begin at diagnosis, when expressions of empathy and affection dominate. Later, this optimism fades, and there is an increase in family anxiety as families struggle to accommodate the sick member's needs into their normal routines. Because of lack of time and energy, family members may neglect social engagements and lose the associated support. Increased isolation may occur, and caregivers may become drained and exhausted. The patient may suffer a loss of autonomy or feel guilty: "I am the reason my wife can't do the things she wants." As patient and caregiver become more involved, they may begin to feel even more distress. The caregiver may begin to feel responsible for the patient's illness and become angry or frustrated. One family member may take on all the caring responsibilities, causing tension in the family.

Many other psychological factors influence the severity of chronic illnesses. Elders differ in how they define and react to illness. One arthritic older woman may insist she is living well while another constantly complains about her stiff joints. Some individuals become angry, deny they are ill, or become compliant and resigned to the patient role. Chronic illnesses can lead to mental health problems such as depression or anxiety. There is much variability in the coping style and level of responsibility the elder assumes for the illness. Some people perceive every minor symptom as a worsening of the disease and seek frequent medical attention, while others take more responsibility for themselves and still others deny the illness.

Caregiving extracts a tremendous toll on family members—financially, socially, and emotionally. Chronic illnesses that seriously impinge on activities of daily living can often result in other social problems. A family member may have to quit work or move to care for a disabled elder. The monthly income or life savings of a couple may be depleted through medical expenses. The chronic illness of one member of a couple can severely impact the other. For example, if one spouse loses his sight and can no longer perform many activities of daily living, the other will have to take on more responsibility.

The Five Major Killers

The remainder of this chapter discusses the five chronic diseases that are most likely to cause death in middle-aged and older adults: heart disease, cancer, stroke, chronic obstructive pulmonary disease, and diabetes.

The following descriptions of each disease do not detail the psychosocial effects of the symptoms or treatment on the individual because they depend on the extent of illness, personality, coping skills, financial situation, and degree of family support. Nevertheless, as you read about each of the chronic conditions, use Box 4.1, "Problems of Daily Living for the Chronically Ill," to consider the particular issues that individuals may have to address as they deal with the disease on a day-to-day basis. For some individuals, treating symptoms may mean popping a pill every day and dealing with minor side effects. For others, the illness becomes a constant companion, and the daily regimen to cope with the symptoms and the treatment modality is life changing.

Heart Disease

In the United States and other industrialized nations, most adults die from heart disease. If they die of something else, heart disease is still almost always present and contributing to their decline. The terms *heart disease, ischemic heart disease, coronary artery disease (CAD)*, and *coronary heart disease (CHD)* are interchangeable terms used for the spectrum of disorders affecting the *coronary arteries*—the blood vessels that carry oxygen and nutrients to the heart muscle to enable it to effectively pump blood through the rest of the body. The coronary arteries undergo progressive damage from years of buildup of fats inside the artery wall, buildup that eventually restricts the free flow of blood to the heart muscle and causes high blood pressure. This buildup is called atherosclerosis and is the common denominator of most types of heart disease.

Heart disease is the end result of a complex cascade of problems in the blood vessels, beginning with *high blood cholesterol* and *high blood pressure,* which progresses to *atherosclerosis,* then causes reduced blood flow to the heart muscle. Reduced blood flow within the coronary arteries may be temporary, causing the heart pain called *angina pectoris*. However, if a blood clot blocks nutrients and oxygen to the heart muscle, the part of the muscle that is deprived of oxygen and nutrients will die, causing a heart attack. Over time, high blood pressure strains the heart muscle, causing it to enlarge, then to weaken. Heart attacks and reduced blood flow further weaken the heart muscle so that it cannot effectively pump blood to the rest of the body. Sometimes the part of the muscle that controls the rate or rhythm of the heart is affected, resulting in abnormal heart rate, called *cardiac arrythmias*. Some people with heart disease die suddenly from a heart attack, arrhythmia, or heart failure; many more suffer a more gradual decline. These conditions, and the factors leading up to them, are described in this section.

As you can see, several diseases and conditions are part of the constellation of heart disease. Combined, they are the leading cause of death among those 65 years and older, the second leading cause of death among those aged 45 to 54, and the third leading cause of death among those 25 to 44. We all must take notice. What are your chances of developing the disease? To answer that question, you need to learn about risk factors.

What is a risk factor? A *risk factor,* as previously stated, is a personal characteristic, a condition, or a behavior that increases susceptibility to a disease. Having a risk factor does not mean that disease is inevitable, but it does mean that one is at a higher risk than someone without the risk factor.

In our country, almost every adult has some degree of cardiovascular damage, but risk factors predict who will have cardiovascular disease and who is most likely to die from it. Extensive research has identified factors that increase the risk of cardiovascular disease and their level of importance. Some risk factors cannot be modified, treated, or controlled; others can be changed.

Some risk factors that cannot be changed are age, gender, race and ethnicity, and family history. *Age* is a very important factor. More than four of five people who die from heart disease are 65 and older. In regard to *gender,* men are at greater risk of heart attack than women at all ages and tend to have attacks earlier in life than women do. *Race and ethnicity* are also significant. Black Americans have more severe high blood pressure than whites and a higher risk of heart disease. Heart disease risk is also higher among Mexican Americans, American Indians, Native Hawaiians, and some Asian Americans. This is partly due to higher rates of obesity and diabetes in these minority populations. *Family history* also plays a role. Children of parents with heart disease are more likely to develop it themselves, whether due to genetics, which can't be changed, or family habits, which can be adjusted. The younger the age at which the parents or relatives developed heart disease, the more likely it is that genetic factors were involved and the higher the risk.

Several risk factors of major importance can be reduced by modifying negative health behaviors or by taking medicine. To reduce our chances of dying or being disabled by heart disease, we should begin with the following:

- *People who smoke* have double the risk of non-smokers of developing heart disease and experiencing a sudden heart attack. Pipe and cigar smoking increase the risk of cardiovascular disease, but not as much as smoking cigarettes. Exposure to other people's smoke increases the risk of heart disease even for nonsmokers.
- As *blood cholesterol rises*, so does the risk for coronary artery disease. When other risk factors

(such as high blood pressure and tobacco smoke) are present, the risk becomes even greater. A person's cholesterol level is affected by genetics, but it is also determined by health behaviors such as diet and exercise. Details on this important risk factor are addressed below.

- *High blood pressure* (hypertension) increases the heart's workload, causing it to stiffen, thicken, and enlarge. Hypertension also increases risk of stroke, heart attack, kidney failure, and congestive heart failure. When high blood pressure occurs with other risk factors (e.g., obesity, smoking, high cholesterol, or diabetes), heart attack or stroke risk increases several times. Hypertension is discussed further below.

- A *sedentary lifestyle* increases the risk of heart disease; regular, moderate-to-vigorous physical activity reduces it. The more vigorous the activity, the greater it benefits the heart. However, even moderate-intensity activities help if practiced regularly. Exercise can help control blood cholesterol, diabetes, and obesity. This risk factor is fully addressed in Chapter 9, "Physical Activity."

- People who have *excess body fat*—especially if it accumulates at the waist—are more likely to develop heart disease and stroke than people who carry extra weight in their buttocks and hips. Excess weight increases the workload of the heart and raises blood pressure. Obesity is associated with diabetes, high cholesterol and triglyceride levels, and lower HDL ("good") cholesterol levels. Losing even 10 pounds substantially reduces blood pressure and lowers heart disease risk. See Chapter 10, "Nutrition," for more information on obesity, its prevention, and treatment.

- *Diabetes* is a major risk factor for developing cardiovascular disease, and the risk is even greater if the diabetes is not under control. About three-quarters of people with diabetes die of some form of heart or blood vessel disease: Those with diabetes need to keep blood pressure, cholesterol, and weight low to reduce the risk. Diabetes in itself is a leading cause of death and is addressed more fully later in this chapter.

Other risk factors have been identified that contribute to heart disease, such as stress and excessive alcohol use, but they are not as important as those listed above. See the American Heart Association Web site for more detail: www.americanheart.org

High Cholesterol

A major risk factor for heart disease is *high cholesterol,* or elevated lipids or fats in the bloodstream. Other terms for high cholesterol are *hypercholesterolemia* and *hyperlipidemia.* Cholesterol and other lipids are necessary for health, but some people have too much of them. It is unclear whether these people eat too much food that is high in cholesterol and fat or whether their high cholesterol level is genetically determined. In any case, the excess lipids circulate through the body, thicken the blood, and accumulate inside the artery walls, causing atherosclerosis.

Cholesterol is a waxy, fatty substance present in all cells of the body. The body needs cholesterol to make hormones, vitamin D, and substances important in digestion. Our bodies can produce cholesterol as needed. In addition, we eat animal products that contain cholesterol. Cholesterol travels in the bloodstream. However, because cholesterol is a fat and blood is watery, the cholesterol is transported in the bloodstream within a protein shell called *lipoprotein.*

Two kinds of lipoprotein carry cholesterol in the bloodstream: low-density lipoprotein (LDL) and high-density lipoprotein (HDL). Low-density lipoprotein (LDL) cholesterol is sometimes called "bad" cholesterol because it is the main source of cholesterol buildup and blockage in the arteries. *The higher the LDL cholesterol level, the higher the risk of heart disease.* In contrast, high-density lipoprotein (HDL) cholesterol is sometimes called "good" cholesterol because its role is to pick up cholesterol throughout the body and return it to the liver, so that cholesterol does not build up in the arteries. *The higher the HDL cholesterol level, the*

Headline News: The Latest Breakthroughs

Health news is big on the Internet and in print media. You have seen the headlines—"Studies show blueberries reduce heart disease" or "Soy is secret to long life, researchers say."

It seems there are advances every day and the secret is simple—eat more blueberries or soy and you can forestall death or disability from heart disease. How appealing! Which would you rather do? Add blueberries to your cereal, or stop smoking? Take a vitamin or exercise 30 to 45 minutes daily at a moderate pace? Drink soy drinks and laugh or eat nine servings of fruits and vegetables and fewer than 25 percent of calories as fats? These headlines appeal to our love of simple solutions by promising a quick fix to the great American problem of heart disease.

When you read the text of the article, often there is a scientific study cited followed by commentary on what it all might mean for the future. If you choose to read the actual study, you will almost always find that the benefits purported are quite small and the media report is overstated. These numbers and percentages sound good, but the fact is that there is no shortcut to prevent heart disease. Good health takes dedication and perseverance.

Although we all would like a magic blueberry–soy–vitamin E–laughter bullet, the overwhelming volume of data supports the less flashy approach. The single most important way to reduce risk of heart disease is to stop smoking. Steer clear of fads and stick to the less exciting headlines: Reduce your risk by regular moderate exercise, control diabetes and high blood pressure, stop smoking, lower cholesterol, and maintain a healthy weight.

---

lower is the risk of heart disease. High HDL levels are associated with being female and/or being physically active. Because there are no symptoms associated with high cholesterol, many people are unaware that they have it.

Diagnostic tools are available to measure the levels of various types of cholesterol in the blood. Cholesterol levels are measured in milligrams (mg) of cholesterol per deciliter (dL) of blood. National surveys show that about one in six U.S. adults has elevated cholesterol, with levels higher among women. High cholesterol is defined as more than 240 mg/dl. Elevated cholesterol is more common in whites than other ethnic groups. Even though obesity is increasing in the United States, the incidence of high cholesterol is declining. This is likely because many adults with high cholesterol take medication to reduce it.

The level of HDL, LDL, and triglycerides that is appropriate for any given person is different based on other risk factors for heart disease. For example, those who do not have diabetes or hypertension may not need to treat moderate elevations in cholesterol as this is their *only* risk factor. In contrast, those with diabetes, hypertension, obesity, and/or inactivity may require treatment at much lower cholesterol levels to reduce their risk of heart attack and stroke. Expert recommendations for the diagnosis and treatment of elevated and abnormal cholesterol, as well as suggestions for particular population subgroups (like those with diabetes or high blood pressure, for example) can be found in the Third Report of the National Cholesterol Education Program.[1]

A national study based on physical examinations of a sample of Americans between 2005 and 2008 reports that 15 percent of the population had high cholesterol (greater than 240 mm/dL). The prevalence of high cholesterol is even higher among elders. Among women 65 to 74 years of age, 21.8 percent had high cholesterol; and among women 75 and older, 19.4 percent. For men, the percentage was lower: 7.9 percent of men 65 to 74 had high cholesterol and 8.6 percent of men 75 and older had it.[5] Continually updated information on elevated cholesterol can be found through the National Cholesterol Education Program Web site.

Elevated cholesterol levels can be treated with diet and exercise or with lipid-lowering medications. When abnormal lipids are diagnosed, the first recommendation is lifestyle changes: reducing animal fats, increasing dietary fiber, losing weight, exercising more, quitting smoking. If lifestyle changes do not reduce cholesterol sufficiently in three months, lipid-lowering medications are prescribed.

There are several classes of lipid-lowering medications, and each class works differently. The choice depends on the levels of LDL, HDL, total cholesterol, and triglycerides. One drug may be prescribed, or drugs may be used in combination. Each class has its benefits, side effects, and risks. Generally, the *statin drugs* are the first line of drug treatment (their generic names end in *statin*). They reduce cholesterol by slowing down the production of cholesterol in the body and by increasing the liver's ability to remove the LDL cholesterol already in the blood. No matter which medication is prescribed, the goal is to increase HDL levels (the "good" cholesterol) and reduce levels of LDL, triglycerides, and total cholesterol. For a list of the many types of cholesterol-lowering medications, their benefits, and side effects, refer to www.mayoclinic.com

No matter how old an individual is, LDL cholesterol and high triglycerides are major risk factors for heart attacks and strokes. Older people have been shown to respond to the cholesterol-lowering drugs, but these drugs have not been tested in the very old or for long-term use. In addition, older people are more likely to experience side effects from the medications, such as muscle aches and drug interactions.

People who have already had a heart attack or stroke derive the greatest benefit, but even those with other risk factors can benefit from cholesterol-lowering drugs. National guidelines recommend that treatment of high cholesterol be based on cardiovascular risk factors (such as diabetes, history of heart disease, and levels of cholesterol) and not age. These drugs are very expensive and are often taken for life: The cost is prohibitive for some individuals.

Even though pills may reduce cholesterol levels, the first line of treatment to reduce cholesterol and other risk factors for heart disease is to develop healthy behaviors. Sidney Smith, MD, the former head of the American Heart Association, stated, "I am continually amazed that patients are willing to take pills, have tubes snaked into their heart, even have their chest sawed open—but aren't willing to change their diet, get some exercise, or stop smoking."

Hypertension (High Blood Pressure)

Hypertension is the medical term for high blood pressure. It is known as the "silent killer" because most of the 50 million Americans with the condition (about one in four adults) have no symptoms and look healthy. The proportion of individuals with hypertension increases with age, and a higher proportion of women have hypertension than men. A large national survey based on physical examinations reported that 48 percent of the males between 65 and 74 years of age had hypertension, and of those 75 years and older, 54 percent had hypertension. Females had a higher rate: 51 percent of women between 65 and 74 years of age had hypertension, and among the 75-plus age group, 63 percent had hypertension.[1] Further, a significantly higher proportion of elder black and Mexican American males have hypertension than do white males. And, a significantly higher proportion of older Mexican American women have hypertension when compared to black and white women.[1]

Reducing blood pressure reduces the risk of many diseases. Treatment of high blood pressure generally begins with lifestyle modifications: losing weight; stopping smoking; reducing salt, fat, and alcohol intake; and increasing physical activity. Of those, the most significant reductions in blood pressure can be realized with weight loss: Even a small amount can result in dramatic blood pressure reductions. Also, potassium and calcium supplements have shown to be effective for some.

If changes in health behaviors do not reduce blood pressure, then medication is prescribed.

Blood Pressure: What Is It and How Is It Measured?

*B*lood pressure is the force exerted by the blood against the artery walls. When the heart *contracts,* a great volume of blood is forced into the arteries, and pressure reaches a maximum point (called *systolic* pressure). After the heart has contracted and pushes blood out, it *relaxes* between beats to refill. During this time, the pressure in the arteries is at its lowest point (called *diastolic* pressure). Systolic and diastolic pressure can be measured by an instrument called a *sphygmomanometer,* commonly known as a blood pressure gauge. The pressure the blood exerts on the arteries is measured as the amount of pressure able to fill a column of mercury in millimeters (mm). Blood pressure readings are expressed as a fraction. The top number is the systolic pressure; the bottom number is the diastolic pressure. The systolic pressure is always stated first

and the diastolic pressure second. For example: 120/80 reads as "120 over 80"; the systolic blood pressure is 120, and the diastolic blood pressure is 80. The following are the current medical guidelines for blood pressure readings.[7]

- Optimal: Blood pressure below 120 over 80 mmHg (millimeters of mercury).
- Prehypertension: A systolic pressure of 120 to 139 mmHg or a diastolic pressure of 80 to 89 mmHg needs to be watched carefully or treated if there are other risk factors.
- Hypertension: A systolic blood pressure reading of 140 or higher or a diastolic blood pressure of 90 or higher. An elevated systolic blood pressure (upper number) is a more important heart disease risk factor than diastolic blood pressure.[6]

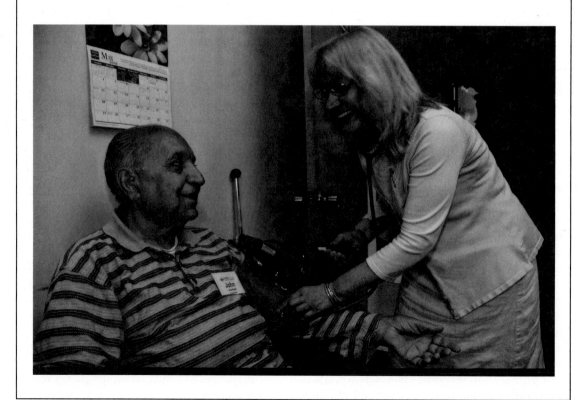

Continued

Blood Pressure: What Is It and How Is It Measured?

Just as with elevated cholesterol, there is no absolute level of blood pressure that is healthy or unhealthy, but a higher blood pressure is associated with higher morbidity (illness) and mortality (death). Because of this, it should be monitored and treated. The physician will treat hypertension more aggressively if the individual has other conditions such as a history of a heart attack, heart failure, high risk of heart disease or diabetes, or chronic kidney disease. In contrast, low blood pressure is not a cause for alarm unless it is exceedingly low, or when blood pressure falls due to shock or blood loss.

Blood pressure readings are highly variable. Anxiety, stress, physical activity, even giving a presentation, may elevate blood pressure. In addition, many people who are borderline hypertensive exhibit a "white coat syndrome," in which their anxiety at seeing a doctor can increase blood pressure. One isolated high blood pressure reading should not be cause for treatment. To increase accuracy, at least three different readings should be taken at different visits and averaged. A more accurate alternative is a mobile blood pressure instrument that is attached to the patient and automatically records hourly blood pressure throughout a 24-hour period.

Many types of medication are available to reduce blood pressure and may be used alone or in combination. The most common first-line therapy is a diuretic (rids the body of excess water) or a beta blocker (reduces the heart rate). Antihypertensive medications have a host of side effects, including erectile dysfunction, chronic cough, and fatigue. If one drug causes a side effect, another drug may need to be substituted.

Because medication for high blood pressure is usually taken for years, or even decades, it is important that a regimen is found that does not significantly affect an individual's quality of life. It is not unusual to try several different medications before finding one that works, or to have to change the medication multiple times over the years. The medications often can be reduced if an individual has lost weight or made other positive lifestyle changes. Because hypertension usually has no symptoms and the medications used to treat it may cause distressing side effects, many individuals do not take their medication regularly.

Despite the availability of effective treatment for the disease, most individuals with hypertension do not have it under control.[6] Uncontrolled high blood pressure causes extensive damage to body organs and blood vessels. Damage to the arteries increases the risk of atherosclerosis, heart attack, irregular heartbeat, stroke, and congestive heart failure. Increased blood pressure also causes irreversible damage to the blood vessels in the kidneys and eyes, causing kidney failure and blindness. Hypertension can affect the brain and is associated with reduced cognitive function as well as increased risk of strokes. All adults need to be educated about the severe consequences of uncontrolled hypertension. No matter what, everyone with hypertension needs regular measurements of his or her blood pressure to ensure that it stays within an appropriate range.

Table 4.3 displays the major drug types used to treat hypertension, the mechanism of action, and common brand names. All drug types have the goal of reducing the pressure on the artery walls, but each accomplishes it with a different mechanism. These medications are also used for other heart diseases. For details on each type or a particular drug, including other uses and side effects, refer to the Mayo Clinic's excellent site on high blood pressure: Click on www.mayoclinic.com and type "choosing blood pressure medications" in the search bar.

TABLE 4.3	Drugs for Hypertension and Other Heart Diseases	
Type of Drug	**Mechanism of Action**	**Examples**
Diuretics	Reduce the volume of fluid in the arteries by ridding the body of sodium and water, thus reducing the pressure on the artery walls.	Zaroxolyn (metolazone), Hydrochlorothiazide, Bumex (bumetanide), Lasix (furosemide)
Beta blockers	Slow the rate and force of the heart, thus reducing work of the heart and consequent pressure on the blood vessels.	Tenormin (atenolol), Coreg (carvedilol), Lopressor (metoprolol), Inderal (propranol)
Angiotensin-converting enzyme (ACE) inhibitors	Prevent the body from producing the hormone, angiotensin II, that stiffens and narrows blood vessels, thus relaxing the vessels.	Lotensin (benazepril), Capoten (captopril), Vasotec (enalapril), Prinivil (lisinopril)
Angiotensin II receptor blockers	Work similarly to ACE inhibitors, but *blocks the action* of angiotensin II instead of preventing the body from producing the hormone, consequently relaxing the vessels.	Atacand (candesartan), Avapro (irbesarta)
Calcium channel blockers	Reduce the flow of calcium into the muscle cells of the heart and artery, relaxing artery walls. Some types also slow heart rate.	Norvasc (amlodipine), Cardizem/Dilacor XR (diltiazem), Calan (verapamil)
Alpha blockers	Some block the hormone norepinephrine from constricting small blood vessels, relaxing artery walls. Others also slow the heartbeat to reduce the amount of blood traveling through the vessels.	Catapres (clonidine), Cardura (doxazosin), Hytrin (terazosin)
Vasodilators	Directly relaxes muscles in vessel walls.	Isordil (isosorbide), Nitrol (nitroglycerine)

Atherosclerosis

Atherosclerosis is a slow progressive condition of the blood vessels that can begin as early as childhood in countries with high-fat diets. Arteries in the body gradually become narrowed due to the buildup of fat and cholesterol on the artery walls, causing inflammation of the arteries. The deposits eventually harden, forming plaques that can eat into the wall of the artery and interfere with the flow of blood. The plaques also stiffen the artery walls so they are less able to expand or constrict as needed. Atherosclerosis can occur anywhere in the body but is most dangerous in the coronary arteries (arteries that supply blood to the heart muscle), in the blood vessels leading to the brain, and in the arteries leading to the kidneys. Pieces of plaque can break away and clog an artery, leading to a heart attack or stroke. In addition, blood may stick to the thickened irregular walls of the blood vessels, forming blood clots, further interfering with blood flow. Sometimes, the clots break off to cause a heart attack or stroke. Scientists also hypothesize that inflammation, hormones, and bacteria may play a role in atherosclerosis.

The development and progression of atherosclerosis are accelerated by the Western lifestyle: inactivity, smoking, obesity, and a diet high in fats. High cholesterol, diabetes, and hypertension are known to aggravate atherosclerosis. Treatment to slow the buildup of plaque in the arteries is focused on reducing dietary fat and lowering blood cholesterol levels, controlling diabetes and hypertension, losing weight, and stopping smoking.

Angina

When the heart muscle does not get enough blood, it hurts and the pain is called *angina*. Angina is generally described as a chest pressure, more than a chest pain, and it may be associated with pain in the left arm or jaw, sweating, a sense of panic or doom, nausea, or dizziness. Angina most often occurs with exertion (this type is called *stable* angina). During exercise, the heart muscle requires more blood and oxygen. If the narrowed blood vessels cannot deliver enough oxygen, pain occurs. When exertion is stopped, the pain subsides. Both physical stress and mental/emotional stress can induce symptoms of angina. Stable angina is a chronic medical condition. A more dangerous and rare condition is when angina occurs at rest, called *unstable* angina. This condition results when plaque breaks away within the narrowed arteries and almost blocks a coronary artery. Unstable angina is an acute condition that needs immediate evaluation because the risk of heart attack and death are very high.

Angina is often treated surgically with procedures to widen or replace the blocked coronary blood vessels. Some procedures are more invasive and dangerous than others. Surgical treatments for angina are the same as those for a heart attack and are discussed below.

Heart Attack

When a coronary artery becomes completely blocked, the part of the heart muscle that the artery previously supplied with blood and nutrients becomes starved. If the heart muscle is without oxygen for more than a few minutes, that part of the heart dies. The person is having a heart attack, also called *myocardial infarction*. Like angina, a heart attack causes chest pain or pressure, generally over the center or left side of the heart. The pain may be felt in the left arm, the neck or jaw, or even the abdomen. The person may become sweaty and anxious (or very calm); the person may feel nauseated or feel as if he or she has "heartburn." In some cases, the symptoms are dramatic, such as a loss of consciousness or sudden death. In many cases, particularly among older people, there are no symptoms.

Most heart attacks are not fatal, but all heart attacks permanently damage heart tissue. The bigger the blood vessel involved, the larger is the section of the heart that is robbed of blood and dies. The extent of the attack depends on how much heart muscle is affected below the coronary artery blockage. This damage can result in cardiac arrhythmias (irregular heart rate) or congestive heart failure. Fatal heart attacks are most common among younger people, the very old, and women.[7] Many studies have attempted to answer why women are more likely than men to die from a heart attack. Whether there are biological reasons or whether the difference is the result of discrimination in diagnosis and treatment is not yet clear.

Anyone with chest pain or pressure for more than 10 minutes should seek immediate medical care. If a heart attack is suspected, an aspirin should be chewed immediately, and aspirin therapy should continue after the attack. Many individuals with heart disease die in the emergency room or before they reach the hospital. The survival rate of a heart attack is increased significantly if hospitalization occurs within an hour of pain onset.

If victims seek care immediately, drugs can be administered to dissolve the clot, thus saving some heart muscle. A new generation of drugs has been developed to break down blood clots after a heart attack or stroke. Tissue-plasminogen activator (TPA) and streptokinase are therapies given intravenously, generally in the emergency room, if a heart attack or stroke is suspected. If given within three hours of the event, these drugs can reduce the extent of disability. Persons who have had a heart attack must stay in the hospital to be monitored for abnormal heart rhythms, a complication that can occur hours or days after a heart attack and can be deadly. About a day or two after a heart attack, one or more diagnostic procedures are performed to find where the coronary artery is blocked (see Box 4.2).

A common treatment for blocked coronary arteries is angioplasty, usually accomplished during

---

Box 4.2

Diagnostic Tools for Heart Disease

There is no single test to diagnose heart disease. Many people do not know they have it until they have a heart attack. Physicians would like to identify those with heart disease earlier so patients can benefit from medications, lifestyle changes, and procedures that can prevent life-threatening cardiac problems. A medical history, a family history, and a physical examination are first and foremost in determining whether the patient has cardiac problems. In addition, the physician may use one or more diagnostic tools to determine the extent and severity of the disease as well as to rule out other causes. Which tools are used depends on the individual's symptoms, risk factors, history of heart problems, and the physician's assessment. Generally, simple tests are done first.

The following tests are commonly performed if an individual is at high risk for heart disease or already has heart disease:

- *Blood tests*: Most common blood measurements are blood sugar and cholesterol. If the individual is taking blood thinners, regular blood tests are needed to determine the correct amount of medication needed. Also, after a heart attack, there is a blood test that measures the level of certain muscle breakdown products. Other common blood tests might include thyroid level and other hormones, levels of electrolytes, tests of kidney function, and the level of some proteins that increase with heart failure.

- *Chest X-ray*: An X-ray is commonly used to measure the size and shape of the heart and the large arteries. It can be used to diagnose congestive heart failure.

- *Electrocardiogram* (ECG, also called EKG): Sticky electrodes are placed on the body to measure the way that electric currents move through the heart. The machine prints out a series of tracings that enables a trained individual to detect abnormal rhythms or abnormal electrical conduction of the heart. A normal ECG does not mean there is no heart disease, but it does mean that the heart is conducting electricity correctly. An abnormal ECG may indicate a heart attack, irregular heart beat, an enlarged heart, or a heart that is working too hard.

- *Stress test:* This test shows how well the heart pumps during vigorous exercise when the heart needs more oxygen. ECG and blood pressure readings are taken before, during, and after exercise to see how the heart responds to exercise. If a patient cannot exercise, chemicals that raise the heart rate and thereby simulate exercise and stress can be injected. The test continues until the heart rate set by the doctor is

---

B O X   4 . 2   *Continued*

Diagnostic Tools for Heart Disease

reached. The exercise part is stopped if chest pain or a very sharp rise in blood pressure occurs. Monitoring continues for 10 to 15 minutes after exercise or until the heart rate returns to baseline. A stress test measures the function of the heart under stress, such as during exercise or when medications that increase heartbeat and workload are given. This test can show if the heart is straining to function and can give hints as to where the blood supply may be partially blocked.

- *Holter monitor*: This portable, battery-operated recording monitor is worn to find out if the heart is beating regularly or has arrythmias from time to time. A Holter monitor uses some of the same electrodes that are used for an ECG on the chest. Heart activity is measured while the wearer keeps a detailed diary of activities pursued and their times. Irregular heart activity is then correlated with activity at the time.

- *Echocardiogram*: Ultrasound of the heart that uses sound waves to create a picture of the heart. The tool can assess how well the heart pumps blood and how well the heart valves are working.

- *Cardiac catheterization*: A thin flexible tube (a catheter) is passed through an artery at the inside top of the leg (groin) or in the arm and is guided, with the help of a special X-ray machine, into the coronary arteries. This procedure allows the physician to examine inside the coronary arteries, to measure the pressure and blood flow in the heart's chambers, and to collect blood samples from the heart.

- *Coronary angiography or arteriography:* This test is usually performed with cardiac catheterization. While the catheter is in the coronary arteries, a special dye is injected, and the blood flow in the coronary arteries can be visualized with multiple X-ray pictures. These X-rays show the location and degree of narrowed coronary arteries.

- *Magnetic resonance imaging (MRI)*: A specialized machine uses magnetic forces to take computer-generated pictures of body organs. An MRI can show the heart muscle, identify damage from a heart attack, and evaluate disease of larger blood vessels and other heart problems. The procedure is also called nuclear magnetic resonance imaging (NMR).

---

cardiac catheterization. *Angioplasty* is a procedure that widens the portion of the coronary artery that has dangerously narrowed. There are several types. *Balloon angioplasty,* also called percutaneous transluminal coronary angioplasty (PTCA), involves passing a deflated balloon into the artery, then inflating the balloon to widen the artery where it was earlier found to be narrowed. Another type of angioplasty, *laser angioplasty,* uses a laser-tipped catheter to vaporize the plaque in the artery. Still another type, *atherectomy,* uses a catheter with a rotating shaver on its tip to shave off the plaque and debris within the vessel (like a Roto-Rooter). During these angioplasties, a wire mesh stent (a tube) may be permanently implanted inside the artery to hold it open.

In contrast to angioplasty and stents, *coronary artery bypass surgery* is a lengthy procedure that removes veins from the chest or leg and grafts them onto coronary arteries around the areas of narrowing. When you hear of someone having a triple bypass or quadruple bypass operation, you know that individual had three or four severely narrowed coronary arteries that were grafted.

Individuals who are recovering from a heart attack generally undergo a program of cardiac rehabilitation that combines exercise, diet, medication, and health education. Cardiac rehabilitation may be continued for months or even years. In cardiac rehabilitation programs, those who have suffered a heart attack are encouraged to begin an exercise program, usually walking.

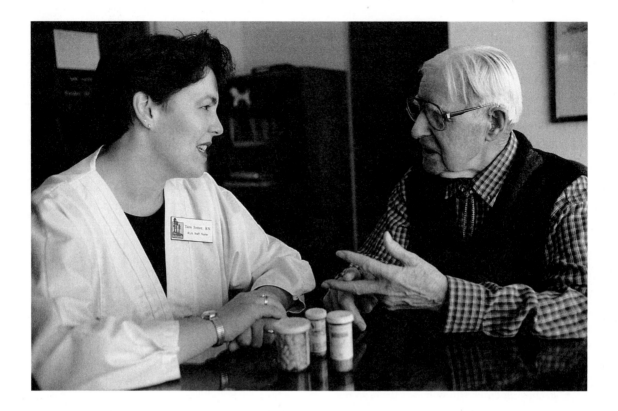

Several drugs are used to reduce the recurrence of a heart attack and the risk of death after a heart attack. One baby aspirin daily reduces the recurrence of heart attack and the risk of death after a heart attack, even in the very old. Beta blockers (drugs that slow the heartbeat and increase pumping efficiency) are extremely effective at reducing death and rehospitalization rates after myocardial infarction but are underprescribed for older persons. Other drugs may be recommended based on other cardiovascular risk factors, such as elevated cholesterol, cardiac arrhythmias, hypertension, diabetes, or congestive heart failure.

Congestive Heart Failure

Congestive heart failure, also called *heart failure,* is a progressive weakening of the heart muscle that reduces its ability to pump blood effectively. Heart failure affected 5.8 million people in the United States during 2006, reducing their quality of life

and limiting their activity. Congestive heart failure can range from a mild condition to a severely disabling condition of fatigue and breathlessness that requires multiple medications and oxygen. The prognosis of heart failure depends on many factors—the severity, the type, and the treatments implemented. Studies suggest that approximately half of those who are diagnosed with it die within five years.

Most causes of heart failure are related to atherosclerosis, although hypertension, diabetes, lung diseases, or other heart diseases may contribute. When the coronary arteries are narrowed from atherosclerosis, the heart has to work harder to pump blood through narrowed vessels, creating a strain on the heart. The heart muscle enlarges with the increased workload, much like any other muscle that is stressed, but the heart tissue can compensate only so much. After prolonged strain, the heart muscle begins to fail as a pump. The heart may have *poor output,* a reduced blood supply to vital organs, such as the brain and kidneys. The consequences of poor output are decreased urine production, fatigue, and confusion. Or the blood in the heart *backs up,* leading to excess fluid in the lungs, veins, and ankles. The most common symptoms of congestive heart failure related to poor output are decreased urine production, fatigue, and confusion. Symptoms related to "backup" include shortness of breath and swollen ankles or fluid-distended abdomen.

Congestive heart failure must be carefully managed since it can be life threatening. Physicians may prescribe medications that increase the pumping ability of the heart, reduce the excessive fluid, and expand blood vessels to decrease pressure so blood can flow more easily. Usually, multiple medications are prescribed. Each of the following medications has significant side effects and must be closely monitored. Note that most of these medications are also used for hypertension (see Table 4.3).

- *Digitalis* increases the strength of the heartbeat and normalizes heart rate.
- *Diuretics* eliminate excess water and salt in the blood, reducing the overload on the heart. Diuretics also reduce the fluid in the ankles, lungs, and other areas where water accumulates.
- *ACE inhibitors* prevent certain hormones from constricting blood vessels.
- *Beta blockers* slow the heart rate and increase pumping efficiency.

In addition to taking medications as prescribed, people with congestive heart failure should significantly reduce their daily salt, fluid, and alcohol intake. An exercise program can also help. A signal that the disease is worsening is shortness of breath or sudden weight gain indicating fluid retention. Because episodes of symptoms may be interspersed with periods without symptoms, elders may have difficulty complying with medical recommendations.

The case study in Box 4.3 shows the complex effects of heart disease on daily life and describes how one woman copes with reduced function.

Cardiac Arrhythmia

Cardiac arrhythmia is the medical term used for an irregular heartbeat. Arrhythmias occur when the electrical impulses in the heart that direct the heartbeat do not function properly, making the heart beat too fast, too slow, or in an irregular fashion. Arrhythmias can be acute and life-threatening emergencies or become chronic (for example, atrial fibrillation). Arrhythmias are the result of damage to the portion of the heart muscle that regulates heartbeat. Arrhythmias may occur after years of other cardiac problems, such as congestive heart failure, or they may occur after a heart attack. Discussion of the multiple types of arrhythmias is beyond the scope of this text; however, two of the most common are addressed: atrial fibrillation and ventricular fibrillation.

Atrial fibrillation is a disorganized beat of the upper heart chambers (the atria) that prevents them from delivering blood efficiently to the ventricles. The elder may complain of palpitations, and the pulse is very irregular. Atrial fibrillation is particularly dangerous if it is associated with a rapid heartbeat. If the beat of the heart has a tendency to change in and out of atrial fibrillation, the individual is at high risk of having a stroke, because during fibrillation, blood pools in the atrial chambers of the heart and may clot. With the next beat, a clot could dislodge and travel to the brain. When this condition is detected early, sometimes medications or an electric shock to the heart (defibrillation) can return the heart to normal.

If the heartbeat cannot be normalized, then medications can be prescribed to maintain the heart rate in the normal range by slowing the heart rate and thinning the blood to prevent blood clots. An implanted *pacemaker* may also be effective in regulating slow heartbeats. The small battery-operated device is placed under the skin of the chest wall, and its wire is permanently extended to the right side of the heart. If the heart rate is too slow or there is no heartbeat, electrical impulses are sent to the heart to stimulate it to speed up or start it beating again. In some cases, a defibrillator is implanted. Many people can live for years with atrial fibrillation.

BOX 4.3

Chronic Illness: Joan Gehrman's Story

Joan Gehrman is a little woman, 4'9" tall and about 80 pounds. Her small size belies her strong will, independence, and spunkiness. Joan graduated from Smith College and was a teacher and an active community volunteer for most of her working life. She is divorced and has lived alone for more than thirty years.

She now lives in a senior apartment that is small enough so she can get around, but filled with enough furniture, photos, and memorabilia to make it "home." Her caretaker sits in the living room, reading the paper while Joan rests in her bed. The caregiver is paid minimum wage by the state to provide care that allows Joan to stay at home. Joan is lucky; the caregiver is gentle, knowledgeable, and a good cook (after Joan taught her to make all her specialties).

Joan tells me of her life with chronic illnesses. She characterizes the last twenty to thirty years as the "tarnished years" rather than the "golden years." She first developed arthritis in her forties, and it still pains her greatly. "It's one pain all over, but I have been able to control it. Just thinking about it [the pain] can kill you sometimes."

She has undergone two total hip replacements and two knee replacements. Recently she suffered a spiral fracture of her left femur (thigh bone), requiring an operation to enable her to walk. After the fracture, she went to a rehabilitation hospital, but left after a week because she thought it was too much like a nursing home and she didn't like the way they were managing her constipation. She gradually increased in strength at home so that she was able to walk a block or two, but then began to weaken again, as the fracture is not healing properly.

In describing her multiple medical problems, she states: "I feel quite surprised and angry. I can't do things that I used to do and see my ability decreasing; I can't live this way." However, as often as she describes the negatives of living with chronic illness, she refuses to give up hope. "I am not going to let my body run me. If my mind can stay in control, then I won't give up. I did not give up before. I had the power to fight it. The power within me allowed me to

continue. Surgeons have been able to patch me, to keep me going."

In addition to long-standing arthritis, Joan has heart disease. While in her sixties, she underwent three coronary artery bypass operations in a single year. "The first two didn't work, so I went for a third," she says, and bears the scar down her chest and the long, serpentine scars down her legs to prove it. After the surgery, she made big changes in her diet—low fat, low cholesterol, and low salt—and has stayed slim for the past twenty years. Nevertheless, her heart disease has progressed to congestive heart failure.

Joan takes quite a few medications. She takes medications to reduce the pain of arthritis. She has a long history of constipation and takes laxatives on a daily basis to "stay regular." She takes a blood thinner because she had blood clots in her legs in the past that went up into her lung and damaged it. She takes nitrates and ACE inhibitors for her heart failure, and has recently begun to require oxygen at home.

Her chest pain has been getting worse, although she does not call it pain, merely pressure. When she gets chest pressure, she takes nitroglycerine under her tongue and some Ativan (a benzodiazepine) and falls asleep, and when she awakens the chest pain is gone. She has recently had episodes of blacking out and falling down when she has chest pain. Her doctors tell her this is because her heart is failing and not enough blood is going to the brain, or perhaps she is experiencing little strokes. In any case, she is too weak to undergo further surgery and doesn't want any more tests, so she lives with it. She looks on the bright side, "It could be worse."

The falls are worrisome. When her physician suggested that she stay in bed or in a chair unless her caregiver is there, she agreed, but invariably she gets up to do things for herself. She now needs help bathing and cooking and sometimes getting dressed.

She has three children, but only keeps in close contact with one, a nurse practitioner who works full-time. She pages him during the day to ask him questions about her condition or medications, and he visits her daily to make sure she is OK. He does the shopping, takes her to the doctor, manages her

B o x 4 . 3 *Continued*

Chronic Illness: Joan Gehrman's Story

caregiver, and helps with her finances. She knows as she becomes weaker that it may be necessary for him to stay at her house overnight, but for now she desires her privacy. He has promised never to put her in a nursing home.

As she has weakened, she is beginning to talk more about the end of her life. "I have been active all my life, and it is time for a rest now. I am listening to my mind, it will tell me when it is time to call this 'all over.' In my mind, when I became eighty, I knew I would not have much time left, and I will be ready to go. I am eighty years old, I don't expect it to keep beating forever. I have had a long, interesting life. The party has to come to an end sometime."

Excerpted from an interview conducted by Joan Gehrman's son, Roger Strong, a nurse practitioner.

In contrast, ventricular fibrillation is a life-threatening emergency. Ventricular fibrillation is a quivering in the bottom chambers of the heart (ventricles), making them unable to pump blood. Ventricular fibrillation is a significant cause of death in the day or two following a heart attack. This is a medical emergency, and the rhythm must immediately be converted to normal with electric shock (defibrillation) or drugs; otherwise, the person will die. If a person is at high risk of developing this condition, the physician may prescribe antiarrhythmic medications on a long-term basis or implant a defibrillator or pacemaker.

A *defibrillator* is a device that stops the heart if its beat is irregular, allowing the heart to restart in a normal rhythm. Although the shock emitted from the device can be painful, even causing the individual to lose consciousness, it saves lives. Because of the unpredictability and deadliness of arrythmias, and the effectiveness of electric shock to the heart, many public places now have AEDs (automated electronic defibrillators) on the walls for use by trained staff on unconscious individuals with fibrillation. The machines have voice commands to assist a passerby who recognizes that an unconscious individual is having fibrillation. For individuals at high risk, a defibrillator may be implanted in a fashion similar to a pacemaker. It senses the abnormal rhythm and delivers a large shock to the heart to correct the rhythm. If an individual does not have an implantable defibrillator, family members are often given an easy-to-use computerized defibrillator so they can administer electric shocks at home.

Cancer

Few words evoke such fear and anxiety as "cancer." Cancer is the second leading cause of death in the United States: One out of four of us will die from it. *Cancer* is a general term that includes many different types of tumors that can affect nearly every body system. Cancers vary widely in their presentation, their symptoms, their treatments, and their ability to kill. Some types are extremely rare, such as cancer of the heart, the small intestine, or muscles; others are much more common (lung cancer, breast cancer). Some types of cancer are almost universally and rapidly fatal (such as pancreatic cancer and some lung cancers). Others tend to grow more slowly (such as prostate cancer and bladder cancer).

A cancer begins with a group of body cells that, for an unknown reason, multiples and grows out of control. This abnormal growth is called a *tumor* or a *mass,* and eventually it can be felt or even seen. The cancer cells use more than their share of nutrients and cause the body to produce new blood vessels to supply their voracious growth. Pieces of the tumor may break off and spread (metastasize) through the blood or lymph to other parts of the body, creating new tumor sites. Not every tumor or mass is cancerous, but masses are a common symptom of cancer. The classic seven warning signals of cancer are:

- Change in bowel or bladder habits
- A sore that does not heal
- Unusual bleeding or discharge
- Thickening or lump in the breast or elsewhere
- Indigestion or difficulty in swallowing
- Obvious change in a wart or mole
- Nagging cough or hoarseness

In addition, general problems such as rapid weight loss without dieting, lack of appetite, and fatigue or weakness should be evaluated promptly, for they may be caused by cancer.

Extensive research is being conducted to determine the causes, prevention, and treatment of various cancers, but there is much to be learned. Genetic factors, hormones, environmental toxins, cigarette smoking, radiation, and stress have all been implicated for some cancers. While many cancers can be very effectively treated if found early and still localized, most advanced cancers that have spread throughout the body cannot be cured. However, for some cancers, treatments may extend life, making "living with cancer" more common than "dying from cancer."

The risk of developing cancer increases significantly with age: More than half its victims are over age 65. The most common cancer deaths among elders are lung, colon and rectum, prostate, and breast cancers. A number of factors may explain the increased cancer risk among older people. The aging process may reduce the ability of the immune system to reject abnormal growths. Some researchers hypothesize that elders lack sufficient DNA for the increased repair demands of an aging body, thereby allowing defective cells to grow unchecked. Another theory is that the elderly have had more time to be exposed to carcinogens such as cigarette smoke and environmental toxins.

Because cancer often has no specific symptoms, it may be difficult to diagnose in elders. In younger patients, cancer is usually the only disease condition present. However, in elders, cancer symptoms are often overshadowed by symptoms of other diseases. Furthermore, physicians may mistakenly attribute warning signals to diseases already present. For instance, the rectal bleeding characteristic of colon cancer may be attributed to long-standing hemorrhoids. Fatigue and weight loss may be attributed to "growing old."

Cancer is often found by an individual who notices a mass, has rectal bleeding, or simply "feels different." Some cancers can be found more easily than others in their early stages. Cancers may be detected by a variety of screening tests, depending on the site. It is not reasonable to scan the entire body to assure oneself that no tiny cancers are growing. On the other hand, many simple screening tests are useful, especially among high-risk groups. These include rectal exams, colonoscopy, blood tests, mammography, chest X-rays, and Pap smears. The different types of cancer screening are discussed in Chapter 12.

Generally, cancer is treated with surgery, chemotherapy, or radiation. Cancer treatments pose more risks and have more side effects than almost any other type of medical treatment. Radiation and chemotherapy both inadvertently damage many normal cells in the process of killing the cancer cells, and treatment is very stressful for the body at any age. In addition, elders are generally less able to tolerate anesthesia or long surgical treatments and suffer more complications from surgery such as wound infections, postoperative heart attacks or strokes, and hospital-acquired infections such as pneumonia or urinary tract infections. Medications to reduce pain, alter mood, and induce sleep may also be used to help the individual with cancer to be more comfortable.

A patient's age, rate of cancer growth, type and extent of treatment, state of health, and the quality and the remaining length of life are important considerations when developing a treatment plan. Studies suggest that older people are more likely to develop cancer but are less likely to be treated than younger people. It is unclear how much of this differential is due to patient preferences and how much is due to physicians not offering treatment to the elderly. If treatment increases survival only slightly, if the procedure has a high complication rate, or if cancer growth is slow, it may be better to limit treatment to symptom relief. However, even those who are very old can benefit from cancer treatments if they increase the quality of life in their remaining years.

The single most effective way to prevent cancer is to quit smoking cigarettes. Cigarette smoking is strongly implicated in cancer of almost all body systems. Although many other health behaviors have been implicated in cancer prevention, including diet, exposure to sunlight, environmental toxins, exercise, and medication use, cigarette smoking is by far the greatest cause.

In 2011, it is estimated that more than 1.5 million people in the United States were newly diagnosed with cancer and almost 600 million (1,500 people a day) died from it. One of four deaths in our country is due to cancer.[8] Lung cancer is the leading cause of cancer death in both men and women. The second leading killer in women is breast cancer, and in men, prostate cancer. Colorectal cancer is third in both genders.[8] In the following paragraphs we look at those cancers. Skin cancer, the most common cancer, is generally not deadly and is discussed in the next chapter.

Excellent information regarding cancer can be found at the Web sites of the American Cancer Society (www.cancer.org) and the National Cancer Institute (www.cancer.gov).

Lung Cancer

As mentioned earlier, lung cancer is the leading cause of cancer deaths for both men and women in the United States. The death rate for lung cancer is currently higher among men than among women. The rates are declining in both sexes because of the decreased smoking rate over the last 30 years. The lung cancer rate increases with age: The average age of those diagnosed with lung cancer is 60.

Ninety percent of all lung cancer is attributed to cigarette smoking (see Box 4.4). The more one smokes, the greater the risk of contracting the disease. People who smoke two or more packs a day have death rates 15 to 25 times greater than those of nonsmokers. While it is true that not all smokers develop lung cancer, lung cancer is very seldom found among those who do not smoke. Other environmental contaminants correlated with lung cancer are asbestos, radon, X-ray exposure, secondhand smoke, and air pollution. A genetic factor, Alpha 1 antitrypsin deficiency, is responsible for a small proportion of lung cancer cases.

Warning symptoms for lung cancer include chronic cough, blood in the sputum, and shortness of breath. Some of these symptoms are similar to those of chronic obstructive pulmonary disease (COPD); however, their onset is more rapid. Lung cancer may be localized to the lung or may metastasize to the lymph nodes, bones, and brain. When it has spread, lung cancer can also cause systemic symptoms such as weight loss, bone pain, or hormonal problems. Lung cancers are generally deadly: Only about 15 percent of those who are diagnosed with lung cancer have survived after 5 years.[8]

There are two types of lung cancer, defined by cell type. *Non–small cell* lung cancer is the most common type and can sometimes be successfully treated with surgery, radiation, or chemotherapy. *Small cell* lung cancer is even more strongly associated with smoking. It grows fast and is more deadly. If cancer is advanced, chemotherapy may be offered, but it may extend life only for months.

Encouraging the public to not start to smoke and to quit smoking is the best way to stem the tide of lung cancer deaths. Although chest X-rays may detect the disease, lung cancer is often advanced by the time it is diagnosed.

Breast Cancer

Breast cancer is the second leading cause of cancer death among women in the United States. It occurs infrequently in men. The incidence of breast cancer among women increases with age: Almost three-fourths of breast cancer cases occur in women over age 50.

The causes of breast cancer are unknown, although studies give us information on risk factors. Breast cancer is associated with a high-fat diet, obesity, alcohol intake, and inactivity. Some breast cancer runs in families and is associated with

BOX 4.4

Cigarette Smoking: A Deadly Addiction

Cigarette smoking is the single most important cause of preventable illness and death in the United States. The most common smoking-related deaths are due to lung cancer, heart disease, and respiratory diseases.[8] Cigarette smoking decreases life expectancy by five to eight years. By age 75, two-thirds of those who smoke are dead compared to only one-third of nonsmokers. Despite the documented dangers of smoking cigarettes, about one in five adults smoke cigarettes in the United States. People who are 65 years and older are less likely to be cigarette smokers: only about one in 10 smoke.[9] Cigarette smoking is more common among men than women.[9] Smoking is less common among Asians and Hispanics than whites, blacks, and Native Americans. Those from South and Midwest U.S. are more likely to be smokers than adults from the West. Smoking is more common among the poor. Education impacts smoking—the more education a person has, the less likely he or she is to smoke. Among adults with only less than a high school education, more than one-third smoke, but less than 6 percent of those with a graduate degree do.[9]

There is overwhelming evidence that cigarette smoking is harmful to every body system. Most important, it is a known cause of cancer, heart disease, stroke, and chronic obstructive pulmonary disease. Smoking doubles or triples the risk of stroke and heart disease. Smoking increases the risk of many cancers: lung, cervix, head and neck, esophagus, stomach, bladder, pancreas, and kidney. It is now known that cigarette smoking is associated with reduced bone density, skin wrinkling, increased cataract risk, and gum disease. Elders are at greater risk for smoking-related disease than younger age groups: They have smoked longer, they tend to be heavier smokers, and they are more likely to be suffering from cigarette-related illnesses.

The most well-known effect of cigarette smoking is that it causes lung cancer. Its negative impact on

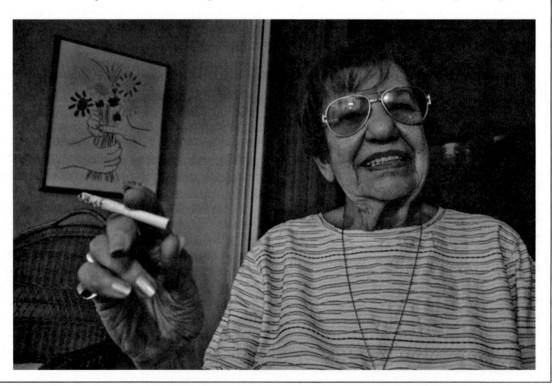

Cigarette Smoking: A Deadly Addiction

lung tissue also causes emphysema, chronic bronchitis, and other respiratory problems. Even in very young smokers, lung tests detect evidence of disease and reduced function. The lungs have a tremendous reserve capacity, so symptoms are not noticed until widespread irreversible damage has been done. Those who smoke have more frequent and severe respiratory infections, chronic cough, and phlegm production. Individuals who are around people who smoke are at increased risk of lung cancer, respiratory disease, and cardiovascular problems.

It is important to note that cigarette smoking is addictive and is classified as a substance use disorder. It is estimated that seven out of ten smokers would like to quit, and many try several times before succeeding, because nicotine is an addictive drug. Two prescription drugs may be used to help individuals stop smoking: Chantix, a smoking cessation aid, blocks the pleasant effects of nicotine on the brain and Zyban, an antidepressant, reduces craving and other withdrawal effects. Also, smoking cessation might include medication that provides nicotine without smoking, skills training (coping with the desire for a cigarette), supportive counseling, and long-term relapse prevention counseling. The more intense and varied the counseling and support, the higher is the success rate.

Experts agree that quitting smoking pays. Within a year after quitting, a person's risk of heart disease is cut in half, and the risk of lung cancer, stroke, and respiratory conditions declines. Even older smokers who quit reduce their risk of death or heart attack. For detailed information, refer to the Surgeon General Reports: *The Health Consequences of Smoking* (2004)*, The Health Consequences of Involuntary Exposure to Tobacco Smoke* (2006), and *How Tobacco Smoke Causes Disease: The Biology and Behavioral Basis for Smoking-Attributable Disease* (2010) at www.surgeongeneral.gov

specific genetic mutations. Women with a family history of breast cancer are at increased risk of developing breast cancer early in life, but the importance of this risk factor diminishes with age. Environmental toxins, particularly pesticides, may also affect risk. Another risk factor may be the length of time estrogen circulates in the body. For instance, women who menstruate early, have a late menopause, or have no children have had more estrogen cycles than those who do not. Although those with the risk factors mentioned above are at increased risk of developing cancer, every woman is considered at risk because many women get breast cancer yet have none of those risk factors.

Currently there is no way to prevent breast cancer: The best way to decrease morbidity and mortality from the disease is to detect it at an early, treatable stage. Clinical breast exams (by physicians) and self-breast exams are widely used, although there is no evidence that they reduce death rates. Mammography is the single most effective means to detect breast cancer early. Mammography uses extremely low doses of radiation to detect abnormalities in breast tissue that are too small to be noticed with self-examination. If a mammogram or breast exam is abnormal, the lump in the breast is biopsied. Although there is not much research documenting the benefits of screening among older women, most organizations advocate that women over 40 get a mammogram every year. Screening for breast cancer is discussed more fully in Chapter 12.

Treatment for breast cancer differs, depending on the type of cancer, whether it has spread into the lymph nodes, and whether it is a cancer recurrence. Unfortunately, many women do not see a physician until the cancer has already spread. Even after treatment, many of these women have a recurrence of cancer in the breast, or the disease metastasizes to other parts of the body. Almost everyone survives five years, but if

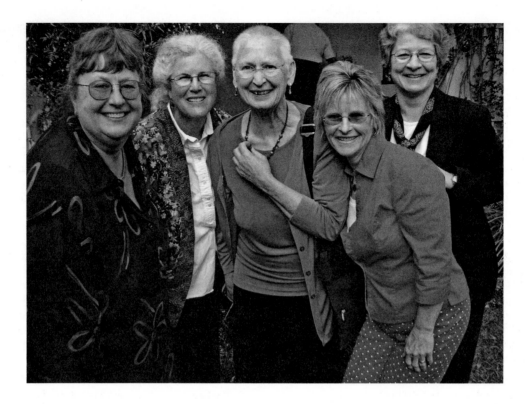

the cancer has spread to the bones or brain, then only about one in four people lives five years past diagnosis.

Treatment may include radiation, surgery, chemotherapy, and hormones. For tumors localized to the breast, surgery or radiation is the first-line treatment. Surgeons may remove only the lump (lumpectomy), the breast (simple mastectomy), or the entire breast, lymph nodes in the armpits, and adjacent muscle tissue (radical mastectomy). When disease is localized, radiation and lumpectomy are as effective as radical mastectomy, but the choice is usually left to the patient. Often radiation or chemotherapy is used before surgery to shrink the tumor. Radical mastectomies can result in long-term consequences of swelling of the arm, which can be ugly and uncomfortable. After surgery, many women elect to have breast reconstruction or wear a prosthesis (artificial breast).

Recurrences are generally treated with a combination of surgery, chemotherapy, and hormonal therapy. Hormonal therapy involves medications, primarily tamoxifen, to reduce estrogens. Older women are less likely than younger women to be treated aggressively for breast cancer. Further, since few research trials include elderly women, there is little evidence on which breast cancer treatment works best for that group.

Research on prevention of breast cancer is progressing. Physical activity, a low-fat diet, weight reduction, and reduced alcohol use may protect against breast cancer. Tamoxifen, a drug that blocks estrogen, used to be used only to treat breast cancer, but now it also is used to reduce the chance of developing breast cancer among those at high risk. Another drug, raloxifene, is similarly used. Since the risk of developing uterine cancer and blood clots in the lungs and major veins is increased when the drug is used, women need to balance the benefits and risk when making decisions about using the drug.

Prostate Cancer

Prostate cancer is the most frequently diagnosed cancer in the United States and is responsible for about 11 percent of all cancer deaths among American men.[10] Only lung cancer has a higher death rate. Each year close to a quarter million new cases are diagnosed and close to 34,000 men die of prostate cancer. Almost all diagnosed prostate cancer cases (97 percent) occur in men aged 50 and older.[8] The incidence of prostate cancer is likely increasing because more men are undergoing screening tests and consequently being diagnosed with the disease. Death rates for prostate cancer are higher in African American men.

Prostate cancer is one of the more complicated cancers. On the one hand, it is a leading cause of cancer death in American men. On the other, it is not uncommon in older men and in many cases is not deadly. Unlike many other cancers, prostate cancer can be relatively slow growing, and some cancers may be insignificant. Prostate cancer may have a varying course. It may affect a man for one to two decades, remain quiescent for years, then recur and spread.

If men are diagnosed with localized prostate cancer through a PSA test and decline to have surgery, radiation, or hormone therapy, they still have a survival rate of 94 percent after eight years.[10] In fact, many men die *with* prostate cancer rather than *from* it. Prostate cancer is easily curable when it is localized to the prostate, and the vast majority of prostate cancers are found in the early stages.

The search for the cause of prostate cancer remains elusive. It is clear that its incidence increases with advancing age, and the majority of men over age 90 have prostate cancer. Black men or men who have a family history of prostate cancer are at higher risk. Some studies suggest that dietary factors may be protective (e.g., tomatoes, low fat, vitamin E, selenium).

The principal screening tests for detection of prostate cancer are the digital rectal examination (DRE) and measurement of the serum tumor marker prostate specific antigen (PSA). All major professional organizations recommend that physicians discuss prostate cancer screening and offer screening with a rectal exam or a PSA test annually to all men with a life expectancy of at least 10 more years, starting at age 50 (earlier for men with risk factors). They also recommend that the physician discuss the pros and cons of these tests with their male patients so that they can decide for themselves whether or not they want to be screened.

Many men with localized prostate cancer are offered a choice between "watchful waiting"—monitoring their disease—and a *radical prostatectomy,* surgery to remove the prostate gland. Many factors influence the decision of the doctor and patient about which is the better course of action: the biology of the tumor, the health of the patient, and the patient's values and preferences.

If surgery is chosen, cancer confined to the prostate can be treated by removal of the prostate, which usually eliminates the cancer. However, surgery may have serious side effects of impotence and incontinence. Men with a life expectancy of less than 10 years rarely benefit from a prostatectomy. If an elder is unable to tolerate surgery, radiation therapy is useful, but the side effects are significant: incontinence, diarrhea, or erectile dysfunction. Radiation may be directed at the entire pelvis, or radioactive seeds may be implanted in the prostate.

Cancer that has spread outside the prostate is more deadly and is managed by hormonal therapy or removal of the testes (castration, also known as orchiectomy). Both procedures stop the production of testosterone and reduce bone pain. Hormonal therapy is a pharmacological castration in which a wide variety of estrogen-like substances may be used to block testosterone production. These treatments cause side effects such as erectile dysfunction, osteoporosis, weight gain, and hot flashes. Much more research needs to be done on how to determine which treatments are effective and how men who may benefit from treatment may be differentiated from those who may not.

Colorectal Cancer

Colorectal cancer is a significant cause of death among both men and women, and it is strongly related to age: Almost 90 percent of the cases are diagnosed after 50.[8] Colorectal cancer is not always deadly if detected early. If it is found when localized, the survival rate is 90 percent; when it has spread to surrounding tissues, the survival rate is 70 percent; and when it has metastasized, the survival rate is only 12 percent.[8] The most common early symptom of colorectal cancer is rectal bleeding. However, constipation or diarrhea, the passage of stools of increasingly narrow diameter (pencil-thin), or systemic symptoms such as weight loss may also occur.

Many factors have been correlated with the development of colorectal cancer. The presence of outgrowths in the colon (polyps), many years of colon inflammation, or a family history of polyps or colorectal cancer increases risk. In addition, there is something about the American lifestyle that predisposes U.S. residents to develop more colon cancer than people from Japan, China, or less-developed countries. A diet high in animal fat and low in fruits, vegetables, and fiber has been implicated, as has alcohol and cigarette use. Some factors may reduce colorectal cancer risk: a high-fiber diet, adequate intake of important vitamins (especially B vitamins), calcium, and regular aspirin use.

Colorectal cancer may be detected through a digital rectal examination, testing of stool for occult (invisible) blood, or direct visualization of the colon through a sigmoidoscope or colonoscope. For the latter two examinations, a tube is passed at varying distances into the rectum, and a physician visually examines the inside of the colon for signs of cancer. Any polyps, where cancers are thought to originate, are removed. It is estimated that one-third of all people over age 50 have one or more polyps. Experts recommend annual testing of stool for occult blood and rectal exams for everyone over the age of 50, as well as undergoing a sigmoidoscopy or colonoscopy exam every ten years (see Chapter 12 for details).

Colorectal cancer, unless it has spread, is almost always treated with surgery. The cancerous bowel is removed, and the intestine is either reconnected or a colostomy is performed. A colostomy is a surgical procedure in which the end of the intestine is routed through the abdominal wall, creating an artificial opening in the abdomen called a *stoma*. Feces are collected in a disposable plastic bag, which is regularly emptied. Because cancer recurs in over 50 percent of the cases, radiation and chemotherapy are commonly used after surgery.

Stroke

Strokes are the third leading cause of death and a major cause of physical and mental disability among elders. Every year, close to 800,000 people in the United States have a stroke and about twenty percent of them die of it. A stroke can be thought of as a heart attack occurring within the brain. Their risk factors and the mechanism of damage are similar. The blood vessels within the brain either become blocked or burst, depriving brain cells of necessary oxygen and nutrients.

There are two types of strokes: ischemic and hemorrhagic. Almost 90 percent of strokes are *ischemic* strokes: Blood clots or clumps of cholesterol break away from inside a blood vessel in another part of the body and travel through the bloodstream to the brain, where they lodge in a small blood vessel, cutting off the blood supply to adjacent brain cells. In contrast, *hemorrhagic* strokes result from bleeding in the brain caused by a broken or leaking blood vessel. Hemorrhagic strokes occur primarily in persons with severe hypertension. No matter what the cause of the stroke, when the brain cells are deprived of the oxygen and glucose carried by the blood, they die. The degree of damage from the stroke depends on the area of the brain affected, the extent of brain tissue damaged, and the level of prior functioning.

A number of factors predispose individuals to strokes. Age is an important variable. About two-thirds of those who experience a stroke are over 65, and the risk of dying increases with advanced age. Blacks are more likely than whites to have a stroke and die from it. The main risk factor for stroke is high blood pressure. Also, other negative health behaviors increase stroke risk: smoking, heavy drinking, high cholesterol, and inactivity. Several chronic diseases such as major depression, diabetes, heart disease, obesity, atherosclerosis, and atrial fibrillation also increase the likelihood of having a stroke. Like heart attacks, strokes can be prevented by modifying behavioral risk factors: maintaining a healthy blood pressure, controlling weight, keeping cholesterol level low, avoiding smoking, controlling diabetes, exercising and eating a low-fat diet. To determine your risk of stroke, an assessment is available at www.yourdiseaserisk.Harvard.edu

Perhaps the most important warning sign for a stroke is a "mini-stroke" or transient ischemic attack (TIA), which is caused by a temporary blockage of the arteries in the brain. These attacks are similar to angina attacks in the heart—blood is cut off briefly causing symptoms. A TIA may result in transient or permanent motor weakness, blackouts, speech disturbances, or personality changes. The attacks may last from a few minutes to 24 hours. People who experienced a TIA are much more likely to have a stroke than the general population.

Warning signs of an impending stroke are:

- Sudden confusion, trouble speaking or understanding
- Sudden weakness or numbness of face, arm, or leg, especially on one side of the body
- Sudden trouble seeing in one or both eyes
- Sudden trouble walking, dizziness, or loss of balance or coordination
- Sudden severe headache with no known cause

Those signs of stroke should be considered an emergency even if the symptoms don't cause pain or go away quickly or seem subtle. Medical evaluation soon after a stroke is crucial and may make the difference between full recovery and permanent disability or death. Unfortunately, nearly half of all stroke deaths occur before the stroke victims get to the hospital, partly because of lack of knowledge about the six warning signs listed above.

Individuals who have had a stroke and quickly go to the hospital may be treated with strong blood thinners called tissue plasminogen activators (tPA). If the drugs are administered promptly after the stroke (up to three hours), they are effective in breaking down clots to reduce the impact of an ischemic stroke.[11] TPA is not used if the blood pressure is too high, if the doctors suspect there has been a hemorrhagic stroke, or if too much time has passed. Other drugs are being tested to be used with tPA drugs to minimize damage to brain cells caused by a cascade of harmful chemical reactions after a stroke.

After a stroke, the individual may be prescribed medications such as aspirin or other blood thinners to reduce the risk of future blood clots. Daily aspirin therapy is prescribed to individuals who are at high risk for stroke or who have had a stroke, to reduce the risk of a subsequent stroke.[12] Control of risk factors becomes even more important for those who have already had a stroke. If the cause of a stroke can be identified, then it can be corrected. For example, if a stroke is caused by a blood clot in the heart from an abnormal heart rhythm (e.g., atrial fibrillation), the cause can be treated. If the stroke is caused by a narrowing of the artery in the neck (carotid artery) that supplies blood to the brain, the narrowing can be treated with surgery (e.g., carotid endartectomy) to widen the artery. However, carotid endartectomy is associated with risks: An individual may have a stroke during the procedure if a piece of plaque breaks off and goes to the brain.

The disabilities people suffer from strokes are highly variable and depend on the portion of the brain affected. Weakness or paralysis of the face, arm, or leg, or even the entire left or right side of the body, is common. Many older people manifest alterations in thought patterns or speech (aphasia). They may lose their ability to comprehend speech, or to speak fluently. They may be able to speak only in obscenities, lose the ability to draw or write, be unable to read, or lose a portion of their vision. Some elders suffer seizures or hallucinations. They may lose sensation in parts of their body, experience lack of coordination or balance, or lose their ability to determine the position of their limbs.

The degree of disability can change during the course of the stroke. While a stroke is progressing, different problems may emerge depending on what parts of the brain are affected. A stroke may start with a tingling in the hand, then the arm becomes numb. Speech starts out slurred, then is lost altogether. As the brain swells or bleeds, more abilities may be lost, even the ability to stay awake. During stroke recovery, part of the brain is damaged and often never recovers, but symptoms get better as the brain around it heals and as other parts of the brain can compensate.

Rehabilitative therapy begins in the acute care hospital after the patient's medical condition has been stabilized, often within 24 to 48 hours after the stroke. The first steps involve promoting independent movement because many patients are paralyzed or seriously weakened. Patients are prompted frequently to change positions while lying in bed and to engage in range-of-motion exercises to strengthen their stroke-impaired limbs. Rehabilitation nurses and therapists help patients perform progressively more complex and demanding tasks, such as bathing, dressing, and using a toilet, transferring from bed to chair, and walking (often with a cane, brace, or walker).

Stroke rehabilitation may continue for weeks, months, or years and can result in significant improvements in mobility, speech and swallowing, and ability to do things for oneself. It may occur in a nursing home, at home, or in a rehabilitation hospital. Its effectiveness depends on the type and extent of the stroke as well as the client's overall health status, motivation, personality, and financial resources. As soon as possible, occupational, physical, and speech therapists should implement a rehabilitation plan to retrain the brain and reduce the disability. However, it is important to realize that rehabilitation, for the most part, does not bring the person back to the state he or she was in prior to the stroke, and much of the physical damage (such as weakness or paralysis on one side of the body) is permanent.

Both cognitive loss and the emotional effects of a stroke are common (e.g., lack of motivation, depression, anxiety, or frustration) and can adversely affect recovery. For this reason, psychological counseling and support are appropriate for both the patient and the family. More information is found at the National Stroke Association (www.stroke.org), the American Stroke Association (www.strokeassociation.org), and the National Institute of Neurological Disorders and Stroke (www.ninds.nih.gov).

Chronic Lung Diseases

Older people are more susceptible to lung infections and chronic lung conditions. Experts attribute their increased susceptibility to many factors: decreased resistance to environmental contaminants, bacteria, and viruses; age-associated decline that reduces pulmonary function; and long-term exposure to substances that could cause lung irritation. However, the greatest single cause of environmental contamination and the largest contributor to chronic lung disease is cigarette smoking (see Box 4.4). Since one of five adults in our country smokes, chronic lung diseases will continue to be a significant cause of illness, disability, and death.

Chronic obstructive pulmonary disease (COPD) is an umbrella term for a number of lung conditions, including chronic bronchitis, emphysema, and asthma. In each condition

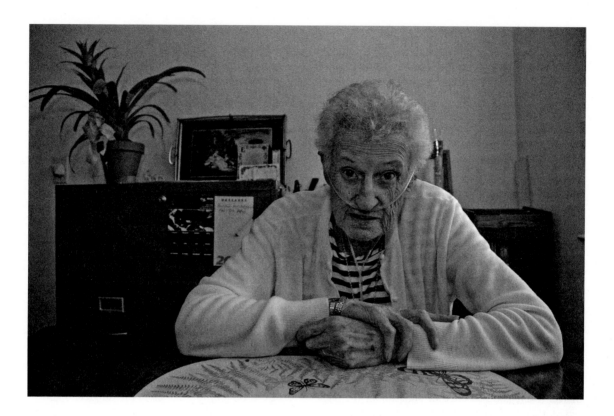

discussed below, an obstruction of air flow in the bronchi of the lungs worsens over time. Although individuals may exhibit no symptoms early in the disease, abnormalities can be detected on tests of lung function. With time (and often more cigarette use), the disease worsens, causing debilitating breathlessness, cough, and weakness. Some individuals eventually need to carry supplemental oxygen. Others must use *corticosteroids,* an anti-inflammatory agent to reduce the inflammation in the lung. Unfortunately, these medications increase the risk of diabetes and lower immune function. Those with COPD are at high risk of acquiring infections (pneumonia and influenza) and other chronic diseases (heart failure, stroke, and lung cancer). For this reason, they should receive the pneumonia vaccine and yearly influenza vaccinations.

The number of individuals who are sick or dying of COPD in the United States has been rapidly increasing in the last 30 years, primarily because of cigarette smoking. Although cigarette smoking is implicated in about 90 percent of all COPD cases, frequent lung infections, pollution exposure, and secondhand smoke also contribute. Men are more likely to suffer from COPD than women because a higher proportion of men smoke. The incidence of COPD also increases with age. The diseases and their associated disabilities develop gradually, sometimes taking 20 to 30 years to become serious or symptomatic. As a result, the disease is usually not diagnosed until it is advanced. In the early stages, symptoms are mild, if present: sputum production and cough. In the later stages, breathlessness is constant, with periods of acute breathlessness. Individuals with

COPD may have emphysema, chronic bronchitis, or both.

Chronic Bronchitis

Chronic bronchitis is a common condition, particularly among individuals who smoke. It is characterized by chronic cough and abundant sputum production for at least three months a year for two consecutive years. Chronic irritation by infections or environmental contaminants overwhelms the respiratory tract. Consequently the mucous cells produce excessive and thickened mucus, further decreasing the airway's ability to clear itself. A persistent cough and expectoration occur as the body attempts to rid the airways of excessive mucus secretions.

Emphysema

Emphysema, an irreversible deterioration of the air sacs (alveoli) in the lungs, reduces the ability to inhale oxygen into the lungs and exhale carbon dioxide. Air trapped behind mucous plugs in the narrowed airways causes prolonged inflation of the air sacs. The presence of stale air in the sacs reduces the amount of fresh air available for oxygen/carbon dioxide exchange. With time, the air sacs, which remain inflated by trapped air, eventually burst. Thus, the small separate air pockets merge to form larger sacs, consequently decreasing the surface area of the sacs available for oxygen/carbon dioxide exchange.

Early symptoms of emphysema include a chronic mild cough with phlegm, fatigue, and loss of appetite or weight loss. Later symptoms include shortness of breath, difficulty fully exhaling, and, still later, a widened chest (barrel chest). Typically, those with emphysema need to make a strong effort to exhale to rid their lungs of trapped air. They may have trouble breathing while lying down. They also have a difficult time exercising. Generally symptoms do not occur until a significant proportion of the lung tissue has been irreversibly damaged.

To diagnose the presence and severity of emphysema, the physician is likely to recommend certain tests. The pulmonary function test is effective and easy to perform. The individual breathes through a tube that measures the flow of air into the lungs and the volume of the lungs. Two other diagnostic tools may be used: a chest X-ray or a CT scan (computerized tomography). However, they are not as effective because even significantly impaired lungs may look perfectly normal. To determine the ability of the lungs to bring in oxygen and release carbon dioxide, a special blood test (called arterial blood gas or ABG) may be taken in the artery of the wrist to measure the amount of oxygen and carbon dioxide in the arterial blood. A simpler test, pulse oximetry, can measure the oxygen in the blood by means of a clip placed on the finger. Supplemental oxygen may be prescribed if the patient's blood oxygen content is low.

The goal of treatment is to improve lung function. Two types of drugs are the mainstay of COPD treatment: bronchodilators (widen the air passages) and corticosteroids (decrease inflammation in the lungs). The physician may also prescribe drugs to liquefy the mucus in the lungs and antibiotics when an infection is present. As a last resort, portable oxygen is prescribed.

Bronchodilators relax the muscles that surround the airways, widening them so that air can travel in and out more easily. These medications often must be inhaled multiple times a day, either with a metered dose inhaler (MDI), which is a small L-shaped device inhaled by mouth, or through a nebulizer, a machine that converts the liquid medications into a mist that is inhaled through a mask.

Corticosteroids expand the airways by reducing their inflammation and consequent swelling. This type of drug is particularly useful during acute stages of COPD but may also be used long term. Steroids can be inhaled in a MDI or taken in pill form. Although corticosteroids are very effective, many side effects limit their use: They suppress immune function, consequently decreasing healing time and increasing infection risk. They also cause thinning of the skin and bones, aggravate cataracts and diabetes, cause weight gain (particularly in the face and abdomen), increase fluid retention, and alter psychological and cognitive function. In some individuals, they can cause a sense of elation, in others, psychosis. When steroids are withdrawn, the dosage must be gradually tapered to prevent symptoms of withdrawal. To prevent steroid-associated osteoporosis, individuals should be prescribed supplemental doses of calcium and vitamin D while on long-term steroid therapy. For these reasons, the lowest dose should be used for the shortest possible time. Steroid inhalers have fewer side effects because the drug is absorbed where needed and less circulates through the body.

Individuals with advanced COPD may need oxygen therapy to lead a normal life. Liquid oxygen in a portable cylinder allows the individual to have oxygen available day and night. An oxygen concentrator that can be used at home makes higher strengths of oxygen by concentrating the oxygen already in the air.

Those who have COPD should eat well and keep as physically active as possible to maintain muscle strength. Elders with COPD can do breathing exercises or moderate physical exercises (such as walking) to reduce the symptoms. Inhalation exercises increase the volume of air inhaled. They should learn ways to clear lung secretions, including tapping on the chest to loosen secretions and lying on one side to help drain them. They often must learn energy-saving techniques for accomplishing daily activities (see Box 4.5). If patients are still smoking, they

---

B O X 4 . 5

Effects of Breathlessness on Lifestyle

A common symptom of emphysema and other COPDs is breathlessness. Some people are breathless only with exertion (e.g., walking a block), while others with advanced disease are breathless at rest or with the slightest activity. People who are breathless lack "reserves" or the ability to exert themselves and breathe faster to get more oxygen with exercise.

Coping with breathlessness and the consequent lack of energy reserves is the central concern of the day for some individuals. Imagine if every breath were a struggle—if all the time you felt as if you had just sprinted a race. What if pulling on your pants or putting a shirt over your head tired you so much you had to rest for 15 minutes afterward? What if taking the forty steps from the bedroom to the living room required five rest periods on the seat of your walker? For some people, even getting a full sentence out can be exhausting. Any exertion can feel like a marathon.

The following two cases enable the reader to better understand the impact of breathing problems on everyday life: One woman who becomes short of breath after a few steps requires two to three hours to get dressed. She arises from bed and goes to the bathroom, rests, washes sitting in a chair with frequent rest periods, walks back to the bedroom, rests, and dresses, always needing to rest every few minutes. Another man worked out an elaborate routing pattern to mop his kitchen every week. He gathers the cleaning paraphernalia and puts it near a chair in the middle of the room—these motions requiring frequent periods of "getting my breath back." He mops a few strokes and rests, sitting in the chair.

Coping with breathlessness and a lack of energy is a daily struggle for many people with COPD and heart failure. Their energy level often varies; they have good days and bad days when even the smallest chore is too difficult. They might need help to carry things or help to place necessary items (water, glasses, pills) within arm's reach. They may need to choose clothing that takes less energy to put on, or not schedule any activities on days they need to bathe or go to the doctor because of their exhaustion. They may have to forgo important activities (having a bowel movement, getting food from the kitchen) because the energy required is too great.

should be strongly encouraged to stop to reduce further lung damage.

Diabetes

Diabetes is a metabolic disorder characterized by difficulty in regulating the production or use of insulin. *Insulin,* a hormone produced by the pancreas, allows the body cells to take up sugar (glucose) from the bloodstream to be used for energy. According to CDC's most recent National Diabetes Fact Sheet, the number of Americans with diabetes continues to increase. So does the number of Americans with prediabetes, a condition that increases their risk of type 2 diabetes, heart disease, and stroke. From 1980 to 2009, the number of individuals in the United States with diabetes has more than tripled to 19.7 million. By the age of 65, 27 percent (more than one in four) of elders have diabetes and more than a quarter of these are undiagnosed. Black Americans, Hispanic Americans, and Native Americans have a greatly increased risk of diabetes.

There are two types of diabetes. Type 1, also called *juvenile-onset diabetes,* occurs in childhood or young adulthood. Only 10 percent of all diabetics are type 1. The pancreas stops producing insulin so these individuals have high blood sugar and no insulin to help the sugar enter the cells where it is needed. Type 1 diabetes is deadly, and those who have it die before old age. Individuals with type 1 diabetes require regular insulin injections to stay alive.

Type 2, or *adult-onset diabetes,* occurs when the pancreas produces sufficient insulin but the body cells become resistant to it. As a consequence, individuals with type 2 diabetes have high insulin levels and high blood sugar levels. Adult-onset diabetes develops gradually and first appears in middle age. Often the disease has no symptoms, and many people are unaware of its presence until they are admitted to a hospital or nursing home for some other condition, such as heart attack or stroke. Risk factors for adult-onset diabetes include obesity, particularly a propensity to store fat on the abdomen, and a family history of diabetes. Individuals can reduce their risk for adult-onset diabetes with weight management and physical activity. Clinical trials have shown that losing 5 to 7 percent of body weight—that's 10 to 14 pounds for a 200-pound person—and getting at least 150 minutes of moderate physical activity each week can reduce the risk of type 2 diabetes.

A blood test that measures the level of sugar in the bloodstream is commonly used to diagnose diabetes or prediabetes. A person who is diagnosed with diabetes will have this condition for life. Individuals may be able to control their blood sugar levels with diet and exercise, but they still have abnormal processing of sugar and insulin and remain at risk for all the complications associated with diabetes.

The first line of treatment for type 2 diabetes is health behavior change: reducing calories, controlling weight, and following the DASH (Dietary Approaches to Stop Hypertension) diet, which is rich in fruits, vegetables, and low-fat dairy products and has very little saturated and total fat. This diet decreases the need for insulin and helps lower blood cholesterol. Exercise is also important for weight loss and to improve the body cells' response to insulin. For about two-thirds of adult-onset diabetics, dietary changes, weight loss, and physical activity can control symptoms. Diabetics are taught to monitor their blood sugar by pricking a finger multiple times a day to determine if the treatments are effective in keeping their blood sugar normal. When blood sugar is kept in a near-normal range, there is a marked reduction in diabetic complications for individuals with either type of diabetes.

Oral medications are almost always prescribed. These medications are of various types: some increase insulin from the pancreas, others make body cells more sensitive to insulin, and still others alter the digestion and processing of sugar. However, the medications need to be monitored closely because the drugs might lower blood sugar too much (hypoglycemia) or cause weight gain.

All type 1 diabetics and about one-third of type 2 diabetics inject insulin. Insulin cannot be taken by mouth because it cannot survive the process of digestion. Those who take insulin must measure their blood sugar, keep detailed records of their measurements, and adjust the dose of their insulin in response to those measurements. Insulin can be long acting with once-a-day injections or short acting with injections right before a meal to allow the body to use the glucose from that meal only. Many people use a combination of insulins and inject them themselves. The insulin is drawn up into a syringe or into a pen device and is injected under the skin in various places. The process can be difficult for those with arthritis or vision problems or dementia. Another method of injection is an insulin pump, which delivers insulin automatically either by using an external pump that can be hooked onto a belt or one that is implanted under the skin. On the horizon is inhaled insulin, which will be a major breakthrough for diabetics.

Diabetes is associated with complications in almost every body system. Diabetics have an increased rate of atherosclerosis, strokes, heart disease, and kidney failure. In addition, diabetics often have high blood cholesterol levels and high blood pressure. Because of poor circulation and peripheral nerve damage, older diabetics are highly susceptible to infections and nonhealing sores, especially on the feet, and too often require amputation. In addition, diabetics suffer neuropathy (nerve damage) in their feet and legs, which can be extremely painful and affect the ability to walk. Diabetes is a leading cause of blindness, kidney failure, and erectile dysfunction. Those with diabetes suffer delayed healing, increased falls, decline in cognitive status, and higher rates of dementia. Diabetics face a higher risk of death from any illness they get and are more likely to be hospitalized or suffer a complication in the hospital. In addition to prescribing one or more drugs to treat the symptoms of diabetes, physicians may recommend other drugs to reduce the many complications listed above, particularly to maintain control of cholesterol and hypertension.

Although diabetes is listed as the sixth leading cause of death among individuals 65 and older in the United States, it plays an even larger role in causing death among older people. Diabetics have nearly twice the death rate of those without diabetes, primarily from heart disease, stroke, and kidney disease. Diabetes doubles men's risk of heart disease and increases women's risk fivefold. It is estimated that a diagnosis of diabetes at age 60 translates into seven to ten years of lost life. Further, the complications of the disease decrease the quality of years remaining.

In addition to the damage the disease does to the individual, diabetes imposes a tremendous financial burden on society as a whole. Diabetes is the most costly chronic disease. Because of the high incidence of complications, the need for regular monitoring, and lifetime use of multiple prescription drugs, people with diabetes are high users of the health care system. It is estimated that one of every four Medicare dollars pays for the health care of people with diabetes.

Luckily, it is possible to prevent or delay type 2 diabetes. Clinical trials have shown that losing 5 to 7 percent of body weight—that's 10 to 14 pounds for a 200-pound person—and getting at least 150 minutes of moderate physical activity each week reduces the risk of type 2 diabetes by nearly 60 percent even for those at high risk for developing the disease. In addition, community based group lifestyle intervention programs for high-risk people, like those established by CDC's National Diabetes Prevention Program that include components like training and outreach for instructors, and evaluation, monitoring, and technical assistance, can be very effective. Please refer to www.cdc.gov for more information.

Metabolic Syndrome

When a person has multiple health risk factors but has not yet developed diabetes, heart disease, or stroke, he or she may have a condition called metabolic syndrome. To qualify as having metabolic syndrome, the person must exhibit at least three of the following risk factors: borderline high blood pressure, elevated insulin levels, excess body fat around the waist, and abnormal cholesterol. Experts disagree on the name of the syndrome (some call it syndrome X or insulin resistance), and others are not sure it is even a syndrome, only a collection of risk factors. Nevertheless, those with this collection of risks are very likely to have a heart attack or a stroke, or to develop diabetes.

What defines metabolic syndrome? Obesity is a large component of metabolic syndrome, especially when the excess weight is carried around the waistline. People who have metabolic syndrome typically have apple-shaped bodies, meaning they have larger waists and carry a lot of weight around their abdomens. Those who are overweight but carry the weight in their hips and thighs (pear-shaped) with a narrower waist are less at risk. You don't have to have full-blown hypertension to have metabolic syndrome—this is defined by "borderline" elevations in blood pressure, which signals that problems are beginning. A systolic (top number) blood pressure measurement higher than 120 millimeters of mercury (mm Hg) or a diastolic (bottom number) blood pressure measurement higher than 80 mm Hg is enough to classify as metabolic syndrome. Those with metabolic syndrome have borderline or high glucose levels and consistently high levels of insulin in their bloodstream. The body cells are less responsive to insulin, so more is made. Increased insulin raises triglyceride level and other blood fat levels and is associated with obesity. Increased insulin levels interfere with the kidneys, causing high blood pressure.

Individuals who qualify as having metabolic syndrome need to make immediate, aggressive, and sustained lifestyle changes, and in some cases take medication, to improve their risk profile. If the problem is not addressed, it will lead to heart disease, stroke, or diabetes. Lifestyle changes include exercising at least 60 minutes a day, losing weight (even as little as 5 percent can make a difference), reducing fat and sugar in the diet, and quitting smoking. Extensive information on nutrition and physical activity recommendations to reduce the risk of disease is found in Chapters 9 and 10.

SUMMARY

Old age is usually accompanied by chronic illness, and many individuals have more than one. Chronic conditions are progressive, generally irreversible, and long-term. Rather than a cure, medical management of chronic illnesses involves treating symptoms and preventing further deterioration. The social, financial, and emotional considerations of chronic illnesses are a critical part of coping with disease. Chronic illnesses are responsible for the majority of deaths among older people in our country.

Although death is inevitable, how long you live and in what state of health depend at least in part on factors that are under your control. A constellation of risk factors (unhealthy diet, obesity, cigarette smoking, and inactivity) place individuals at high risk for many of the killer diseases in the United States. Modification of these risk factors can slow the onset of a disease, reduce its effects and complications, and extend life. Prevention of chronic illness requires a personal, lifelong effort to improve health habits. However, for many, both young and old, the benefits are too distant and the short-term costs too great.

This chapter explores the five chronic diseases that are responsible for the majority of deaths and disability in our country: heart disease, cancer, stroke, chronic lung disease, and diabetes. The discussion of each illness includes a description of the disease, its risk factors, methods to diagnose and treat its symptoms, and ways to prevent its occurrence or at least reduce its symptoms. In the next chapter, we explore other chronic diseases common among older people. The discussion of chronic diseases is intended to help individuals who work with older people to understand the diseases that afflict their clients in order to serve them effectively. Even more important, this information may motivate men and women with poor health habits to improve them before a chronic disease develops.

ACTIVITIES

1. Choose a chronic disease discussed in this chapter. Then, refer to Box 4.1, "Problems of Daily Living for the Chronically Ill," and discuss what an individual with that disease must deal with, given the nature of the disease, the symptoms, and treatment.

2. You have been asked to coordinate a health fair for older adults in your community. You have 10 booths to fill with health education materials. Considering the information gathered in this chapter, list what you think are the 10 most important educational topics for this age group.

3. Locate the smoking cessation classes in your area, and find out what treatment is used. Ask the director of smoking cessation classes in your area what percentage of older people attend. In the director's opinion, what is the success rate with elders? How does it compare with success rates for other age groups?

4. Visit a shopping mall, drugstore, supermarket, or some other public place, and tally how many individuals have visible health problems, as well as their approximate ages. What health problem seems most common? Can you detect any difference in types and numbers of problems with age?

5. Create a brief case study of an older individual who has one or more of the chronic health problems described in this chapter. Include the impact of the disease on the overall quality of the person's life. Be sure to include the psychological, social, and economic effects. Assuming the individual in the case has a spouse, describe the impact on that family member. If you have a family member with one of the diseases discussed in this chapter, ask her or him for permission to conduct an interview and write up her or his case experience with chronic illness.

BIBLIOGRAPHY

1. Centers for Disease Control and Prevention. 2010. *Health, United States, 2010.* Special excerpt: Trend tables on 65 and older population. Hyattsville, MD: National Center for Health Statistics.

2. Katz, S., Ford, A.B., Moskowitz, R.W., Jackson, B.A., and Jaffe, M.W. 1963. Studies of illness in the aged. The index of ADL: A standardized measure of biological and social function. *Journal of the American Medical Association* 185:914–919.

3. Lawton, M.P., and Brody, E.M. 1969. Assessment of older people: Self-maintaining and instrumental activities of daily living. *The Gerontologist* 9(3): 179–186.

4. Strauss, A. L. 1975. *Chronic illness and the quality of life.* St. Louis: C.V. Mosby.

5. Parsons, T. 1958. Definition of health and illness in the light of American values and social structure.

In Jaco, E. G. (Ed.), *Patients, physicians, and illness.* Glencoe, IL: Free Press.

6. Chobanian, A.V., Bakris, G.L., Black, H.R., et al.; National High Blood Pressure Education Program Coordinating Committee. 2003. The seventh report of the joint national committee on prevention, detection, evaluation, and treatment of high blood pressure. *Journal of the American Medical Association* 289(19):2560–2572.

7. Marrugat, J., Sala, J., Masia, R., et al. 1998. Mortality differences between men and women following first myocardial infarction. *Journal of the American Medical Association* 280:405–409.

8. American Cancer Society. 2011 Cancer Facts and Figures 2-11. Atlanta: American Cancer Society.

9. Centers for Disease Control and Prevention. 2010. Vital signs: Current cigarette smoking among

adults aged $\geq$ 18 years—United States, 2009. *Morbidity and Mortality Weekly Report* 59(35):1135–1140.

10. Lu-Yao, G.L., Albertsen, P.C., Moore, D.F., et al. 2009 (September 16). Outcomes of localized prostate cancer following conservative management from the Cancer Institute of New Jersey in New Brunswick. *Journal of the American Medical Association*, 302(11): 1202–1209.

11. Albers, G.W., Bates, V.E., Clark, W.M., et al. 2000. Intravenous tissue-type plasminogen activator for treatment of acute stroke: The Standard Treatment with Alteplase to Reverse Stroke (STARS) study. *Journal of the American Medical Association* 283(9):1145–1150.

12. Tran, H., and Anand, S.S. 2004. Oral antiplatelet therapy in cerebrovascular disease, coronary artery disease, and peripheral arterial disease. *Journal of the American Medical Association* 292(15):1867–1874.

CHAPTER 5

Other Chronic Diseases and Conditions

Old age is no place for sissies.

Bette Davis

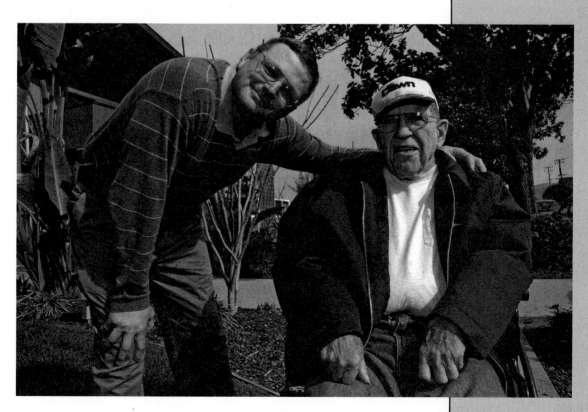

Chronic diseases persist for years, although medication and nondrug treatments can reduce or eliminate the symptoms. In the previous chapter, we discussed the five major chronic diseases that cause the majority of deaths among older adults: heart disease, cancer, stroke, chronic lung diseases, and diabetes. In this chapter, we describe chronic diseases or conditions that are not as deadly but are common in elders. These diseases also occur in the middle and younger years. The longer a person lives, the more likely it is that she or he will confront these health problems. In combination, the aging process, the growing number of health problems and medications to counteract them, and the disability that accompanies many of these disorders take their toll. Although most of these chronic illnesses do not cause death, many cause disability and reduce functional status and quality of life. The presence of multiple chronic illnesses increases frailty and deaths from other causes.

In this chapter we discuss common chronic conditions that are not major killers but can be disabling, demoralizing, or just plain annoying. For each condition we describe the common symptoms, why they occur, and common treatments. The conditions are grouped according to the body system they affect. Acute conditions caused by a virus or by bacteria are covered in Chapter 6, "Acute Illnesses and Accidents."

Musculoskeletal Disorders

Musculoskeletal disorders are by far elders' most frequent complaint because the diseases are painful and restrict movement, making it especially difficult to conduct activities that require strength or stamina. Musculoskeletal disorders cause similar symptoms (aches, pains, limited movement, and stiffness).

Arthritis and osteoporosis are the most common skeletal disorders affecting the older population. Arthritis is the number-one crippler of all ages in the United States. Two major types of arthritis are discussed here: osteoarthritis and rheumatoid arthritis. Osteoporosis or its precursor

osteopenia is a major cause of fractures in the later years. It can cause spinal deformities, loss of height, and chronic back pain. The extent of these disorders varies: Some afflicted elders are severely disabled, while others face few or no limitations on their daily routine.

In general, treatment is geared to prevent further degeneration, control pain, and encourage as much independence as possible. Prevention of accidents is another important goal of therapy because individuals with skeletal problems are at high risk for falls and fractures.

Osteoarthritis

Osteoarthritis is the most common type of arthritis in the world, the most reported chronic illness, and a major cause of disability in the United States. An estimated 50 million U.S. adults (about one in five) report doctor-diagnosed arthritis. About 50 percent of those aged 65 and older report arthritis symptoms. As the U.S. population ages, these numbers are expected to increase sharply. Arthritis is more common among women than men in every age group, and it affects members of all racial and ethnic groups, but non-Hispanic blacks are most affected. Other risk factors are inactivity, obesity, and current or former smoking.[1]

Osteoarthritis is characterized by the gradual deterioration of the bone and cartilage within a joint. Normally the ends of the joints are covered by cartilage that cushions the joint. Wearing of the cartilage puts bone on bone and causes pain and inflammation.

Osteoarthritis may affect any joint in the body, including joints in the fingers, hips, knees, lower back, and feet. People with osteoarthritis have a decreased range of motion, swelling, deformities, and stiffness and pain in the finger joints, knees, and hips. In general, pain is mild to moderate and gradual in onset. It worsens when the joint is moved and improves with rest. Diagnosis can be made through examination or X-ray.

There is no cure for osteoarthritis so the treatment focuses on reducing symptoms. In general, treatment involves analgesics (low doses of aspirin, acetaminophen, or other nonsteroidal anti-inflammatory agents), hot/cold compresses, and weight loss. Steroid medications injected into the joint can provide long-term relief, but the side effects are significant. Capsaicin, an extract of hot pepper, placed on the affected joint affords some relief. Alternative treatments, such as acupuncture, ginger, glucosamine-chondroitin, avocado-soybean oils, and tai chi and yoga have shown preliminary evidence of some effectiveness in osteoarthritis.

Orthoses (splints or braces) that are properly fitted to help align joints may reduce pain and disability associated with arthritis. Physical therapy can strengthen muscles and keep joints flexible. Weight loss relieves pressure on joints. Aerobic exercise, muscle strengthening, and range-of-motion exercises are effective (see Chapter 9, "Physical Activity"). When pain or disability is severe, surgeons may operate to correct deformities or replace joints. Viscosupplementation injects hyaluronic acid into the joint to replace missing fluid and add lubrication. Joint replacements (arthroplasty) use plastic and metal joints in place of worn-out bones—these last up to 20 years. Surgery to realign joints can relieve pain, and bones can even be fused together to stabilize a joint, but the fusion will limit range of motion and flexibility. The most common operations are total hip replacements and total knee replacements.

Rheumatoid Arthritis

Though not nearly as common as osteoarthritis, rheumatoid arthritis is more likely to cause pain, crippling, and disfigurement. It affects not only the joints but also may cause damage to the eyes, the lungs, the heart, and the nerves. The disease usually occurs between the ages of 20 and 50, so many people enter old age with a history of the disease. Rheumatoid arthritis is two to three times more common in women than in men.

Rheumatoid arthritis is caused by persistent inflammation in the tissue lining the joints, particularly the bones of the hand and foot. However, it can also spread to the larger joints. Without treatment, joints and ligaments are destroyed, producing permanent stiffness, joint dislocation, and deformity. What causes the inflammation is not completely understood, but it is believed that the immune system attacks its own cells. There is also a genetic component.

People with rheumatoid arthritis experience joint swelling, inflammation, and morning stiffness that lasts from one to five hours. In some cases, systemic symptoms like weight loss, weakness, and fatigue occur. The disease is characterized by flare-ups and remissions. Just as the pain leaves one joint, it may reappear in another. In some cases, the disease is inactive, and the individual has no symptoms. Older adults may already have deforming nodules on the joints and permanent joint damage because of lack of treatment in earlier years. Today, early aggressive treatment can prevent severe crippling in most cases.

Nonsteroidal anti-inflammatory drugs, including aspirin, are the mainstays of therapy, along with corticosteroids and a variety of disease-modifying antirheumatic drugs (DMARDs), which use different mechanisms to reduce pain and prevent loss of joint function. More information is available through the John Hopkins arthritis center at www.hopkins-arthritis.org

Besides medication, there are other ways to reduce symptoms. Experts recommend a balance of rest during flare-ups and frequent exercise during remission to achieve the fullest possible range of motion in each joint. Applying moist heat to afflicted joints temporarily reduces pain, swelling, and stiffness and makes exercise easier. Surgery to repair joints and tendons and to correct deformities may be performed when immobility and constant pain occur. Physical or occupational therapists can assess the extent of disability, suggest devices to assist in tasks of daily living, and teach ways to protect the joints from further destruction.

Osteoporosis

Osteoporosis is an age-related disorder that reduces bone mass and increases susceptibility to fractures.

Anti-inflammatory Drugs to Reduce Musculoskeletal Pain

Anti-inflammatory medications reduce joint swelling, stiffness, inflammation, and pain for people suffering from osteoarthritis or rheumatoid arthritis or other chronic musculoskeletal conditions. These drugs have often been recommended to be taken for years, and they do improve pain and joint mobility. Recent studies, however, are identifying significant risks posed by anti-inflammatory medications for long-term use. Patients face the difficult decision of whether or not to take a medication that reduces pain and increases ability to move but may increase the risk of gastrointestinal bleeding, ulcer, heart attack, or death.

The umbrella term *nonsteroidal anti-inflammatory drugs,* or *NSAIDs* (pronounced en-sayds), is used to describe a plethora of chemicals that work by inhibiting prostaglandin production. *Prostaglandins* are a specialized group of hormone-like compounds found in all body tissues. Prostaglandins have a variety of functions. They may regulate nerve impulses, protect the lining of the stomach, sensitize pain receptors, produce a fever, and inhibit blood clotting, to name a few. The main types of over-the-counter analgesics are aspirin (Anacin, Bayer, Bufferin), naproxen sodium (Aleve), ketoprofen (Orudis KT, Actron), and ibuprofen (Advil, Motrin IB, Nuprin). Acetaminophen (Tylenol, Pandol) is also used as an analgesic, although it works differently.

Aspirin is a widely used medication that reduces pain, reduces inflammation, and makes blood less likely to clot. Not only is it sold as a single product, but it is also an active ingredient in over 200 different over-the-counter (OTC or nonprescription) products. Aspirin effectively reduces pain, fever, and inflammation. It is inexpensive and generally safe, and the body does not build up tolerance for the drug. Physicians prescribe aspirin in high doses for arthritis and in low doses for prevention of blood clotting, heart attacks, and stroke. (It is recommended that an individual experiencing symptoms of a heart attack chew an aspirin immediately.) Aspirin is quite effective for joint, bone, or muscle pains that accompany arthritis, osteoporosis, and fractures, even for the bone pain of advanced cancer.

Though widely used, aspirin is not benign. Its most well-known side effect is the potential to damage the lining of the stomach, causing pain, bleeding, ulcers, and anemia. Although this side effect is more common in elders taking high dosages, it can also occur with very low doses. In addition, high doses of aspirin may cause nausea, hearing and vision disturbances, abdominal pain, confusion, or dizziness. Elders with reduced kidney function have a higher risk of toxicity. Finally, because aspirin reduces the ability of the blood to clot, it can be detrimental if taken before surgery.

The other NSAIDs have similar uses and side effects. Some are now sold over the counter in lower doses than earlier prescription-only products. These medications may be even more effective at reducing fever, pain, and inflammation than aspirin. However, they also irritate the stomach, causing bleeding or ulcers, and can cause kidney disease or confusion in elders. They cause thousands of deaths each year, mostly among the elderly.

Newer drugs called *COX-II inhibitors* were thought to be the solution because they had similar effects on reducing inflammation and pain but reduced the likelihood of ulcers and gastrointestinal bleeding. Physicians were excited about a product that was effective and safe, and patients found the one-a-day dosing and the low side effect profile ideal. Then, unfortunately, study results pointed to a higher rate of cardiovascular problems and even death among people taking COX-II inhibitors (e.g., Celebrex and Vioxx). Strict warnings were placed on packaging, many lawsuits are pending, and some drugs were removed from the market. In fact, the same studies also suggested an increased risk of heart attack and death in people taking the older NSAIDs for prolonged periods of time. Bottom line: Anti-inflammatory drugs have great benefits and high risks. The individual and the health care practitioner need to balance these risks and benefits for the person's particular needs and values.

Although gradual bone loss occurs in everyone with advancing age, the bone loss due to osteoporosis is more severe. Bones in the back, hips, and forearm are most likely to be affected. Osteoporosis is the major cause of fractures in the later years. It can also cause collapsed vertebrae, leading to spinal deformities such as dowager's hump, loss of height, and chronic back pain. Severe postural deformities result in reduced lung function. Oftentimes osteoporosis is not discovered until the patient has suffered a fracture and the disease is very advanced. Individuals with advanced osteoporosis are so fragile that even a minor fall might result in a severe fracture and subsequent disability and dependence.

Ten million Americans have osteoporosis, and it is estimated that three times that number have *osteopenia* (less severe loss of bone mass). Although osteoporosis frequently affects the spine, the most serious consequence is hip fracture, which has a much greater impact on a person's life. Experts believe that one-third of the hip fractures among women and one-sixth of hip fractures among men are caused by osteoporosis. Individuals who have an osteoporotic hip fracture take longer to heal, and the accompanying immobilization causes further bone loss. A significant number of elders who fracture a hip die within the year. Many of those who survive do not regain their previous function and may have to be admitted to nursing homes.

People at increased risk for osteoporosis are older, smoke cigarettes, consume excessive alcohol, and have a sedentary lifestyle. Women are four times more likely to have osteoporosis than men. Those who are underweight or have a slight build have an increased risk; those with heavier bones have a reduced risk. Individuals with a family history of fractures or osteoporosis are at increased risk. High caffeine or carbonated soda intake increases the risk of osteoporosis; consumption of milk products reduces risk. White and Asian women have higher risk of bone loss than black or Hispanic women.

Research shows that estrogens play a role in osteoporosis, although the exact mechanism is not known. It is clear that osteoporosis worsens after menopause, and that estrogen replacement therapy reduces bone loss and incidence of fractures.

Women who have completed menopause before age 45, had their ovaries removed without estrogen replacement, and have a low-calcium diet are at high risk of osteoporosis and consequent fractures.

Although bone loss is progressive throughout life, it has no symptoms, and many people do not know they have it until they break a bone. Even after getting a fracture, many elders are not prescribed medications and supplements to prevent further bone loss.

Standard X-rays are not very good at quantifying how much bone is lost or even whether a person has osteoporosis. A common technique for measuring bone density is dual X-ray absorptiometry (DXA), known as a "DEXA scan." A newer device uses ultrasound to measure bone density. It can be used during a routine examination and is faster and less expensive than a DEXA scan. Chapter 12 describes screening recommendations for elders.

Sufficient calcium, vitamin D, and regular weight-bearing physical activity are the most effective ways to maintain bone health. In 2010, the Institute of Medicine reviewed the existing literature and made new recommendations for calcium and vitamin D dietary intake. Women ages 19 through 50 and men up to 71 require on average 800 milligrams daily of calcium. Women over 50 and both men and women 71 and older should take in 1,000 milligrams per day on average to ensure they are meeting their daily requirement for bone health. Depending on sun exposure, which is highly variable, the vitamin D requirement changes, which makes recommendations harder to determine. Recommendations are based on minimal sun exposure. North Americans need on average 400 International Units (IUs) of vitamin D per day. People age 71 and older may require as much as 800 IUs per day because of potential changes in their bodies as they age.

There is such a thing as too much vitamin D; once intakes surpass 4,000 IUs per day, the risk for harm, particularly to the kidneys, begins to increase. Once calcium supplement intakes surpass 2,000 milligrams per day, the risk for harm—for example, kidney stones—also increases.[2] High calcium intake in the younger years, through diet or supplements, is

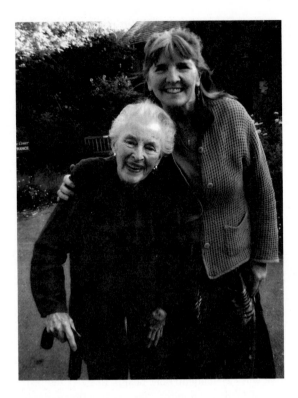

associated with reduced rates of bone loss and fractures in later years.

A person with osteoporosis should begin a gradual physical activity program of weight-bearing exercises to increase muscle and bone strength. Several medications also may be prescribed either to reduce bone loss or to stimulate bone formation. In the past, physicians routinely prescribed hormone replacement therapy because it was shown to be very effective. However, the risk of hormone replacement therapy and the rise of other drugs that treat osteoporosis have reduced its popularity. A newer treatment that acts like estrogen is raloxifene.

Bisphosphonates are used to treat those who have a low bone density or who already have a vertebral fracture—these medicines reduce the incidence of fractures and improve the quality of life. They do not seem as effective in those with osteopenia (low bone density) who have not had a fracture. They decrease fracture rate in the first five years of use and decrease bone rate resorption (the breaking down of bones), but they can last more than ten years in the bones and long-term effects are not known. They are used for certain categories of people who have a high fracture risk such as women with vertebral compression fractures or low bone density, and men with non-traumatic fractures. Bisphosphonates can also be used for bone cancer. Some are oral, which must be administered in an upright position with water so as not to burn the esophagus, and some are intravenous.

Calcitonin, a calcium-retaining hormone, is taken by injection or nasal spray. Another medication is terparatide, the only medication that actually builds bone. A daily shot is prescribed for people with a history of fractures or at high risk for fractures.

Experts debate who should be screened and who should be prescribed drugs for osteoporosis because many people with osteoporosis never suffer any adverse effects and bone density is not the only predictor of fracture risk. The U.S. Preventive Services Task Force recommends screening for osteoporosis in women aged 65 years or older and in younger women whose fracture risk is equal to or greater than that of a 65-year-old white woman who has no additional risk factors (www.uspreventiveservicestaskforce.org). Even though the drug treatments are often prescribed for years, there are few studies that look at their long-term effectiveness. Finally, all drug treatments have side effects.

Low Back Pain

Backs are complicated and delicate structures made of bones, muscles, ligaments, tendons, and disks, which act as cushions between vertebrae. The legendary Atlas carried the world on his back and reportedly suffered back pain. Although we don't support the earth, strains, structural problems, and arthritis (among other things) can cause pain in our backs. In some people, the specific causes for their back pain can't be found.

B o x   5 . 1

Proper Lifting Techniques to Prevent Back Injury

- Check out the load. Lift a corner to see how heavy it is. Is it easy to get a good grasp?
- Make sure your footing is secure. Do not lift objects that are so big that you can't see where your feet are and where you are going.
- Bend your knees when lifting, not your back.
- Bring an object close to your body before lifting it, and center yourself over it to balance the load.
- Lift straight up and smoothly.
- Avoid twisting or turning your body when lifting.
- Put the load down by bending your knees, not your back.
- Know your limits: Don't try to lift more than you can easily handle.
- Get help with large loads, or use a dolly to avoid lifting altogether.

Factors that increase the risk of developing back pain include smoking, obesity, old age, being female, stress, anxiety, depression, or a physically taxing or sedentary job. The most common source of back pain is strained muscles and ligaments, which can result from improper heavy lifting, bad posture, or a sudden movement like a muscle spasm. See Box 5.1 for the correct technique for lifting and bending. Back pain also can be caused by structural problems, like skeletal irregularities, arthritis, or bulging or ruptured disks. It is natural for a spine to curve, but if the curve becomes exaggerated or curves to the side (*scoliosis*), it can lead to back pain. Arthritis is common in the lower back and can result in a narrowing of the space around the spinal cord called *spinal stenosis*. If a bulging disk presses on a main nerve, it can cause *sciatica*, which is a sharp pain through the back of the leg. Another condition is osteoporosis, where bones become porous and brittle and weak, and can collapse, causing painful or painless compression fractures. In addition to these painful structural problems, there are a few rare but very serious conditions that should be mentioned. *Cauda equina* syndrome is a neurological problem that causes weakness or numbness in the leg or groin area, which can lead to loss of bladder or bowel control. Tumors on or near the spine can cause severe back pain. Infections are also a danger.

In general, the cause of the back pain doesn't affect the prescribed treatments. Over-the-counter treatments like acetaminophen (Tylenol, others),

aspirin, ibuprofen (Advil, Motrin, others), and naproxen (Aleve) can relieve acute pain. Prescription pain medication can also be used, but many people don't need the more powerful dosage. In addition to medication, the application of ice or heat can often help. Exercising with the help of a physical therapist or chiropractor (or solo) can relieve stiffness and back pain. Surgery is looked at only as a last resort.

To reduce the risk of back pain, it is important to make good lifestyle choices, such as participating in regular exercise, strengthening the muscles in the core of the body such as the back and abdomen, having good posture, using safe-lifting techniques, quitting smoking, or maintaining a healthy weight. A Web search can find many different exercise programs for preventing back pain, many adapted for frail elders.

Foot Problems

Feet are remarkable. They carry our full weight every day, sometimes traveling many miles. The average person walks more than 100,000 miles in the course of a lifetime. Walking is the "ideal exercise," a safe way to get fit for almost everyone. However, foot problems can derail physical activity to the point of immobility. We generally take our feet for granted, until we have a foot problem. Then, our daily routine is affected. Foot problems can arise from bones, joints, muscle, skin, and nails. Systemic diseases such as circulatory disorders, heart or kidney disease, diabetes, arthritis, and nerve conditions can cause foot pain. Obesity and inactivity also aggravate pain. Breaks in the skin of the feet—ulcers—can be painful and can result from poor arterial circulation (not enough blood), poor venous circulation, edema or swelling, or from diabetes. Wearing shoes that fit poorly can cause foot pain.

Foot problems increase with age. Skin is thinner and less resilient to injury. Skin becomes drier and more likely to have corns or calluses—a buildup of dead skin from continual friction or pressure. The fat pads on the foot become thinner, making the feet tender. Toenails may become more brittle. Aging increases fungal infections of the toenails, resulting in thick, hard-to-cut nails that eventually may loosen and fall off. The bones in the foot may change shape, joints lose some flexibility, and ligaments, tendons, and muscles may weaken, causing loss of movement. In the following paragraphs we look at foot problems likely to occur with age, although they are not necessarily due to the aging process.

Calluses and corns are hard, thick areas of skin caused by friction or pressure. They occur when foot bones are out of alignment or shoes are rubbing too hard on the skin. Treatment involves relieving the pressure, generally by wearing comfortable shoes. Pads that relieve the pressure are available, but they must be positioned carefully. In some cases, surgery is necessary to remove a bony prominence that is causing the corn or callus.

Some individuals have a big toe that leans toward the second toe instead of pointing straight ahead. Over the years, the bones of the big toe become out of alignment, and the joint at the base of the big toe becomes enlarged. The characteristic bump on the side of the toe is called a *bunion*. Since the big toe carries a lot of the body's weight during walking, bunions can cause extreme pain if left untreated. Bunions cause pain, stiffness, and swelling around the joint. They are not hereditary, but the foot structure that promotes them is hereditary. Wearing shoes that are too tight and arthritis can promote the formation of bunions. Treatment includes pain relievers, properly fitted shoes, use of a protective moleskin pad, and shoe inserts. A permanent treatment is surgery. There are many different procedures, but all realign the toe joint, relieve pain, and correct deformity.

A *hammertoe* is a deformity of the toe joint that most often affects the toe next to the big toe. The toe bends up and curls at the middle joint. Hammertoes may be hereditary, or they may be caused by arthritis. Most commonly, they are due to ill-fitting shoes. If the problem cannot be helped with roomier shoes, toe pads, exercises, splints, and orthotics (a shoe insert to place the foot in a certain position), an in-office procedure can be accomplished to remove a small piece of bone so that the toe can return to a normal position.

Two types of professionals specialize in treating foot problems: orthopedists and podiatrists. *Orthopedists* complete four years of medical school and five years of hospital training, most of it in orthopedic surgery. They are physicians who are trained to treat musculoskeletal problems, including bones, joints, tendons, and nerves in the body. They can treat bone disorders medically and surgically. *Podiatrists* are specialists in foot disorders. They complete four years at a podiatric medicine college followed by one to four years of hospital residency. Podiatrists are doctors of podiatric medicine who are trained to perform surgery and prescribe medications for foot and ankle disorders only. For more information on foot problems, click on the American Podiatric Medical Association site at www.apma.org

ENDOCRINE DISORDERS

Diabetes and thyroid problems are the most significant problems of the endocrine system. Although these chronic conditions may begin in early or middle adulthood, they are lifelong conditions and must be continually monitored. Diabetes, a significant cause of death and disability in the older population, is discussed in the previous chapter.

Thyroid problems are common among elders. It is estimated that 10 percent of older people have abnormal thyroid hormone levels. Elders can suffer from either a deficiency (hypothyroid) or an excess (hyperthyroid) of the thyroid hormone, thyroxin, although a deficiency is more common. Whites, women, the middle-aged, and those over 75 are at higher risk for thyroid problems. Because of the high prevalence of the condition, many groups recommend routine testing of all elders for thyroid disease.

Hypothyroidism can be subtle among elders. It appears as slowed thought processes, reduced ability to respond to stress, constipation, weight gain, decreased cold tolerance, depression, or hallucinations. These symptoms are so common that it is difficult to determine whether they are due to medications, disease, or old age. If left untreated, hypothyroidism is lethal. Hypothyroidism is also associated with abnormalities in cholesterol levels. Regular administration of thyroid hormone pills reverses the condition, but the dose should be regularly monitored by blood tests.

Hyperthyroidism is an excess of thyroid hormone and causes the opposite symptoms of hypothyroidism: increased heart rate, increased sensitivity to heat, sweating, diarrhea, weight loss, irritability, and tremors. This condition also can be dangerous in older adults because they may suffer a heart attack due to the excessive strain on the heart. Elders may not show typical symptoms but may manifest rapid heart rate, fatigue, and weight loss. Because hyperthyroidism can be caused by a number of mechanisms, the treatment varies but may include drugs or procedures to destroy thyroid cells.

DIGESTIVE DISORDERS

Indigestion, abdominal pain, heartburn, constipation, and diarrhea are very common complaints among older people. Some problems are serious and need immediate attention; others are bothersome at times but not life threatening. It is often challenging for elders and their physicians to identify the cause of many abdominal complaints. The digestive system extends from the mouth to the anus and also includes the glands that provide enzymes and acid for the digestive system. It is a large system in which much can go wrong. Here we discuss the most common digestive conditions among older people.

Tooth, Gum, and Mouth Conditions

Oral health is an important part of overall health and well-being. Oral health problems include missing teeth, ill-fitting dentures, dental cavities, gum disease or infection, and dry mouth. Many dental problems accumulate over the years—broken teeth and cracked fillings, loss of bone supporting the teeth, missing teeth, gum disease. Teeth and gum problems cause acute or chronic pain and general discomfort. Further, the ability to chew is impaired, limiting consumption of some types of foods, especially fiber. Finally, tooth loss and untreated dental and gum problems may affect appearance and the ability to speak clearly, reducing self-esteem and social interactions. Problems related to the mouth are complicated when elders become too frail to care for their teeth and gums. Bad teeth can lead to a poor diet. Those with broken or painful teeth or gums might eat less fiber, fewer vegetables, seeds, or nuts, and instead gravitate toward soft foods that need less chewing. In addition, there is increasing evidence that the bacteria from the mouth play an important role in overall health and may even be responsible for some cardiac diseases, making dental hygiene even more important.

Until the 1950s, most older people were edentulous (had none of their natural teeth). Since that time, water flouridation and improvements in dentistry and the initiation of health eduction in the schools have led to a continuous decrease in the number of elders who are edentulous. The latest Nutrition and Health Examination Survey reports that less than 30 percent of elders are edentulous. Those who are older, black, current smokers, lower income and less education are more likely to have no teeth.

Tooth loss is not due to advancing age but from poor diet and dental hygiene. *Dental caries,* or *cavities,* are localized areas of tooth destruction that dentists treat by drilling out the decayed portion of the tooth and rebuilding it with a filling material. Only 5 percent of Americans have no cavities. Among the young, most cavities develop on the biting surfaces of teeth. With advancing age and gum recession, cavities are more likely to develop along the roots because they are less protected by enamel. Up to 70 percent of elders with natural teeth develop root cavities. Elders are also susceptible to cavities around old fillings. Good oral hygiene with fluoridated toothpaste and regular dental care reduce the risk. Although the prevalence of dental caries has declined over the last few years in the United States, it has not declined among the most socially disadvantaged elder group: poor blacks.

The most important contributor to tooth loss among elders is *periodontal (gum) disease,* a chronic bacterial infection of the gums (gingivitis) that may eventually destroy tooth roots and even erode the jawbone. The disease significantly increases with age because of bone loss and recession of gums from the teeth. Periodontal disease begins when bacteria collect at the base of the teeth and form plaque, a sticky substance composed of food debris and bacteria. If not removed daily, the plaque hardens into calculus, which must be removed by a dental professional. Symptoms of periodontal disease include swollen, red, or bleeding gums, gums that bleed during brushing or eating, gums that are separating from the teeth, bad breath, and loose teeth. Gum disease in elders is aggravated by medications that dry the mouth.

If, during a routine dental exam, gum pockets are found to be 4- to 5-mm deep or more, that individual has periodontal disease. It is effectively treated with antibiotics, deep cleaning, antibacterial mouthwashes, and surgery. Surgery may be recommended when the tissue around the teeth is unhealthy and cannot be saved with other treatments. The types of surgery include cutting away the gum pockets, rehaping the gum tissue around the tooth, and soft tissue grafts.

Tooth loss and periodontal disease can be reduced with regular brushing and flossing, dental checkups, and smoking cessation. A soft-bristled toothbrush and fluoride toothpaste should be used twice daily. Elders with coordination problems may use aids such as floss-on-a-stick, sponge-on-a-stick (toothettes), or electric toothbrushes to assist in dental hygiene. An oral rinse called "Answer" is designed for elders, those who are frail, and those with problems with dry or sore mouths to clean the teeth (www.theanswer2oralcare.com). Frail elders, whether homebound or in institutions, need caretakers who are trained in providing oral health care daily.

It is expected that fewer people in the future will enter their later years with poor oral health, for they will have been better educated about dental hygiene. On the other hand, since a greater number of older people will be keeping their teeth, more dental services will be needed.

Older adults have the lowest rates of dental visits of all age groups. Visits are especially low among minorities, the oldest-old, and elders in institutions. The greatest barrier to receiving dental services is financial. The ability to pay for dental care decreases after retirement, both from loss of income and loss of dental insurance. Medicare does not cover dental care, so most elders are responsible for their own dental expenses. Few elders carry dental insurance.

For those poor enough to qualify, states may elect to provide dental services to their adult Medicaid-eligible population or elect not to provide dental services at all as part of its Medicaid program. Most states provide at least emergency dental services for adults. However, few dentists participate in that program. Go to www .oralhealthamerica.org to see how well your state is meeting the oral health needs of its elders.

Saliva is very important to oral health. It breaks down carbohydrates into simple sugars and helps to neutralize acids, produced by bacteria in our mouths, that otherwise would destroy tooth enamel. Antibodies in the mouth also fight the bacteria that cause cavities and gum disease. Saliva enables us to eat and swallow with ease and is important to our senses of taste and smell. The average adult produces about three pints of saliva a day.

Dry mouth is often related to dehydration (not enough fluids) or medication side effects. Medications that dry the mouth include many blood pressure medications, antihistamines, painkillers, bladder agents, antidepressants, and chemotherapy. A dry mouth increases the risk of cavities, gum disease, and denture irritation. There are several ways to increase saliva production. The first step is to change medications, if possible. Over-the-counter artificial saliva products are available. Individuals with symptoms also might limit sugar, chew sugarless gum, increase water intake, avoid alcohol, caffeine, and tobacco, and practice good oral hygiene. An oral rinse containing xylitol (e.g., Answer) can moisten the mouth and assist in maintaining proper acid balance.

Stomach Disorders

Heartburn is a misnomer as the heart is not involved at all. The "burning" pain experienced behind the breastbone is related to stomach acid. When the lining of the stomach is irritated, pain occurs with eating, after eating, or at night. When the muscular valve between the esophagus and the stomach does not tighten fully, acidic stomach contents back up into the esophagus. The lining of the esophagus cannot tolerate the acids, it becomes irritated and inflamed, causing pain. Sometimes gastric juices and small amounts of food are brought all the way back to the mouth or respiratory tract.

Acid-related abdominal pain can be caused or aggravated by smoking, alcohol, an infection (caused by a bacteria called *H. pylori*), or from medications like nonsteroidal anti-inflammatory drugs, aspirin, or steroids. Garlic, onions, and spicy or fatty foods can worsen the condition. Heartburn symptoms occur in almost everyone at some time or another but are most common among individuals who are elderly, overweight, or pregnant.

If heartburn occurs more than twice a week, *gastroesophageal reflux disease (GERD)* may be present. In this case the acid has progressively destroyed the lining of the esophagus, creating a premalignant condition. Individuals with continuous bouts of heartburn from gastroesophageal reflux disease are at high risk for ulcers and cancer of the esophagus.

Overeating, lying flat, or coughing increases the discomfort. The condition is also aggravated by obesity, straining when defecating, and wearing clothes too tight at the waist. Heartburn may be relieved temporarily by sitting upright, taking antacids, belching, eating smaller meals, and avoiding tight clothing. More permanent solutions are losing weight; reducing or avoiding alcohol, coffee, and fatty foods; and increasing physical activity.

A *hiatal hernia* occurs when part of the stomach protrudes into the chest cavity through the valve in which the esophagus passes through the diaphragm. Experts believe a hiatal hernia is caused by a weakness in the diaphragm. Hiatal hernia, like GERD, causes inflammation of the esophagus because stomach acid is regurgitated into the lower part of the esophagus. Many older people have some degree of hiatal hernia.

Ulcers are small holes or wounds in the lining of the the esophagus, stomach, or first part of the intestine. Ulcers are caused by medication use (steroid and nonsteroidal anti-inflammatory medications) or can be associated with a type of bacteria called *Helicobacter pylori*. The bacteria secrete enzymes that neutralize the stomach acid long enough to allow them to burrow into the protective mucous layer of the stomach lining. The small holes made by the bacteria weaken the stomach lining, allowing the stomach acid and bacteria to eat through the lining, producing an ulcer. Most people with the *H. pylori* bacteria do not have ulcers.

Ulcer disease affects up to one in ten Americans. The most common complaint is abdominal pain that comes and goes for several days or weeks. It often occurs in the middle of the night or two to three hours after a meal, and it may be relieved by food or antacids. Those with ulcers may have anemia or microscopic blood in the stool. Ulcers can be self-limiting (disappear without treatment), or they may erode through the stomach or intestinal wall to cause a surgical emergency. In a few cases, an ulcer is a sign of cancer. Various studies can diagnose the cause of stomach pain. Commonly, an individual drinks a chalky liquid that makes abnormalities of esophagus and stomach visible on an X-ray. Also, an endoscope (lighted tube) may be inserted down the throat to inspect the lining of the esophagus and stomach, and samples can be taken if needed. Blood tests can detect the presence of *H. pylori,* and if this is found, antibiotics can treat the infection. Stool tests detect if there is hidden bleeding.

Treatment of stomach disorders should begin with behavior changes: losing weight, sitting up or taking a leisurely walk after meals, avoiding tight belts, and avoiding foods that irritate the stomach (tomatoes, coffee, soda). However, if medication is needed, several types of drugs are successful, including over-the-counter medications that neutralize stomach acid or reduce the production of stomach acid.

Antacids relieve symptoms of upset stomach, heartburn, and indigestion by neutralizing excess stomach acid. There are over a hundred different antacid products on the market, and they come in many forms: pills, lozenges, gum, powder, and liquids. Some popular brand names are Alka-Seltzer, Tums, Pepto-Bismol, and Maalox. These antacids generally begin acting immediately and may be effective for up to 40 minutes. All antacids contain one or more of 13 active ingredients, each with its own side effects. Aluminum hydroxide has a constipating effect, magnesium salts may cause diarrhea, and antacids with high sodium content can cause fluid retention. Antacids may decrease the absorption of some drugs, aggravate symptoms of upset stomach, or mask symptoms of an ulcer. Nevertheless, antacids are a very effective treatment for sporadic or daily symptoms of heartburn and GERD by providing short-term relief. They do not promote healing, however, and are best used for mild occasional symptoms of heartburn.

Histamine 2 (H2) blockers (Tagamet, Zantac, Pepcid) provide short-term relief by blocking the production of stomach acid and promoting healing of the lining of the esophagus. Tagamet has also been associated with increased rates of confusion in elderly patients. H2 blockers are available over the counter and at higher doses by prescription.

A third type of drug, proton pump inhibitors (PPI), shuts off the chemical pump that moves acid into the stomach. PPIs suppress nearly all production of stomach acid and allow healing of ulcers and irritations. Drugs in this family include Prilosec, Prevacid, and Nexium. It may take as much as four days to realize an effect. Proton pump inhibitors are available over the counter, and, in higher doses, by prescription. PPIs are some of the most widely used and widely advertised drugs in the United States. Some believe these drugs are overused, especially in the elderly. They may be started for mild symptoms or in the hospital to protect the stomach, and then continued long after they are needed. Proton pump inhibitors can increase the risk of pneumonia and fractures and can cause a rebound when stopped suddenly after long-term use.

Surgical procedures are available. For GERD, the valve between the esophagus and stomach can be repaired to keep acid from backing up. In the case of hiatal hernia, surgery can return the stomach to its proper place, the diaphragm can be repaired, and a valve can be constructed around the esophagus to prevent the backflow of stomach acid. Ulcers can be treated surgically through repair or removal of part of the stomach or intestine.

Constipation

Constipation is the most common digestive complaint in our country, and its incidence increases with age. Constipation is responsible for millions of physician visits, thousands of hospitalizations, and several hundred million dollars spent on laxatives each year. Though seldom life threatening, constipation can be all-consuming. Older people commonly report that it interferes with their quality of life and feeling of well-being. The five most common complaints linked to constipation are (1) straining to pass feces, (2) hard stools, (3) inability to defecate when desired, (4) infrequent bowel movements, and (5) abdominal discomfort. People who are constipated also complain of nausea, depression, bloating, abdominal pain, and diminished appetite.

Medically, *constipation* is defined as the inability to evacuate stool completely and spontaneously three or more times per week. There is tremendous variability in frequency of stool passage. The range of normality is between three times daily to once every three days. It is not necessary to have a daily bowel movement for ideal health. Many elders, however, prefer to have daily bowel movements even if they must rely on laxatives. It is estimated that one-third to one-half of the elder population uses laxatives, and the percentage is higher in nursing homes.

There are several types of constipation, but the majority of those complaining about being constipated really are not constipated: Their stool travels normally through the colon, and the frequency of evacuation is normal. The misperception is likely due to perceived difficulty with evacuation or the presence of hard stools.[3] Differences in perception of constipation make it difficult to accurately assess the prevalence of constipation because the medical definition differs so radically from the layperson's view.

Although complaints of constipation increase with age, constipation is not part of the aging process. The increased incidence of constipation among the older age group is more likely the consequence of reduced physical activity, low-fiber diet due to poor chewing ability, medication side effects, poor straining ability, and chronic diseases. A low level of mobility or immobility is one of the most significant causes of constipation because it reduces intestinal motility. Some drugs (e.g., antidepressants, painkillers) and dietary supplements (e.g., calcium and iron) have a constipating effect. Long-term laxative use, particularly stimulant laxatives, may damage the nerve cells in the colon wall, promoting further constipation and dependence on laxative therapy. Many chronic illnesses are associated with increased risk of constipation, including cancer, depression, spinal cord lesions, Parkinson's disease, and hypothyroidism.

Modifying the diet and participating in daily physical activity are the two simplest and most effective ways to treat constipation. Constipated elders should be encouraged to increase their intake of fluids, especially fruit juices, and of foods containing fiber such as bran and prunes. Ten to 20 grams of fiber daily are recommended, as well as at least 6 cups of fluid daily. If elders are not able to consume enough fluids, fiber supplementation can aggravate constipation and alternatives need to be explored.

Sometimes changes in daily routine reduce constipation. Importantly, elders need to respond to the natural urge to have a bowel movement rather than ignoring it. Elders should set aside time each day to have a bowel movement, preferably after a meal, to take advantage of the physiological reflex to empty the bowels after a meal. The use of a footrest while on the toilet can be helpful.

Many experts assert that laxatives are the worst choice to treat constipation because they can reduce the natural functioning of the bowels. Instead, the source of the problem needs to be identified. Checking to see if prescriptions are causing

constipation, increasing fluid and fiber intake, increasing physical activity, and going to the toilet after eating should be the first line of treatment. Laxatives should be used only temporarily and after serious causes of constipation are excluded. Dried fruits like prunes, raisins, figs, and prune juice can have laxative effects. Bulk laxatives, which increase fiber, are generally safe, and osmotic laxatives are safer than stimulants. See Box 5.2 for an overview of laxative types.

Constipation may be a transient event due to travel, change in activity level or diet, medication use, or emotional stress. Or constipation may be a sign of a serious physical problem, such as bowel blockage, fecal impaction, or colon cancer. When someone suffers from constipation alternating with diarrhea or the passage of stools of increasingly narrow diameter, colon cancer or inflammatory bowel disease may be the cause, and a physician should be contacted.

Fecal impaction is a consequence of untreated constipation, resulting in the accumulation in the rectum of hard, dry stools that cannot be passed. The diagnosis may be difficult because individuals sometimes have watery diarrhea as liquid stool passes around the impacted stool. A manual digital rectal examination is critical for accurate diagnosis of fecal impaction. Recommended treatment is extraction of the fecal mass, either manually or by using an enema.

Once an individual has suffered from impaction, bowel abnormalities persist. For example, a larger stool volume is required to stimulate contractions of the colon before an urge to defecate is felt. Sufficient fiber intake and use of laxatives to produce regular bowel movements should be instituted to prevent future events.

Fecal Incontinence

Few symptoms are more distressing to elders and their families than *fecal incontinence*, the loss of bowel control causing unintended passage of liquid or solid stool. The problem may range from partial soiling due to gas or liquid stool, to lack of control of normally formed stool. Estimates vary, but as many as 15 percent of women and 10 percent of

---

BOX 5.2

Laxatives

Products that promote bowel movement are frequently used—some would say overused—by elders. Laxatives are helpful for occasional use by many elders and routine use by those with chronic health problems. They are also useful for individuals who must take medications with a side effect of constipation (such as codeine and morphine). There are many types of laxatives, and each type works differently.

Perhaps the safest are *fiber or bulk laxatives,* which increase the volume and water content of stools and move waste through the colon more quickly. Common names are bran, psyllium (Metamucil), methylcellulose (Citrucel), and calcium polycarbophil (FiberCon). Bulk laxatives are most useful for people with a low-fiber diet and should be taken with a lot of water to avoid intestinal obstruction. Their common side effects include bloating and flatulence (passing gas).

Oral osmotics are not absorbed by the body, but as they pass through, they draw water into the colon. These include nonabsorbable sugars like Sorbitol, Lactulose, Miralax, and Go-Lytely. *Stool softeners* increase salts and water inside the intestines. When stools are very hard, they may be useful to reduce straining. The most commonly used stool softener is Colace.

Lubricant laxatives, including mineral oil, are effective in softening the stool, but they prevent absorption of fat-soluble vitamins by the intestine and may cause fecal leaking or incontinence.

Stimulant laxatives increase intestinal motility by increasing fluid excretion into the gut and irritating the nerves supplying the intestines. They are some of the most commonly used and abused laxatives among the elderly. Examples include Dulcolax, Sennakot, and Peri-Colace. Prolonged use can lead to laxative dependency, fluid-salt imbalance, severe cramps, malabsorption, diarrhea, and dehydration.

Some laxatives are taken rectally. Rectal stimulants such as dulcolax/bisacodyl or gycerine suppositories irritate the rectum and can produce stool. Enemas may be concocted from a variety of substances, including mineral oil, tap water, phosphate (Fleet), or soapsuds. They soften and lubricate the stool in the rectum and assist evacuation by distending the rectum.

---

men over 50 have some degree of fecal incontinence. It is estimated that almost 50 percent of nursing home residents have fecal incontinence. It is a major reason for institutionalization.

Affected individuals seldom talk to their friends, physicians, or even their families about this embarrassing problem. An accident can be a significant blow to self-confidence and to the ability to freely interact with family, friends, and coworkers. Those with fecal incontinence often reduce social interaction, especially outside the home, because of the fear of embarrassing accidents.

There are many possible causes of fecal incontinence. The most common reversible cause is diarrhea. Many other causes are less reversible. Nerve or muscle damage to the area (from spinal problems, childbirth, or stroke) and advanced dementia can be associated with fecal incontinence. Those with advanced dementia may no longer recognize the need to go to the bathroom and lose their ability to control defecation. With strokes, people can develop a similar phenomenon with a decreased ability to detect when they have to pass a bowel movement and reduced or slowed ability to use the toilet. Some people maintain the ability to tell when they have to go, but have a "functional" incontinence. With functional incontinence, individuals use a brief because they are weak, in pain, or unable to get help to get to a toilet.

Treatment for fecal incontinence depends on the cause. Adding fiber to the diet, using the toilet at the same time every day, practicing Kegel exercises to strengthen the anal sphincter, and surgery to repair the anal sphincter are effective. For those with dementia, having them sit on the toilet after meals may prompt defecation in the toilet. For those with physical disabilities, there are special lifts that can hold people in a comfortable position over the toilet to have a bowel movement. A prosthesis is available that keeps the anus closed until the person opens the anus to defecate by squeezing a pump in the genital area. For some, a colonostomy is performed that diverts fecal matter to a bag outside the body. The most common treatment, however, is no treatment: Disposable underpants are worn and changed frequently.

To help individuals cope with short- or long-term fecal incontinence, the International Foundation for Functional Gastrointestinal Disorders offers information and practical advice online (www.aboutincontinence.org).

CIRCULATORY CONDITIONS

Chronic illnesses related to the heart and blood vessels are the most common causes of death in the United States. Both heart disease and stroke are related to atherosclerosis and difficulties with circulation to the brain and heart. Heart disease and stroke were discussed in the previous chapter. In contrast, the three conditions related to the circulatory system are less likely life threatening but impact quality of life and functional status. Claudication reduces mobility and independence, and varicose veins and hemorrhoids can cause much discomfort.

Claudication

When the arteries in the leg become narrowed by atherosclerosis, a condition called *intermittent claudication,* or simply *claudication,* may develop. Elders with this condition complain of severe crampy pain in one or both legs whenever they walk a certain distance. The pain is triggered by exercise when not enough blood is getting to the leg muscles. After a brief rest, the pain disappears but recurs when walking resumes. Some individuals may also experience numbness and coldness in their legs. There is no effective medication for this disorder. Since inactivity causes further deterioration, the individual is encouraged to walk to the point of pain, rest, then walk again, gradually building up circulation to the muscles. In severe cases, artery bypass surgery is performed. A vein is taken from the leg and grafted

or attached to the narrowed artery in the leg to allow blood to flow more freely.

Varicose Veins

Almost everybody has seen *varicose veins,* distended ropelike blood vessels that commonly appear on the inside of the leg and the back of the calf. Although they rarely cause serious problems, they are considered unsightly and often cause physical discomfort after prolonged standing or sitting. Varicose veins are a common condition, affecting more than half of all Americans. Women, especially older women, are more likely than men to have this problem.

With advancing age, the valves within the blood vessels, primarily in the lower legs, become defective, causing blood to back up and damage

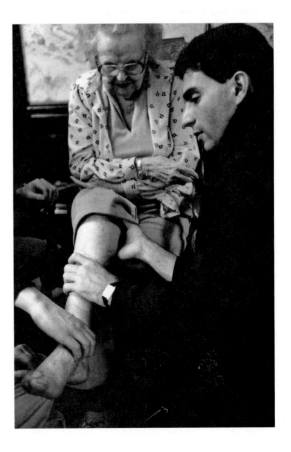

the vessel walls. The veins lose their elasticity and become distended and twisted, reducing the flow of stagnant blood back to the heart. Symptoms include leg aches, swelling in the lower legs, and sometimes persistent itching. Very rarely, if damage to the vessels is severe, a blood clot, inflammation of the vein, or even ulcers may occur.

In most cases, the following activities are helpful: keeping legs elevated, wearing stockings that compress the veins, increasing exercise, avoiding excessive standing or sitting, losing weight, avoiding high heels and tight clothing, and avoiding sitting with the legs crossed. Sometimes, medical treatment is needed to close or remove varicose veins. *Sclerotherapy* involves injecting medium-size varicose veins with a solution that scars those veins and forces the rerouting of blood to healthier veins. The scarred veins fade within weeks, although the procedure may need to be repeated. Laser surgery can also destroy veins without an incision. Or a small tube can be placed into a vein to destroy it with heat. In severe cases, varicose veins can be removed surgically (a procedure called *stripping*). No matter what procedure is used, other veins take over to bring blood from the legs back to the heart.

Hemorrhoids

Hemorrhoids are the most common problem of the anal area, and Americans spend over $100 million annually on over-the-counter medications to relieve their symptoms. *Hemorrhoids* are swollen and distended blood vessels clustered just beneath the mucous membranes lining the lowest part of the rectum and the anus. They may be internal (in the lower rectum) or external (under the skin around the anus). Internal hemorrhoids cannot be seen or even felt because they are inside the rectum. Occasionally internal hemorrhoids become so enlarged that they protrude through the anal opening. External hemorrhoids are visible around the anal opening. They may fill with blood and become engorged, painful, or itchy. Hemorrhoids may occasionally bleed, causing streaks of bright red blood on the stool after straining.

Hemorrhoids have many possible causes. The condition is related to chronic constipation, straining during bowel movements, and prolonged sitting on the toilet. Individuals who must sit or stand for long periods are at increased risk. The best prevention is to reduce constipation by eating a high-fiber diet, engaging in physical exercise, and going to the toilet when the urge to defecate occurs.

There are several treatments for hemorrhoids. The least invasive is the application of ointments to the anal area to decrease pain, itching, and irritation. These may contain a local anesthetic or numbing agent (e.g., xylocaine), a steroid cream (e.g., hydrocortisone), or lubricating agents. Witch hazel also reduces the symptoms, and soaks in the tub can provide relief. Internal hemorrhoids can be pushed back into the anus to reduce pain and discomfort. A diet high in fiber or the use of a bulk laxative and stool softeners can reduce irritation from hemorrhoids associated with hard bowel movements (see Box 5.2). Weight loss, regular exercise, responding to the urge to defecate, and increased fluid intake are also helpful.

Internal hemorrhoids may be tied off at their base with elastic bands until they eventually fall off. Hemorrhoids may also be destroyed by chemicals, light, electric current, or laser. However, there is no guarantee they will not return. If the hemorrhoids are persistent or large, the veins may be cut out surgically.

UROGENITAL DISORDERS

Older adults are at greater risk than younger adults for a number of chronic problems of the urinary and genital systems. Kidney failure, enlarged prostate, and urinary incontinence are the most prominent. Although both kidney failure and urinary incontinence may also occur as emergencies, they are more likely to be chronic in nature.

Kidney/Renal Disease

The main functions of the kidneys are to cleanse, filter, and purify the blood, and to produce the waste product, urine. The kidneys need blood to do their job effectively, and they become damaged if their blood supply is too weak (e.g., from heart failure) or too strong (e.g., from hypertension). In addition, the kidneys are very sensitive to the chemicals and hormones circulating in the body and can be injured by antibiotics, toxins, or prolonged high levels of hormones. Kidney failure, also called renal failure, can be sudden (acute), such as might occur after an auto accident when there is no blood to the kidney, or gradual (chronic).

Acute kidney failure (acute renal failure) causes fluid retention and swelling, internal bleeding, confusion, seizures, and coma. It is a life-threatening emergency that needs immediate hospital-level treatment. Many times, acute kidney failure is reversible. Therapy is aimed at treating the injury or illness that damaged the kidneys and supporting the body until the kidneys can heal. Some people need to be hooked onto a kidney dialysis machine that cleans the blood for days to months; others may improve on their own. Often the kidneys are damaged and are susceptible to further injury.

In contrast to acute kidney failure, *chronic kidney/renal disease* usually develops slowly, with few signs or symptoms in the early stages. Many people with chronic kidney disease don't realize they have a problem until their kidney function has decreased significantly. High blood pressure and diabetes are the most common causes of chronic kidney disease. In addition, long-term use of medications, particularly pain medications and some antibiotics, can increase the risk. Over time, chronic kidney disease can lead to congestive heart failure, weak bones, stomach ulcers, and damage to the central nervous system.

According to the National Health and Nutrition Examination Survey, over 40 percent of elders have chronic kidney disease. Many of these individuals have *renal insufficiency:* They may feel fine, but blood tests reveal that the body is not adequately filtering the blood. These people are very vulnerable. If they develop an infection, or take certain medications, or have other health problems, they may develop *end-stage renal disease,*

in which the kidneys are working at less than 10 percent of normal capacity. At this point, the body cannot function. To stay alive, people with end-stage renal disease need either dialysis or a kidney transplant.

Chronic kidney disease has no cure, but treatment can help control symptoms, reduce complications, and slow the progress of the disease. The first priority is controlling the condition responsible for kidney disease and its complications. Those with diabetes or high blood pressure (hypertension) need to keep their blood sugar and blood pressure under control through medications, diet, and exercise. Those with kidney disease need to follow a special diet low in protein, salt, potassium, and phosphorus. By the time end-stage renal disease develops, dietary measures are no longer enough: The kidneys cannot support life on their own, and dialysis or a kidney transplant become the only options.

Dialysis is an artificial means of removing waste products and extra fluid from the bloodstream when the kidneys are unable to filter the blood and produce urine. It is not a cure, but it may be the only option to remain alive. Dialysis is a significant hassle. At least three times a week the person has to sit for hours at a dialysis clinic while the blood is being filtered, or multiple daily treatments are done in the home. Surgery is required to insert devices to enable the dialysis machine to be used. People with end-stage renal disease experience many complications, particularly infections. The patient experiences discomfort as waste products and fluid build up in the body.

For those who are otherwise healthy, a kidney transplant may provide a better quality of life, but many more people need a kidney than there are donors to provide one. The donor can be living or dead but must be a good match, having cell proteins that match those of the patient. A sibling is likely to be the best donor, or another blood relative may give up a kidney. If there are no suitable or willing relatives, a kidney from an accident victim or individual who has just died may be used.

What Is Your Opinion?
Should there be an age limit on dialysis treatment?

The use of dialysis for individuals who are very old raises many ethical issues. Since so many younger individuals are awaiting transplants, should elders have the same opportunity as younger people to have a transplant? Should taxpayer dollars fund dialysis for everyone who needs it? What if they damaged their kidneys due to failing to care for themselves or poor habits like drugs? What if they are demented, more than 80 years old, or frail and ill? When should dialysis be discontinued? If a person on dialysis develops other debilitating diseases, should dialysis be continued? Who should decide whether someone gets dialysis: The person who needs it? His or her family? The physician? The insurance company? The government? Taxpayers?

Urinary Incontinence

Urinary incontinence—the inability to control urination—ranges from the occasional passing of a few drops of urine while sneezing to the inability to control the voiding of urine at all times. The National Association for Continence (www.nafc.org) estimates that 25 million adult Americans experience transient or chronic urinary incontinence. The prevalence of urinary incontinence increases with age. Women are much more likely to become incontinent than men. As expected, the percentage of individuals who are incontinent is high in hospitals and nursing homes. More than half of all nursing home residents have some degree of incontinence, and incontinence is a common reason for placement in a nursing home.

Causes of incontinence include neurological problems that affect the central nervous system (such as strokes, dementia, or spinal injuries), medication side effects, infection of the genital or urinary system, and weakening of the pelvic muscles from childbirth. The National Association for Continence asserts that about 80 percent of those with incontinence can be cured or improved. However, too few people are evaluated, particularly those who are demented and institutionalized. The patient may be embarrassed to bring the topic up, or the physician is reluctant to broach it. Physicians should evaluate and treat all patients with incontinence because its physiological and psychosocial effects are serious.

There are various types of incontinence, each with different causes and treatments:

- *Stress incontinence* occurs when abdominal pressure, caused by coughing, sneezing, laughing, or jumping, triggers leakage of urine. It is commonly due to weakness of the muscles supporting the bladder and urethra. This predominantly occurs in women and is caused by childbirth, estrogen deficiency, or previous pelvic surgery.
- *Urge incontinence* occurs when an individual suddenly feels the urge to urinate but cannot wait long enough to reach the toilet. Local irritation or infection or neurological problems, commonly occurring in dementia and stroke, can trigger involuntary bladder contractions and cause leakage. Urge incontinence may be the consequence of an overactive bladder—a bladder that is very sensitive to urine and frequently contracts, causing an intense need to urinate. People with an overactive bladder have to urinate more than eight times a day and more than twice at night.
- *Overflow incontinence* occurs when a person's bladder fills to capacity and a small amount of urine flows out even though the individual does not feel an urge to urinate. The most common cause of overflow incontinence is prostate enlargement. Other causes include nerve injury and medication use.

- *Functional incontinence* occurs when a continent elderly person is unable or unwilling to urinate normally. Causes might be mobility impairment, use of sedative medication, or psychological disturbances.

Many elders have *mixed* incontinence, particularly a combination of urge and stress incontinence. Because incontinence is a symptom of a disease, not a disease in itself, the treatment selected is dependent on the diagnosis. A variety of treatments are available.

Scheduling a trip to the toilet every two to three hours reduces accidents, particularly in the hospital and nursing home. People generally urinate when they arise and after meals, but the schedule can be individualized based on normal habits and drinking patterns.

Kegel exercises are known to reduce or eliminate stress incontinence (and fecal incontinence) by strengthening the pelvic floor muscles to improve the function of the sphincter muscles that control the flow of urine (see Box 5.3). Avoiding alcohol, caffeine, or carbonated beverages may also help. Other supportive measures include having accessible toilets and avoiding excessive sedation. All prescription and over-the counter medications should be assessed by a pharmacist to ensure that urgency of urination is not a side effect.

Various devices are available to delay urine flow. Urethral tampon-like devices can be worn and removed when urination is desired, and vaginal inserts called pessaries can help reduce stress incontinence. Nerve stimulation of the pelvic nerves or the tibial nerves in the leg can be used to improve muscle control of urination.

For patients who never regain continence, catheters or disposable underpants are the major means of management. Catheters, tubes inserted through the urethra and into the neck of the bladder, allow the urine in the bladder to be drained. Elders can learn to catheterize themselves every few hours rather than have a permanent catheter that drains into a bag. Occasionally catheters are placed through the abdomen. Because catheters provide a direct route for bacteria to get into the bladder, individual using catheters have a high rate of urinary tract infections.

If other treatments do not work, surgical procedures are available. The "sling" procedure lifts the urethra, creating a narrower passage that helps it to close. Newer procedures include collagen injections around the urethra to help it to close, implantation of an artificial urinary sphincter, and implantation of an electrical device that stimulates the sacral nerve to fire, contracting the urethral sphincter.

Urinary incontinence has widespread social and psychological implications for elders and those

---

B O X 5 . 3

Kegel Exercises

Kegel exercises are effective in reducing or eliminating stress incontinence in both men and women. It is important to use the proper technique and to be consistent in performing the exercises three times a day.

To locate the pelvic floor muscles, it is recommended that the individual sit on the toilet, begin to urinate, then try to stop the flow by contracting the pelvic floor muscles. The exercise should be repeated until the person is familiar with the feel of contracting the correct muscle group. The abdomen, thigh, or buttocks muscles should *not* contract. After someone learns how to contract the pelvic floor muscles, the exercises can be done anywhere. The bladder should be empty.

Tighten the pelvic floor muscles and hold for a count of 10. Then release completely for another count of 10. Do 10 repetitions of tightening and releasing three times each day (morning, afternoon, and night). Some individuals notice an improvement in four weeks. Others may see no improvement for as many as three months.

around them. In our culture, the act of urination is considered a private activity. Any loss of continence in public is considered socially unacceptable and may be cause for worry, embarrassment, chastisement, or ostracism. Because urinary incontinence is difficult to manage at home, it plays a role in the decision to place an elder in a nursing home. Some nursing homes refuse incontinent applicants because of the increased workload they generate. The costs of labor, laundry, and supplies used to manage incontinence and its complications contribute significantly to the growing costs of nursing home care. Because of its wide-ranging physical, psychological, and social effects, every effort should be made to treat this disorder.

Enlarged Prostate

With age, almost all men experience *benign prostatic hyperplasia (BPH),* a gradual enlargement of the prostate gland. Half have an enlarged prostate by age 60, about 90 percent by age 85. Because the prostate surrounds the urethra, its growth often compresses the urethra, producing a host of urinary symptoms. However, only some men with BPH have symptoms.

The most common symptoms of BPH are that it takes longer to start urination and the force of the urinary stream lessens. Further, there is increased frequency, dribbling of urine after urination, and an inability to fully empty the bladder despite an increased urge to urinate. Men may feel they must "bear down" to urinate. Because many need to use the toilet every two hours, sleep is disturbed. Urine remains in the bladder after urination, increasing the risk of urinary tract infections.

Symptoms of an enlarged prostate develop gradually and though bothersome are not life threatening. Certain medications may cause urinary retention (e.g., many over-the-counter cold medications,

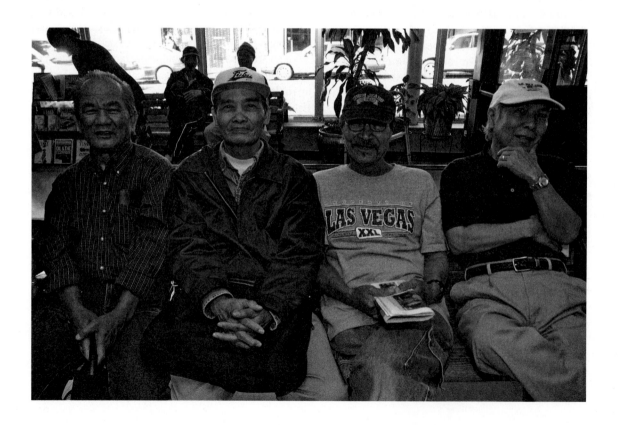

pain medications, antidepressants) and should be avoided. Alcohol, caffeine, and carbonated beverages also should be avoided.

BPH can be diagnosed by means of a medical history, a rectal examination, lab tests of kidney function and urine, and a testing of the flow of urine. A test called "postvoid residual" uses a catheter or ultrasound machine to check how much urine is left in the bladder after urinating. Sometimes a catheter is inserted into the bladder after voiding to determine whether urine is remaining in the bladder.

An enlarged prostate requires treatment only if the patient is suffering urinary blockage, urinary tract infections, or damage to the urinary system from the prostate. Medications (e.g., Proscar) are available that slightly shrink the prostate and allow easier passage of urine, but they are not very effective in reducing other symptoms. Another type of drug relaxes the smooth muscles of the bladder and the urethra, allowing the urine to pass more freely.

Surgical treatment is offered to men whose symptoms disrupt their lifestyle. The most common operation for an enlarged prostate is a *transurethral resection of the prostate* (TURP). A small loop is inserted through the penis, and the part of the prostate causing the obstruction is scraped to widen the urethra. This procedure can be done on an outpatient basis, is relatively low risk, and has few side effects. However, not all men experience relief after surgery, and most have "retrograde ejaculation"—the passing of semen into the bladder during ejaculation. Also, the prostate tissue may grow back. Up to 20 percent of the operations must be repeated. TURP is the second most common surgical procedure (after cataract surgery) covered by Medicare.

A more radical surgery that is less commonly used for an enlarged prostate is a prostatectomy, removal of the entire prostate through the abdomen. This operation has more side effects than TURP and requires a longer convalescence. The effects of prostate surgery on erectile function are discussed in Chapter 11, "Sexuality."

If surgery is not an option, an indwelling urinary catheter or self-catheterization when needed is recommended in some cases. An indwelling catheter is kept in the bladder, and a bag attached to the leg collects the urine and is emptied a few times a day. The catheter can be changed at home by a nurse or in the physician's office. Another alternative is catheterization only when needed. In this treatment, the man inserts a straight tube into the urethra to the bladder and drains off the urine every few hours. Catheterization used on demand is less likely to cause infection than indwelling catheterization, but it requires more work and may not be possible if the prostate is very large. Another alternative to surgery is dilation of the urethra with a balloon catheter, similar to the one used to widen blood vessels. Although symptoms may recur faster than with surgery, this procedure is simple and effective.

SKIN CONDITIONS

Older people are susceptible to the same skin disorders as younger groups. Senile pruritis and skin cancer, however, are more common in the later years.

Senile Pruritis

Senile pruritis (literally "itching in old persons") is the most common skin condition of elders. Pruritis is caused by a great number of factors and varies widely in severity. The disorder may cause mild discomfort, or it may cause acute mental distress.

The most common reason for itching is skin dryness. In addition to itching, the skin looks abnormally dry and may be cracked in a grid pattern, often with skin scaling. Frequent bathing and use of hot water are not recommended. Treatment consists of lukewarm baths with minimal soaping followed by application of an oil-based moisturizer while the skin is still wet. Aloe vera gel may also be effective. Topical and oral medications to treat itching are also available over the counter and by prescription.

In as many as half of all elders, there is an underlying cause for the itching. Pruritis may be caused by lice or mite infestation; fungus; an allergic reaction; emotional upset and tension; drug reaction; or a chronic disease such as diabetes, kidney disease, liver disease, or cancer. Because itching may be a symptom of other medical conditions besides simple dry skin, a medical evaluation should be conducted to rule out other possibilities.

Elders may have chronic lower extremity swelling and poor circulation leading to a condition called stasis dermatitis. The skin of the legs is red, may be weepy wet, and may have less hair growth. This is treated with topical moisturizers and stockings, wraps, and elevation of the legs to reduce the swelling.

Skin Cancer

Skin cancer is the most common type of cancer with more than three million new cases occurring annually in the United States. There are threee main types: basal cell cancer, squamous cell cancer, and melanoma. Basal cell cancers are by far the most common (80 percent of all skin cancers), followed by squamous cell cancers (15 percent), melanoma (4 percent) and unusual skin cancers (1 percent). Despite the high incidence of skin cancers, the vast majority are highly curable. Melanoma is the most deadly. Even though melanoma comprises less than 5 percent of all skin cancers, it is responsible for almost three-fourths of all cancer deaths.[4]

In general, the incidence of skin cancers increases with advancing age because these cancers are related to total lifetime sun exposure. These skin cancers are usually diagnosed after age 60. Ultraviolet light damages the skin's genetic material and increases the likelihood of skin tumors. People who are at high risk for skin cancer are those who have endured much sun exposure and have blue eyes and light skin. Skin cancers are on the rise in the United States and now appear at younger ages. This increase is blamed on increased sun exposure through tanning and depletion of the protective ozone layer that filters ultraviolet light.

Basal and squamous skin cancers are most common among whites and are generally located on the face, eyelid, scalp, forearm, or shoulder.

Forty percent of these cancers start on or inside the ears. *Basal cell cancers* are limited to hair-bearing areas (e.g., scalp, face, back). They appear as flat, firm, pale areas or as small raised pink or red shiny waxy areas that may bleed from injury. In contrast, *squamous cell cancers* are common in sun-exposed areas but may occur anywhere on the skin, including the mucous membranes. They appear as growing lumps, sometimes with a rough surface, or as flat reddish patches that grow slowly. Squamous cell cancers are much more lethal than basal cell cancers.

Basal and squamous skin cancers grow slowly and are almost always curable by simple procedures. Basal and squamous cancers and precancerous growths known as actinic keratoses generally are removed in the physician's office by burning and scraping, by freezing with liquid nitrogen, or by being dissolved with a laser. They may also be treated at home with chemical ointments. People with skin cancer or precancerous lesions are advised to protect their skin from further sun damage and to use broad-spectrum sunscreens.

Although not common, *melanoma* is the most serious skin cancer because it is capable of metastasizing and causing death in a relatively short period of time. Melanoma primarily occurs among whites; it is 10 times more common in whites than in blacks. Among the elder population, its incidence is twice as common in men as women.[6] People at highest risk for melanoma have a large number of brown moles (50 or more); have fair skin, freckles and blond or red hair; have a history of severe sunburn as a child or adolescent; or have lived or vacationed in sunny climates.

Symptoms of melanoma include a noticeable change on the skin, either a new spot or one changing in size, shape, and color. Melanomas appear most often on the lower legs and feet in women and the trunk in men, although they may occur on the face, on the nails, or in the mouth. The lesions usually start as small, dark molelike growths that increase in size, change color, become ulcerated, and bleed with slight injury. A molelike lesion that changes size, has irregular borders, is multicolored, is surrounded by reddened skin, becomes softer or harder, or is associated with pain or itchiness should be checked by a physician. To help you remember the appearance of melanoma, the letters ABCD are used: **A**symmetry, irregular **B**order, uneven **C**olor, and **D**iameter greater than 6 mm.

Treatment for melanoma is to remove all parts of the growth as soon as possible. In advanced cases, a nearby lymph node is removed to determine if the cancer has spread. Removed tissue is examined under a microscope. Advanced cases are treated with chemotherapy or therapy to increase the immune system defenses. However, once melanoma spreads, it is usually fatal.

Individuals who have any risk factors should thoroughly and regularly check their skin for suspicious moles. There is controversy regarding whether sunscreens are effective at preventing melanoma. Sunscreens may incompletely protect against damage and provide a sense of false security, although newer broad-spectrum sunscreens may be helpful. Experts recommend sun-protective clothing such as broad-brimmed hats and long sleeves. The American Academy of Dermatology maintains a Web site (www.skincarephysicians.com) that provides information and resources related to skin cancer, including photos of each type of skin cancer.

NEUROLOGICAL DISORDERS

In this section we present three chronic neurological disorders that are more likely to appear in older people than those under 65: Parkinson's disease, dizziness, and tinnitus. Alzheimer's disease, a neurological disorder that reduces cognitive function, is discussed in Chapter 7, "Mental Health and Mental Disorders."

Parkinson's Disease

Parkinson's disease is caused by a shortage of a particular neurotransmitter, dopamine, in the nerve cells in the part of the brain controlling muscle movement. The disease begins gradually but almost always becomes disabling over a period of years. Approximately 3 percent of the elder population has the disorder. Symptoms generally include involuntary shaking of the extremities (tremors), which occurs at rest; slowness in movement; body rigidity; a mask-like facial expression; and speech and gait disturbances. Some people with Parkinson's disease develop slowed thought processes and dementia.

Parkinson's disease is more common with advancing age, and men are more likely affected than women. There is at least some genetic component and some association with pesticide exposure, but these effects are small.

The symptoms of early Parkinson's disease are treated with lifestyle modifications. A high-fiber diet prevents the constipation that accompanies the disorder. Exercise and physical therapy can help people with Parkinson's disease by improving their ability to walk, increasing their range of motion, muscle tone, and strength, and improving balance and thereby reducing falls. Speech therapy can improve the quality of speech and ability to swallow.

The drug levodopa, commonly known as L-dopa, has been used for decades to replace the dopamine in the nerve cells of the brains of individuals with Parkinson's disease because it effectively reduces the symptoms. But L-dopa can cause side effects, and it becomes less effective as the disease worsens. For that reason newer drugs are used, generally alone or in combination with levodopa. Some of these drugs work by extending the effectiveness of L-dopa in the brain; others work more directly on the dopamine nerve receptors or slow the breakdown of L-dopa. Many of the drugs used to treat Parkinson's disease cause side effects such as hallucinations, dry mouth, sedation, and confusion.

Another treatment that has had encouraging results is deep brain stimulation (DBS). A brain stimulator, similar to a heart pacemaker, is implanted in certain areas of the brain. For some people, DBS controls symptoms so well that medications can be greatly reduced. Surgery on the brain is an option for some individuals when symptoms cannot be controlled by medications.

Essential Tremor

When a person's hands tremble with movement but not at rest, the culprit is generally not Parkinson's disease but *essential tremor,* a benign condition that becomes more common in advanced age. The hands tremble about six to ten times a minute. The trembling may start in the dominant hand (the one used for writing) then spread to the other hand, the head, or the voice. Tremor of the head (in a yes-yes or no-no motion) is also common. At times, the symptoms are mild and not bothersome, but they can become so severe that they interfere with activities of daily living. This tremor runs in families and decreases after alcohol ingestion. Drugs are available to control the symptoms (some beta blockers and anticonvulsants). Rarely is surgery needed.

Dizziness

Dizziness is a common nonspecific complaint that can have a myriad of causes. Serious illnesses, medication reaction, dehydration, infections, and other conditions may cause dizziness. Elders with persistent dizziness should visit a physician because a thorough exam often reveals its cause.

Vertigo is a particular type of dizziness characterized by a sensation of movement felt in the head—the room seems to be spinning. A common cause is a viral infection that has disturbed the balance mechanism of the inner ear. Vertigo may also occur as a side effect of medication or injury to the head. In contrast, *disequilibrium* causes unsteadiness in the body, not the head. The individual may feel he or she is about to faint. This sensation could be caused by low blood pressure or a medication side effect.

One type of vertigo is *benign positional vertigo.* Some people develop short episodes of vertigo, lasting less than a minute, after changing the position of the head. This is thought to be caused by tiny granules of calcium that build up in the semicircular canals of the inner ear. Although the problem is temporary, it can be disabling and unpleasant.

Treatment is accomplished by a 5- to 10-minute repositioning procedure (called the Epley maneuver) that involves moving the head and body through a series of positions to restore the calcium granules to their normal position. These simple movements reposition the granules and provide permanent relief. Fortunately, symptoms of benign positional vertigo usually subside in two to three months, even without treatment.

Not all causes of dizziness are neurological. Dizziness can be due to sudden drops in blood pressure, to medication side effects, and to panic or anxiety reactions. *Orthostatic* or *postural hypotension* is a sudden, temporary drop of blood pressure that occurs on rising from a sitting or lying position. It results in light-headedness or dizziness. Some drop in blood pressure on rising is normal because gravity causes blood to flow away from the head, but if it commonly occurs, the cause should be determined by a physician. This condition is very common, affecting one-third to one-half of elders. It often lasts just seconds and resolves. It is easy to diagnose—just take the blood pressure and heart rate when lying, sitting, and standing and compare the measurements. If low blood pressure persists, this needs to be evaluated. Sitting up in bed before attempting to stand allows the body to acclimate to an upright position and reduces the risk of falls.

Medication side effects are the greatest cause of orthostatic hypotension, particularly from high blood pressure drugs, diuretics, and some types of antidepressants. Dehydration may also be to blame. Although orthostatic hypotension is not dangerous in itself, it can result in a loss of balance that may lead to falls. The condition can be easily remedied by changing medication type, adjusting dosage and timing, drinking more fluids, and avoiding sudden changes in posture. Further, learning to respond to the first sign of dizziness by sitting down will reduce fall risk.

Light-headedness, sometimes accompanied by heart palpitations and panic, might occur during stressful circumstances. Many people can induce this state by breathing deeply and rapidly for a few minutes (hyperventilating). Hyperventilation triggered by anxiety or depression may be the underlying cause of many patients' complaints of dizziness.

Tinnitus

Tinnitus is described as a roaring or ringing in the ears when no external physical sound is present.

Most people experience tinnitus occasionally, but some experience an incessant ringing or buzzing. For some, tinnitus is only a nuisance, but it can be so severe that it interferes with the ability to hear, sleep, and work. Tinnitus increases with advancing age.

The most common cause of tinnitus is exposure to excessively loud noise. However, there are many other causes, including medical conditions (hypertension, ear infection, nutritional deficiency) and obstruction of the ear canal with wax. Tinnitus also may be a side effect of medication, such as aspirin. It can worsen with loud noises, caffeine, nicotine, excessive alcohol, and stress.

The first line of treatment should be to improve the underlying medical condition, if possible. Other treatments include medications, stress-reduction techniques, and masking units, which create neutral noise to block out the tinnitus. Medications, such as antidepressants, anticonvulsants, anti-anxiety agents, and antihistamines can be helpful. Masking devices that create white noise may be helpful in blocking out the ringing noise. Techniques to control stress, such as biofeedback and relaxation exercises, may also help. In many areas, support groups are available to help sufferers cope with their symptoms.

VISION DISORDERS

Vision impairment and blindness are leading causes of disability in our country. Both have a profound effect on the ability to perform daily activities and result in a decreased quality of life. In this section we explore three disorders that significantly impair vision and become more prevalent with advanced age: cataracts, glaucoma, and macular degeneration. Diabetic retinopathy, a complication of diabetes that gradually deteriorates visual acuity, even causing blindness, is mentioned in the previous chapter. Presbyopia, an age-associated change, is described in Chapter 3.

Cataracts

Cataracts are considered to be the leading cause of *reversible* blindness in the United States. In our country, more than three-fourths of all adults over 60 have some degree of cataract formation. Cataracts are related to age: The older someone is, the more likely he or she is to have them. Women are more likely than men to have cataracts, and blacks are more likely than whites to have them. Diabetes, cigarette smoking, alcohol use, some medications, and sun exposure can cause or accelerate cataract formation.

A cataract is the consequence of gradual changes that occur in the lens of the eye. It thickens, yellows, clouds, and becomes less elastic, and the amount of light that can pass through it is reduced. Although any clouding of the lens is considered to be a cataract, it may or may not impair vision. Some individuals are unaware that they have a cataract; others are unable to enjoy activities of daily living such as reading, driving, and watching television. When cataracts interfere with daily activities, surgery is usually recommended.

Cataract surgery is the most frequently performed operation in the United States. It takes less than an hour, and almost all procedures are done on an outpatient basis. The operation improves vision in the vast majority of cases, and complications are rare. If both eyes need surgery, they are done at separate times. Cataract surgery has become quite sophisticated, and procedures vary. The lens is removed from the lens capsule, and an artificial lens—a plastic disk—is implanted in its place. After surgery, some patients need to wear glasses or contacts for optimal vision. Not only is vision improved with cataract surgery; most elders also report an enhanced quality of life.

Factors other than poor vision affect the likelihood of undergoing cataract surgery. It is documented that race, gender, geographic location, and type of medical reimbursement plan play a role. For instance, women are more likely than men to undergo the surgery, and whites are more likely than blacks. Since blacks are four times more likely to become blind from cataracts, this disparity is of special concern. Nursing home residents are more likely to have untreated cataracts, perhaps because they are thought too frail to bene-fit from the surgery. However, cataract surgery should be considered as it can significantly im-prove quality of life.

Glaucoma

Glaucoma is a disease characterized by increased pressure within the eyeball due to a buildup of flu-ids. Because the drainage system for optical fluids is blocked, or because excessive fluid is produced, pressure builds up and progressively deteriorates receptor cells in the retina and the optic nerve. Ultimately, untreated glaucoma results in vision loss. It is a leading cause of *irreversible* blindness among older people.

Acute glaucoma comes on suddenly with nausea, vomiting, and eye pain. Much more com-monly, glaucoma comes on gradually, affecting peripheral vision first. Glaucoma is often called the "sneak thief of sight" because the vision loss is so subtle that significant damage may occur be-fore glaucoma is diagnosed. Headaches, blurred vision, and the appearance of halos or rainbows around lights are signs of glaucoma. African Americans, people who have a family history of glaucoma, or people who are diabetic, hyperten-sive, or anemic are at increased risk.

There is no cure for glaucoma, but eye drops eliminate pressure buildup or encourage drainage. These medications are recommended to be contin-ued for life, although many elders have difficulty adhering to the regimen.

Treatments include laser therapy to enlarge the drainage channel and ultrasound to create small holes in the eyeball to reduce pressure buildup. The elderly should be regularly screened for glaucoma (see Chapter 12).

Macular Degeneration

Age-related *macular degeneration* is a chronic eye disorder that deteriorates the part of the retina (macular area) that is responsible for cen-tral vision. The disease can cause blurred vision,

even a blind spot, in the center of what we see. People who have the disorder may complain that the shape of objects seems distorted or that they are unable to see fine detail. Much of what we do requires central vision: reading, driving, watch-ing TV, doing detail work, and recognizing faces.

There are two types of age-related macular degeneration: dry and wet. The *dry form* is the more common and is related to the aging process. When the central part of the retina (the macula) does not get supplied with enough nutrients, the cells are damaged. This results in blurring and blind spots in the center of the visual field. In contrast, the *wet form* is less common, but causes more blindness. The wet form is caused by new blood vessels growing from underneath the retina, leaking blood, and causing rapid and se-vere deterioration of vision.

There is still much to learn about the causes of macular degeneration, but we know that age, race, and family history play a role. Women, indi-viduals with blue eyes, members of the white race, and smokers are at higher risk. There is some evidence that sunlight exposure increases the risk of macular degeneration and that supple-ments of antioxidants, zinc, and copper may reduce the risk or slow the progression of the disease.

Special low-vision aids such as magnifying eyeglasses help elders with macular degeneration. Other helpful strategies are to install bright lights in their homes and to increase light-dark contrast—for example, by placing dark furniture against white walls.

There is no recommended treatment for age-related macular degeneration. Laser therapy to seal off leaky blood vessels can be used only in the early stages to prevent further vision loss. How-ever, many people cannot undergo the procedure, and only about a third of those who do are perma-nently cured. The drug verteporphin slows vision loss and even restores some lost vision among a small percentage of people with age-related macu-lar degeneration.

Web Resources

There are many excellent sites where you can learn more about the diseases presented in this book. The National Institutes of Health Web site (www.health/nih.gov). NIH also offers a site specifically for older people, providing information on selected diseases and much other health information. The site allows the user to click for large print, more contrast, and sound (www.nihseniorhealth.gov).

The National Institutes of Health and the National Library of Medicine support Medline, an online service that enables professionals to access abstracts of articles from professional refereed journals (www.pubmed.gov). Access can be by author, keyword, or journal. Those agencies also support MedlinePlus, a less technical source of health information (www.medlineplus.gov).

The Mayo Clinic has an extensive Web site of accurate medical information that includes symptoms, causes, mainstream and alternative treatments, and prognosis in easily understandable language (www.mayoclinic.com).

Many organizations and foundations focus on particular diseases and can be accessed by keying in the disease and perusing the sites. Sites with an *org* or *gov* suffix are generally the most dependable.

SUMMARY

Rarely does anyone get through old age without at least one chronic disease, and many older people have several. The symptoms of chronic diseases worsen over time and cannot be cured. However, treatments are available to reduce the symptoms and in many cases delay progression of the disease. This chapter describes the many chronic diseases that commonly appear in the later years. Some may cause only a minor limitation of daily routine while others may be disabling. Lifestyle factors are prominent in the development and treatment of most of the illnesses explored in this (and the previous) chapter.

The most effective way to prevent or reduce the progression of the majority of them is through a lifelong effort to improve health habits. Unfortunately, for many, both young and old, the benefits of a healthy lifestyle are too distant and the short-term costs too great.

The information presented here is intended to educate individuals who work with elders about the chronic diseases that their clients might have, so that they can serve them effectively. Even more important, this information may motivate individuals with poor health habits to improve them before a chronic illness develops.

ACTIVITIES

1. Create a case study of an older individual who has a chronic health problem. Include the impact of the disease on the overall quality of the person's life. Be sure to include psychological, social, and economic effects. Assuming the individual in the case has a spouse, describe the impact on that family member.

2. After studying the common chronic health problems of elders, make a list of the diseases that you will likely have to deal with as you grow older, either because of heredity or because of

your current health behaviors. Be complete. Remember that many chronic diseases and conditions are extremely common. What might you do to prevent or reduce the impact of one or more of them? Are you trying to modify any dubious habits? If so, which ones? If not, discuss the factors keeping you from doing so.

3. Visit the campus library and peruse recent medical journals. Choose an article that presents new information on some aspect of a common disease

of elders. Write a brief summary of the findings, and discuss the implications of this new information on the outcome of the disease and its effect on the individual.

4. Read the health section of your local newspaper, and cut out an article describing a new treatment for a particular chronic illness. Bring the article to class for discussion. Compare the newspaper article with the article in the professional journal from which the news article is based. How do the two differ?

5. Interview a family member who has a vision loss. How does the loss affect his or her lifestyle? How has this person compensated for the loss?

6. Develop a list of resources for visually impaired elders and their families in your community. Go to the local library to find the resources offered for the visually impaired.

7. Collect fliers, booklets, brochures, and newsletters geared for elder use, and analyze the suitability of paper color, typeface, content, and layout. Ask several older people which items they find easiest to read.

8. Choose one chronic disease and view at least five reputable Web sites (with the suffixes *.org, .edu,* and *.gov*) offering information about it. Which site is the best and why?

BIBLIOGRAPHY

1. Mortality and Morbidity Weekly Report. 2010. Prevalence of doctor-diagnosed arthritis and arthritis-attributable to activity limitation—United States, 2007–2009. 59(39):1261–1265.

2. Institute of Medicine. 2010. Dietary reference intakes for calcium and vitamin D. Washington DC: Food and Nutrition Board.

3. Lembo, A., and Camilleri, M. 2003. Chronic constipation. *New England Journal of Medicine* 249(14):1360–1368.

4. American Cancer Society. 2011. *Cancer facts and figures 2011.* Atlanta, GA: American Cancer Society.

Acute Illnesses and Accidents

Age seldom arrives smoothly or quickly. It's more often a succession of jerks.

Jean Rhys

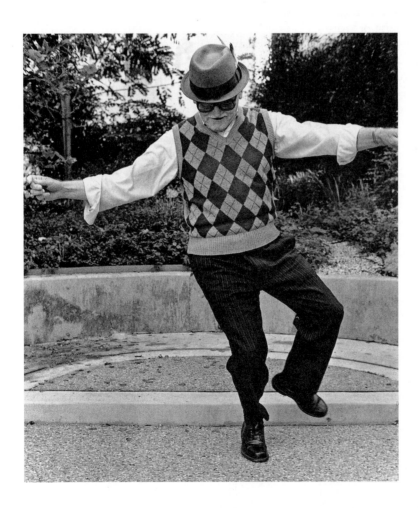

Long-standing chronic illnesses account for the largest proportion of death and disability among elders. However, acute illnesses and accidents are also responsible for a significant amount. For example, pneumonia, an acute respiratory infection, is the seventh leading cause of death among older people, and accidents—including falls, car and pedestrian accidents, and burns—are the ninth most common cause of death. Acute illnesses and accidents are major reasons for hospital admissions and consequently are a major part of health care expenses for those 65 and older. This chapter provides information about the acute illnesses that commonly appear in older people, including the cause, treatment, and prevention of each.

Acute illnesses have a rapid onset, are short-term, are generally caused by bacteria or viruses, and generally the individual recovers completely. For a number of reasons, frail elders are more likely to suffer complications from an infection than their healthier cohorts. In this chapter we explore the most common acute conditions among older people, including infections and conditions induced by temperature extremes.

Accidents, also called *unintentional injuries,* cause significant disability and death among the older population. Older people are more prone to accidents, take longer to recover, and are more likely to die from them. Old age in itself is not the reason for increased accidents; many other factors increase susceptibility among older people. This chapter addresses the common types of accidents among elders, factors that increase susceptibility to accidents, and suggestions to prevent accidents.

ACUTE ILLNESSES IN ELDERS

In younger populations, a pneumonia begins with a cough, a urinary tract infection begins with urinary discomfort of burning or frequency—the symptoms experienced by the illness guide the individual and the doctor toward the correct treatment. In elders, especially those with underlying conditions or those who take multiple medications, the "presentation" of illness is often vague and nonspecific, which makes it more difficult for elders, caregivers, and health care professionals to know what exactly is wrong.

Acute illnesses in the older population often begin with subtle, nonspecific symptoms, such as feeling more tired than usual, feeling a little groggy or confused, having a reduced appetite, even an incident of incontinence. These symptoms can occur whether the elder has a bladder infection, pneumonia, heart failure, or a medication side effect. An elder or the family may miss these symptoms, attributing them to "overexerting themselves" or "just being tired." Ideally, the person recognizes the symptoms, seeks medical attention, the problem is identified, and treatment is initiated.

If vague symptoms are ignored, a cascade of events may occur that lead to a life-threatening emergency. For instance, lack of interest in eating and drinking, fever, an increased rate of breathing, or diarrhea can lead to dehydration. Medication levels build up in the bloodstream—the medications can cause more toxic effects. Blood pressure drops and heart rate rises. The increased heart rate adds stress to the body and can lead to risk of heart attack or arrythmia. The lowered blood pressure causes dizziness, increasing the risk of falls. The dehydration leads to more confusion, perhaps to nausea and even less fluid intake. At this point, an elder may begin to show worsening signs of cognitive troubles—confusion, forgetfulness, lethargy, or perhaps becoming agitated. As the cascade continues, an elder is at higher risk of a fall. In addition, reduced physical activity may promote deconditioning or the development of sores or pressure ulcers. Functional status begins to decline, and a person is less able to complete the necessary activities of daily living. Again, in most elders, this cascade is reversible. If the underlying problem is treated and secondary dehydration is corrected, the elder may be able to return to previous levels of functioning.

As symptoms worsen, a condition called delirium can result. Delirium is a relatively sudden onset of confusion, causing agitation, poor attention span, and insomnia alternating with sleepiness.

Delirium can develop over a few days or over a few weeks. Some elders may develop hallucinations or psychotic symptoms when delirious. They become paranoid, withdrawn, or frightened. Delirium can result from a variety of physical problems—infections, dehydration, pain, abnormalities in blood salts and sugar, toxic levels of drugs in the system, medication side effects, inability to urinate, and constipation, to name a few. Delirium is a highly dangerous state, causing great psychological and physical stress. It must be recognized quickly and treated to prevent further serious damage and possibly even death.

Delirium often involves problems with multiple body systems—cognitive, renal, cardiac, immune—and an individual who is less alert is not able to tell the health care workers about the symptoms, what they are usually like, what they are sensitive to, and what their goals of care are. It becomes important for someone to be available to be the person's advocate and to communicate with the health care team. The diagnosis and treatment of delirium is fraught with hazards. Diagnosis begins with blood and urine tests, X-rays, urinary catheters, and intravenous fluid and antibiotics. In an emergency room or hospital setting, often antibiotics and fluids are started before doctors even know exactly what is wrong. Fluids reduce dehydration but can overload a person with fluid, leading to congestive heart failure. Antibiotics treat infections but can also cause significant complications. Necessary catheters and intravenous tubes can provide an entry point for bacteria resistant to multiple antibiotics and other hospital-acquired bacteria infections. The ill person may be restrained for safety reasons with bed rails, wrist restraints, or lap belts and discouraged from getting out of bed. Elders who are ill can rapidly decondition without exercise. Their days and nights can get mixed up in the disorienting, unfamiliar, loud, and constant light of the hospital environment where something is happening 24 hours a day. Elders may experience medical errors or side effects from medications, medication interactions, new infections, or even pressure ulcers.

However, if all goes well, the diagnostic therapies find a cause, unnecessary treatments are stopped, and the treatment becomes focused. The condition gradually improves with the appropriate treatment.

Acute Infections

Infections occur when a foreign invader, generally a bacteria, virus, fungi, or parasite, enters the body and begins to replicate, using the resources of the human host. The immune system intervenes to fight off the infection, often causing fever, chills, inflammation, swelling, redness, and the production of pus, which can collect (abscess) or drain from the infection. Infections are usually local, but sometimes they infect the whole body via the blood (called septicemia or sepsis). When invaders enter the bloodstream, the bacteria get a free trip around the body to find other places to set up their dangerous activities—such as the heart, the lungs, the kidneys, the joints, or even the brain. Most infections are caused by bacteria, but viral infections (influenza, for example) or fungal infections of the skin, mouth (thrush), and blood can also occur.

Older persons generally are no more likely to acquire an infection than younger people, but when they do, they are at higher risk for complications or death. Mortality from pneumonia and influenza is particularly high in the older population. When considered together, the two are the seventh leading cause of death among people 65 and older in the United States.

A number of factors, including age-associated physiological changes, the prevalence of chronic illnesses, and environmental influences, play a role in placing older people at higher risk of illness or death from common infections. Susceptibility to viral or bacterial infections increases when immunity is reduced. Diminished pulmonary function, especially the ability of the lungs to clear foreign matter, increases the risk of pneumonia and other respiratory tract infections. In addition, age changes in the skin, such as a reduced supply of blood and subcutaneous fat, and thinning of the outer layer of skin increase susceptibility to skin and wound infections.

The high prevalence of chronic illness among the older population plays a role in their high rate of infections. For example, chronic bronchitis increases susceptibility to pneumonia and to other respiratory infections. Further, elders with diabetes are more likely to develop urinary tract infections or foot ulcers.

Chronic disease may also indirectly promote infection. Some medical instruments used to treat chronic illnesses (e.g., catheters and intravenous equipment) predispose the user to infections. Malnutrition, common among cancer patients, is also thought to lower resistance to illness. Many drugs used to treat a chronic disease (e.g., corticosteroids used to treat asthma and lung diseases) lower resistance to infection. In addition, the immobility caused by some chronic illnesses can predispose individuals to pneumonia, urinary tract infections, and pressure ulcers (bedsores). Finally, those who have a chronic disease are more likely to become sicker and to take longer to recover when faced with an acute illness than others without such diseases.

Certain environmental factors increase the opportunity for acute illnesses. Extremes of environmental temperature may cause hypothermia or hyperthermia, especially among those who are frail. A hospital or nursing home setting encourages infection because confining many ill people in a small area increases their chances of contracting an infection. It is estimated that more than one in five nursing home residents acquire an infection, most commonly an infection of the urinary tract or pressure ulcers.

The Role of Antibiotics

Treatment of infections is much simpler than treatment of chronic diseases. For the vast majority of bacterial infections, antibiotics are prescribed. The first antibiotic, penicillin, was discovered in the middle of the twentieth century by Dr. Alexander Fleming. *Antibiotics* are medications designed to destroy disease-producing bacteria that invade the body. Since sanitation, nothing has been more effective in preventing death and disability from infection. Penicillin and the dozens of antibiotics discovered since then have revolutionized treatment for bacterial infections and have been responsible for dramatic reductions in infection-related deaths.

A tremendous variety of antibiotics are used alone or in combination to treat a wide range of bacterial infections. With the exception of ointments for wounds, all antibiotics in the United States are available only by prescription. The choice of antibiotic depends on the location of the infection and the bacteria most likely causing that type of infection.

Often body fluids such as urine, vaginal secretions, or sputum may be "cultured" to determine the type of bacteria causing the infection so the appropriate antibiotic may be prescribed. Culturing bacteria involves taking a sample of body fluids and growing it in the laboratory for a couple of days, then classifying the type of bacteria. Which antibiotic is best also depends on the way the drug is metabolized, how it is administered, and its potential for toxicity. Some antibiotics are metabolized by the kidney, others by the liver. Most antibiotics can be taken orally (liquids or pills) but some can be given only intravenously or by injection.

Antibiotics have many possible side effects. When killing the invader bacteria, they inadvertently kill some of the good bacteria in the body, and this can lead to stomach upset, diarrhea, and fungal infections of the skin, mouth, and vagina. Each class of antibiotics has a different list of possible side effects including nausea and vomiting, lack of appetite, hearing loss, increased sensitivity to sunlight, severe muscle damage, and kidney problems. All antibiotics carry a risk of allergy, ranging from a rash to airway constriction.

Over the years, many strains of bacteria have become resistant to particular antibiotics. As a result, newer and stronger antibiotics are needed to treat infections. What causes this increased resistance? There are many reasons. Antibiotics are prescribed too often. Sometimes they are prescribed for viral infections even though antibiotics are ineffective against them. Nevertheless, when patients feel poorly, they demand an antibiotic and some physicians prescribe them. Also, because there are many resistant strains of bacteria and physicians want to be sure an infection is stopped, physicians prescribe new and stronger antibiotics, called "broad-spectrum" antibiotics, which are effective against a wide variety of bacteria for common infections. They are generally easier to take, so the patient is more likely to complete the treatment. For instance, Zithromax is taken once daily for five days and penicillin must be taken four times a day for ten days. In most cases, treatment is started before the physician knows exactly which bacteria are causing the infection.

Another reason for increased bacterial resistance is human habits. Patients are not taking antibiotics properly. Instead of finishing a prescription, some people discontinue antibiotics when their symptoms subside. The antibiotics kill off 90 percent of the bacteria, but the 10 percent that remains is less sensitive to the antibiotic, and sometimes the infection returns even stronger than

Nosocomial Infections

Sometimes the environment makes you sick. Unfortunately, the same places you go to get better can make you sicker, sometimes a lot sicker. A sickness (generally an infection) that an individual contracts in a hospital or nursing home is called a *nosocomial infection*. Nosocomial infections can be passed from patient to patient, but most often they pass through a hospital on the hands of health care workers or on surfaces or equipment used by more than one person. They can be respiratory infections such as flu, viral infections, tuberculosis, SARS, or pneumonia; they may be diarrheal infections, skin infections, or bloodstream infections. The most common sites of infection are the urinary and respiratory tracts, in the blood, and in wounds.

Why are nosocomial infections so dangerous? They often involve bacteria that are highly resistant to antibiotics, and they are likely to attack the most vulnerable patients. Patients in nursing homes and hospitals often have multiple coexisting chronic illnesses, suppressed immune systems, and wounds, and they use medical devices such as catheters, tubes, and IVs that allow entry of bacteria or viruses into the body. Nosocomial infections can increase the time spent in the hospital or nuring home, due to complications, and they can cause death.

How can nosocomial infections be reduced? One of the most important ways to prevent them is for health care workers to practice good hand hygiene before and after every patient contact (see Box 6.1). In addition to handwashing, standard precautions should be used for everyone: wearing gloves if there is to be any contact with potentially infectious material (such as nasal secretions, blood, tears, sweat, or urine), wearing gowns, masks, and goggles to ensure that no potentially infectious material enters the worker's body through the skin, eyes, nose, or mouth. Health care workers caring for a patient with an infection, particularly one that is highly infectious, and visitors in contact with such a patient should use stringent precautions. Precautions are recommended based on the type of infection but may include putting on a mask or gown or gloves when in contact with the individual or sometimes even special isolation rooms.

Other ways to reduce the risk of these infections include minimizing the use of catheters, IVs, and other invasive treatments that provide a way for bacteria to enter the body; carefully observing patients and staff for signs of infection; screening for disease upon entry into a facility; vaccinating against influenza or pneumonia or whooping cough; and using antibiotics carefully.

The Centers for Disease Control and Prevention operates a voluntary program, National Nosocomial Infections Surveillance Systems, in which hospitals report and investigate nosocomial infections at their site and participate in studies and programs to reduce them. Extensive information on nosocomial infections, precautions, antibiotic-resistant infections, surveillance, and recommendations to reduce nosocomial infections can be found at www.cdc.gov

before. Also, concern is growing that giving antibiotics to farm animals contributes to bacterial exposure to and resistance to antibiotics in humans.

All these practices contribute to the development of "super bacteria," which are resistant to (not killed by) even the strongest antibiotics. Super bacteria are common in hospitals, where the patients are already sick and weakened. There is evidence that super bacteria are spreading into the community as well. The key to prevention and control of bacterial infection is judicious cleanliness and handwashing, isolation of patients with serious illnesses, and the appropriate use of antibiotics by physicians and patients.

Respiratory Infections

Acute respiratory illnesses are a significant problem for older people, especially those who are frail. They face a higher risk of complications and death from pulmonary infections than younger people. The risk increases for those who smoke, inhale secondhand smoke, have chronic lung diseases, are immobile, or are in institutions. This section explores the major respiratory infections among older people: pneumonia, influenza (flu), the common cold, and acute bronchitis.

Pneumonia

Pneumonia is a major cause of illness and death among older people. They are more likely to get pneumonia, more likely to be hospitalized, and more likely to die of it than younger people. It most commonly occurs among those who are critically ill and those living in institutions. The increased risk of pneumonia with age is due not to age itself but to coexisting medical problems that weaken the immune system. Pneumonia is a frequent complication of the flu. Individuals who smoke, have respiratory diseases or heart failure, or are malnourished are at increased risk. Individuals who use drugs that suppress stomach acid have a higher risk of pneumonia because the reduced acid allows pneumonia bacteria to multiply easier in the mouth and esophagus.[1] People who are bed-bound or immobilized after surgery are likely to develop pneumonia in the lower lobes of their lungs unless

they are encouraged to breathe deeply and cough. Institutionalization places individuals at risk because of increased exposure to bacteria.

Pneumonia is an inflammation of the tiny sacs (alveoli) within the lungs where oxygen and carbon dioxide gases are exchanged. Most cases of pneumonia are caused by bacteria or viruses. Pneumonia caused by bacteria is most common and deadly among the older population. The immune system of a healthy person is able to control the bacteria that enter the respiratory tract, but when the body is weakened from another respiratory infection, such as influenza, pneumonia gains a foothold. Inflammation of the alveoli increases the production of mucus, which interferes with sufficient oxygen entering the bloodstream, usually causing shortness of breath. Before antibiotics were discovered, over half the deaths among those over 60 were due to pneumonia. In his medical text written over a century ago, Sir William Osler defined pneumonia as "a friend of the aged" because it produced a relatively quick and often painless death among the frail old.[2]

Symptoms of pneumonia are fever, chills, and pain during inhalation. Elders, however, often do not exhibit such symptoms. They are less likely to be feverish and more likely to be confused, weak, and lethargic. Usually pneumonia subsides after a week or two, but it can last longer in those with reduced immunity. The common tests to diagnose pneumonia are blood tests to measure white blood cell count, cultures of the blood to determine type of microbe present, microscopic examination of the sputum, and chest X-rays.

Antibiotic therapy has significantly reduced the number of people dying from pneumonia. Sometimes antibiotics are prescribed after determining the type of invading bacteria that is usually diagnosed from the blood, lung fluid, or sputum. Because it may take days for bacteria to be cultured from these fluids, physicians generally have to guess what type of bacteria is causing the pneumonia and begin treatment with broad-spectrum antibiotics that can kill many types. Antibiotics can be provided orally, intravenously, or by injection.

Most cases of pneumonia are caused by more than 20 strains of pneumococcus bacteria. A vaccine has been developed that effectively fights about 90 percent of the strains. The vaccine is recommended for all adults over age 65: Most only need one shot for life. However, the vaccine is the subject of many debates. First, the older you are when you get the vaccine, the more you need it, but the less effective it is. The reason age 65 is chosen is because doctors want to immunize about five years before someone becomes frail and ill—when the immune system can mount a good response and "remember it" later when it is needed. However, the age at which people become frail is dependent on many variables. In addition to this dispute, there is debate about who should be revaccinated and when. Some experts recommend revaccination after five years for elders with some conditions. Some ethicists recommend against vaccinating those who have end-stage dementia because of pneumonia's reputation as the "old man's friend" because it provides a relatively quick and often painless death among very frail elders.[3] Then there is the concern that vaccination doesn't actually reduce the incidence of pneumonia.[4] Finally, although a study conducted in 1977 reported a 40 percent reduction in mortality with the vaccine, no study since then has shown the same benefit.[5] The cost of the pneumococcal vaccine is covered by Medicare, and nursing home regulations encourage vaccination.

Significant ethnic and racial differences have been reported among those who are vaccinated. In a national survey of those 65 and older, pneumococcal vaccination coverage among adults 65 years and older was stable at 60 percent, with non-Hispanic white older adults (65 percent) more likely to be vaccinated than non-Hispanic black older adults (45 percent) and Hispanic older adults (40 percent).[6] Older people who have a regular health care provider were more likely to have been vaccinated.

A particular threat to elders is *aspiration pneumonia,* which occurs when sputum, stomach contents, or food is sucked into the lungs. The stomach acid causes damage to the lung tissues, and the bacteria introduced into the lungs can cause an infection. Elders at particular risk are frail elders who have trouble swallowing or coughing, are bedridden, confused, semiconscious, or sedated, and are fed with a nasogastric tube. Individuals who have Parkinson's disease or Alzheimer's disease, or have had a stroke, fit into this risk category. As a preventive measure, bedridden patients should be seated upright when eating or drinking and should not be prescribed drugs that depress respiration or produce sedation. The textures of food and liquids can be modified to assist those with difficulty chewing and swallowing. Some people have more difficulty with solid foods, so their foods are moistened, chopped up, or even blended to a puree form without lumps. Others have more difficulty with liquids, and they can use thickeners to make their liquids more like nectar. Speech therapy can help provide techniques to strengthen the mouth and also strategies and positions that will reduce the chance for aspiration.

Influenza

Influenza—the flu—is a viral infection that affects the respiratory tract and skeletal muscles. Uncomplicated influenza is characterized by the abrupt onset of fever, chills, headache, muscle aches, confusion, weakness, and respiratory symptoms. On the basis of symptoms alone, it is difficult to distinguish the symptoms of the flu from other respiratory viruses and bacteria.

Even though the rate of infection is highest among children, the rates of serious illness and death from the flu and its complications are highest among persons older than 65 and persons of any age who have medical conditions that place them at increased risk. For the majority of persons, influenza typically resolves after a limited number of days, although cough and weakness can persist for longer than two weeks. Among individuals with underlying medical conditions (respiratory or cardiac diseases), the flu can lead to bronchitis or pneumonia.

An annual flu shot, given in the fall before flu season starts, offers some protection against influenza and its complications. Because the virus mutates quickly, the influenza vaccine is reformulated by the Centers for Disease Control each year to target the strains that are predicted to be most likely to cause an infection in the upcoming winter. The individual is injected with the vaccine so that the body is exposed to just enough of the inactivated virus to enable the immune system to set up a defense against it. A yearly vaccination is required because the immunity protects only against one type of virus and lasts only a few months. Higher doses of the flu shot have been recommended for the elderly. Older people, particularly those who are frail or who have chronic medical problems, the institutionalized, and those who have significant contact with elders are advised to be vaccinated each year in October or November before flu season starts. A national survey reported that 66 percent of elders in the United States got flu shots in 2009: white elders were much more likely to get a flu shot (66 percent) than blacks or Latinos (both 41 percent).[6]

To encourage more individuals to get flu vaccinations, the nonprofit organization, SPARC (Sickness Prevention Achieved through Regional Collaboration), developed a public health initiative called Vote & Vax. The program goal is to expand protection from influenza by helping public health agencies and other licensed immunizers provide flu shots at or near polling places on Election Day. Since Election Day is early in the flu shot season, and

more than 120 million Americans go to the polls in Presidential election years, and two-thirds of voters are over 50, the program has a potential to reach many who otherwise would not get flu vaccinations. Thus far, a higher proportion of blacks and Latinos than whites are participating. For more information, see box below and www.voteandvax.com

Although immunization of the elderly is recommended worldwide, the influenza vaccine provides imperfect protection. Sometimes the elder cannot mount an immune response to the vaccine, and sometimes the virus strain that occurs that year is not part of the vaccine. However, multiple studies show that the vaccine reduces complications from influenza, such as pneumonia, hospital admissions, and deaths, by 20 to 60 percent, both in elders living in the community and in those living in nursing homes.[7]

When an individual has influenza, the over-the counter medicines to reduce its symptoms are the same as those used for the common cold (analgesics, antihistamines, decongestants). Flu complications, such as pneumonia, are treated with antibiotics. Several types of antiviral drugs are useful if taken after exposure to the flu but before symptoms develop. These drugs reduce the symptoms, the duration, and complications of influenza.

Vote and Vax

V ote & Vax is a public health initiative directed by the nonprofit organization SPARC (Sickness Prevention Achieved through Regional Collaboration). This initiative is funded by the Robert Wood Johnson Foundation and AARP, and SPARC works in partnership with the Centers for Disease Control and Prevention (CDC). Vote & Vax is focused on expanding protection from influenza by helping public health agencies and other licensed immunizers provide flu shots at or near polling places on Election Day. There are 186,000 polling places across the U.S. and these facilities are statutorily required to be accessible to persons with disabilities. Election Day is early in the flu shot season, and more

than 120 million Americans go to the polls in Presidential election years. Approximately two-thirds of these voters are age 50 and older, a priority group for influenza vaccination.

In 2008, 21,434 persons received influenza vaccinations at 331 Vote & Vax Clinics in 42 states and the District of Columbia on Election Day; 62 percent of vaccine recipients were age 50 and older. Results indicate that 60 percent of African-American and 65 percent of Hispanic participants were not regular flu shot recipients, as compared with 42 percent of white participants—suggesting that these clinics reached underserved populations not otherwise likely to be immunized (see www.voteandvax.com).

The Common Cold

Though generally not disabling, the common cold is by far the most prevalent acute infection in the United States, costing billions of dollars in cold remedy purchases and immeasurable losses in productivity each year. It is a small consolation that each individual is susceptible only once to a particular cold virus because more than 200 types of viruses have been identified. The sheer number of different viruses makes the development of a vaccine very unlikely. Older people are less likely to get colds and the symptoms are milder because they have already been exposed to many of the cold viruses. However, among older people, a cold is more likely to lead to complications, such as sinusitis, ear infections, acute bronchitis, and pneumonia. Signs of an infection that require medical care are an extended fever, a bloody discharge from the nose or mouth, recurring chest pains, greenish or thickened nasal discharge or phlegm, persistent cough, earache, sinus pain, and severe sore throat.

The *common cold* is a viral infection of the cells that line the nose and throat. In response to the virus, the mucous membranes lining the respiratory passages secrete large amounts of fluids. These fluids contain virus particles that are infectious. Viruses that cause colds are more likely to be spread by contaminated hands touching the eyes and nose than through the air. The best way to prevent a cold is by frequent handwashing with warm water and soap, avoiding touching the eyes and nose, and avoiding people with colds (see Box 6.1).

Symptoms of a cold appear one to three days after infection. Stress, poor general health, lack of sleep, and smoking predispose a person to a cold. The most common symptoms are familiar to all: nasal congestion, runny nose, scratchy or sore throat, sneezing, and coughing. Since colds are self-limiting (they go away on their own), the treatment is to drink plenty of liquids and rest. There is truth to the adage "If untreated, a cold will last about seven days; if treated, a cold will last about a week."

Although colds are self-limiting infections, medications are available to reduce the symptoms. It is best to treat each symptom with a different drug, for the highly advertised combination cold remedies are not as effective. Box 6.2 displays the various drugs that treat cold symptoms. Combination drug products likely contain ingredients to reduce symptoms that are not even present in many people. Further, the more drugs that are taken, the greater is the risk of drug interactions and side effects. For example, you may not realize that the two medications you are taking have the same or similar ingredients, resulting in a drug overdose. Finally, the drugs in the combination products often are in doses that are insufficient to reduce symptoms effectively. It is important to note that upper respiratory infections are caused by a virus so antibiotics (drugs that fight bacteria) are ineffective. The excessive prescribing of antibiotics for viral infections is a significant problem in the United States. The practice results in unnecessary side effects, increased health care costs, and increased antibiotic resistance.

B O X 6 . 1

Handwashing: Too Important to Ignore

Handwashing is the best way to prevent a respiratory or gastrointestinal infection. Although some bacteria and viruses are spread through the air from one individual to another with a cough or sneeze, it is much more common for the germs to land on a phone receiver, doorknob, hand, or pencil and be picked up by someone else's hands. Once the germs are on the hands, they have a free ride to infect multiple objects in the home, public space, or the hospital. We touch things, then touch our noses, or rub our eyes, or put our fingers in our mouths, and the germs gain a foothold and multiply. Hands can be washed with soap and water, scrubbing vigorously for at least 20 seconds (try singing the happy birthday song to keep time). Alcohol-based waterless hand gels are also highly effective in sanitizing hands.

Drugs That Reduce Cold Symptoms

- *Cough suppressants* are useful to control coughs that cause chest pain or interfere with sleep or breathing. Since coughing due to colds is usually caused by postnasal drip, a nasal decongestant, in addition to relieving nasal congestion, will ease the coughing. Although products with codeine work well, they cause constipation, are available by prescription only, can cause confusion, and can be habit-forming.

- *Decongestants* unclog blocked nasal passages and sinuses (stuffy nose) and prevent postnasal drip in the throat by constricting blood vessels in the nasal passages. They may be taken by pill or by nasal drops or sprays. Nasal drops or sprays are safer, work faster, and are more effective than pills. However, their use is restricted to only a few days because rebound congestion may occur, requiring higher and more frequent dosages for the same effect. In fact, these products can cause serious addiction. Decongestants may cause side effects of nervousness, dizziness, urinary retention, dry eyes, or insomnia, particularly among elders. In addition, these medications can aggravate hypertension (high blood pressure) and glaucoma and interact with other medications.

- *Expectorants* thin and loosen the excessive phlegm common in the airways of a cold

sufferer. Although these results are desirable, most over-the-counter products have low doses and are not very effective.

- *Analgesics,* such as ibuprofen, aspirin, and acetaminophen, reduce the aching feeling that may accompany a cold or flu and reduce a fever. These need to be taken with plenty of liquids, for they may cause kidney problems, and with food to reduce the chance of stomach irritation and ulcers.

- *Medicated lozenges and sprays* ease the minor pain of a sore throat that accompanies a cold. Since a sore throat is caused by postnasal drip, a decongestant can reduce the soreness.

- *Antihistamines* reduce the production of histamine and the symptoms of allergy such as sneezing, itching, watery eyes, and itchy nose and throat. These include older medications such as Clortrimaton and Benadryl, and newer medications such as Allegra and Claritin. The older medications cause drowsiness and are actually a major ingredient in many sleep aids. The older drugs can be dangerous for elders because they can cause confusion, agitation, and, in men, urinary retention and an inability to fully empty the bladder.

Acute Bronchitis

What begins as a cold or flu can develop into *acute bronchitis,* characterized by a productive cough that brings up a large amount of phlegm. Other symptoms that may occur are chest pains, wheezing, chest congestion, shortness of breath, and mild fever. If the infection is from a virus, antibiotics are not recommended. Even if it is bacterial, the infection may clear on its own. However, elders with preexisting lung diseases might be prescribed antibiotics because they may have more difficulty clearing the phlegm due to lung damage. Antibiotics may also be prescribed

to reduce the secretions. Generally, this infection runs its course in a week or two. If a cough persists, pneumonia or pertussis (whooping cough) needs to be ruled out by a health professional.

Inhalers can open the airways and reduce coughing and shortness of breath. Prescription cough suppressants may be helpful for those whose coughing is severe and interferes with sleep, but these have significant side effects. Over-the-counter cough preparations are generally ineffective and often contain sleep agents, which can cause confusion and urinary retention in elders. Increased fluid intake, humidifiers, or steamy showers can also help.

Acute Gastrointestinal Infections

Gastrointestinal symptoms such as indigestion, abdominal pain, heartburn, diarrhea, and gas are very common complaints among older people. Some problems related to the gastrointestinal tract (e.g., appendicitis) are serious and need immediate attention; others are bothersome at times but not life threatening (e.g., diarrhea). Because gastrointestinal symptoms are so common in all people, it can be challenging for elders and those who care for them to tell which complaints are serious and which are not. This section discusses the most common acute gastrointestinal illnesses among older people: ulcer disease, gallstone disease, appendicitis, diverticular disease, and diarrhea. Gallstone disease and diverticular disease are chronic diseases, but they are not bothersome until the acute stage, so they are placed in this chapter.

Gallstone Disease

Gallstones consist of calcium or cholesterol deposits in the gallbladder that can be as small as a grain of rice or as large as a golf ball. People may develop one large gallstone or hundreds of small ones. Most people never even know they have gallstones, only experiencing indigestion, belching, bloating, nausea, vomiting, and episodes of pain after eating high-fat foods. However, if a gallstone blocks a duct entering or exiting the gallbladder, it can cause a *gallbladder attack* (cholecystitis), an abrupt onset of severe cramping pain below the rib cage or in the right shoulder. Sometimes nausea and vomiting accompany the pain. For some individuals, the symptoms occur often; others may go months or years between episodes. If the symptoms are frequent, the best diagnostic tool to determine if surgery is needed is ultrasound.

The incidence of gallstones increases with age. Gallbladder removal operations are one of the most common surgeries performed in the United States. Three times as many women suffer from gallstones as men: Native American women have the highest incidence of gallstones in the United States. Other identified risk factors are obesity, rapid weight loss or fasting, a diet high in cholesterol and fat, and a family history of gallbladder disease.

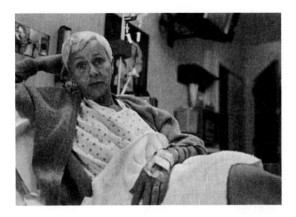

Physicians have differing opinions regarding the best treatment for gallstones. Some advocate a *cholecystectomy* (removal of the gallbladder) before an acute attack to prevent complications. This surgery can be performed with a large incision or with several small incisions by using a long thin tube with a scope on its end that is used to see the inside of the body (*laparoscopic cholecystectomy*). The latter procedure causes less discomfort, decreases recovery time, reduces complications and scarring, and is less expensive than traditional surgery. The procedure is so successful that the number of laparoscopic surgeries on the gallbladder is on the rise, and there is concern that many are unnecessary.

Some physicians advocate a more conservative approach for older people: not removing the gallbladder unless the patient develops a gallbladder attack that does not subside. However, older people needing an emergency gallbladder removal have a much greater risk of death than those who have elective surgery. Conservative treatments include losing weight, taking antacids, and avoiding fatty foods.

Nonsurgical treatments are available for those at high risk from surgery although they are not permanent. A bile salt tablet dissolves small cholesterol stones when ingested. However, the medication is expensive and must be taken indefinitely. Another alternative is *sound wave therapy* (also called extracorporeal shock wave lithotripsy) that is available in some locations. The patient is placed in water, and shock waves are focused on the gallstones to break them into smaller pieces, eliminating the need for surgical removal. After the treatment, the individual must take a bile salt tablet to dissolve the fragments.

Appendicitis

Appendicitis, an inflammation of the appendix caused by bacteria, usually progresses rapidly. Classic symptoms of appendicitis are fever, nausea, pain in the central abdomen that moves to the right side. If surgery to remove the appendix is not accomplished promptly, the appendix may rupture, causing life-threatening complications. Appendicitis is most common in the teen years, and most cases are reported in those under 30.

Although patients over age 60 account for a small proportion of all cases of appendicitis, when they do suffer from it, they are more likely to have complications and die from the disease.

Appendicitis is more risky in the elder population for a number of reasons. They may have a reduced immune function and several coexisting chronic diseases that make diagnosis, surgery and recovery more difficult. Since one of four older people does not exhibit the classic symptoms of appendicitis, they may not be diagnosed properly, increasing the chance of an abscess or a ruptured appendix. Appendicitis is treated by surgical removal of the appendix (appendectomy). Complications can include an infection in the peritoneal cavity or a wound infection, increased incidence of blood clots, pneumonia, or heart attack.

Diverticular Disease

Diverticular disease, rare in the past, is now the most common disorder of the colon in the United States. When the mucous membrane that lines the colon protrudes through the muscular layer of the bowel wall to the outside of the intestine, a pea-size pouch, or *diverticulum,* is formed. These small, distended sacs increase in size and number with age: About 10 percent of people in their 40s and half of those 65 and older have the condition diverticulosis.

The cause of *diverticulosis* is thought to be insufficient dietary fiber intake leading to reduced stool bulk. Consequently, the stool takes longer to pass through the lower gastrointestinal tract. Pressure in the colon is created by increased straining and more forceful contractions of the colon. This elevated pressure eventually weakens the muscle wall of the colon, allowing the inner mucosal lining to slip through. Constipation, obesity, and emotional tension also play a role. Researchers believe that physical activity and high fiber intake may prevent diverticulosis, for both health behaviors increase the speed at which the food passes through the gut. Most people do not even realize they have diverticulosis unless a diverticulum becomes infected or ruptures, causing abdominal pain, bloody stools, and change in bowel habits.

Diverticulitis occurs when a piece of undigested food or hardened particles of fecal matter become trapped in a diverticulum, preventing it from emptying properly. As a result, a bacteria-laden mass forms in the pouch, blocking the blood supply and causing the pouch to become infected and swollen. If it ruptures, an abscess (collection of pus) can erode surrounding tissue, creating a fistula, or passageway, between the bowel and bladder or vagina. If the fecal matter spills out of an infected diverticulum into the abdominal cavity, it can cause an infection of the abdominal lining or throughout the body. Fortunately, diverticulitis occurs in less than 10 percent of those who have diverticulosis.

Symptoms of diverticulitis vary from slight discomfort to severe abdominal pain and fever. The usual treatment for mild cases is a clear liquid diet, stool softeners, and antibiotic therapy. If symptoms do not improve, hospitalization with intravenous feeding and broad-spectrum antibiotic treatment are necessary. When inflammation is controlled, a gradual increase in fiber is prescribed to prevent a recurrence. In most cases, a high-fiber diet and increased fluid intake will both prevent and treat this condition. For those who have chronic attacks, or whose condition worsens despite treatment, the affected part of the colon is surgically removed.

Diarrhea

Nearly everyone has experienced a bout of *diarrhea,* or loose, watery stools. Diarrhea has many causes. Diarrhea can be a side effect of a variety of medications (e.g., antibiotics) or the overuse of laxatives, or it can be the consequence of a temporary infection from unclean water or food.

Shingles

Herpes zoster, also called *varicella zoster* virus, but most commonly called *shingles,* is characterized by an extremely painful blistering red rash caused by reactivation of the virus that was responsible for chicken pox earlier in life. Since the body does not destroy all the viruses from the chicken pox infection, those that remain migrate to the nerve tissue near the spinal cord and remain in a dormant state, usually for many years. Stress, declining immunity, and disease and treatments that suppress the immune system may reactivate the virus, producing shingles. For this reason, shingles is called a *latent infection.*

Most adults carry the latent virus, but only 10 to 20 percent get shingles. Although shingles may occur among all age groups, it is more commonly reactivated in those aged 50 and older. It is believed that half those who live to be 85 will have at least one bout of shingles. Upon reactivation, the virus travels from the spinal nerves to the skin, causing a very painful rash of pea-size blisters, usually on a band clustered on one side of the trunk but sometimes on the arm, leg, or face.

Some people experience only mild discomfort; others experience excruciating pain, especially where clothing touches the skin. The rash and pain usually disappear after two to three weeks. Shingles is highly contagious; however, individuals who have had *varicella* (chicken pox) or who have received the varicella vaccine do not have to worry about acquiring a second infection from a person who has shingles.

The most common and feared complication of shingles is *postherpetic neuralgia,* a burning stabbing pain that persists a month or more after an acute attack. The pain can be constant or intermittent and can last for months or years because of nerve damage from the virus. The likelihood of postherpetic neuralgia becomes more common with advanced age: Up to three-fourths of people over 70 have postherpetic neuralgia after a bout of shingles. There is often a deterioration of the quality of life. Some individuals reduce social interaction and cannot even stand the feeling of clothing on the skin. For some, the extended period of severe pain may be so demoralizing that it leads to prolonged depression.

An antiviral drug, if prescribed within three days after the rash appears, heals the rash more quickly, slows the replication of the virus, and reduces the severity of postherpetic neuralgia. For those with mild shingles, talcum powder, cornstarch, calamine lotion, wet compresses, painkilling skin patches, and analgesics are helpful. It is important that the rash is kept clean and dry and a loose dressing placed on it so there is no direct contact with clothing. For postherpetic neuralgia, painkillers are often required.

A vaccine for shingles has been approved by the FDA. Studies report that the vaccine halved the chance of getting the infection, and if infection still occurred, the chance of getting postherpetic neuralgia was reduced by two-thirds.[8]

Overexposure to Heat and Cold

Age-associated changes and the presence of disease make elders more susceptible to accidental death from hyperthermia (too high a body temperature) or hypothermia (too low a body temperature). Because of increased sensitivity, elders should be monitored closely when temperatures are very high or very low.

The normal body temperature fluctuates by 2 or 3 degrees Fahrenheit within a 24-hour period, generally decreasing at night and increasing during the day. Both hyperthermia and hypothermia are more common and serious in the frail, the poor, and those who live alone.

Hyperthermia

Hyperthermia occurs when the core body temperature is 100°F or more because of infection or high environmental temperatures. Hyperthermia can result in illness, injury, even death. Most episodes of hyperthermia occur when the temperature is over 90°F with humidity over 50 percent.

The most common heat-related illnesses among elders, especially the frail, are heatstroke and heat exhaustion. A life-threatening emergency, *heatstroke*, is characterized by a high internal body temperature (at or above 105°F). This temperature rise is associated with insufficient sweating; hot, dry skin; and altered mental status that can result in disorientation, convulsions, or coma. Heatstroke may be caused by exposure to high environmental temperatures or by excessive exertion among healthy persons who work in hot environments. To treat heatstroke, the body temperature must be reduced rapidly by ice water washes or baths. Medical personnel should be contacted as soon as possible. Even with medical care and aggressive cooling, heatstroke can cause brain damage, even death.

More common is *heat exhaustion,* which is slower in onset than heatstroke and is not life threatening. This condition is due to excessive loss of water and salts. Heat exhaustion often occurs in elders who use diuretics. Thirst, fatigue, and light-headedness are common symptoms. Treatment includes resting in bed away from the heat, drinking cool liquids to replace fluid, and taking alcohol sponge baths or applying wet towels to the body.

Heatstroke and heat exhaustion can be prevented by drinking plenty of fluids, keeping cool, and avoiding heavy exertion. Elders should stay in air conditioned places when the outside temperatures rise. Taking cool baths or showers, increasing home ventilation, forgoing vigorous exercise, and dressing in lightweight clothing will reduce the effects of heat.

Access to air conditioning is the most effective intervention to reduce the effects of hyperthermia. Because the effects of high temperatures are more extreme among frail elders, it is important that they be closely monitored during hot weather.

Hypothermia

Hypothermia occurs when the body temperature drops below 95°F because of exposure to a cold environment without sufficient protection. Hypothermia can also occur in mild conditions over a period of time. For example, a frail person might get hypothermia after spending an extended period of time indoors at temperatures at 60 degrees Fahrenheit without sufficient warm clothing.

When the body temperature lowers, metabolic rate decreases, heart rate slows, pulse weakens, and blood flow decreases to the brain. Common signs of hypothermia are shivering (the body's way of generating heat by increasing muscle activity) and the "-umbles"—stumbles, mumbles, fumbles, and grumbles. The victim may not complain about feeling cold. Treatment for accidental hypothermia involves warming the person with hot water bottles, electric blankets, or another person's body heat. If conscious, the victim should be given warm fluids. The person may have to be hospitalized and may need transfusions of warm blood. Hypothermia can worsen preexisting chronic conditions and can damage internal organs. The most serious problem during hypothermia and rewarming the body is irregular heartbeat that can lead to death.

Hypothermia can be prevented by keeping the house warm in cold weather, wearing warm clothing, using an electric blanket, maintaining fluid and calorie intake, refraining from alcohol consumption, and keeping active. Elders should be encouraged to dress warmly in cold weather even if they don't feel cold. It is especially important to protect the head, hands, and feet. For the poor, subsidizing fuel costs and financial support for home weatherization programs reduce the incidence of hypothermia.

ACCIDENTS

Unintentional injuries are the ninth leading cause of death among persons 65 years of age and older. Even though that group constituted 13 percent of the total population, they comprised almost one-third of all accidental deaths in 2009.[9] As a group, elders are more than twice as likely to suffer accidents as younger people, and they are more likely to become seriously injured during an accident, to be hospitalized, and to die from an accident. Further, accidents in older people are more likely to result in increased dependence, permanent physical damage, institutionalization, and death. Even when there may be no lingering physical effect, often self-confidence is reduced, causing excessive cautiousness because of the fear of a future accident. Accidents are responsible for a significant proportion of hospital care expenses. The average hospital stay for accident victims over age 65 is longer than the stay for most diseases.

Contrary to popular opinion, an accident is not due to fate, chance, or luck; instead, it is the outcome of a combination of individual susceptibility and environmental hazards. Although the effects of aging vary considerably, older people are particularly susceptible to accidents because of reduced vision and hearing, and other declines associated with aging. Also, a number of chronic and acute conditions play a big role in accident risks, particularly the medication prescribed and the conditions that make walking difficult.

Psychological status also affects susceptibility to accidents. Slowed reaction time, poor conditioning, impaired balance, bad vision, and worsened flexibility all combine to increase risk of accidents. Medications affecting blood pressure and alertness can make things worse.

As changes in vision, balance, and reaction time can occur slowly, elders may not be aware of limitations and believe they can do things just as well as they always used to. If there is any cognitive decline, it makes it even more likely that an elder will not be realistic about what he or she can and cannot do. This denial can place older persons at risk of falling because they may refuse to ask for or accept

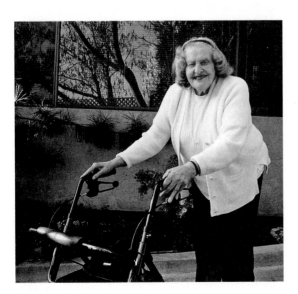

assistance, may insist on living alone when it is no longer safe for them to do so, or may engage in activities that put them in danger. Denial of physical limitations may also increase the risk of driving accidents because of refusal to give up a driver's license.

Although it is important to try to be as independent as possible, sometimes the desire for independence outstrips an individual's physical capacity. In this situation, the person needs assistance in developing alternative ways to perform daily tasks that maintain dignity. The sense of helplessness in those who are dependent can produce unconscious feelings of rage and fear. These individuals may take risks because they no longer have goals or a strong will to live.

Despite family support and counseling, some older people refuse to alter an unsafe living situation. If they are capable of making that decision for themselves—if they understand the possible consequences of their behavior—there is nothing to be done except to encourage them to accept support in the home.

It is possible to reduce an individual's susceptibility to accidents. For instance, the types of drugs or their dosage can be changed, vision and hearing impairments can be improved, and symptoms of some chronic illnesses can be reduced. However, some health conditions cannot be corrected, and the individual must learn to adjust to them.

Most experts assert that the number of accidents could be reduced significantly if environmental hazards were eliminated. Unlike individual factors that increase susceptibility to accidents, environmental hazards are simple to find and correct. Several types of home checklists are available for that purpose. These lists are valuable for individuals to assess their living space to prevent future accidents. A list should be used when a human service worker does a home visit, and deficiencies should be remedied. This type of accident prevention in the home may save the life of a frail elder.

Common Types of Accidents

The majority of accidental deaths among elders result from falls and vehicular and pedestrian accidents. Falls are the most common cause, accounting for one-half of all accidental deaths. The second most common cause of accidental death is from motor vehicles, both as an occupant and as a pedestrian. Accidental deaths from poisoning and exposure to noxious substances and from fires and burns are responsible for most of the remainder of the unintentional injury deaths among those 65 and over.[10]

Falls

Of the nagging, minute-by-minute worries of old age, none seems to eclipse the fear of falling. Every mundane act—taking a bath, scrubbing the floor, shopping for groceries—appears fraught with peril. If you go down, what then? A bruise? A fracture? Or could this be the big one, the one that sends you to the nursing home with no return passage?[11]

Falls are the most common cause of injury, disability and death among elders, both at home and in institutions, and the numbers drastically increase with advanced age. Although falls are common, it is important to note that most do not result in injury. Among older people, when an injury does occur, it is commonly a bone fracture. Fractures in the elderly are serious and are often followed by declining health, decreased mobility, reduced independence, and premature death.

Hip fracture is the most serious fall injury, accounting for most of the disability, death, and medical costs associated with falls. This is due to both hospital and nursing home admissions and the cost of complications. Hip fractures occur about twice as frequently among older women as among older men. Women with osteoporosis are most susceptible. The incidence of hip fractures increases exponentially with age.

The effects of hip fracture on the individual are tremendous, often causing disability, dependence, nursing home admissions, and premature death. Since mortality increases significantly after a hip fracture, it is important to start rehabilitation soon afterward. Because of the trend toward shortened length of stay in the hospital setting, home and nursing home rehabilitation programs are becoming more important after a hip fracture.

A great many physical conditions are associated with an increased risk of falls. The stooped posture and shuffling walk of some older people make them more susceptible to tripping and decrease their ability to catch themselves when they begin to fall. Many elders have increased body sway, further increasing the tendency to fall. Not surprisingly, these postural limitations are most common in the very old and frail. *Orthostatic hypotension* (blood pressure drop when a person gets up quickly) causes transient light-headedness because of reduced blood flow to the brain. Many falls are associated with an urgent need to use the bathroom, so those individuals with urinary urgency may be more likely to fall. Problems in walking and balance may be due to foot conditions affecting bones, muscles, ligaments, and skin. Diabetics have reduced blood flow to the feet, resulting in reduced pain and pressure sensation. Elders with such conditions are more likely to wear loose-fitting shoes or floppy slippers, causing further gait disturbances and increased risk of falls or other injuries. Decreased visual acuity is a significant factor in falls among elders. Those with vision problems have a higher risk of falling. There is also some evidence that bifocals and trifocals increase fall risk because the lower lens reduces depth perception: When an individual looks down at his or her feet, the floor is not in focus.[12]

Musculoskeletal disorders (e.g., arthritis, osteoporosis, and Parkinson's disease) often cause walking difficulties that increase the likelihood of falls. Arthritis can reduce joint flexibility so that when balance is lost, it is difficult to recover quickly enough to avert a fall. Further, a significant number of falls may be due to "drop attacks," a condition in which an elder experiences a sudden weakness of the legs, loses control, and falls. The elder does not lose consciousness but needs assistance in rising. Drop attacks are thought to be due to arthritic changes in the neck that impair blood-flow to the brain, especially when the head is tilted backward. Individuals who rely on walking aids, such as canes and walkers, are even more susceptible to accidents than those who do not use them.

Mental illnesses and emotional state can increase susceptibility to falls. For instance, people with organic brain disorders may experience disorientation, memory loss, poor judgment, poor comprehension, or emotional imbalances that affect awareness and appropriate response to the environment. Individuals with diseases of the central nervous system also increase accident risk. Behavioral characteristics such as impulsivity, lack of attention to detail, being in a hurry, and unsafe behaviors can also increase fall risk. Individuals who are unaware of their own limitations are also at increased risk of falls. For example, someone who recently had a stroke and is weak on one side of the body may "forget" he or she cannot stand without help and try to do so. Being in new situations or environments also increases fall risk.

The side effects of many medications increase the likelihood of accidents. Mood-altering drugs, such as tranquilizers, antidepressants, sleep medication, and anti-anxiety agents, are consistently shown to be related to increased falls and hip fractures. Also, sedatives and alcohol are an important cause of falls because they commonly produce drowsiness, distort judgment, and impair motor response. Many medications may induce lightheadedness, dizziness, and possible falls; these include mood-altering drugs and medications for diabetes and high blood pressure.

Environmental conditions such as loose rugs, cluttered hallways, poor lighting, and slippery floors increase the risk of falls. Tripping over the edge of a rug, slipping on scatter rugs and highly waxed floors, and moving from one type of flooring to another are common causes of accidents. Staircases, especially those that are poorly lighted and lack handrails, can be hazardous because it is easy to miss the first or last step. Environmental dangers alone, however, seldom cause accidents among healthy and active elders. New or unfamiliar environments can be more risky. Individuals who are physically or psychologically vulnerable are much more likely to be injured.

Institutionalization, even with its increased surveillance of patients, does not decrease the risk of falling. In fact, severe falls are much more common among the institutionalized than among individuals

When Did My Daughter Become My Mother?

I remember nursing her, dressing her, teaching her to use the potty.
Making the house baby-proof, telling her what to watch out for,
Walking her to school, making sure the babysitter knew her particularities,
Giving her advice, lots of it, mostly good.
So when did the tables turn? When did she have to help me with my coat?
Talk to me about answering the door to strangers,
Remind me to go to the bathroom, take my medication and wipe my face?
When did she get so smart about money, and knowing what to do
And telling me, too, in an exasperated tone which sounds suspiciously like my own sometimes.
When did she get so bossy about grab rails, and throw rugs and nightlights?
So worried I might fall, or get scammed, or burn down the house?
"I can do it myself," I tell her
Just like she did to me so many years ago.
And we were both right.

living at home. Why are institutionalized patients at higher risk of falling? They are more likely to have many underlying illnesses, to be confused and disoriented, to have problems moving about, and to take medications that affect brain function. Furthermore, patients with a history of falling and those with visual problems are more likely to fall.

Although the frequency of falling is highest among the frail, when vigorous older people fall, they are more likely than the frail to have serious injuries. Older people who are strong and mobile may create situations where significant damage might occur (e.g., participating in sports, carrying heavy items, or climbing a ladder).

What is the best way to keep frail elders from falling? Is it by restraining their movements? Should a seat belt be attached to a wheelchair to keep someone from standing and falling—perhaps a seat belt that buckles in the back? Should side rails be attached to a bed to prevent someone from falling out of bed?

Studies consistently show that physical restraints do not prevent falls and may cause severe injury and even death. Restraints make people struggle to remove them. Restraints keep people from moving around, thereby deconditioning their muscles and increasing the risk of pressure sores and incontinence. When someone who is strapped into a wheelchair falls, he or she may be injured by the wheelchair itself. A fall over bed side rails is a fall from a greater height than one from an ordinary bed, with the additional chance of entanglement in the rails.

Restraining devices may be appropriate in some instances. An elder who is very forgetful and impulsive and not able to stand on her own may need a self-release seat belt on her wheelchair that gives the caregiver time to see what she is doing and get near her when she undoes the belt and tries to stand up. Some people with severe problems holding themselves in

an upright position benefit from devices that position them correctly in a wheelchair. In general, however, restraints do more harm than good.

Physical and occupational therapists can help elders reduce their risk of falls by improving their strength and balance and by teaching them techniques to compensate for their reduced abilities. Rehabilitation specialists can provide excellent assessments of the elder and the home and recommendations on how to prevent accidents.

Elders who have problems walking may be prescribed a cane, walker, or wheelchair. Although assistive devices are meant to help with mobility, they can be hazardous. A walker can help with walking, but what if the individual does not use its brakes when getting up from a sitting position? What if he or she misses the seat when trying to sit down? A cane can help steady an elder, but if it drops and the person must bend to pick it up, this can cause a fall! Further, elders who lean too far forward in their wheelchairs can tip them over and the wheelchair may fall on top of them. Also, the wheels of walkers

Falls and Their Consequences

These two case studies illustrate the impact of accidents on the daily life and independence of elders. How might these accidents have been prevented?

- A 90-year-old woman has been living independently since her husband died 15 years ago. Although her daughter helps her with shopping and she no longer drives, she is able to do everything for herself and is fiercely independent. After suffering a stomach flu, she becomes dehydrated and dizzy and falls in her apartment. The first time, she is bruised; the second time, she catches the side of her leg on the table and develops a laceration. The third time, she fractures her hip and is unable to get to the phone to summon help. She is discovered about eight hours later after her daughter notes she does not answer the phone. She is taken to a local

hospital where the hip is repaired surgically. She recovers somewhat but requires a stay in a nursing home because she has become weaker. She dies of pneumonia three months later.

- A 76-year-old woman is nearly blind but can get around her tiny apartment by feel. When she develops an episode of heart failure, she is hospitalized. The medication she is given for sleep causes confusion, and when she awakens at night to go to the bathroom, she forgets she is not at home. She stumbles to the bathroom and falls, and the IV pole lands on top of her. Her confusion worsens, and she cannot remember to stay in bed. Drugs given to sedate her worsen the confusion and delirium; she becomes agitated and is restrained in the bed. Her recovery is delayed, and she loses the ability to ambulate because of bedrest.

and wheelchairs must be locked in place before an elder tries to stand. Anyone beginning to use a mobility aid needs careful instruction and monitoring.

Appropriate footwear increases balance and stability. Loose-fitting slippers or socks or stockings alone should not be worn. Shoes that fit well, are lightweight and somewhat flexible, without slippery bottoms, are preferred. Hip protectors (foam pads or plastic shields that are held in place at the hips with specially designed undergarments) were designed to divert the impact of a fall away from the hip bone. It is not clearly established whether hip protectors prevent fractures after a fall.[13]

Modifying the environment is an effective strategy for preventing falls. Ridding hallways of clutter, providing adequate lighting, raising the toilet seat height, installing grab bars in the shower, and ensuring that there are no trip hazards are just a few ways to prevent falls.

A home safety checklist (Box 6.3) is a good tool to determine the safety of the environment. It can identify changes to be made to reduce accident risks. An excellent checklist for elders themselves to use was developed by the National Center for Injury Prevention and Control. "Check for Safety: A Home Fall Prevention Checklist for Older Adults" points out potential fall hazards in each room of the home and describes what to do to reduce each hazard. The brochure is printed in large type and is available in English and Spanish at www.cdc.gov and type Home Fall Prevention in the search box.

B O X   6 . 3

Home Safety Checklist

GENERAL CONSIDERATIONS
Can the person climb the stairs to enter and exit?
Is the neighborhood safe?
Is the house clean?
Is the house insulated and well ventilated?
Are there signs of neglect (old food, dirty clothes, unwashed dishes)?
Is the food supply sufficient?

EXTERIOR
Are step surfaces nonslip?
Are step edges visually marked to avoid tripping?
Are steps in good repair?
Are stairway handrails present? Are they securely fastened to fittings?
Are walkways slip-and trip-free?
Is there sufficient outdoor light available to provide safe walking at night?
Are the stairways and landings free of stored items?
Are garden hoses and tools out of the walkway?
Is the walkway free of leaves and snow?

INTERIOR
Are lights bright enough to compensate for limited vision?

Are light switches accessible upon entering rooms?
Are night lights strategically placed throughout house, especially on stairs and routes from bed to bath and bed to kitchen?
Are lights glare-free?
Are stairway carpets and molding edges securely fastened and in good condition?
Are throw rugs at the head or foot of the stairs?
Are throw rugs secured with nonslip backing?
Are handrails present and secure on both sides of staircases?
Are step edges outlined with colored adhesive tape and slip-resistant?
Are carpet edges taped or tacked down?
Is the floor material in good repair?
Are rooms uncluttered to permit unobstructed mobility?
Do low-lying objects (coffee tables, step stools, etc.) present a tripping hazard?
Are telephones accessible?
Are any phone or electrical cords located in walkways?
Is furniture secure enough and nontrippable to provide support if leaned upon for mobility assistance?

Continued

BOX 6.3   *Continued*

Home Safety Checklist

Are chairs of proper height and equipped with armrests to help in getting in and out?

Are wheelchairs and other walking aids in good working condition? Can they be safely used in all areas of the house?

Are there any overloaded electrical outlets or frayed electrical wires?

Is the hot water heater set at 120°F or below?

Does the resident have an escape plan in case of fire?

KITCHEN

Are storage areas easily reachable without having to stand on tiptoes or chairs?

Are the linoleum floors slippery?

Is there a nonslip mat by the sink area to soak up spilled water?

Are chairs wheel-free, equipped with armrests, and of proper height to sit down and get up?

If the pilot light goes out on the gas stove, is the odor strong enough to alert the person?

Are step stools strong enough to provide support? Are their treads in good repair and slip-resistant?

Is a smoke alarm present and functional?

BATHROOM

Are doors wide enough to provide unobstructed entering with or without a device?

Does door threshold present a tripping hazard?

Are floors slippery, especially when wet?

Are skid-proof strips or mats in place in the tub or shower?

Are tub or grab bars available? Are they securely fastened to the walls?

Are toilets low in height? Is an elevated toilet seat available to assist getting on and off the toilet?

If a throw rug is used, does it have a nonslip rubber backing?

BEDROOM

Are night lights and/or bedside lighting available for getting up at night?

Is the path from the bed to the bath clear?

Are beds of appropriate height for ease in getting in and out of bed?

Are bed mattresses sag-resistant at the edges to provide good sitting support?

Are floors nonslip and trip-free? Can the person easily reach objects on closet shelves?

Is a smoke alarm present and functional outside the bedroom door?

Treating diseases and closely monitoring medications can reduce the risk of falls. For diabetics, better control of blood sugar means less chance of losing vision, feeling in the feet, and the ability to balance. Monitoring the effect of medication on blood pressure can reduce orthostatic hypotension (dizziness on rising from the bed or chair). Health professionals can reduce accident susceptibility by correcting vision and hearing disorders, diagnosing acute illnesses and bringing them under control, reducing the symptoms of chronic illnesses, and regularly reviewing medication to lessen the side effects of drowsiness and dizziness.

Falls may create psychological consequences among older people. *Fallophobia* is the abnormal fear of falling by a person who has fallen before.

Fallophobia may occur even when the previous fall was not serious. It is estimated that one of four of those who have fallen limit their daily activities because of fear of falling again.[14] The fear of falling is the most commonly reported anxiety among older people, even more common than fear of robbery or financial difficulties.[15] Although being cautious is a rational response to a potentially serious event, unnecessary restriction of activity leads to a downward spiral of physical and mental deterioration and to an increased risk of falling.

In 2010, The U.S. Preventive Services Task Force reviewed thousands of scientific articles to identify which interventions by physicians best reduced the risk of falls among elders living in the community. The best evidence supported physician recommendations for exercise or physical therapy, Vitamin D supplementation and a "multifaceted assessment" of elder patients to identify their particular risk factors followed by individualized and comprehensive interventions.[16] Federal law mandates that Medicare cover treatments recommended by the U.S. Preventive Services Task Force. Because of their findings, the Affordable Care Act health care reform plan includes a provision for Medicare and other insurance plans to cover annual health risk assessments and customized prevention plans.

Aside from the government-supported work of the U.S. Preventive Services Task Force, two prominent geriatrics organizations conducted similar research, with similar findings. In 2010, the American Geriatrics Society and the British Geriatrics Society Panel on Fall Prevention published the results of an extensive literature search on fall prevention in the elderly by physicians. The revised guidelines focus on two major recommendations: screening/assessment and intervention. The components of screening/assessment include: a *fall-risk assessment* to include history of falls, review of medication, and identification of relevant risk factors for falls; a *physical examination* to include gait, balance, mobility levels, neurological function, muscle strength, cardiovascular status, vision, and examination of feet and footwear, and a *functional assessment* to include assessment of activities of daily living, how an individual perceives their functional ability and fear of falling and an *environmental assessment* including home safety. These experts concluded that the best way to reduce fall risk was for the physician to assess each individual situation and focus on correcting the risks identified. For example, if the patient has weak legs, poor balance and poor vision, interventions may focus on strengthening, balance exercises, installing grab bars, improving lighting and updating the glasses prescription. Interventions that were the most helpful for the most people included an exercise program to include flexibility endurance strength gait and balance, keeping the home safe, and vitamin D supplements of at least 800 IU/day.[17] A summary of the practice guidelines for physicians can be found at www.americangeriatrics.org

There is a great need for physicians to work with patients to reduce the risk of falls. Not only do accidents cause unnecessary deaths, but those who survive may have serious disabilities and be dependent on others for the remainder of their lives.

Motor Vehicle Accidents

Motor vehicle accidents are the second leading cause of accidental death among elders aged 65 and over.[10] Overall, older drivers account for the fewest miles driven, the fewest crashes, and the lowest crash rate of all age groups. They are less likely to drink and drive, speed, or drive without a license, and they are more likely to wear seat belts. Compared to other age groups, elder drivers are involved in a small percentage of all accidents. But when the data are analyzed on a per-mile basis, drivers aged 75 and older have the worst record. Further, elders are more likely to sustain serious injuries, be hospitalized, and die from motor vehicle accidents than younger age groups.[18] Although there is a clear association between increasing risk and advancing age, there is wide variability among elders in miles driven and driving skills. Just as in other age groups, some persons are excellent drivers while others should not be on the road.

Vision problems are associated with an increased risk of driving accidents among older people. Vision problems include presbyopia, glaucoma, macular degeneration, diminished night vision, and cataracts. Cataracts increase susceptibility to glare and reduce color contrast; surgical repair is associated with improvement in vision. Because most vision problems have a gradual onset, often elders are unaware of the extent of their vision loss. Unfortunately, the simple vision chart used to apply for or maintain a driver's license does not pick up all vision problems.

Many chronic illnesses and the medications used to treat them affect the ability to drive safely. Dementia, strokes, and other illnesses cause lapses of attention, impaired memory, impaired judgment, diminished reaction time, and slowed information processing, all of which impact driving skills. Arthritis and osteoporosis make it more difficult to turn the head in order to directly note traffic patterns.

Parkinson's disease and other diseases affect the ability to drive by reducing the use of the hands or feet.

Antihistamines, sedatives, painkillers, and many other prescription drugs may cause confusion, drowsiness, and impaired reflexes, consequently reducing driving skill. In addition, many driving accidents are caused by a health crisis that results in loss of consciousness or distraction of attention; heart attack, stroke or transient ischemic attacks, arrhythmias, and seizures, among others.

Certain driving patterns are characteristic of elderly drivers: They are less likely to yield the right of way, less likely to observe signs and signals, and more likely to have turning violations. On the other hand, older people are less likely to be cited for reckless driving or drinking while driving. In urban areas, elderly drivers are overrepresented in accidents involving turns, parking, and head-on crashes. Elders often drive with a spouse or "copilot" in the car for assistance. Although two may see some hazards more easily than one, two partially impaired individuals cannot react to an emergency situation with only one behind the wheel.

The ability to drive represents competence and independence and sends a message to others that the driver is a functional and capable adult. In our culture, giving up driving not only mean a loss of status but also a lessening of social contacts, which is made worse by a lack of public transportation in many areas. Elders no longer able to drive safely start to feel old and dependent. Nevertheless, families, medical personnel, and elders themselves concerned about safety must take into account both the benefits and the risks of an elder driver remaining behind the wheel.

Most older people are aware of their decreasing abilities and make adjustments by driving only in daylight, traveling short distances, avoiding heavy or fast traffic, or having another person drive. And most decide to stop driving on their own. Most stop driving on their own due to medical conditions, declining vision, or worry about abilities and accidents. A few older people discontinue driving because of a sudden disabling event. The most dangerous situation arises when elders with cognitive problems, such as from Alzheimer's disease or stroke, continue to drive because they are unaware of their reduced capabilities.

How can it be determined whether an individual can still drive safely? Because physicians are aware of the physical and mental limitations of their patients, and because their views are respected, they are in a position to recommend driving limitations to protect elders as well as

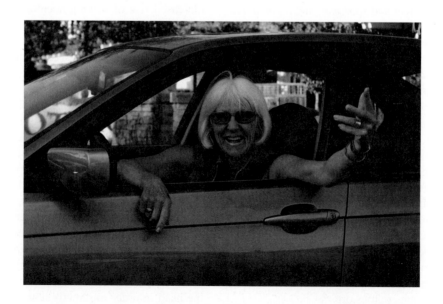

other drivers and pedestrians. For example, driving only in town during nonrush hours and only in daylight may be a reasonable compromise. Box 6.4 lists safe-driving tips for drivers of any age. The Department of Motor Vehicles, the American Medical Association, the American Automobile Association as well as others have developed informational brochures, videos, and other courses for senior drivers and screening tools to be used by elder drivers and those who care for them to assist in improving driving, compensating for losses, and determining when driving needs to cease.

When family members or friends voice concern or when an elder accumulates traffic citations, reducing or eliminating driving altogether should be considered. Referral to a doctor, to the department of motor vehicles, or to an occupational therapist for an evaluation may be helpful.

Educating elders about factors that increase their risk of car accidents likely reduces the incidence of future accidents. Older people must be cautioned about driving when they are using drugs that interfere with driving skill, such as those affecting perception and reaction time. Keeping elders updated about the current driving rules might also increase their confidence and reduce accidents. The American Association for Retired Persons (AARP)

offers a community education program for drivers over age 55 to help older people understand physical changes that come with aging and their effect on driving skills. Elderly drivers who complete driver education courses have significantly fewer accidents and traffic violations, and attendance is often rewarded with reductions in car insurance premiums. To find out more, go to www.aarp.org/life/drive

The United States is experiencing a rapid growth in the number of older drivers and the number of drivers over 75 is increasing the most rapidly and the vast majority will rely on cars for their transportation. Although many elders escape physical and cognitive disorders, as a group they are more likely to exhibit such impairments that compromise driving safety. Because many areas lack public transportation, many elders continue to drive (either from necessity or by desire) despite these limitations. The effect this will have on driving statistics in our country may be significant.

Many states are responding to the increase in elder drivers by improving roadways to prevent common driving accidents. Wider lanes, intersections that give drivers a longer view of oncoming traffic and more time for left turns, road names displayed well in advance of intersections, street signs with larger letters and numbers, bigger orange construction-zone cones, reflective pavement markers,

---

B O X   6 . 4

Safe Driving Tips

- If possible, limit driving in bad weather, during rush hours, and on high-speed freeways.
- Limit night driving if it is a problem for you.
- Drive close to the speed limit: not too fast or too slow.
- Wear your seat belt correctly.
- Keep one car length for every ten miles of speed between you and the vehicles around you.
- Do not use cell phone or text while driving. Do not try to do other tasks, like read a map, smoke, apply makeup, or eat as these can distract you.

- Don't rely only on mirrors. Instead turn your head to look for other cars.
- Never drink alcohol and drive.
- Do not drive when you are taking medication that makes you drowsy, such as antihistamines, sedatives, anti-anxiety drugs, and some painkillers.
- Optimize your vision and hearing while driving: Wear your hearing aid and clean eyeglasses or contact lenses.
- Keep your car in good repair.
- Clean windshields and mirrors and replace ineffective windshield wiper blades.

and larger lettering on stop, yield, and warning signs are improvements that should decrease accidents for all driving-age groups. The California Department of Motor Vehicles provides a site specifically for older adults: www.dmv.ca.gov/about/senior/senior_top.htm

Most state governments enforce stringent regulations for older people to try to reduce the number of impaired elders renewing driver's licenses. Despite the added cost to the state and increased red tape for the older driver, there is little evidence that this effort results in fewer traffic fatalities among elders.[19] One problem is that written tests do not accurately measure how drivers behave on the road, especially in an emergency situation. An elder who knows the rules of the road and is able to drive safely in most conditions may have diminished sensory and reaction capabilities that limit his or her ability to respond to an unexpected situation, unusual weather, the distraction of passengers, an accident, or heavy traffic. Today, there is no unified approach to assess the driving skill of older drivers, and tests currently in use have not been documented to reduce traffic fatalities.

It is generally agreed that individuals with advanced Alzheimer's disease should not be on the road. According to a study by the American Academy of Neurology, people with early or possible Alzheimer's disease have a mild impairment that is no greater than impairments tolerated in the general population, but individuals with advanced Alzheimer's disease pose a significant safety problem—evident in tests measuring their driving performance and in their crash rates—and should not drive.[20] To that end, the Alzheimer's Association offers several suggestions to assist families at www.alz.org and type Driving in the search bar.

Pedestrian Accidents

Death rates for pedestrians struck by vehicles increase after middle age. Elder pedestrians not only are more likely to be hit by a motor vehicle but also are more likely to be injured severely and die from their injury.

Although older pedestrians are generally more cautious than younger groups, hearing and vision impairments, problems in walking, and other disabilities increase their susceptibility to pedestrian accidents. Also, the extra energy needed to run out of harm's way decreases with age and disability. Box 6.5 lists tips for reducing pedestrian accidents.

BOX 6.5

Tips for Reducing Your Risk of Pedestrian Accidents

- To guarantee plenty of crossing time, wait for a new green light before starting across the street.
- Whenever possible, wait to cross with other pedestrians.
- Look both ways before stepping into a crosswalk, even when the light indicates you may walk.
- Be alert for drivers who are turning. Before crossing the street, get their attention by making eye contact.
- Cross only at intersections. Do not jaywalk, and do not walk between parked cars or in front of or behind a stopped bus or truck.
- Wear reflective or white clothing or reflector patches if out at night. Carry a flashlight.

- Stand on the curb, not on the street, while waiting to cross.
- Whenever possible, walk on sidewalks, not on the road. If you must walk on the road, use the left side facing the oncoming traffic.
- Concentrate on the traffic around you as well as what you are doing and where you are going.
- If you are on medication or have used alcohol, be wary of their side effects.
- Do not carry umbrellas or packages in a way that blocks your vision or hampers your ability to walk.

Pedestrian accidents frequently occur at intersections, especially those without lights, crosswalks, or stop signs. Even when there are crosswalk lights, they may not be long enough for a frail elder to cross the street. Safety interventions such as crosswalk signals that are large, loud, and clear (e.g., some have a countdown feature and verbal cues) can maximize safety. Well-marked and lighted street crossings are also helpful. Curb cuts, ramps, and maintaining roads to minimize rough bumps or high curbs can also reduce accidents. A campaign to increase the walkability of a neighborhood might include these as well as other changes to make streets and sidewalks safer. The majority of accidents involving older pedestrians occur at crosswalk intersections, particularly those with no traffic lights or stop signs.[21] Crosswalks are so hazardous because some older people are less able to judge the speed and distance of oncoming vehicles. This is problematic because crosswalk lights often do not stay green long enough for slow-moving elders to safely cross the street. One study found that less than 1 percent of people 72 years of age and older has a normal walking speed sufficient to cross the street in the time typically allotted at average intersections. Even in neighborhoods with lights adjusted for elders, only 7 percent can get across before the light changes.[22] Crossing times that reflect an elder's range of abilities would not only decrease injuries but also reduce the stress of crossing a busy intersection. Another way to help elders cross busy intersections would be to install a wide median strip at signalized intersections. Difficulty in ascending and descending street curbs also increases the risk of pedestrian accidents. In this case, ramps or curb cuts would make crossings more accessible.

Most fatal pedestrian accidents among older people occur in early evening. Whether the driver is unable to see the older pedestrian or vice versa is not clear. One community significantly reduced pedestrian accidents after lengthening traffic signals, installing pedestrian signals on traffic islands, making signals and crosswalks more visible, increasing enforcement of speed limits, and

making educational presentations to seniors. Some communities are developing "walkable neighborhoods" for older people to increase walking among older adults. This is accomplished by identifying obstacles that keep adults from walking and overcoming those obstacles. See www.walkscore.com for details.

A good safety education resource for older people, "Stepping Out—Mature Adults: Be Healthy, Walk Safely," is available from the National Highway Transportation Safety Administration, at www.nhtsa.dot.gov The site also includes an excellent powerpoint workshop on line, "Pedestrian Safety Workshop: A Focus on Older Adults" for professionals to educate elder groups.

Choking

Choking occurs when an obstruction (food, vomited matter, mucus, or even water) enters the windpipe instead of the esophagus and blocks air passages. Suffocation, or choking, occurs mainly among the very old and the very young. Elders, especially those 75 and older, are much more likely to die from suffocation than other age groups. Suffocation by choking is more likely among people who have difficulty swallowing, such as those with neurological problems (e.g., stroke, Alzheimer's disease, and Parkinson's disease). Other factors that contribute to the unintentional breathing of food or fluid into the lungs are overmedication, alcohol intoxication, poor eating position, poorly fitting dentures, missing teeth, and emotional excitement.

The typical choking victim is unable to speak, makes high-pitched sounds when gasping, grabs the throat, turns pale, and then turns blue. If the individual can speak or cough, the obstruction is likely partial, and you should not interfere with his or her own attempts to dislodge the object. Sometimes people who are choking show no evidence of distress; they suddenly stop eating and talking, then collapse, and the problem may be misinterpreted as a heart attack. In any case, a choking person will sustain permanent brain damage from lack of oxygen unless the object is removed within minutes.

If it looks as if the individual is not able to cough up the object—if the person cannot speak, cough, or breathe—get someone to call an ambulance, and then work quickly to unblock the airway.

The American Heart Association recommends administering a series of abdominal thrusts (also called the Heimlich maneuver) to force air out of the lungs to dislodge the object from the airway. To perform abdominal thrusts, the rescuer stands behind the victim and wraps her arms around the victim's waist (above the naval and below the rib cage). A fist is made with one hand and grabbed with the other hand. Subsequent quick inward and upward thrusts into the abdomen should be continued until the airway is cleared or the victim becomes unconscious. If the victim is unconscious or if the victim is too big to reach around for abdominal thrusts to be effective, he or she should be brought to the floor to administer chest thrusts.

The American Red Cross recommends a series of five back blows to the choking victim, followed by five abdominal thrusts. To give back blows, the responder should put her arm diagonally across the victim's chest and lean the person forward. Then, with the other hand, the rescuer should firmly strike the person between the shoulder blades with the heel of the hand. The rescuer continues to give sets of back blows and abdominal thrusts until the victim can cough forcefully, speak, or breathe. The recommendation for rescuing the unconscious victim and the victim who is too big for the rescuer's arms to encircle is the same as that of the American Heart Association: Chest thrusts should be administered on the floor.

The two organizations agree that there is no evidence to support one technique over the others: Back slaps and abdominal thrusts are similarly effective. If one method doesn't work, trying another method increases success. Resources for education on CPR are found at the University of Washington Web site, http://depts.washington.edu/learncpr/ index.html or www.redcross.org or the American Heart Association at http://guidelines.ecc.org/

Fires and Burns

Accidents due to fire and burns are not nearly as common as falls among elders, but when they occur, they are more likely to cause serious injury or death. Most deaths from fire are caused indirectly, from smoke and gas inhalation. Careless personal behaviors, especially leaving lighted cigarettes untended, are the primary causes of fire accidents in younger adults. Among older adults, faulty electrical products such as electric blankets or electric heaters more commonly cause fires. Cooking accidents are the second most common causes of fires and burns. One type of preventable accident occurs among elders wearing clothes with dangling sleeves while they are cooking. Severe burn injuries are caused as the sleeve ignites when it drags across a lighted burner while the person is reaching for a pot on the back burner. Accessible fire extinguishers in the kitchen would reduce the consequences of cooking accidents.

When a fire occurs, older persons, particularly those who are frail, are more susceptible to injury or death than the young because they are less able to respond quickly enough to prevent injury. Many times, fire-related injuries are due to cognitive impairments. Furthermore, many older people live alone and have nobody to alert them and get them to safety. Not uncommonly, elders trap themselves in their homes because they have installed multiple locks that are difficult to open when an emergency arises. The risk of accidents from fires and burns can be greatly reduced by installing smoke detectors and checking them twice a year to be sure that they work. It is also helpful to devise a fire escape plan.

Though less serious, burn injuries due to hot liquids, or scalding, are much more common than burns due to fire. Elders are particularly vulnerable to scalding because of their reduced perception of pain and temperature changes. Many elders, especially those with diabetes or other health problems, soak their feet in hot water then later realize they have severely burned themselves. Water temperature and duration of exposure affect the severity of the burn. Tap water at 140°F will cause a serious

Caring for Elders During a Natural Disaster: We Can Do Better—But Are We?

Editor's Note: This article was originally published in the July–August 2011 issue of *Aging Today,* the bimonthly newspaper of the American Society on Aging.

By Jenny Campbell

As I write this, the waters of the Mississippi are lapping over the levees in Louisiana and Mississippi. It seems impossible that so many disasters could befall one area: following the devastation of hurricanes Katrina and Rita, there was Gustav, Ike, an oil spill, biblically fierce tornados and now a river that will not be contained. And it's not just this region. According to FEMA, the United States has experienced 381 disasters since Hurricane Katrina. Since 1954, every state has experienced a disaster—an average of 34 per state. Everyone has a stake in disaster planning.

Some disasters happen in slow motion. Some happen quickly. Some are repeat offenders. But no matter the venue, the results will be exponentially more devastating to older adults. When it comes to needing to move quickly and strategically out of harm's way, frailty can instantly become a terminal condition. In New Orleans, older adults made up only 15% of the population, but accounted for more than 71% of the dead. In Japan, the images of crowds running for high ground, and the trail of older adults inexorably lagging behind, haunt us.

It is the most marginalized—older minority adults with few fiscal resources—who bear a disproportionate burden in disasters. But disaster planning is challenging, not unlike playing multidimensional Sudoku. What works in one set of circumstances may not work in another.

LEARNING FROM KATRINA

So what have we learned since Katrina? In a brave challenge, AARP issued a post-Katrina report, *We Can Do Better.* It cited the failings of disaster preparedness at all levels that resulted in the death, devastation and long-term trauma for older adults that was Katrina's legacy. Six years later, are we doing better?

One of the major failings in the case of Katrina was a lack of coordination between federal, state and community entities. On the federal level, planning has made great strides. Legislatively, the Pandemic and All-Hazards Preparedness Act of 2006 opens the door for requiring organizations involved in disaster planning to include State Units on Aging with financial incentives. Another two laws—each enacted after Katrina—encourage greater coordination of services (National Response Framework, January 2008; Homeland Security Presidential Directive 8).

But in a discouraging development, a new FEMA directive issued November 2010, *Guidance on Planning for Integration of Functional Needs Support Services in General Population Shelters,* lacked input from the professional aging network. FEMA admirably sought membership in its workgroup from the disabilities network, and included the Administration for Children and Families. But the needs of older adults are not subsumed under these agencies. The prevalence of multiple chronic diseases and a high degree of frailty result in older adults having distinctly different risks and needs than the disabled population.

An elder who is evacuated may be fully independent and functional on day one, with diabetes and hypertension well under control, but by day three, in the heat, noise and chaos of a shelter, can quickly become fatigued and dehydrated. Lack of proper medications or access to medical records can exacerbate issues. Add to the mix emergency meals typically high in salt, and suddenly both diabetes and hypertension spiral out of control.

Despite setbacks, there is progress. In May 2011, *The New York Times* ran this headline on a tornado story: "Government's Disaster Response Wins Praise from Those Affected." In that article, a victim whose house was in shambles is quoted saying, "It ain't like Katrina . . . we're getting help."

After Katrina, Shirley Laska, from the University of New Orleans Center for Hazards Assessment and Technology, organized an interdisciplinary group to identify and address problems with cross-systems

Continued

Continued

Caring for Elders During a Natural Disaster: We Can Do Better—but Are We?

evacuation for older adults. The evacuation of New Orleans in the face of Gustav demonstrated there had been vast improvements.

Progress is also being made on restoring a sense of community after a disaster; this is both more important and more difficult to achieve than we had previously understood. HelpAge International has developed a model that establishes support and structure for older adults to rebuild their sense of community, which is arguably as important as food and shelter in the healing process.

But we haven't made much progress in providing trauma-informed care to address the emotional impact of a disaster. Although we know a good deal about how elders respond to disasters, we lack systems to provide ongoing trauma-informed care. Two federally funded endeavors focus on the needs of children who have been traumatized in a disaster, and provide a template for resources that could be developed for older adults (National Child Traumatic Stress Network, The Children's Health Fund).

LOOKING AHEAD

So what can be done to prepare? Plan for an all-hazards disaster: although your area may be prone to flooding, you need a plan that will also work in a fire, or a tornado. Use one of the toolkits to develop a disaster plan for your family, including regularly updating medications and contact information. Sign up with the Red Cross or a VOAD (Voluntary Organizations Active in Disasters) and get training. Inquire with your Area Agency on Aging about disaster planning, and volunteer to participate in drills. Encourage elected officials to hold community-based disaster drills, where specific scenarios are explored. All are designed to heighten preparedness and promote inter-agency communication.

Since Katrina, it has become clear there is no one point of ultimate responsibility for older adults in a disaster. There are roles for everyone: individuals; community groups; and local, state and federal government agencies. But the professional aging network has to be included in planning. And elected officials must find the courage to invest in disaster preparedness services we hope to never use. To answer AARP's challenge, are we doing better? Yes, we are. And there is still work to be done.

Jenny Campbell, Ph.D., teaches social work at Bryn Mawr's Graduate School of Social Work and Social Research in Pennsylvania, and consults for nonprofits. She was the director of the Hurricane Fund for the Elderly, an initiative of Grantmakers in Aging that raised money to help rebuild senior services after Hurricane Katrina. Contact her at jwcampbe@brynmawr.edu

---

burn after only a few seconds, whereas water at 120°F will cause the same burn in 10 minutes. Almost all scald injuries could be prevented by adjusting the temperature of the household water heater to 120°F or below.

Assessment after an Accident

After an accident, the first concern of medical personnel is to treat the injury. Look at the body— is there any bruising, pain, broken skin, or swelling? It is important to check not only right after the accident, but over the next hours to days as signs of injury are often not immediately apparent. After the acute problem is under control, the circumstances surrounding the accident should be explored to reduce the risk of a future accident. A careful accident history includes these questions:

1. What was the person doing at the time?
2. Were physical symptoms present before the accident?
3. What was the person's state of mind before the accident?
4. Were there any environmental hazards that contributed to the accident?

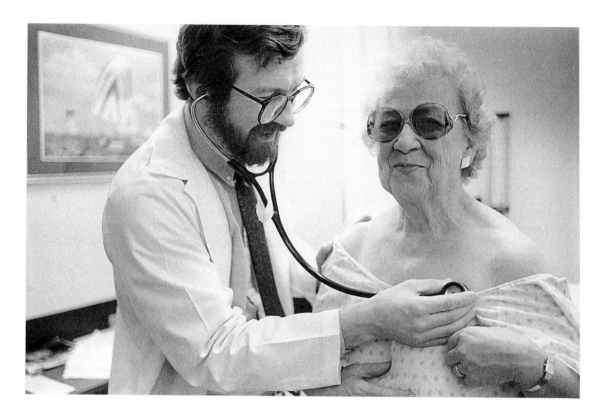

5. Were any new medications taken recently?
6. Was there something else different about today that may be related to the accident?

It is seldom easy to determine the circumstances leading up to an accident. People may be vague about how it happened, or they may not remember any symptoms preceding it. People who fall may be unwilling to disclose how they fell because they were doing something dangerous or foolish. If witnesses were present, they should be questioned.

Physical assessment after a fall can identify medical problems that might otherwise go unnoticed. Estimates vary, but as many as two-thirds of the accidents occurring among elders might be prevented by treating underlying medical conditions and reducing environmental hazards. Many problems can be corrected with physical therapy or strengthening or balance exercises. The environment can be changed to improve safety or more assistance

or supervision can be provided. The pharmacist should review the medications to see if any might contribute to falls and suggest alternatives.

Accident Prevention

There is a great need for both health professionals and elders to learn how to prevent accidents. Many resources are available to help older people reduce their accident risk in the home and when walking or driving. Education is important for health and social service professionals so they can spot environmental hazards when they visit elders in their homes. It is their responsibility to advocate for elders' safety in the community and beyond. Among the most important issues are the inclusion of safety features in housing for the elderly, the timing of crosswalk lights, laws regarding elder drivers, and the design of cars to ensure safety.

The families and friends of frail elders, especially those living alone, are concerned about their safety. But overprotectiveness can undermine self-confidence, produce unnecessary cautiousness, and promote anxiety. There are many constructive ways in which families can assist an older person to continue living at home: monitoring drug intake, being aware of symptoms that may increase the risk of falls, scheduling regular visits to physicians (including vision and hearing specialists), eliminating hazards in and around the home, encouraging elders to attend classes for drivers over age 55, and making daily phone calls or visits, to name a few. Some communities offer services such as daily visits, phone calls, and monitoring devices. Further, providing an older person with a cell phone is a simple way to have immediate access to family or emergency personnel when needed.

SUMMARY

Although chronic conditions account for the majority of deaths and disabilities among elders, infections and accidents remain an important cause of illness and death. For a number of reasons, older people are more likely to suffer from infections and accidents than other age groups.

Infections may be difficult to diagnose in elders because symptoms may be vague or absent. Common infections and acute conditions in the 65 and older age group include pneumonia and flu, gastrointestinal conditions, urinary tract infections, and acute crises in response to heat and cold (hypothermia and hyperthermia).

Even though elders comprise less than 13 percent of the population in the United States, they comprise almost half of all accidental deaths. The three most common types of accidents are falls, motor vehicle accidents, and pedestrian accidents. Because so many factors can contribute to an accident, health professionals should conduct a thorough assessment to prevent further accidents and to treat underlying conditions. Accident prevention programs are effective in reducing accident susceptibility among elders.

ACTIVITIES

1. Question elders on their knowledge of the prevention and treatment of acute illnesses. How do they determine whether their conditions are severe enough to see a doctor? What methods do they use to prevent or treat minor acute illnesses?

2. Find out how nursing homes cope with patients with colds, the flu, or other infectious diseases. How is the spread of disease prevented in nursing homes?

3. Design a pamphlet or information sheet for elders discussing one of the acute illnesses discussed in this chapter.

4. With a partner, devise a list of routine errands (e.g., buying milk at the grocery, visiting the bank or post office, attempting to find a specific book at the library) that elders may need to do in the course of daily life. Then do them, without driving yourself. You must walk or take public transportation or persuade someone to drive you. Try to act as if you were a frail elder with reduced mobility, hearing, and vision. To simulate being in a wheelchair, you can push a stroller (remember not to step off curbs, climb into a car or bus unaided, or go up or down steps on your own). Make a list of the physical barriers you encounter and your concerns. Also list the steps merchants have taken to reduce barriers.

5. Using a checklist for home safety, assess the safety of the home of an older family member. (Be sure to ask permission first.) Discuss your findings with the occupant. Use the list to assess the safety of your home. What areas need improvement?

6. Attend a senior nutrition site, senior center, or local drugstore and look for environmental hazards that may cause falls. Write a letter to the manager outlining the problems and suggesting solutions.

7. What programs in your community reduce accidents among elders (e.g., driver education for those over 55, safety checks of homes)? Compile a list of ways in which your community could further decrease accidents among elders.

8. Debate: Should states consider mandatory testing of drivers at age 75?

BIBLIOGRAPHY

1. Laheij, R.J., Sturkenboom, M.C., Hassing, R.J., et al. 2004. Risk of community-acquired pneumonia and use of gastric acid-suppressive drugs. *Journal of the American Medical Association* 292(16):1955–1960.

2. Osler, W. 1892. *The principles and practice of medicine*. New York: Appleton.

3. Zimmerman, R.K. 2005. If pneumonia is the "old man's friend," should it be prevented by vaccination? An ethical analysis. *Vaccine* 23(29):3843–3849.

4. Jackson LA, Neuzil KM, Yu O, et.al. 2003. Effectiveness of pneumococcal polysaccharide vaccine in older adults. *New England Journal of Medicine* 348(18): 1747–1755.

5. Riley, I.D., Tarr, P.I., Andrews, M., et al. 1977. Immunisation with a polyvalent pneumococcal vaccine. Reduction of adult respiratory mortality in a New Guinea Highlands community. *Lancet* 1(8026):1338–1341.

6. Centers for Disease Control and Prevention. 2011. 2009 Adult vaccination coverage, NHIS. www.cdc.gov/vaccines/stats-surv/nhis/2009-nhis.htm

7. Jefferson, T., Rivetti, D., Rivetti, A., et al. 2005. Efficacy and effectiveness of influenza vaccines in elderly people: A systematic review. *Lancet* 366(9492):1165–1174.

8. Oxman, M.N., Levin, M.D., Johnson, G.R., et al. 2005. A vaccine to prevent herpes zoster and postherpetic neuralgia in older adults. *New England Journal of Medicine* 352(22):2271–2284.

9. Kochanek, K.D., Xu, J.Q., Murphy, S.L., et al. 2011. Deaths: Preliminary data for 2009. *National Vital Statistics Reports*. 59(4):1–51 Hyattsville, MD: National Center for Health Statistics.

10. Minino, A.M., Murphy, S.L., Xu, J., and Kochanek, K.D. 2011. Deaths: Final data for 2008. *National Vital Statistics Reports*. 59(10):1–152.

11. Kleinfield, N.R. 2003, March 3. For elderly, fear of falling is a risk in itself. *New York Times*.

12. Lord, S.R. 2006. Visual risk factors for falls in older people. *Age and Ageing* 35 Suppl 2:ii42–ii45.

13. Gillespie, W.J., Gillespie, L.D., and Parker, M.J. 2010. Hip protectors for preventing hip fractures in older people. *Cochrane Database Systems Review* (10):CD001255. *New England Journal of Medicine* 343(21):1506–1515.

14. Tinetti, M.E., Speechley, M., and Ginter, S.F. 1998. Risk factors for falls among elderly persons living in the community. *New England Journal of Medicine* 319:1701–1707.

15. Howland, J., Lachman, M.E., Peterson, E.W., et al. 1998. Covariates of fear of falling and associated activity curtailment. *The Gerontologist* 38(5):549–555.

16. Michael, Y.L., Lin, J.S., Whitlock, E.P., et al. 2010. Interventions to prevent falls in older adults: An updated systematic review. Rockville (MD): Agency for Healthcare Research and Quality.

17. Panel on Prevention of Falls in Older Persons. American Geriatrics Society and British Geriatrics Society. 2011. Summary of the updated American Geriatrics Society/British Geriatrics Society clinical practice guideline for prevention of falls in older persons. *Journal of the American Geriatrics Society* 59(1):148–157.

18. Massie, D., Campbell, K., and Williams, A. 1995. Traffic accident involvement rate by driver, age and gender. *Accident Analysis and Prevention* 27:73–87.

19. Grabowski, D.C., Campbell, C.M., and Morrisey, M.A. 2004. Elderly licensure laws and motor fatalities. *Journal of the American Medical Association* 291(23):2840–2846.

20. Dubinsky, R.M., Stein, A.C., and Lyons, K. 2000. Practice parameter: Risk of driving and Alzheimer's disease (an evidence-based review): Report of the quality standards subcommittee of the American Academy of Neurology. *Neurology* 54(12):2205–2211.

21. Koepsell, T., McCloskey, L., Wold, M. et al. 2002. Crosswalk markings and the risk of pedestrian-motor vehicle collisions in older pedestrians. *Journal of the American Medical Association* 288(17):2136–2143.

22. Langlois, J.A., Keyl, P.M., Guralnik, J.M., et al. 1997. Characteristics of older pedestrians who have difficulty crossing the street. *American Journal of Public Health* 87:393–397.

Mental Health and Mental Disorders

Body and soul cannot be separated for purposes of treatment, for they are one and indivisible. Sick minds must be healed as well as sick bodies.

C. Jeff Miller

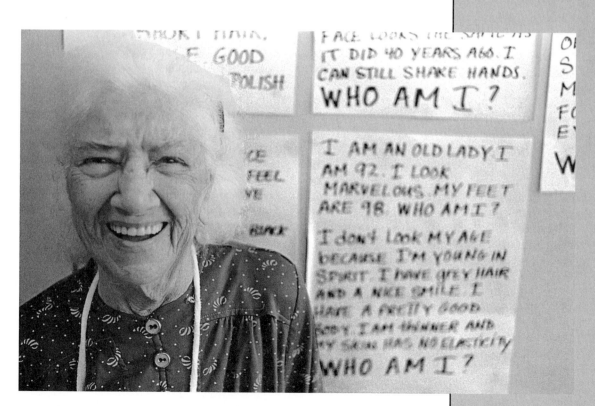

Most people as they grow older continue to function well and lead meaningful lives, just as they did in their younger years. The ability to adapt and be fulfilled in later life is related to a number of physical, psychological, and situational variables.

Failing to adapt to change and loss at any age can result in physical and emotional illness. The nature, prevalence, and treatment of mental disorders that are common in the later years are addressed. Although the majority of older people are able to adjust on their own or with support from family and friends, a few need professional assistance. Various mental health services are discussed. Unfortunately, most mental health services serve only a fraction of older people who need help. This chapter explores barriers that reduce the opportunities for elders to effectively use mental health services.

MENTAL HEALTH

Mental health is generally described as the ability to engage in productive activities and fulfilling relationships and to cope successfully with change and adversity. What characteristics are associated with good psychological health? Is there a set of "ideal traits?" Are any particular characteristics necessary? What kind of balance between positive and negative traits is consistent with mental health? Are any traits really "all good" or "all bad"? When examining seemingly opposite traits, such as independence and dependence or introversion and extroversion, is one extreme better than the other, or is it "best" to be somewhere in the middle? Although we may say that independence is a sign of mental health, how do we characterize individuals who express this trait to an extreme, remaining socially isolated and refusing needed help? Conversely, what about those elders or disabled individuals who are fully dependent yet mentally healthy? To what extent are our definitions of what is "healthy" determined by our culture or even our situation?

Behaviors that are normal or adaptive in one situation may be abnormal in others. For instance, sadness or melancholy following the death of a friend is quite different from severe, prolonged depression. What constitutes abnormal or normal behavior also depends on the individual's personality and past actions. Lethargy may be normal in an elder who has always moved at a slow pace, but abnormal when suddenly appearing in another elder who usually is self-motivated and energetic. Further, healthy behavior is culturally defined. For example, Asian cultures place more importance on the family and on individuals' responsibilities to family members, stressing interdependence within the family. In contrast, American culture puts more emphasis on the desires and rights of the individual to achieve success and independence.

Over the years, psychologists have attempted to determine what constitutes mental health and wellness in later life. Some people seem to age well, maintaining physical and mental vitality throughout their life span, while others appear to age poorly, with their later years characterized by poor physical health, unhappiness, or profound disability. Although there is no consensus among experts regarding what defines "successful aging," the prevailing frontrunner is the model develoed by Rowe and Kahn in 1998. They assert that three conditions are necessary for an older person to age successfully: (1) avoidance of disease and disability, (2) high cognitive and physical functioning, and (3) active engagement with life, including maintaining interpersonal relationships and sustaining productive activity.[1] More recently, Holstein and Minkler examined the values, assumptions, and consequences of the Rowe and Kahn model. They emphasize that because many important variables (e.g. sufficient income and access to affordable and accessible housing, nutrition and medical care) are beyond the control of many older people, especially older women, minorities, the uneducated, and the poor, the choices that individuals can make for themselves are reduced.[2]

With aging, there is inevitable decline in abilities and progression toward the unavoidable end of life. The way in which the individual adapts to these changes and declines may determine how "successfully" he or she ages. Concepts of adaptation, compensation, and resilience are thought to be important in healthy aging. *Adaptation* is the ability to redefine oneself in terms of independence and autonomy; *compensation* is the ability to change one's lifestyle to accommodate physical changes. Adaptation and compensation result in *resilience*—the ability to bounce back, to change, to be flexible, and to age successfully.[3] As an example, an elder notes that her vision is worse and she cannot read the novels she has always loved. She feels stiff in the mornings, her endurance is lower, and she believes that her thinking is not as "sharp" as it was. She may first have to adapt to the idea that her body is changing. She can compensate for the difficulties she is experiencing. Maybe she purchases reading glasses and leaves them around the house, or switches to large-print or audio books. She could start doing crossword puzzles and let her nephew teach her to use Facebook to stretch her mind. She decides to drive only in the daytime. She plans a walk when the morning chill wears off to limber up and makes sure not to

schedule events before noon as she has more pain in the mornings.

Models of successful aging often include concepts of physical health and vitality, active engagement with life, and psychological and cognitive fitness. But what about a person who is ill and/or disabled? A bedridden elder living in a nursing home with advanced dementia and heart disease may lack the cognitive, social, or physical resources to experience what we might call "mental health." Does this mean this elder is not mentally healthy? When poor health, disability, or financial circumstances force elders to give up activities that formerly fulfilled their needs for autonomy and self-esteem, individuals must satisfy their needs through a more restricted set of alternatives. Perhaps, then, mental health is best defined as maximizing satisfaction and future potential in the face of changing strengths, abilities, challenges, and resources.

Clearly, what constitutes mental health varies throughout the life cycle, for individuals have different expectations and priorities as they age. Although each individual's life is unique, psychologists suggest that certain patterns and needs are universal for each period of the life cycle. Whereas young adults look toward their future possibilities, elders may look more at their past achievements.

One critical developmental task of old age is acceptance. Elders must modify previous goals and accept the limitations of an aging body. They must accept the inevitability of their own death and the deaths of loved ones. They must also accept, without shame, their increased dependence, decreased physical health, and increased spectator role. However, they must also continue to develop and master new goals to maintain self-respect and self-esteem. Psychologist Erik H. Erikson described old age as ushering in the culmination of the life cycle, a time when the individual develops "ego integrity," mature judgment, and satisfaction with a life well lived. Poor adjustment is characterized by despair, the fear of death, and dissatisfaction with one's life.[4]

TRANSITIONS IN LATER LIFE

Growing old in a youth-oriented society that places primary value on independence, competence, energy, and productivity is not easy. It is the primary adaptive task of old age to find satisfaction and self-esteem when role loss, social status loss and physical ailments are more noticeable and decrements more likely than ever before.

—Iris Winogrond

Just like any other period in life, the transition into old age requires adapting to change. However, the life transitions faced by each age group differ. In general, the young are preparing for employment, finding a mate, and setting up a home, and the middle-aged are raising children, maintaining a job, and caring for aged parents. In the later years, many of the transitions are characterized by loss:

Physical losses: chronic illness and increasing disability, the loss of previous strength and endurance, and the loss of youthful appearance.

Psychological losses: forgetfulness, impaired cognitive ability, reduced status, reduced independence, loss of control, facing one's own mortality.

Social losses: changing residences, loss of job status, loss of driving abilities, loss of social status.

Economic losses: loss of employment, reduced income from retirement, living on a fixed income despite increased costs of medical expenses and inflation.

Interpersonal losses: death of spouse, friends, and family members.

Even though old age is accompanied by multiple losses, it has many benefits. Many older people experience the joy of seeing their children grow up into healthy, successful adults. Many elders have grandchildren, and, if bumper stickers and T-shirts are any indication, they are an important part of

their identity and happiness. For those who are still in good health and can afford it, travel opportunities provide an important part of their later years, especially among the young-old. And, although retirement is a loss for some who have not developed social networks or hobbies, retirement finally gives those who have many interests the free time to read, garden, socialize, and volunteer. For some, it is the beginning of a new career. Good health, sufficient income, and a network of family and friends can truly make the later years "golden."

Retirement

A sufficient income is an important factor in the ability to cope with the transitions of old age. The elderly used to be the most vulnerable segment of our society. When they were no longer able to work because of physical disability or illness, they had to rely on charity or their families for help. The Social Security Act of 1935, enacted during the Great Depression, provided a universal, stable income for retiring elders starting at age 65. These Social Security benefits have been increased over the years, and medical care benefits were added through Medicare (see Chapter 13). During this same period, more employers began to offer pensions, and individuals began saving for retirement through individual retirement accounts (IRAs). These changes completely revolutionized the financial situation of many elders. Now, for a greater proportion of older people, retirement symbolizes an achievement and the beginning of a life of leisure. However, others, particularly women living alone, minorities, and the very old, may have no pensions, are in poor health, and are likely to live in poverty. Many will not have the opportunity to experience the "golden years."

Although many people look forward to retirement, it is a major transition and all changes engender conflict. The majority of elders cope very well with this transition, reporting high levels of life satisfaction. There are vast differences in what older people do after retirement. Some travel, go back to school, volunteer their time, begin new hobbies, and spend time with grandchildren. However, a few elders have difficulty coping. Those with poor health or lower incomes may realize that they are not able to do all they had hoped in retirement. Retirement can cause emotional stress on marriages as roles change and couples spend more time together.

Relationships with Adult Children and Grandchildren

In general, elders derive much strength and support from relationships with adult children. Many elders live near adult children and visit frequently. Elders and their adult children may communicate through telephone calls, visits, and written communication. However, the amount of contact is not necessarily predictive of the quality of the relationship. In fact, contact may increase in times of trouble (such as the divorce of the adult child or the illness of the aged parent).

The quality of interaction between older adults and their children is important. With age, the relationship between adult parents and their children may change. Instead of parent-child interaction, many elders and their adult children are more akin to friends. In contrast, parent-child relationships focusing on economic dependency are not as satisfying. With advanced age and increased disability, there is often a change in roles as adult children attempt to "parent" their parents.

In addition to alterations in relationships with their adult children, elders may experience new or different relationships with their grandchildren. Grandparenting can be a source of joy and satisfaction to elders in their later years. Adult grandchildren can become friends to elders, or even provide caregiving. Elder grandparents may provide child care for their grandchildren when their own children are employed.

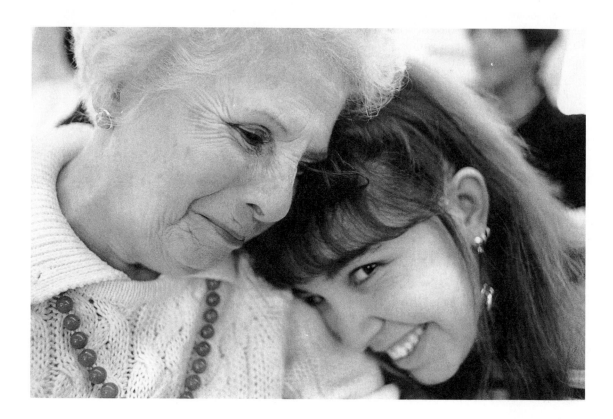

At times, elders may be called upon to care for their grandchildren in their later years, either temporarily or permanently. In 2009, there were 475,0000 elders who had primary responsibility for one or more grandchildren who lived with them. There are many reasons why the parent may not be able to care for the child: abandonment, physical or mental illness, death, teenage pregnancy, drug abuse, incarceration, child abuse, and neglect. Many grandparents faced with raising a grandchild experience ambivalent feelings. It is a big responsibility to care for a child, and their lives are changed significantly. Some grandparents are grateful for the opportunity to raise a grandchild, while others may fear or resent the parenting role and associated responsibilities late in life. Some grandparents are revitalized; others experience adverse health effects.

Marital Transitions

Marital transitions are common in later life. Relationships between partners evolve over the years, some becoming more dissatisfied with the relationship, others becoming more satisfied. In the 1800s, couples had children early in a marriage; therefore, many men and women had very little time as a couple before the first child arrived (generally less than two years). Further, they were often widowed before their children were grown. These days, more couples delay having their first child, some have no children at all, and people are living longer. The combination of these trends means that about one-third of married life is spent simply as a couple. Although a good number of relationships last for decades, many couples cannot tolerate this much togetherness and decide to divorce.

Studies of educated elders report a high degree of marital satisfaction as well as fewer arguments and more shared activities than younger couples.[5] However, studies analyzing the characteristics and success of older marriages rely on self-report rather than observation and do not take into account the changing expectations of marriage. For example, your grandparents may be satisfied with a very different kind of relationship than the kind you would desire.

It is clear that expectations of marriage vary by generation. Many of today's elders look at marriage differently than young adults. They are more likely to believe that divorce is not an option. Further, there are obvious cohort differences. Someone who is currently old may be satisfied that his or her spouse engages in traditional sex-specific roles and is a "good wife" or a "good provider." Many elders do not expect a spouse to be their best friend, lover, and partner. It will be interesting to study how the marital relationship of those who are old now compares with the marital relationship of members of the baby boomer generation as they grow older.

Coping with the illness of a spouse is also a considerable transition, especially if the illness is prolonged and the spouse needs constant care.

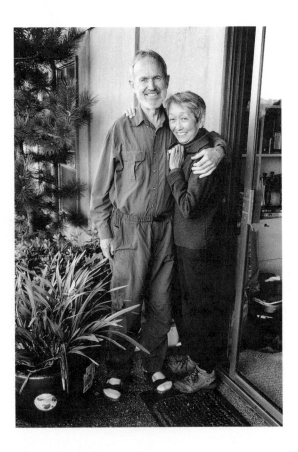

Illness can prompt many changes in the relationship, most of them negative. When one partner becomes ill, the other must adapt to more responsibility, altered relationship roles, and less personal time. The well spouse often must assume caregiving responsibilities while simultaneously receiving little support and encouragement. Illness may also impact elder sexuality and the ability to engage in other activities that the couple previously had enjoyed. The following vignette illustrates some of the changes that can occur in a relationship with illness.

> Mrs. Smith had always been known to their friends and their two daughters as "the strong one" who took care of everything. She was the hub around which the family revolved; she arranged social interactions, cooked and cleaned and shopped for her husband, Mr. Smith. She was on the phone frequently with the couple's daughters, assisting them with their problems. When Mrs. Smith suffered a stroke that left her unable to speak and paralyzed on one side of her body, Mr. Smith was abruptly cast into a care-giving role. First, he lived alone for almost a month while Mrs. Smith was in the hospital and then in a nursing home for rehabilitation. When she came home, she was unable to do any of her normal activities and required assistance in eating, bathing, and dressing herself. Mr. Smith threw himself into the role of caring for his wife, but found that he missed all the things she used to do. Now he felt he had to do his old jobs and hers as well. He missed the affectionate banter that was so characteristic, the sexual relations, and the easy way she had with their daughters. Sometimes Mr. Smith felt more like his wife's nurse than her husband and he longed to talk about his troubles, but the only person he was used to talking to about these things was his wife.

Despite its stresses, most elder spouses do not shy away from the strains of caregiving, and some of them report that the experience heightens their sense of love and commitment. This commitment is confirmed by national figures: the majority of frail elders in the United States are cared for by family members, most often by the spouse.

Widowhood

Deaths of family members are commonly experienced in the later years. Often the most traumatic death that elders must face is the loss of a spouse. Not only is there a loss of a long-time companion, but also there is a change in their social and financial situation, a loss of someone to care for them when illness strikes, and additional responsibilities. The loss of a spouse prompts grief and mourning reactions called *bereavement*.

It appears that women adapt better to the loss of a spouse than men. Although both men and women experience psychological distress, newly widowed men have a significantly higher rate of death and illness compared to their married counterparts. A widowed man maintains a higher risk of dying than a married woman throughout his life, but his risk drops if he remarries. This same trend is not apparent in women. One possible explanation for this differential is that women's role in relationships is to watch over the physical, emotional, and social well-being of both partners. Others suggest that this difference occurs because women, in general, maintain closer and wider networks of social support—whether through friends, family, or co-workers—and men rely much more on their spouses for social support. Although there are clear differences in physical health, some studies suggest that men's and women's psychological responses following the death of a spouse are relatively similar. Women generally suffer more of a decline in financial status than men upon widowhood and must cope with those associated stresses. Support groups for widowed persons are helpful for many.

Widowhood can be associated with other transitions. Often friendships broaden and deepen with other widows, widowers, or adult children. Widowhood may also result in a change in living situation. The majority of widows and widowers do not want to move in with their adult children, although some do. Often an adjustment must be made to a change in financial status. Finally, widowhood can have dramatic impact on sexual expression. Depending on their past sexual and marital satisfaction and present mental state, widowed men and women adapt

...easing the frequency of sexual fantasies and ...oeroticism, developing an interest in seeking out a future partner, channeling sexual energy into other pursuits, or losing interest in sexual activities altogether.

Factors Affecting Adjustment

The ability to cope successfully with the losses accompanying old age depends on many factors: personality traits, health status, financial situation, social support, and the ability to cope with stress.

Personality traits profoundly influence how people adapt to the physical and social transitions that occur with advancing age. Those who are extroverted, flexible, and expressive of their feelings generally cope better than those who are introverted and inflexible. A sense of control or mastery over one's environment is associated with positive physical and mental health in all age groups.

Health status may affect the ability to cope with the aging process, both physiologically and psychologically. When elders suffer reduced energy, diminished mobility, sensory decrements, and increased dependence and disability, they may be less likely to handle stress and adapt to changes. Both the symptoms of illness and the treatment regimen strain adaptive capacity.

The pain, debilitation, and dependence that often accompany illness impact elders' emotional health, particularly when the illness worsens over time. Physical illnesses are often accompanied by mental distress, especially anxiety and depression. Furthermore, the treatment of physical problems may cause mental symptoms (e.g., depression, insomnia, and hallucinations) and may restrict a person's customary lifestyle. Even the age-related decline in sensory abilities, especially vision and hearing, can result in withdrawal from social contacts, confusion, depression, and impaired orientation and mobility if not corrected.

Oftentimes, elders' perception of their health status is a more important predictor of coping ability than is their actual health. In fact, elders' perception of their physical health is one of the strongest correlates with life satisfaction, adjustment, self-esteem, and mental health. Despite physical decrements, the majority of elders think their own health is better than that of their peers.

Financial situation can also affect psychological health. Persons with sufficient income are able to meet their food, shelter, recreational, and health needs. Conversely, individuals who are poor have the additional stress of maintaining their health with limited resources. As income declines after retirement, many older people must deal with poverty and its associated problems for the first time. Poverty and the fear of poverty affects an individual's sense of security and increases anxiety and depression at any age.

It is well established that the presence of social support promotes health. Isolated adults have a significantly higher death rate than those with social ties; the more ties, the lower the death rate. The presence of social support not only buffers stress but may also reduce the symptoms of physical illness. Pets may provide social support by improving coping ability. Pets often lavish their owners with attention, stimulate laughter, encourage regular exercise, and make owners feel safe and needed.

The ability to cope with stress is an important factor in determining how successful adults will be when adapting to old age. Stress is any physiological or psychological situation that challenges the individual's capacity to adapt. For instance, extreme temperatures, radiation, noise, and starvation cause physical stress, while life events such as the death of a loved one, change in residence, and retirement cause psychological stress. An individual's response to stress is more important than the amount of stress experienced. Certain personality types are able to adapt more easily to stress than others: Some people are debilitated by it, while others are challenged.

Even though older people experience a number of life changes, they report less stress than any other adult age group. It is difficult to imagine, however, that elders, with their multiple health problems and the associated losses of old age, feel less stressed than younger groups.

Perhaps elders do not identify feelings of worry, frustration, irritability, isolation, or anxiety as stress. Or perhaps elders may cope more effectively with stress for a variety of reasons: They have learned to anticipate the changes; they allow themselves more time to adapt to their stressors; they minimize the total number of stressors to those they can control; or they adapt effective coping strategies. It remains to be seen what the reported stress level of today's baby boomers may be when they reach their later years, after growing up during the decades in which "stress" was a household word.

At any age, stress demands adaptation, and adaptation demands energy. Stress management techniques such as relaxation, meditation, supportive counseling, social interaction, exercise, good diet, humor, and setting new goals may help people cope more effectively with emotional and physical stressors. When the stress becomes unmanageable, temporary mood disturbances or even more serious mental illness may result.

MENTAL DISORDERS

A *mental disorder* is a condition that affects changes in thought, mood, or behavior (or a combination of these) that result in distress or impairment in function. Through the years, psychiatrists and other mental health professionals have collaborated in categorizing, defining, and developing criteria for the recognized mental disorders in order to properly diagnose a mental condition.

The most widely recognized classification schema utilized by the mental health profession is the *Diagnostic and Statistical Manual of Mental Disorders (DSM),* first published in 1952 by the American Psychiatric Association. The fourth edition of this comprehensive manual was published in 1994, called DSM-IV-TR. An updated version is scheduled to be published in 2013.[6] The *DSM* is based on the majority opinion of professionals, and cultural influences are evident. What is considered to be a mental illness has changed in the last 50 years. For example, homosexuality, listed as a mental disorder in the second edition, is now considered a normal sexual orientation. The *DSM* is surprisingly easy to read and provides a wealth of information. An online version can be found at www.behavenet.com/capsules/ Keep in mind that the proper use of the diagnostic categories requires clinical training and skills and that only licensed professionals can diagnose mental illness.

Mental problems in older people may have begun in their younger years or may appear for the first time late in life. Problems that appear for the first time in the later years are generally due either to an inability to adapt to stresses or to a physiological disorder in brain function that may have taken years to develop. Elders who have sustained multiple losses over a short time period, who have little or no social support, or who adapted poorly to stress in the past are particularly vulnerable to the onset of mental disorders in later life.

Although diagnoses of common mental illnesses such as depression, schizophrenia, and alcohol or drug abuse decline among elders, the prevalence of severe cognitive impairment increases with age. Elders living in nursing homes have higher rates of mental illness, particularly dementia and depression, than elders living in the community. Estimates vary, but one-half to three-quarters of nursing home residents have dementia.

Although mental disorders are common, the good news is there are a variety of effective treatments for those who have access to mental health professionals. Most mental disorders among elders are usually treated with psychoactive (also called psychotropic) medications that act on the central nervous system to alter behavior. Psychoactive medications fall into three major drug classes: antidepressants, antipsychotics, and antianxiety agents. Although psychotherapy, either individual or group, has been documented to be effective in helping people alter their negative thoughts and feelings, few elders utilize this treatment option.

In this section we present an overview of the most common mental disorders among elders, their symptoms, prevalence, and the basics of their treatment: depressive disorders, anxiety disorders,

Warning

When I am an old woman I shall wear purple
With a red hat which doesn't go, and doesn't suit me.
And I shall spend my pension on brandy and summer gloves
And satin sandals, and say we've no money for butter.
I shall sit down on the pavement when I'm tired
And gobble up samples in shops and press alarm bells
And run my stick along the public railings
And make up for the sobriety of my youth.
I shall go out in my slippers in the rain
And pick the flowers in other people's gardens
And learn to spit.
You can wear terrible shirts and grow more fat
And eat three pounds of sausages at a go
Or only bread and pickle for a week
And hoard pens and pencils and beermats and things in boxes.
But now we must have clothes that keep us dry
And pay our rent and not swear in the street
And set a good example for the children.
We must have friends to dinner and read the papers.
But maybe I ought to practice a little now?
So people who know me are not too shocked and surprised
When suddenly I am old, and start to wear purple.

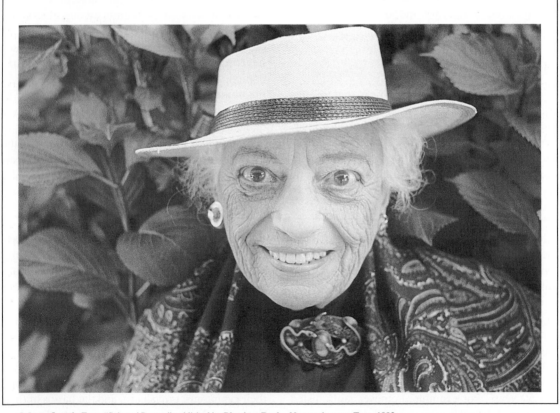

© Jenny Joseph. From "Selected Poems," published by Bloodaxe Books, Newcastle-upon-Tyne, 1992.

sleep disorders, substance use disorders, dementia, and delirium.

Mood Disorders

Classification of mood disorders can be complicated because these illnesses run the gamut from normal sadness associated with bereavement to depression severe enough to result in admission to a psychiatric hospital. Matters are complicated further by the common usage of the word "depression" to encompass everything from transitory feelings of sadness to incapacitating despair resulting in suicide. Mood disorders include *depressive disorders* (such as major depression or moderate depression) and *bipolar disorders,* which are characterized by fluctuations between extreme excitability (mania) and depression. Bipolar disorders are not common among older adults and will not be discussed.

We usually think of depression as feeling sad, blue, unhappy, miserable, or down in the dumps. Most of us feel this way at one time or another for short periods. Clinical depression, or depressive disorder, is distinctly different from transient feelings of unhappiness or sadness following a loss. To meet the criteria for *major depression,* an individual must experience five of the following symptoms all day nearly every day for at least two weeks: either depressed mood nearly all day for most days or loss of interest or pleasure in everyday activities; and several of the following; unintentional weight loss or gain; insomnia or excessive sleepiness; agitation or slowed movement; fatigue or loss of energy; feelings of worthlessness or inappropriate guilt; diminished ability to concentrate or indecisiveness; recurrent thoughts of death and suicidal thoughts.

There are other depressive disorders besides major depression. *Dysthymia* is emotional depression of moderate intensity that persists for most of the day for most days for at least two years and includes two or more of these symptoms: poor appetite or overeating; insomnia or sleepiness; low energy or fatigue; low self-esteem; poor concentration or difficulty making decisions; feelings of hopelessness. Individuals with *seasonal affective disorder* have depressive symptoms only during certain times of the year, most commonly the winter in northern latitudes. These individuals may be especially sensitive to lighting patterns so they are often treated by extended exposure to bright lights during winter days. *Reactive depressive disorder* is depression that follow a loss, such as the death of a loved one.

Major depression is the leading cause of disability in the United States. The prevalence of major depression among elders in the United States is approximately 6 percent and women are more likely to be affected than men. Although the number is less than other age groups, for those who are affected, not only can it impair physical, mental, and social functioning but it can also increase the risk of heart disease, cancer, and death. The vast majority of individuals who commit suicide are depressed.[7] See Box 7.1 for a discussion on suicide.

Older people who are depressed may withdraw from social participation, refuse to speak, and become unable to care for themselves. In addition, depressed elders commonly are cognitively impaired, are disoriented, move slowly, have angry outbursts, and have a shortened attention span. Some elders exhibit symptoms of depression and symptoms of psychosis, such as loss of contact with reality or hallucinations. This condition is called *psychotic depression.*

Depression is most often diagnosed by the patient's primary care physician. When evaluating a patient for depression, the physician rules out other conditions that may cause or aggravate depressive symptoms: some diseases, medications, and excessive alcohol use. Differentiating between dementia and depression can be particularly difficult, for severe depression can mimic dementia, and the two diseases often coexist. In general, dementia has a gradual onset, whereas depression develops more rapidly.

Several screening tools are available to diagnose depression. One very simple screening tool asks two questions: Over the past two weeks, have you felt down, depressed, or hopeless? Have you felt little interest or pleasure in doing things?

> **B O X   7 . 1**
>
> ## Suicide
>
> Suicide is a serious problem at any age. Even though the national focus is on preventing teen suicides, older adults are more likely than teens or young adults to kill themselves. The highest suicide rate occurs among middle-aged adults, particularly those between 45 and 54. Among older adults, those who are 75 and above are more likely to commit suicide than those between the ages of 65 and 74.[8]
>
> Who commits suicide? Gender plays a large role in suicide rates in the United States. Men account for the majority of suicides among all age groups. Race is also important: whites kill themselves at higher rates than nonwhites.[8] Other factors that increase the risk for suicide among elders are depression, multiple severe chronic illnesses, terminal conditions, and severe pain.[9]
>
> Elders who attempt suicide are more likely to succeed than are younger adults. Younger persons often act impulsively, but older people are more likely to plan their suicide attempts and to use highly lethal methods. The majority of the suicides among elders are accomplished with a gun.
>
> Suicide rates may be underestimated among older people because many suicides are reported as other causes of death (e.g., drug overdose, refusal of life-sustaining drugs, intentional starvation, and accidents). Some people take the controversial viewpoint that elderly suicides are more often "rational" suicides: Individuals choose to take their own lives rather than live out their final days ill, in pain, disabled, or as burdens to their families.
>
> Most elders provide behavioral and verbal clues to suicide prior to the act. Previous suicide attempts, preoccupation with suicidal thought, agitation, or expression of hopelessness are important indicators. An older person who is planning suicide may purchase a firearm, stockpile pills, make funeral arrangements, or give away valued possessions. Verbal clues may be direct (e.g., "I'm going to kill myself") or indirect (e.g., "I'm tired of life. What's the point of going on?"). Family, friends, and professionals should be alert to prolonged depression or hints about suicide and should openly discuss the topic.
>
> Talking about suicide will not increase suicidal intentions. Many suicides could be prevented if high-risk elders were identified and referred to appropriate help.
>
> Prevention programs can be offered to older people living in the community and to those residing in sheltered living situations.
>
> Suicide has a great impact on the survivors, who often feel guilty for not having noticed the victim's trauma or for not intervening soon enough. Many survivors feel responsible for the victim's action. For these reasons, those close to suicide victims may need counseling and support to allay their feelings of guilt, depression, and self-blame. A useful resource for both professionals and laypersons is the American Association of Suicidology at www.suicidology.org

Elders may not exhibit the classic symptoms of depression, so the diagnosis may be missed, particularly among those with multiple health problems. For example, elders may complain of aches and pains or note forgetfulness and reduced weight, but they may not complain of "feeling blue." When symptoms are present, many times the physician, family member, or even the older person may mistakenly attribute the symptoms to another chronic illness or to "old age."

Many people who are depressed are never diagnosed or treated. Their symptoms may gradually improve without help, but improvement may take months or even years. Treatment of depression speeds recovery, but even treatment is not immediate. Treatment of depression may be accomplished through medication, individual or group psychotherapy, or electroconvulsive therapy. In general, mild depression may be treated with drugs or psychotherapy. Moderate to severe depression is generally treated with medications or electroconvulsive therapy initially, with psychotherapy offered when the depression begins to lessen. If depressed individuals present a danger to themselves or others (e.g., they have a plan for committing suicide), then medical professionals are legally obligated to place them in a secure hospital setting for 24 to 72 hours until treatment can be initiated and the danger is resolved.

Antidepressant medications work by affecting the balance of neurotransmitters, the communication links within the brain (e.g., seratonin, dopamine, and norepinephrine). These medications are useful for treating both depression and anxiety disorders, sleep problems, and even pain. They are among the most prescribed drugs in the nation.

The first choice of antidepressant medications to treat depression is selective serotonin reuptake inhibitors (SSRIs). They work by increasing serotonin, a neurotransmitter, within the brain. Common names are fluoxetine (Prozac), paroxetine (Paxil), and sertraline (Zoloft). Other similar reuptake inhibitors are venlafaxine (Effexor) and nefazodone (Serzone), but they also increase the availability of another neurotransmitter, norepinephrine. Another type of medication also increases the neurotransmitter dopamine in the brain: bupropion (Wellbutrin, Zyban). Other drug types are tricyclic antidepressants, MAO inhibitors, and stimulants. A wide variety of side effects have been reported for all antidepressant types, including constipation, anxiety, excessive sedation, sexual difficulties, and alterations in weight or appetite. Further discussion regarding psychoactive drug use for mental disorders appears later in the chapter.

Medication combined with psychotherapy works better than either treatment alone in treating depression.[10] However, because of insurance issues, most elders do not undergo psychotherapy for depression.

The most controversial and misunderstood therapy for major depression is electroconvulsive therapy (ECT), also called shock therapy. Studies continue to show it to be a safe, well-tolerated, and effective treatment for major depression, even among older people. It has been endorsed by the National Institutes of Health as effective when antidepressants have not helped or cannot be given for a medical reason. It is especially useful for those who are suicidal or not functioning because it works immediately whereas antidepressants take weeks for a full effect. ECT appears to be equal, even superior, to medications to treat both major and moderate depression.[11]

ECT is very different from the memorable scene in the movie *One Flew over the Cuckoo's Nest*. After a patient receives a light general anesthesia and muscle relaxant, an electrical current is passed through the brain for one to three seconds. This produces a small, controlled seizure that lasts for about a minute. The patient awakens in 5 to 10 minutes, then rests for a half hour. Most people are confused after the treatment and suffer short-term memory loss, but the side effects clear up in an hour. The usual course of treatment is three times a week for three to four weeks. Relapse of depression after response to ECT is high unless antidepressants are used.

No matter what treatment is used, treatment of depression (and other mental illnesses) is optimized if there is collaboration among the professionals caring for the patient, adequate education and support for the individual and family members, and a case manager or advocate to be sure the person is receiving good care. One randomized, controlled study of this "collaborative care model" that included almost 2,000 elder patients with mild or severe depression reported that those with access to a case manager were more than twice as likely to reduce depressive symptoms when compared with a similar group of depressed elders who participated in usual care.[12]

Anxiety Disorders

Anxiety is characterized by a combination of psychological symptoms, such as excessive worry, a sense of foreboding and doom, or nervousness and physical symptoms such as dry mouth, restlessness, sweating, upset stomach, heart palpitations, insomnia, diarrhea, hyperventilation, shortness of breath, feeling faint, obsessive eating, or loss of

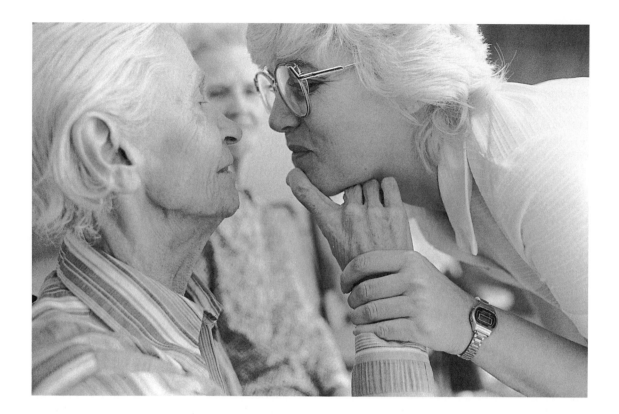

appetite. Individuals may report a sense of dread or may fear they are dying, losing control, or going crazy. Anxiety can be a feeling we all experience from time to time in normal life, or it may be a symptom of a mental disorder. How do you tell the difference?

Transient mild or even moderate anxiety is a normal reaction to a stressful situation. For example, it is normal to be anxious prior to taking a test or before a job interview. Anxiety can be a helpful motivator to study. But when an individual becomes disabled by excessive and irrational fear of everyday situations that affects social function, interpersonal relationships, or work effectiveness, then the symptoms indicate an anxiety disorder.

People can be anxious all the time for no apparent reason (*generalized anxiety disorder*) or have discrete, disabling attacks of anxiety, accompanied by rapid heart rate, breathlessness, and a feeling of doom (*panic disorder*). People can have obsessions where they cannot get certain thoughts or ideas out of their head, and compulsions where they feel compelled to repeat behaviors over and over when there is no need for the repeated behavior (*obsessive-compulsive disorder*). Anxiety can be related to specific situations. For instance, *agoraphobia* means literally "fear of open spaces." Most people with the disorder avoid leaving their homes for fear of developing panic symptoms in public places. Anxiety may be associated with a physical illness, or it may be associated with dementia, depression, or psychosis. Individuals with dementia may have symptoms of anxiety: They may worry that they forgot something or lost something, and they may wander and fuss all day trying to find it (*anxiety disorder due to general medical condition*).

Even though anxiety is common, most individuals with anxiety disorders are never diagnosed or treated. Symptoms of anxiety mimic symptoms of illness: heart palpitations, shortness of breath, weakness, and appetite changes. A comprehensive history and examination is necessary to determine if the person's anxiety is caused by disease, drug reactions, psychological problems, mental illness, or transient life events.

The symptoms of anxiety can be relieved by several types of antidepressant medications. Benzodiazepines or sedatives such as Valium, Ativan, and Xanax can be very effective and useful short-term by creating a drowsy, calming effect. However, many experts believe these drugs are not appropriate for elders. They are habit-forming, they have never been shown to be effective for long-term use, and they cause multiple side effects in elders (an increased risk of falling, constipation, driving accidents, and impaired memory and confusion). Another antianxiety drug, BuSpar, is less habit-forming and may be particularly effective in anxious, demented elders. Beta blockers, prescribed to those with cardiovascular disease, are sometimes prescribed for anxiety to slow the heart rate and reduce feelings of anxiety.

Psychotherapy can be effective in treating anxiety disorders. Therapists can help individuals to learn new ways to cope with anxious thoughts by teaching them to use statements and phrases to calm themselves and break the cycle of anxiety. Desensitization therapy, which involves gradually increasing exposure to the object of fear, can also be effective. Therapists may also recommend relaxation techniques, meditation, imagery, stress management, and biofeedback.

Psychotic Disorders

Psychosis is the inability to distinguish what is real from what is not. Psychosis may include *delusions,* which are false beliefs about who one is and what is taking place (for example, "I am Jesus Christ" or "My wife is trying to poison me"), *paranoia* (unrealistic fears), *hallucinations* (hearing voices that others do not hear or seeing things that others do not see), incoherent thoughts or ideas, inability to sustain relationships, and

difficulty with personal hygiene. Psychosis is a major part of some diseases, such as schizophrenia, but psychotic symptoms may also occur with other disorders, such as depression, mania, dementia, or delirium.

Schizophrenia affects only 1 percent of the population, and its incidence lessens in the later years. Most elders with schizophrenia have suffered the illness from a very young age and must contend with reduced intensity of symptoms coupled with side effects from long-term use of antipsychotic medications. The majority of schizophrenics need a structured environment for survival—they are unable to provide for their own needs or care for themselves. Those with schizophrenia have a significantly reduced life expectancy with a high rate of smoking, high blood pressure, dementia, diabetes, obesity, and suicide. One in ten schizophrenics commits suicide.

Unfortunately, there is no cure for schizophrenia. Antipsychotic medications are prescribed to reduce the symptoms, and they often need to be taken for life. Psychosis can also occur in other conditions, including depression, mania, dementia, and delirium. Antipsychotics can be used in these conditions as well to treat the symptoms of paranoia, hallucinations, and delusions. See Box 7.2 for a discussion on antipsychotics.

Sleep Disorders

There are more than 100 known sleep disorders, and most of them are associated with *insomnia,* the inability to achieve and sustain restful sleep. Insomnia can be transient, short-term, or chronic. Transient insomnia lasts at most a few nights and is generally associated with a specific stressful event (e.g., anxiety regarding the results of a medical test). Short-term insomnia lasts from days to months and is often precipitated by a more significant life stressor (e.g., death in the family). Chronic insomnia persists for longer than a month and is generally related to an underlying medical or psychological condition.

Sleep disorders are extremely common, affecting about one-third of all adults. Elders

---

B O X   7 . 2

Antipsychotics

Various antipsychotic medications (also called major tranquilizers) are available to treat psychosis or behavioral problems associated with depression, dementia, and bipolar disease, each with differing uses and side effects. The earlier antipsychotics worked by depleting the dopamine levels in the brain, thereby reducing the symptoms of psychosis. Unfortunately, the success of the drugs came with a price: short-term side effects such as sleepiness, slowed thinking, and constipation, and a serious and irreversible long-term side effect, tardive dyskinesia.

Tardive dyskinesia is a chronic movement disorder characterized by tremors, or repetitive movements of the face, arms, or legs, similar to symptoms of Parkinson's disease. Unfortunately, this side effect may not appear until after the drugs are stopped, and it is very difficult to treat. Women, elders, and African Americans are at higher risk, and the disorder used to afflict up to one-half of those using the drugs. The best way to prevent

tardive dyskinesia is to use lower doses and short durations of therapy.

Newer antipsychotics significantly reduce the risk of tardive dyskinesia but have a multitude of other side effects: sedation, weight gain, agitation, dizziness, urinary retention, and many more. In fact, these drugs may even cause diabetes, strokes, or cardiovascular disease, and, when used in elders with dementia, they are associated with an increased risk of death.

Antipsychotics are no longer used only for the pyschosis of schizophrenia. They are more commonly used for severe depression, for bipolar disease, and even, in lower doses, for elders with dementia with symptoms of agitation, wandering, aggressive behavior, or screaming due to dementia. It is not clear how effective these drugs are for these conditions, but they are widely used. The medication chosen to reduce behavioral problems should be selected with the side effect profile most acceptable to the patient, and doses should be kept as low as possible.

---

report more sleep complaints than any other age group: difficulty falling asleep, periods of wakefulness in bed, restless sleep, and early-morning awakening. Estimates vary, but it is generally agreed that up to one third of older people living in the community and two-thirds of elders in nursing homes have some kind of sleep disturbances. Insomnia at night can lead to sleepiness during the day. Those who report sleep disturbances have a higher rate of auto accidents, reduced ability to concentrate, memory impairment, interpersonal problems, decreased immune function, and increased risk of serious illness compared to those who sleep well. Despite these consequences, most people do not seek medical care for sleep disturbances.

Some elders' sleep disorders are due to age-associated changes in sleep patterns. With advancing age, the time it takes to fall asleep lengthens. Older people spend more time in light sleep and less time in deep-sleep stages. Although the

number of times an individual awakens at night increases with age, elders are generally able to fall back to sleep. Further, elders spend more time in bed for less actual sleep.

Besides age, sleep disturbances can have a number of physiological and psychological causes. For example, sleep problems are commonly associated with a variety of physical problems: depression, dementia, anxiety, heart disease, urinary frequency, severe pain, itching, and alcoholism. Many prescribed medications cause insomnia. Further, caffeine in coffee, tea, soft drinks, and some over-the-counter medications can also have a significant effect.

When an elder complains of insomnia, a thorough history should be undertaken to determine whether an underlying cause of the problem can be treated. Many sleep disorders can be improved by changing the sleep environment and modifying behaviors and attitudes that are counterproductive to sleep (see Box 7.3). If the sleep disorder is not

BOX 7.3

Have Insomnia?

Tips to Help You Sleep

- Limit the use of your bed to sleep and sexual activity.
- Make sure your bedroom is dark and quiet and at a comfortable temperature.
- Try blocking out light and sound in the bedroom.
- Limit alcohol, caffeine, and nicotine.
- Limit excessive liquid intake before bedtime.
- Don't go to bed too full or too hungry.
- Go to bed only when you are tired.
- Establish a regular bedtime, and avoid late-afternoon naps.

- Get relaxed before bedtime with calming bedtime rituals.
- Regular exercise can aid sleep, just not right before bedtime.
- Before bedtime, try muscle relaxation exercises and think relaxing thoughts.
- If you can't sleep, read for 20 minutes, turn out the light, and try again.
- Ask the pharmacist if your medication causes insomnia.
- See your physician if your insomnia does not improve after following the preceding tips.

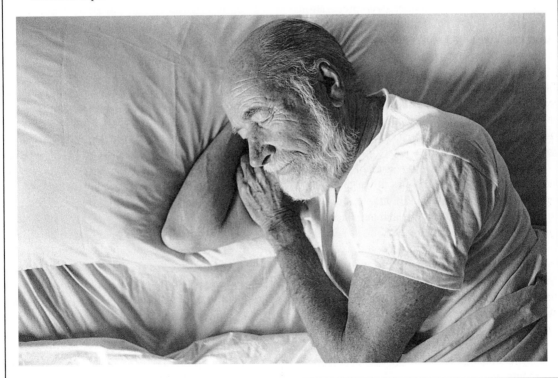

improved with such behavioral changes, observation of sleep/wake patterns in a sleep laboratory provides further information. Sleeping medications may be prescribed.

As a group, elders are high users of sleeping pills. The majority of prescription sleeping medications are "central nervous system depressants" that work by depressing brain activity. These include new, short-acting medications such as Ambien, Lunesta, or Sonata; older, short-acting benzodiazepines (such as Halcion or Restoril); and even older, long-acting benzodiazepines (Valium) or barbiturates (Dalmane). Sleep medications cause drowsiness, but most have serious side effects, especially among elders: confusion, disorientation, dizziness, falls, anxiety, urinary retention, sleepiness the next day, reduced ability to do tasks, and memory loss. The side effects are fewer from the shorter-acting drugs and worse from the longer-acting drugs. These sleep medications are approved only for short-term use (7 to 10 days). Although they provide a short-term fix for insomnia, it is better in the long run to develop good sleeping habits.

Some sleep medications and supplements are available without a prescription. Antihistamines are found in most over-the-counter sleep preparations (e.g., benadryl/diphenhydramine) and are used because they cause drowsiness. However, they also cause dry mouth, constipation, difficulty urinating, confusion, disorientation, and dizziness. Melatonin is a popular supplement that is thought to decrease the time it takes to fall asleep. Melatonin, a brain hormone that regulates sleep-wake cycles, is thought to be a "natural" alternative to prescription drugs.

A relatively common sleep disorder among older people is the condition known as *restless legs syndrome,* the irresistable urge to move the legs because of uncomfortable and unpleasant sensations in the legs and can only be relieved by moving the legs. Unfortunately, the symptoms recur when the individual goes back to bed. The symptoms worsen at night, particularly when lying down or sitting. In rare cases, the arms are affected, or the individual has symptoms at other times, such as during a car trip. It is thought that as much as 10 percent of the population has restless legs syndrome, with incidence increasing with advancing age. The problem may be treated with several types of medications: painkillers, muscle relaxants, sleep medications, and drugs used for epilepsy and Parkinson's disease.

Many elders may suffer from another sleep disorder: sleep apnea. *Sleep apnea* is characterized by brief periods during sleep when breathing stops. Cessation of breathing may last from seconds to more than one minute and may occur hundreds of times a night. Each time the breathing is cut off, the elder awakens to breathe. Although this awakening is life preserving, it is also a severe disrupter of sleep. The common symptoms of sleep apnea are disruptive snoring, breathing pauses during sleep, exhaustion, morning headaches, difficulty concentrating, and excessive daytime sleepiness. The lack of oxygen at night puts these individuals at a higher risk of cardiac arrhythmias, heart attacks, and auto accidents from falling asleep while driving. In addition, individuals with sleep apnea suffer cognitive decline.

Sleep apnea may be caused by problems in the part of the brain that regulates breathing, but it is more often due to mechanical problems related to excess fat and tissue in the throat that cuts off breathing during sleep. Among elders, particularly those who are overweight, the muscle tone in the throat and neck may be more lax, causing the tissue to sag into the airway. Those who snore are also at higher risk because snoring is often related to excess fatty tissue in the throat. Diagnosis of sleep apnea may require time in a sleep laboratory so that vital signs can be monitored during sleep.

Treatment for sleep apnea may include weight loss, sleeping on one's side, quitting smoking, and reducing alcohol consumption. Some individuals gain relief from using tape to widen the nostrils to improve airflow, or dental devices to push the jaw forward to increase airflow in and out of the throat. Surgery to remove excess tissue in the nose, mouth, or throat area or the use of radio-frequency energy to shrink the tissue in the back of the upper mouth (soft palate) are viable options. However, information on long-term effectiveness of various treatments is limited.

The most effective treatment for sleep apnea is to provide continuous air pressure to keep the air passages open to improve breathing while the individual sleeps. This is accomplished by a machine that is composed of a nosepiece or mask and a pump working together to improve breathing by continually blowing air through the trachea and into the lungs. Although the treatment is very effective, some people find it cumbersome and discontinue its use.

Substance Use Disorders

Substance use disorders include two categories. *Substance abuse* is the use of a substance despite negative health and social consequences. *Substance dependence* is the prolonged use of a substance that requires a higher dose for the same effect or results in withdrawal if the substance is not provided. The substances included in these disorders are commonly alcohol, tobacco, illegal drugs such as marijuana, cocaine, methamphetamine, and heroin or other opiates, and prescription painkillers or sedatives. The *DSM-IV-TR* defines substance dependence as "a cluster of cognitive, behavioral, and physiological symptoms indicating that the individual continues use of the substance despite significant substance-related problems." To meet the *DSM* criteria, at least three of the following symptoms need to occur over a 12-month period:[6]

- Needing an increased amount of the substance to achieve the desired effect
- Using the substance to avoid or relieve withdrawal symptoms
- Often taking the substance in larger amounts than intended
- Inability to reduce or stop substance use, even when desired
- Spending much time seeking the substance, taking the substance, and recovering from its effects
- Reducing or giving up important activities because of use

The two most important substance use disorders among elders are alcohol and nicotine. Although dependencies on sedatives and painkillers likely exist among older people because they are prescribed those drugs more often than other age groups, there is not much information regarding the extent of prescription drug dependency among the older population. However, there is ample evidence regarding their dependence on alcohol and nicotine.

Alcohol Abuse and Dependence

Alcohol use is common in American society, although it declines with age. The national Drug Use and Health Survey conducted by the Substance Abuse and Mental Health Services Administration reported that, in 2010, the percentage of individuals aged 26 to 29 who had at least one drink in the last 30 days was 65 percent; of those aged 60 to 64, it was 52 percent; and only 38 percent of those questioned who were 65 and older reported having had at least one drink in the past month. At all ages, women were less likely to drink alcohol than men.[13] The majority of individuals who drink are able to drink in moderation. Alcohol becomes a problem only when it is abused or when individuals become alcohol dependent.

Alcohol abuse occurs when an individual engages in excessive drinking that affects his or her health or social life but the person is not dependent on the drug and has not lost control over its use. In contrast, *alcohol dependence (alcoholism)* involves a preoccupation with alcohol and inability to control alcohol intake. Alcoholics are physically dependent on the drug, and their alcohol use continues despite its negative impact on personal health, work, family life, and financial stability. There may be a genetic predisposition for alcoholism, and psychological and social factors are contributors.

Alcohol dependence is a progressive, debilitating chronic illness. The disease is often fatal and can cause health problems in nearly every organ system. Alcoholism is associated with multiple physical and psychological problems. Studies show that excess alcohol consumption shortens life expectancy, contributes to high suicide rates, worsens many chronic illnesses (especially diabetes), and creates nutritional deficiencies. Additionally, heavy alcohol use can induce dementia, cognitive deficits, depression, and psychosis. Individuals who abuse alcohol and also have a poor diet may get Korsakoff's syndrome, a memory disorder caused by a dietary deficiency of thiamine. The symptoms are memory loss, inability to concentrate, disorientation, and vision impairment. Alcohol affects muscular coordination, reaction time, and equilibrium, increasing susceptibility to accidents. Alcohol adversely affects the quality of sleep. Alcohol abuse is known to be associated with car accidents, suicides and homicides, and physical abuse of family members. Older alcoholics are also at high risk for adverse reactions when medications are taken with alcohol in the blood.

Because of changes in the distribution and metabolism of alcohol with age, persons become more susceptible to intoxication by alcohol with advancing age. Older adults usually have a lower proportion of water content in the body than younger adults, which increases the alcohol concentration, potentially causing more damage to organs and tissues. It is now known that women and older people break down less ethanol in the stomach, allowing a higher proportion of alcohol to circulate in the bloodstream. This occurs because, when compared to young men, they have a reduced amount of alcohol dehydrogenase, the stomach enzyme that breaks down alcohol. Also, elders often take medications whose effect is heightened when alcohol is also used.

The majority of elder alcoholics have suffered from drinking problems throughout their lives, but a few begin drinking to excess late in life. Estimates vary, but it is generally agreed that the proportion of elder alcoholics is about 2 to 4 percent of the elder population, considerably lower that the 10 percent usually quoted for the population as a whole. There may be fewer elderly alcoholics for a number of reasons. Those who drank heavily in earlier life may have already died from alcoholism or its complications. Elders may have reduced their alcohol consumption because they have become more sensitive to the effects of alcohol. Or, because of physical problems stemming from alcohol, a higher proportion of elder alcoholics can be found in hospitals and nursing homes and are not counted in community studies.

Diagnosis of alcoholism is complex in elders because they may exhibit fewer visible signs of intoxication and withdrawal than middle-aged people. Further, elders' alcohol dependence is less likely to be detected by an employer or spouse, since many are already retired, live alone, and are not socially disruptive. An older person with an alcohol problem may often go unnoticed and untreated by medical personnel because the physical signs of alcoholism (depression, dementia, poor grooming, incontinence, susceptibility to accidents, malnutrition, and general physical deterioration) may be mistakenly attributed to chronic illness and old age. Older people may be less willing to seek help because they are afraid of being stigmatized.

Several instruments have been developed to help doctors diagnose alcoholism in their patients. One of the simplest and most widely used is the CAGE questionnaire consisting of four items.[14] Answering yes to two of the questions is suspicious for alcoholism:

> Have you ever felt you should **C**ut down on your drinking?
>
> Have people **A**nnoyed you by criticizing your drinking?
>
> Have you ever felt bad or **G**uilty about your drinking?
>
> Have you ever had a drink first thing in the morning to steady your nerves or get rid of a hangover (**E**ye-opener)?

This screening instrument has been criticized because it doesn't address the quantity (amount) or frequency (how often) of drinking.

Some older people who have been drinking heavily and consistently throughout their lives need to go to the hospital to "detoxify" from alcohol, but most are able to stop drinking without being detoxified. If alcoholism is accompanied by other mental illness, psychiatric treatment of both simultaneously may be helpful. There are medications that reduce alcohol cravings or cause those who drink to vomit, but these are not used by the majority of elders who quit drinking.

Treatment programs are commonly recommended to assist the individual to stop drinking alcohol. Some programs emphasize cognitive-behavioral therapy, and others use regular group meetings, a spiritually based framework, and mentors to achieve sobriety. Most treatments emphasize lifelong abstention. Research comparing treatment programs is needed to determine which programs are more effective for elders.

Alcoholics Anonymous (AA) is a popular choice for elders because it is free and easily accessible and the members offer social support. The purpose of Alcoholics Anonymous is to help alcoholics to become sober and to stay sober. This is accomplished by regular attendance at meetings where men and women with alcohol dependence share their experiences with each other. AA membership is free, voluntary and anonymous. The interventions focus on admitting that you cannot control your addiction; recognizing a higher power that can give strength; examining past errors and making amends; learning to live a new life with abstention from alcohol; and helping others who suffer from the same addictions or compulsions. It is estimated that there are more than 100,000 AA groups and over 2 million AA members in 150 countries. For more information on Alcoholics Anonymous, refer to www.aa.org

Although Alcoholics Anonymous has helped many people stop substance abuse habits, it has not been studied or shown to be effective. Some can quit on their own without any program; others benefit from other approaches. Brief interventions by health care professionals, focusing on the problem, offering advice to quit, and follow-up have been repeatedly shown to be effective at reducing problem drinking. An alternative to Alcoholics Anonymous is SMART Recovery. SMART stands for "self management and recovery training" and uses cognitive-behavioral therapy techniques to help people recover from addictions. These services, like AA, are free and focus on four areas: enhancing and

---

The Twelve Steps of Alcoholics Anonymous

1. We admitted we were powerless over alcohol—that our lives had become unmanageable.
2. Came to believe that a Power greater than ourselves could restore us to sanity.
3. Made a decision to turn our will and our lives over to the care of God as we understood Him.
4. Made a searching and fearless moral inventory of ourselves.
5. Admitted to God, to ourselves, and to another human being the exact nature of our wrongs.
6. Were entirely ready to have God remove all these defects of character.
7. Humbly asked Him to remove our shortcomings.

8. Made a list of all persons we had harmed, and became willing to make amends to them all.
9. Made direct amends to such people wherever possible, except when to do so would injure them or others.
10. Continued to take personal inventory and when we were wrong promptly admitted it.
11. Sought through prayer and meditation to improve our conscious contact with God, as we understood Him, praying only for knowledge of His will for us and the power to carry that out.
12. Having had a spiritual awakening as the result of these Steps, we tried to carry this message to alcoholics, and to practice these principles in all our affairs.

The Twelve Steps are reprinted with permission of Alcoholics Anonymous World Services, Inc. ("AAWS") Permission to reprint the Twelve Steps does not mean that AAWS has reviewed or approved the contents of this publication, or that AAWS necessarily agrees with the views expressed herein. A.A. is a program of recovery from alcoholism only—use of the Twelve Steps in connection with programs and activities which are patterned after A.A., but which address other problems, or in any other non-A.A. context, does not imply otherwise.

maintaining motivation to abstain; coping with urges; managing thoughts, feelings, and behavior and problem solving; and finally, balancing momentary and enduring satisfactions. More information is available at www.smartrecovery.org

Nicotine Abuse and Dependence

Although people may not think of tobacco use as a mental disorder, nicotine or tobacco dependence is perhaps the most commonly diagnosed mental illness in the U.S. today. Individuals with nicotine dependence are usually aware of the severe health consequences of their habit but are unable or unwilling to stop smoking. The Centers for Disease Control and Prevention estimate that one of four adults in the United States smokes cigarettes, but among the 65 and older age group, that percentage drops to one in ten.[13]

Even though most older people no longer smoke, smokers should be urged to quit to reduce the health consequences. Tobacco use is the number-one cause of premature death and disability in our country, and more than one-half of those who smoke die prematurely. Smoking is associated with a plethora of health problems, including cardiac disease, lung disease, cancer, stroke, and accidents. For an excellent literature review, refer to the Surgeon General's report, *The Health Consequences of Smoking.*[15]

Because the majority of smokers visit a physician every year, the physician is in a good position to intervene and promote the treatment of tobacco dependence. A panel of medical experts convened by the Public Health Service researched the literature and published clinical practice guidelines to be used by physicians with their patients to reduce tobacco use in the United States.[16] The panel asserted that the physician should identify all patients who are smokers and should offer treatment, both counseling and medication, and follow-up.

The panel developed the "5As" to be used to approach patients: ASK if they use tobacco, ADVISE them to quit, ASSESS their willingness to quit, ASSIST those who are willing to quit, and ARRANGE for follow-up. For those unwilling to quit, the panel advised physicians to provide a motivational intervention using the "5Rs":

> RELEVANCE: Ask patients why quitting is relevant to them.
>
> RISKS: Ask patients to identify negative consequences of tobacco use.
>
> REWARDS: Ask patients to identify potential benefits of stopping tobacco use.
>
> ROADBLOCKS: Ask patients to identify barriers to quitting.
>
> REPETITION: Repeat the motivational intervention every time a patient returns to the office.

The panel asserts that these interventions are brief, taking about three minutes of the physician's time, but are cost-effective when compared to other disease interventions. For more details on the guidelines, refer to www.surgeongeneral.gov

Many other programs are available to assist individuals to stop smoking. Health educators may provide brochures or fliers and literature about the health consequences of smoking, the costs and benefits of smoking, particular health consequences that matter most to specific individuals, and how to quit. They may implement telephone-based and Web-based programs to help people to quit. Generally, the programs encourage people to set a date to quit and stick to it. They offer medication, education, and follow-up, reinforce successes, and provide reassurance that failures are common and that the participant needs to try again. Some counselors specialize in smoking cessation, both with individuals and in groups.

Drugs are available to help smokers quit. Prescription nicotine delivery systems (e.g., patch, gum, nose spray, inhaler) deliver a small controlled dose of nicotine that diminishes the nicotine craving and reduces the symptoms of sudden withdrawal. These medications are taken when the individual feels a craving to smoke and are gradually withdrawn. They have been shown to be safe and effective. Also, Zyban (also known as the antidepressant Wellbutrin—two names for the same medication!) and Chantix have been shown to reduce craving, withdrawal symptoms, and relapse. These drugs may double or even triple the quit rate, but many people do relapse. Unfortunately, the drugs are associated with side effects, including a risk of suicide. Medications are most effective when used in combination with a comprehensive behavioral smoking cessation program.

Several resources are available for individuals of all ages who want to quit. The Department of Health and Human Services' toll-free tobacco quitline, 1-800-QUIT NOW, routes callers to state-run quitlines that help individuals to find the nearest programs. Also, the Web site www.smokefree .gov provides advice and information on how to quit smoking.

Cognitive Disorders

Cognition is the mental ability that enables us to know about and function in our world. Cognition includes many mental processes: memory, problem solving, attention, comprehension, language, perception, and reasoning, to name a few. A cognitive disorder is manifested by significant problems in one or more of these mental tasks. The two most common cognitive disorders among elders, dementia (including Alzheimer's disease) and delirium, are discussed below.

Dementia and Dementia of the Alzheimer's Type

Dementia is a progressive brain impairment that interferes with memory and normal intellectual functioning. If not treated, it causes further physical impairment, debility, and death. The most common cause of dementia is Alzheimer's disease; the second most common is multi-infarct dementia (a series of small strokes). Dementia can also be caused by alcoholism, depression, brain tumors, AIDS, head trauma, environmental toxins, chronic lung disease, drugs, and Parkinson's disease. Although dementia can occur in midlife, the vast majority of cases are diagnosed after age 75, and its incidence increases with advanced age.

Some dementias are reversible and include those resulting from depression, hearing loss, thyroid disease, pneumonia, electrolyte imbalances, syphilis, and nutritional deficiencies (especially thiamine deficiency, which occurs in alcoholism). Multi-infarct dementia is often a result of a series of small strokes, called mini-strokes or TIAs (transient ischemic attacks). The symptoms of a TIA often are very slight (weakness in arm or leg,

---

Clock Test for Dementia

Although a layperson cannot diagnose dementia, there is a simple test that seems to rule out the disease, called the clock drawing test. Research has documented that a person who can accurately draw a clock must have at least some memory, ability to perceive objects in space, ability to plan and accomplish a task, and ability to take in and follow instructions. Here's how it works. Ask a person to draw a clock and set the hands at half past ten.

The Alzheimer's disease cooperative scoring system is based on a score of five points: 1 point for the clock circle, 1 point for all the numbers being in the correct order, 1 point for the numbers being in the proper spatial order, 1 point for the two hands of the clock, and 1 point for the correct time. A normal score is four or five points.

If the person cannot draw a clock, this doesn't mean he or she has dementia—it may be a physical problem with vision or arthritis. However, this test is often revealing: Even though a person seems normal, he or she may draw an unusual clock face, indicating that the brain is not working properly.

slurred speech, dizziness) and do not last long. Symptoms of dementia may not be noticed until several small strokes occur. Since no treatment can reverse the damage, it is important to reduce the risk of future strokes.

Dementia is characterized by decreases in memory, attention, language, and problem solving that persist at least six months. It can progress slowly or rapidly. Those with dementia are commonly disoriented to time and place—knowing what year or month it is, where they are, or the season, and later, even knowing their own name and recognizing their family. They have difficulty with executive function—the ability to plan and sequence tasks, keep track of a calendar, control their emotions, solve problems or answer "what if?" questions. They often have difficulty in naming or recognizing items (called agnosia) and/or working on tasks (apraxia). This is not due to physical difficulty but rather due to a cognitive difficulty of being able to master the many steps needed to get dressed, write a check, or clean the house.

When symptoms of dementia occur, a thorough medical evaluation is needed to determine whether or not the dementia is reversible. The evaluation should include a complete medical history, office and lab tests to determine blood pressure, thyroid function, cholesterol levels, and heart function, and brain scans. Generally, a sudden onset of symptoms signals a reversible drug reaction or treatable condition, whereas a progressive deterioration that does not respond to therapy is likely to be irreversible.

No matter what causes dementia, the symptoms are the same. Most people slowly lose their memory and their language skills, they have unusual behaviors, and they lose the ability to care for themselves. Short-term memory is much more affected than long-term memory; thus, demented individuals may not be able to recall who made a

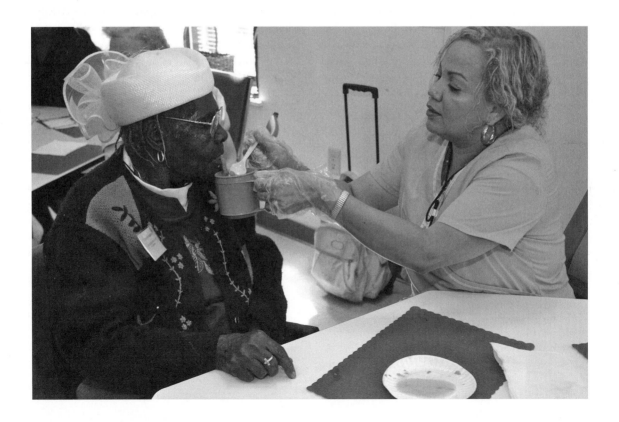

Dementia: A Case Study

Ms. N is an 85-year-old retired nurse who has advanced dementia. She spends the day in constant motion, wandering around the nursing home, appearing to check things. She tries the door-knobs, fiddles with the fire alarm, picks up papers off desks and tables, rearranges the bulletin boards, fiddles with the cloth of her dress, and intrudes on others. She engages in conversations, but her speech is often rambling. She goes into other residents' rooms and seems to be checking on them. At times her presence irritates them, and residents who want her out of their rooms have hit her. She enjoys contact and will smile and converse briefly but is always on the move. When her speech is understandable, she says that she "has to go and check on" or "I'm worried about the baby." In the evenings, she gets more confused and agitated and worried and will not even sit to eat. She stays up late at night, falling asleep only for a few hours at 3 a.m., only to arise at 6 a.m. to begin her "rounds."

visit earlier that day but are able to recall events in the distant past with clarity. They may have difficulty understanding directions, they may get lost in previously familiar places, and their speech may become less coherent. Elders with dementia may start to lose complex living skills, such as grocery shopping, the ability to balance the checkbook, and the ability to drive. They may have difficulty recalling the names of familiar objects. In the early stages, those with dementia may try to hide their disability or compensate. They may become depressed, moody, irritable, or apathetic.

In the advanced stages, individuals with dementia often manifest behavioral problems. They may cry without stopping, become agitated, and try to get out of bed even though they are too weak to walk. They may be verbally abusive or violent toward their caregivers, they may wander out of the house and get lost, or they may be very anxious and panicky, pacing or ruminating incessantly (see Box 7.4). A common phenomenon called "sundowning" is a worsening of symptoms in the evening hours.

As dementia advances, physical declines become evident, such as incontinence of bowel or bladder, inability to walk, and, in the very end stages, inability to hold one's head up. The progression of the disease is accompanied by a variety of physical conditions that cause further disability and death: nutritional disorders, septicemia (blood poisoning), respiratory illnesses (such as influenza and pneumonia), pressure ulcers, and fractures due to falls.

By far the most common type of dementia is Alzheimer's disease. It is estimated that 5.4 million individuals in the United States have Alzheimer's disease, and its incidence increases rapidly with advanced age.[17]

Finding out if an elder has Alzheimer's disease or another type of dementia can be challenging and may take time. Often the individual must undergo a series of mental tests and a careful monitoring of symptoms to exclude other causes. Diagnosing dementia involves blood tests for thyroid disease, anemia, or other illnesses, a CT scan of the head to look for evidence of old strokes, and often a spinal tap to ensure there are no other treatable causes of cognitive changes. When dementia is diagnosed and no reversible or other cause can be found for it, it is diagnosed as Alzheimer's disease.

No one is exactly sure what causes Alzheimer's disease. Alzheimer's disease can be definitively diagnosed by a brain biopsy (taking a tissue sample from the brain), but this is rarely done. The brain loses size and mass. Under the microscope, dead cells and "plaques," clumps of protein that occur outside brain cells, are seen. In addition, tangles or twisted-up proteins are found inside the nerve cells in the brain. Alzheimer's disease can also be diagnosed at autopsy.

Like other dementias, Alzheimer's disease is deadly. Although people can live for as many as 20 years after diagnosis, the usual time from diagnosis to death is 8 years. Early Alzheimer's disease is often missed by both medical professionals and the families of those afflicted because those with mild dementia are still able to function.

Certain risk factors increase the likelihood of developing Alzheimer's disease. Age is the most powerful predictor. Beween the ages of 65 and 74, the risk of developing Alzheimer's disease is 6 percent but by age 85 and older, the risk is increased to 45 percent.[17] Gender also plays a role: Almost two-thirds of those with Alzheimer's disease are women. Level of education is another factor: Those who have completed more years of education are less likely to get Alzheimer's disease than those less educated. It is debatable whether it is due to "cognitive reserve" or that those with fewer years of education have less access to medical care.[17] Another risk factor is family history. Those who have a parent or sibling with Alzheimer's disease are two to three times more likely to develop the disease than those who do not. Scientists are pinpointing some genes associated with the disease but have not found a definitive genetic cause at this time. Severe head injury also increases the risk of Alzheimer's disease. Those who have diabetes, heart disease, or high cholesterol are at increased risk.

Some of the risks mentioned above, such as age and family history, cannot be modified. However, we do know that some health behaviors reduce the risk of Alzheimer's disease: eating well, exercising, staying active, and not smoking cigarettes. Further, keeping the mind active and stimulated seems to reduce the risk or delay the onset of symptoms of dementia.

Most treatment for Alzheimer's disease is supportive; the emphasis is on treating complications as they arise and providing a protected and safe environment. Although there is currently no cure for Alzheimer's disease, a drug class called cholinesterase inhibitors slows the breakdown of acetylcholine, a chemical messenger in the brain that is important for memory and other thought processes. It is estimated that the drug delays the progression of dementia for a few months at most. Unfortunately, the drugs work in only about half the people, and the improvements in mental symptoms are modest. These medications are more effective very early in the disease and become markedly less effective as the dementia becomes more severe.

In addition to the medications that attempt to slow the progression of mental decline, medication for behavioral disturbances may be prescribed. Antidepressants and antipsychotics may be somewhat helpful in treating the most troubling behavioral disturbances that accompany dementia: sleeplessness, violent behavior, depression, and paranoia. Psychoactive medications should be used very carefully as they carry very high risks and limited evidence of effectiveness. Medications work for psychosis and depression, but don't work well for symptoms of dementia such as wandering, pacing, confusion, repeating the same question over and over again, and most agitation. Elders who receive antipsychotics for the first time in their later years are highly sensitive to them and should be given very low doses and be carefully monitored. Doses of antipsychotics used for dementia are much lower than those used for younger people or for other psychotic illnesses, and the treatment is often needed only for a very short time.

Nondrug treatments are also vital in reducing the symptoms. In the early stages of Alzheimer's disease, patients may need counseling to cope with stress and depression. As the disease progresses, it is important to provide a safe environment with adequate nutrition and body care. Although Alzheimer's is not curable, those with the disease may have it for years, and physical problems need to be addressed as they appear. Further, keeping the individual as healthy as possible is crucial (e.g., proper nutrition, good hygiene practices, adequate exercise, annual flu immunizations, and regular vision, hearing, and dental checkups). For individuals residing at home, enrollment in day care programs can offer stimulation and recreation while providing respite for the caregiver.

Common Behavioral Symptoms in Dementia and How to Deal with Them

Many elders with dementia exhibit unusual behaviors, which may be a way for the elder to communicate an unmet need or emotion. Demented individuals can no longer rely on words to express what they need and may not even know themselves. Those who care for people with dementia need to try to figure out what the need or emotion is. The elder may need rest, quiet, reassurance, the underwear changed, food, a trip to the bathroom, or merely something to do. Caregivers must act as detectives to find out what makes the behaviors worse and what makes them better. They need to structure the person's day to include adequate rest, supervision, and activity, much like new parents do for very young children.

- Agitation: Agitation is a general word for getting upset, irritable, restless, or anxious. Sometimes agitation is due to worry—the person thinks he or she is supposed to be doing something and cannot figure out what. Other times it may be physical—they have to go to the bathroom or stretch their legs; they may be too hot, cold, hungry, overstimulated, or tired. Be careful that you do not appear impatient or angry as the person may pick up on your tone and body language more than your words, and this may make the symptoms worse. Be sure to keep your words to simple statements that are reasonable and kind. Redirecting the person's attention or listening without disagreeing can also be helpful.
- Aggression: Some people with dementia become aggressive. They may strike out, bite, or scratch suddenly or without warning. It is important to try to figure out what might cause aggression and minimize this—sometimes people get aggressive when they feel threatened (someone in their space) or when they are confused (perhaps you are changing a soiled pair of pants and they do not understand and fight to protect themselves). Sometimes when you disagree with them they can become violent—it is best to be agreeable as much as possible as those with dementia have a

hard time hearing the word "no." Focus on the feeling and validate that. For example, the elder may state, "You are not my daughter. I don't know who you are but you need to get out right now." You might respond, "You want me out right now! You're angry! I am not welcome!" Keeping the environment calm, maintaining a safe distance when the person is angry, slowing down speech and movements, and redirecting their attention can also be effective.

- Repetition/Perseveration: A challenging symptom is perseveration. This is when the person continually states the same thing over and over again. This may be a sign of confusion or memory loss as they truly do not recall asking the question, or it may be a way to make social contact despite their limited abilities to do so. Sometimes people perseverate on an action—for instance, repeatedly rolling a ball of yarn. It is best to be patient and realize that the person is not trying to annoy you, and this is a sign of the injury to the brain. Often repeating the statement back to the person makes him or her feel heard.
- Hallucinations and delusions: Some older people with dementia hallucinate—they see or hear something that is not really there. Since these hallucinations seem real to the person, telling him or her the hallucinations are not real generally doesn't help. If the hallucination is not bothering the person, then action is unnecessary. However, if the hallucination is frightening, this may be something to treat with medication or distraction, validation of the feelings ("That sounds so scary!"), and social contact.
- Suspicion, delusions, or paranoia: As the brain becomes damaged and memory and function worsens, people tend to have misperceptions. They can become suspicious or paranoid or start to believe strongly in things that you know are not true. It can be tempting to try to set them straight on their facts, but this is rarely effective—the feelings are real and true to the patient even if the facts don't match. Try to

Continued

Continued

Common Behavioral Symptoms in Dementia and How to Deal with Them

validate the feeling—"Oh, how upsetting that things are always missing!" and then offer to help. Use simple statements.

- Apathy: When those with dementia lose interest in doing things, this is called apathy. They may be depressed, or fearful, or perhaps lack motivation or the cognitive ability to get involved in something or in staying focused. Trying to find ways to keep those with dementia engaged can be challenging. A related term is abulia—where people are perfectly happy doing nothing. Sometimes people are apathetic because they are depressed, but other times it is just part of the disease, and it is very hard to get them to do anything because they are happy as they are.

- Confusion/disorientation/memory loss: Those with dementia often do not know where they are, what year it is, the date, the season and even, at the later stages, their caregivers and their own name. They may not be able to find the words they are looking for or be unable to name objects. They may forget where they put things or what they ate for breakfast. They usually maintain their long-term memory (at least until the end stages of the disease). Reminding people that they are losing their memory or are confused is not helpful; asking elders with dementia questions that they cannot answer can be unsettling. It is best to kindly remind them of essentials, but not to correct—enjoy their ability to live in the moment.

- Apraxia: One aspect of dementia is apraxia—the inability to do certain things or use objects. People may maintain the use of their arms and hands, but be unable to dress themselves, put on a coat, get their shoes on, pull up their pants, button, or coordinate eating. It is important to remember that this is part of the illness and it is not stubbornness or willfulness; the elder simply has lost the ability.

- Sundowning: When the behaviors worsen in the evening, this is called sundowning. It is thought that fatigue builds up as the day goes on, then as it gets darker, the tired elder cannot see as well any more and becomes frustrated. To reduce sundowning, decrease stimulation and provide good lighting during the evening hours.

- Wandering: Some people with dementia are active and tend to walk or pace all day, increasing the opportunity to wander off and become lost. This can be very dangerous if the climate is hot or cold, and if the person is unaware of the dangers of traffic and has no sense of direction. Those who wander may need near-constant supervision, redirection, and monitoring, and this is one reason for placement in nursing homes that are secure or locked. If they live at home with a caretaker, installing locks, gates, or alarms may make the house safer. Elders who wander outdoors need to wear identification.

Estimates vary, but from 15 percent to 50 percent of the people in nursing homes have a form of dementia. However, less than one-third of elders with the disease reside in a nursing home; the majority are cared for at home by a spouse or other family member. The absence of a caregiver is one of the most common reasons for institutionalization.

Caring for elders with dementia, particularly those with behavioral problems, can be extraordinarily difficult. In many ways, the patient with dementia becomes a large child, dependent in many activities of daily living, exhibiting poor judgment, and needing constant supervision. Many caregivers are elderly themselves and have to deal with their own health problems. Elders with dementia often require 24-hour care: changing diapers and assisting with bathing, feeding, getting to the toilet, moving from bed to chair, and

I Miss My Mother

As I sit next to her, she twists her shirt in her hands and appears worried. "Why isn't he coming?" she asks me, "He said he'd come." She walks unsteadily and sits down by the door and I follow. I try to distract her attention elsewhere—"Look at that, that looks fun!" or "Do you want to watch television?" "It's a beautiful day outside today, can you see out the window? Do you want to go out?" she shakes her head, "No, I'm waiting, waiting for Cliff. He said he'd come. "

Mom developed Alzheimer's about 10 years ago when she was about 77. My dad Cliff had died about two years before. At first, you could barely notice, she just became forgetful and misplaced things and she talked a little less. She didn't seem worried about it, just took it in stride. I had a woman look in on her at first. I had to do her shopping and help her with bills and such, and I would bring her dinner. After a while, I got worried that she just couldn't be alone so much. She would leave the door unlocked, the food out, eat on dirty dishes, leave the stove on, and I think she skipped meals when I wasn't there. She could do things, but only if you told her to and watched to make sure she did it right. Sometimes she would not be wearing a sweater when it was pretty cold out. So, I talked with my brother, and we decided that it was just easier to bring her to live with me. She was a good walker, so she went everywhere with me then. I found a nice senior center where she could go in the hours when I was working.

Just this last year, things have gotten worse. Ever since her 87th birthday, she seems worried, anxious, and maybe not all there, in the present moment, like she is thinking of things far away. She doesn't talk that much and tends to repeat things. She doesn't always answer questions either. She has accidents where she urinates in her pants and she doesn't even seem to notice. Her walking is more shaky and she

usually forgets to use the walker. Sometimes the senior center people just put her in a wheelchair. She is just less motivated—there is lots to do there, but she tends to just sit and stare and even if you try to convince her, she just doesn't want to do anything!

I think that when she is staring there, she is thinking about her life. I know she keeps thinking about dad, waiting for him, talking about him and fretting about why he isn't there with her. I think she misses him, and I wonder if maybe she is even seeing him somehow in her mind? I tried to tell her he died, but she just started crying and crying and then, when she stopped crying, she went back to the same statements over and over "Why isn't he coming? He said he would come." It didn't do any good to tell her the truth. The worrying is worse in the evenings, but at least she still sleeps the night, well, usually. I have a little alarm on her bed so if she gets up at night, I get up too, because she fell twice at night a few months ago. I can't take her as many places anymore, she gets tired and can't seem to keep track of what is happening or remember what we are doing.

The worst thing of all is that she sometimes doesn't recognize me. She will ask me "Who are you?" or a few times she called me by her sister's name and once or twice she even called me "mom"! If I call her "mom," sometimes she looks puzzled, so sometimes I just call her Edith. When I showed her pictures of me as a child, she thought they were her pictures! She doesn't recognize herself in the pictures—she thinks she is the young one and I am the old one! Sometimes that is how it feels to me too, like she is becoming a little child again, like she is going backwards at the end of her life. I try not to take it personally, I know it is just her "disease" and she cannot help it. She is right here in front of me, and I am holding her hand, but my mother is already lost—I miss her.

walking. Caregivers must remain vigilant for changes in behavior or worrisome behaviors such as wandering, operating appliances, and trying to drive, and must devise ways to keep an elder safe in the home. Altered sleep patterns or worsened behavioral problems occur at night, adding sleep deprivation to the list of trials of the caregiver. When the disease becomes advanced, patients cannot recognize family members, lose control over their bowel and bladder, and cannot speak, walk well, or feed themselves. Family members must witness the slow, progressive physical and mental decline of a loved one, often for several years, with no hope of treatment or cure.

Many communities offer group support and education for families of those with dementia to increase knowledge of the disease and families' feelings of competence in caring for family members with dementia. Many experts recommend psychotherapy for caregivers to reduce their own depression. Providing them with counseling and support can reduce the incidence of nursing home placement.[18]

The elderly with dementia, and those who care for them at home, may receive assistance from a variety of health and social services in the community such as homemaker assistance, home health care, respite care, and adult day care. However, the presence of these services and the payment mechanisms vary significantly among communities, and formal assistance to remain in the home may not be available for many. This subject will be fully discussed in Chapter 14.

Delirium

Delirium, the sudden appearance of a state of confusion, is more common among frail elders, but it may occur among healthy individuals under certain situations. Delirium is often due to infections (usually urinary tract infections or pneumonia), new medications, surgery, or dehydration. However, a variety of other conditions may cause delirium: malnutrition, alcoholism, heart attack, anemia, fever, head trauma, diabetes, or thyroid disease. Generally, delirium is the result of a vulnerable patient dealing with many physical and environmental insults.

The symptoms of delirium include agitation, confusion, disorientation, memory loss, decreased attention span, and insomnia alternating with excessive sleepiness. Visual hallucinations, such as seeing a deceased relative in the room, and paranoia are other common symptoms. A hallmark of delirium is its constant fluctuation: One moment, an elder may be clear mentally and able to respond appropriately; then the next moment, the person is quite confused or agitated. Patients with delirium have difficulty concentrating even for a few moments. They may pick at their bedclothes and not want to stay in bed. Some people mistake delirium for dementia; but dementia comes on gradually over months or years, while delirium occurs suddenly, often within hours. If an elder has an abrupt change in personality, thinking, or level of alertness, it is always important to consider delirium.

Delirium is often life threatening and requires prompt medical evaluation to determine the cause so that treatment can be started to reverse the condition. Treatment of delirium varies, depending on the cause (e.g., antibiotics for infections, fluid for dehydration, blood transfusion for anemia). Although delirium is often treated with antianxiety medication to calm the patient, the drug may increase confusion and agitation in some individuals. Unfortunately, many delirious and agitated elders are physically restrained to prevent injury, although the use of restraints often could be avoided. Imagine how you might feel if you were confused and fearful and the nurses tied you to your hospital bed.

Ways to prevent delirium include reducing all medications to the bare minimum, maintaining a calm environment while an elder is hospitalized, encouraging family members to stay with confused elders, and providing medical treatment at home instead of in the hospital whenever possible. Taking the older person to visit the hospital or intensive care unit prior to hospitalization can reduce the risk of delirium. See page 263 for a case study on delirium.

PSYCHOACTIVE MEDICATIONS

Psychoactive (also called psychotropic) medications work within the brain to affect thinking, mood, and behavior. This category includes medications specific to treat depression (antidepressants), anxiety (anxiolytic or antianxiety), and psychosis (antipsychotics), and medications that work for multiple disorders and symptoms.

When psychoactives first were discovered, they were hailed as a miracle—imagine that there were diseases so serious that had no known treatment except locking people away in institutions. When medications were discovered that changed behavior, it changed the way people looked at mental illness. Now mental illness was seen as worthy of scientific study, a brain imbalance, something to treat and maybe even cure. Individuals who had lived in institutions could be released and moved to the community. Their mood and behavior improved, both from the perspective of the individual suffering and those around him or her. The medications also reduced the symptoms that affect others, such as aggression or violence, paranoia, or homicide or suicide.

The advances in psychoactive drugs have dramatically improved the quality of life for many people. And many mental disorders formerly believed to be treated with psychotherapy alone can now be effectively treated with medications. In most cases, the combination of psychotherapy and medication is more effective than one or the other. Currently, because of the lack of reimbursement for "talk" treatments by private insurance companies and Medicare, physicians are relying more on medication to solve psychological problems.

How do these drugs work? Psychoactive medications improve thinking, mood, and behavior by affecting the balance of neurotransmitters in the brain, primarily dopamine, serotonin, and norepinephrine. Each type and class of medication affects slightly different neurotransmitters. Experts do not know how the drugs reduce the symptoms or exactly where or why they work, but multiple studies show they do work, especially for those with serious mental illness. For those with less serious mental illness, studies suggest that at least some of the effectiveness of the medications is likely due to a placebo effect (see Chapter 8).

How do you know which drug is best for which person? There is no easy answer regarding which medication is ideal for which symptom, and many times there is a period of trial and observation, dose change, or even medication change in an attempt to relieve symptoms while keeping medication side effects to a minimum. First the disease is diagnosed, and then the doctor begins with a class of drugs—perhaps one that works for many people, or one that is covered by their insurance plan. If the symptoms get better and the side effects are tolerated, the drug is continued. When symptoms abate, it can be tapered off. However, if one drug doesn't work, the dose can be increased, changed, or another drug or drugs can be added in various combinations until the maximal success is achieved.

It is not clear why some drugs work better for some people—it may be the neurotransmitters affected or perhaps the side effect profile. No matter which psychoactive drug is used, the dosage needs to start low for older people to compensate for age-associated physiological changes. If necessary, the dosage can gradually be increased as long as the side effects are tolerated. Some psychoactive drugs work immediately (such as benzodiazepines or antipsychotics), while others take up to six weeks to take effect (most antidepressants). Unfortunately, the side effects often start right away. In general, these drugs should be continued for at least six to twelve months to prevent relapse. Many of these medications need to be "tapered" with gradual dose reductions because stopping them suddenly can worsen psychological symptoms.

Psychoactive medications have significant and serious side effects—they are associated with many and varied symptoms: constipation, diarrhea, weight gain, weight loss, sleepiness, insomnia, increased interest in sex, decreased interest in sex, upset stomach, nervousness and more. More concerning are long-term irreversible effects (suicide, sudden death, movement disorders, massive obesity, diabetes, cataracts). Table 7.1 outlines the concerns of the common medications to treat mental disorders. If an individual is so ill that he or she cannot function outside an institution, then the person is often willing to deal with side effects, even serious ones. However, many times when the symptoms of the illness get better, the person then tends to focus on the side effects. When psychotropic medications are used for milder symptoms of mental disorders, the side effects are less tolerable.

TABLE 7.1	Common Medications to Treat Mental Disorders		
Chemical Classification of Medication	**Examples**	**Used For**	**Concerns and Comments**
Older antidepressants (some are called *tricyclics*)	Elavil (amitriptyline), Aventyl (nortriptyline)	Depression, anxiety, obsessive compulsive disorder, chronic pain, sleep	Takes 4–6 weeks to see effect, may have side effects particularly for elders (called "anticholinergic"), which include dry mouth, confusion, constipation, and difficulty urinating
Newer antidepressants (some are called SSRIs, selective serotonin reuptake inhibitors)	Prozac (fluoxetine), Celexa (citalopram), Zoloft (sertaline), Paxil (paroxetine), Wellbutrin (buproprion), Effexor (venlafaxine),	Depression, anxiety, obsessive compulsive disorder, pain, sleep	Risk of suicide increases, takes 4–6 weeks to see effect, Wellbutrin can be used for smoking cessation
Antianxiety	Buspar (busipirone)	Anxiety, dementia	Effective for only a few people
Benzodiazepines	Xanax (alprazolam), Valium (diazepam), Ativan (lorazepam)	Anxiety, muscle spasms	Habit forming, associated with confusion, sleepiness, and falls in elderly
Older antipsychotics (Typical)	Haldol (haldoperidal), thorazine, trilaf on	Psychosis, nausea, hiccups, schizophrenia, behavioral problems in dementia, aggression	Abnormal movements and tics that can be permanent, constipation
Newer antipsychotics (Atypical)	Risperdal (risperidone), Seroquel (quetiapine), Abilify (aripiprazole), Geodon (ziprasidoneHCl), Zyprexa (olanzapine)	Mania, psychosis, schizophrenia, behavioral problems in dementia	Increased death rate in elders with dementia, obesity, diabetes, weight gain, abnormal movements that can be permanent
Mood stabilizers (some also antiseizure)	Depakote (valproic acid), lithium	Bipolar disorder, depression, agitation, psychosis, schizophrenia	Many need blood tests to make sure they are not toxic

Many experts believe that psychoactive drugs are overmarketed, overprescribed, and overused. They point out that antidepressants are prescribed for people with mild sadness rather than severe depression. They are concerned that medications are used instead of psychotherapy or exercise or other less risky treatments.

More importantly, mental health professionals cite concerns that antipsychotics are being used for behavioral annoyances instead of being reserved for severe illnesses such as schizophrenia. Antipsychotics are powerful drugs designed to treat those who lack contact with reality, who hear voices and have paranoid thoughts about the world that are not true. However, increasingly these drugs are being used for those with depression or behavioral problems, and too often are prescribed for elders with dementia. Antipsychotics are often prescribed for wandering, repeating things, anxiety, restlessness, or aggression. Uses of these medications for such behaviors is not approved by the Food and Drug Administration as studies have shown these antipsychotic drugs to be ineffective and to carry a heightened risk of death. These medications are highly regulated in nursing homes by the federal government as experts fear they are too risky and don't work well for agitation in dementia. See Table 7.1 for the major classes of psychoactive medications, their uses, and major concerns when prescribed for elders.

PSYCHOLOGICAL THERAPY

Individuals engage in psychological therapy to help themselves better understand and reduce their negative thoughts, to relieve troubling symptoms and emotions, and to help change their harmful behaviors. Sometimes medication is used to augment the therapy. Psychotherapy may occur individually or in a group. The goal of therapy is to recognize patterns of distorted thoughts and feelings and to learn ways to effectively respond to them. The effectiveness of the therapy depends on the individual's cognitive ability, emotional state, and motivation. Unfortunately, because of elders' negative

beliefs about therapy, the biases of therapists, and system barriers, most elders do not undergo formal psychotherapy, instead relying on medications to solve psychological problems. Alternatively, a variety of informal therapies hold promise for the elder population.

Psychotherapy is a type of structured relationship between a client and a mental health professional with the purpose of improving the client's mental health. It is effective for individuals with many of the disorders discussed above: anxiety and mood disorders, schizophrenia, substance abuse and sleep disorders, and the early stages of dementia.

There are several types of psychotherapy, but most rely on structured conversation designed to foster understanding of the problem and to facilitate change in the client's ways of thinking or acting. Clients may interact one-on-one with a psychotherapist or be part of a group. Group therapy is less expensive and has the added benefit of social interaction. The techniques used depend on the state of the impaired individual and the nature of the problem. When there are difficulties within the familial or marital relationship, family or marital therapy is indicated. With older people, as with any other age group, the fit between client and therapist is crucial to the success of the therapy. Most therapists use a combination of approaches to help the client to better understand the causes and to develop strategies to effectively deal with the mental problem.

Several types of mental health professionals are qualified to offer psychotherapy. *Psychiatrists* are physicians who specialize in treating mental disorders. *Clinical psychologists* have a doctorate in psychology and diagnose and practice psychotherapy. *Marriage and family counselors* have a master's or doctorate in marriage and family therapy and focus on promoting healthy relationships. *Clinical social workers* have a master's or doctorate in social work. *Clinical nurse specialists* are nurses with special training in psychiatry. *Pastoral counselors* are clergy with special training in emotional disorders and primarily assist individuals and families in their congregation.

Research documenting the effectiveness of various types of therapy is sparse for the adult population and is almost nonexistent for elders. There are even fewer data on the optimal type, duration, and focus of therapy among the elderly. It is generally believed that older adults respond as well to therapy as other adult age groups do.

Many experts believe that therapy for elders should be brief and focused more on problem solving than on restructuring personality. Researchers Hayslip and Kooken developed eight goals for therapists who counsel older adults: (1) Aid insight into behavior. (2) Provide symptom relief. (3) Provide relief to relatives. (4) Delay deterioration. (5) Aid in adaptation to the present situation. (6) Improve self-care skills. (7) Encourage activity. (8) Facilitate independence. They assert that the most effective treatment a therapist can offer to alleviate a client's stress is to coordinate family, friends, and community resources to assist the client.[19] Because institutionalized elders commonly have cognitive deficits

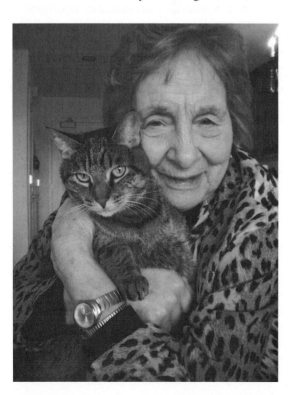

and physical and psychological limitations, the main goals of psychotherapy in nursing homes and other institutions are to maximize physical and psychological function through environmental stimulation and to increase morale.

Alternative psychosocial approaches that do not use trained psychologists are commonly used with groups of older people. Many encourage self-expression and social interaction. Some therapies involve the use of art, music, or dance to express deep-seated feelings and increase self-efficacy; others encourage elders to reminisce and review their life's accomplishments. For institutionalized elders, therapy may involve frequent orientation to where they are and what is going on in the world—so-called reality therapy—or activities designed to facilitate social interaction. Pet therapy among the elderly and disabled is gaining in popularity. In nursing homes, pet visitation has been reported to expand conversation topics, increase sociability and animation, calm residents, and increase self-esteem. Activity directors, occupational therapists, and recreational therapists are the major professionals used for these approaches.

Sometimes therapy is accomplished through self-help groups or peer counselors. Self-help or support groups generally arise spontaneously in response to a specific need expressed by persons who share mutual concerns. Self-help assumes that people who share the same situation or health problem can help themselves and others with the condition by sharing their experiences and helping each other. Typically, these groups are initiated by individuals who want them, although agencies and organizations may facilitate their formation. Most groups meet regularly. They are generally informal, free, voluntary, and confidential, and they focus on sharing experiences, on mutual support, and on providing education.

It is difficult to estimate the number of self-help groups in the United States—according to some estimates, there are more than a million. Self-help groups are available for a wide range of problems or situations. Some, such as Alcoholics Anonymous, smoking cessation, and weight reduction groups, focus on controlling negative behaviors by working on techniques that members can use to help themselves. Often, groups bring together individuals who are in a similar situation, such as bereavement groups for those who have lost a spouse or support groups for those who are caring for a loved one with Alzheimer's disease. Some groups stress medical care or rehabilitation from a specific illness. For instance, there are groups for people with diabetes, people with colostomies, and people coping with the aftermath of breast cancer surgery. Also, there are self-fulfillment and self-improvement groups designed to maximize personal potential.

Elder peer counselors offer informal, nonthreatening interactions by establishing a personal relationship between the counselor and the elder in need. Elder peer counselors may work with individuals or groups of elders. They may visit elders in their own homes or in community centers or institutional settings. They may provide education, social support, counseling, and referral to appropriate community agencies. Peer counselors may be as effective as professional mental health workers in many instances. Elder peer counseling can benefit both the trained elder and the client. Additionally, peer counselors are usually responsible and motivated workers, willing to become friends as well as helpers. This therapy reinforces the belief that elders are capable of solving their own problems.

MENTAL HEALTH SERVICES

Mentally ill elders have been affected by changes in treatment philosophy and in treatment settings over the years. Before the eighteenth century, the mentally ill were kept at home, allowed to wander around the community, housed in almshouses, or confined to jail with criminals. In the mid-1800s, reformer Dorothea Dix was instrumental in establishing institutions solely for the mentally ill. These institutions were large and supported by the states. Though established in the belief that they would provide humane treatment for the mentally ill, these institutions became human warehouses where treatment was the exception.

In 1956, the first of many antipsychotic drugs (also called major tranquilizers) was released and was effective in reducing the major behavioral symptoms of serious mental illnesses. The combination of effective drug treatment and the deplorable conditions in mental hospitals again spurred reformers and resulted in legislative action to reduce the number of patients living in mental hospitals by moving them into community settings where, reformers believed, they could lead more normal lives. The Community Mental Health Act, passed in 1963, provided federal funding for community mental health centers in which mental patients could be treated with medication and therapy as outpatients.

During the deinstitutionalization process, half of the patients discharged were elders who had spent most of their lives in controlled, institutional environments. Many of these patients were "transinstitutionalized"—transferred from mental institutions into nursing homes, even though nursing homes were not (and still are not) equipped to deal with mentally ill patients. Mentally ill elders who were not moved into nursing homes often wound up living in single-room-occupancy hotels or board and care homes or were homeless. Communities did not have the resources to provide the mental health and social services they needed, and many elders could not coordinate and negotiate for those services.

The great promise that drugs would make the mentally ill well enough to live in the community was not completely realized. Although antipsychotic drugs dramatically reduced symptoms in many, they caused irreversible side effects and didn't work perfectly. Becoming dissatisfied with their treatment, the mentally ill began demanding more services, better treatments, and an end to the stigmatization of mental illness.

In the 1960s, consumers of mental health services and advocacy groups joined forces to increase their political influence and press for changes in policies and laws regarding mental illness. Many angry ex-patients charged that they had been given drugs that caused serious side effects, had been overmedicated so they could not think straight, and either had been hospitalized against their will or not provided the services and care they needed. They wanted more rights and more services for the mentally ill, and they wanted to be in charge of how these services were delivered. Many of them disagreed with the treatments utilized by psychiatrists and believed that better treatments were available but not offered. Their efforts prompted legislation to mandate informed consent for medications and treatments and laws safeguarding the rights of mentally ill patients.

By the 1980s, that movement had mellowed, and patients focused on a grassroots, consumer-oriented "whole person" approach to care. Consumers advocated for a "biopsychosocial model" of disease, which recognizes the multiple factors—biological, psychological, and social— that contribute to the development and treatment of mental illness. Efforts of these groups resulted in the right to informed consent and other patient rights.

On another front, in 1972, a group of committed lawyers and professionals in the mental health field formed the Mental Health Law Project specifically to advocate for people with mental disabilities. Since 1993 the organization has been called the Judge David L. Bazelon Center for Mental Health Law. The Bazelon Center is the leading legal advocate for people of all ages with mental disabilities. Bazelon attorneys use litigation, policy advocacy, and public education and focus on four areas: (1) enabling mentally ill individuals to participate equally in the community, (2) promoting self-determination, (3) ending the punishment of individuals who are mentally ill, and (4) preserving the protection and entitlements for people with disabilities in housing, health care, education, and civil rights. They have won many precedent-setting cases that support the right to treatment, the right to services in the least-restrictive setting, the right to education, and the right to federal entitlements. See the Bazelon Web site for more information: www.bazelon.org

Meanwhile, families of the mentally ill were advocating as well. In 1979, the National Alliance for the Mentally Ill (NAMI) was founded. NAMI is the nation's largest grassroots mental health organization dedicated to improving the lives of persons living with serious mental illness and their families. The organization advocates for better care for individuals with mental illness, education and reduction of the stigma of mental illness, research, community-based services, work programs, parity in insurance coverage, and access to both drug and nondrug treatments. They have been lobbying Congress for decades and have played a big role in changing legislation. The organization has a helpline (1-888-999-6264), conducts public awareness campaigns, provides educational programs for laypersons and professionals, and offers support groups. For more information, go to the NAMI Web site: www.nami.org

In 1999, in *Olmstead v. L.C.,* the U.S. Supreme Court ruled that people with mental disabilities should be placed in the least-restrictive community setting possible and should not remain in institutions. This decision and subsequent legislation called the Olmstead Act have increased the availability of community-based services for those with a disability due to mental illness. The focus of the Supreme Court case was two female mental patients whose treatment team recommended community placement but who remained in an institution. The Court ruled that these patients, and others like them, must be offered community alternatives if the benefit of such placement outweighs the harm. Essentially, the Court told the states and other providers of services that they needed to invest as many resources for care outside institutions as were invested for care within them.

Mental health services are of two types: institutional care and community-based care. *Institutional care* includes care in nursing homes, mental institutions, and mental wards of general hospitals. *Community care* encompasses care received at community mental health centers, private psychiatrists and psychiatric outpatient clinics, halfway houses, and a variety of other support services that enable mentally frail elders to remain at home or in a more homelike environment in the community. Whether the individual is cared for in the community or in an institution depends on the extent of the mental problem, prognosis, physical status, current living situation, availability of community services, presence of family members, motivation to improve, and income.

Nursing Homes

Nursing homes house many elderly people with mental illnesses—either those with illnesses that appear late in life (such as dementia) or those who have had mental disorders through adulthood and are too physically and mentally impaired to care for themselves. The 2004 National Nursing Home Survey estimates that two-thirds of adults in long-term care facilities have a mental disorder.

The process of deinstitutionalization of mental hospitals and the advent of Medicare and Medicaid have inadvertently made nursing homes the primary place for mentally ill elders needing long-term care and supervision. Unfortunately, nursing homes may not be the ideal place for that group.

Nursing homes are designed to provide care for medical problems and support activities of daily living. Nursing homes are not set up to deal with people with mental illness because they do not employ staff trained in behavioral management, they do not have appropriate programming for mentally ill people, and they do not employ mental health specialists to provide care. There is a shortage of mental health professionals who will travel to nursing homes to provide care, particularly psychiatrists and psychologists. Federal regulations promote the correct diagnosis and treatment of mental disorders of nursing home residents. They specify the frequency of physician visits, assessment of mental disorders, prescribing and monitoring of psychotherapeutic drugs, and screening for depression, further cognitive loss, and anxiety. They also mandate reductions in psychotherapeutic medications and physical restraints. Nevertheless, many experts feel that psychiatric care for elders with dementia in nursing homes falls far short of ideal.

A number of interventions have been implemented to improve the care of demented elders in nursing homes. Many states require a certain number of hours of dementia training annually for nursing home personnel. The "person-centered care movement" has resulted in multiple interventions to improve dementia care including strategies to bathe demented elders, environmental modifications to make the facility more home-like, fewer staff rotations, and particular interventions to reduce the use of psychotropic medications, physical restraints, and falls. A few facilities have developed units for demented patients with trained staff.

The Alzheimer's Association recently developed research-based recommendations for effective dementia care in nursing homes and assisted living residences. In 2006, the organization began a multiyear Campaign for Quality Residential Care with the goal of making a significant difference in the quality of life of individuals with dementia who live in residential facilities. The association is encouraging adoption of their recommendations by nursing home personnel, advocating that public policy makers incorporate the recommendations into state and federal law, offering training and education programs for personnel working with individuals with dementia, and offering an online guide for elders and caregivers to choose the best care option and to advocate for quality within the residence. A different part of the recommendations is focused upon each year. For further information, go to www.alz.org

An advantage of nursing homes is that they provide 24-hour care and supervision for their residents, and this may be exactly what is needed for both the resident and the family. Nursing homes, however, are institutions and can actually aggravate mental illness, promote increased dependence and decreased motivation and choice by their very nature. Chapter 14, "Long-Term Care," discusses the pros and cons of nursing homes in more detail.

Public Mental Institutions

Even though the number of elders in state and county mental institutions has substantially declined in the last 30 years, these institutions still play a significant role in providing mental health care to this group. Older people are overrepresented in public mental health institutions, comprising almost one of three residents; many have resided there since their early adult years. Half of those admitted to mental hospitals for the first time are over age 65. The majority of institutionalized elders have schizophrenia, although significant numbers of residents have alcoholism and major depression.

Psychiatric Units of Hospitals

Hospitals are the primary providers for patients with acute mental problems or patients who are in a temporary crisis that needs to be managed. The type of crises treated at hospitals include severe depression where a person no longer will eat or interact; severe psychosis where a person is fearful, aggressive, or antisocial; or a person with behavioral problems such as wandering, restlessness, sleeplessness, or mood swings. If a family is unable to care for an elder at home and a nursing home is unable to manage the behavior, an admission to an acute psychiatric hospital can often help. Many units are designed for geriatric patients and have locked areas for safer wandering and medical staff to collaborate with the psychiatric staff to assure diagnostic and therapeutic interventions are appropriate. Medicare Part A finances the stay at acute hospitals, which generally last a few days to a few weeks. The units are not designed for long-term treatment, counseling, or rehabilitation of chronically ill mental patients. Some hospitals have special units for geriatric patients with dementia and other mental disorders.

Community Mental Health Centers

Federally legislated and funded by the Community Mental Health Centers Act in 1963, community mental health centers have been set up in communities with populations between 70,000 and 200,000. The centers offer five services: (1) inpatient and outpatient care, (2) 24-hour emergency services, (3) partial hospitalization, (4) consultation, and (5) education. Many provide additional services. The centers are available to all ages and have no restrictions regarding ability to pay or current and past health condition. Each state sets

up community mental health centers differently. In publicly funded mental health centers, such as those run by state, county, or city governments, the cost of many services is calculated according to what a client can afford to pay. This is called a sliding-scale, or sliding-fee, basis of payment.

Community mental health centers are mandated to offer services to elders including diagnosis, treatment, liaison, and follow-up. Despite the mandate, these centers generally are not effective in meeting the mental health needs of elders. Even though about half the nation's older population has access to these facilities, older people comprise a small percentage of the patient load. There is insufficient programming for this group and insufficient federal and state support for mental health programs for elders, for the services are seldom reimbursed by Medicare and Medicaid. In addition, many of these centers exclude individuals with dementia.

Private Therapists and Psychiatric Outpatient Clinics

Older people comprise less than 5 percent of the clients seen by private psychotherapists. Their services are seldom reimbursed by Medicare and Medicaid. Generally, elders who do participate are those in good health who are financially secure, are highly educated, and have a positive attitude toward their treatment.

The American Association for Geriatric Psychiatry established a nonprofit educational group called the Geriatric Mental Health Foundation. Their Web site (www.gmhf.org) has up-to-date mental health information for elders and their families and the locations of geriatric psychiatrists in the United States.

Halfway Houses

Most elders who have mental illness also have dementia and medical problems as complications from their lifestyle (higher rate of alcohol abuse or smoking, for example) and side effects from their medications or treatments. Those who are still able to walk and care for themselves might live in halfway houses, also called board and care or group homes. These can be licensed or not licensed and are often established in neighborhoods. Some are large with many beds and others are in a home with only a few people living there. Psychiatric halfway houses provide a home environment for the mentally ill who are able to meet many of their own needs yet need some support and supervision to be able to live in the community. These homes have great potential for serving the needs of mentally impaired elders since they prevent or postpone institutionalization for many.

Halfway houses are of varying quality. Some are excellent, while others have many problems. Physical, mental, or financial abuse of residents may occur; cleanliness may be substandard; staff is poorly trained; and there are far fewer homes than are needed. Most elders rely on Social Security, Supplemental Security Income (SSI), or disability benefits to pay their bills. Homes located in community neighborhoods often face problems from neighbors who fear the mentally ill. Currently, board and care facilities and single-room-occupancy hotels house many mentally ill individuals. However, treatment, rehabilitation, or adequate supervision is rare.

Case Management Services

Case management services, often run by county mental health systems, provide trained individuals to help mentally ill individuals navigate the mental health system. These case managers may be nurses or social workers or even laypeople who have been trained to know the local services available and the qualifications for using them. The case manager monitors a caseload of mentally ill individuals in order to meet their needs and delay the need for institutionalization. Further, the case manager provides education and psychological support and advocates for clients when necessary.

Patient Protection Programs

The individuals who are most vulnerable to neglect and abuse are those with mental illness and serious emotional disturbances who reside in public or private residential facilities, such as hospitals, group homes, homeless shelters, residential

treatment centers, jails, or prisons. To ensure that these vulnerable individuals get the care and treatment they need, each state is required to implement the federal *Protection and Advocacy for Individuals with Mental Illness (PAIMI) Program,* which is funded by the federal Center for Mental Health Services. Services include information and referral, investigation of neglect, abuse, and violation of rights, and use of hearings and litigation to remedy documented incidents. Program information and eligibility standards are available at www.mentalhealth.samhsa.gov/cmhs/P&A/

The *Lanterman-Petris-Short (LPS) Act conservatorships* were designed to ensure that disabled mentally ill individuals get appropriate care in an appropriate setting when it is needed, even if they do not want it. An LPS conservatorship is initiated in a state court proceeding when an individual is determined to be a danger either to him- or herself or to others (a risk of suicide or homicide) or is gravely disabled and unable to provide the basics of food, clothing, or shelter. This type of conservatorship often begins in a hospital emergency room when an elder with a mental illness is at high risk of suicide or is very demented and was found in a very unsafe situation on the street or in the home. Under these situations, the hospital can hold a person against his or her will if certain criteria are met. A court hearing is held, and the hospital personnel can hold the person in a psychiatric treatment unit for a specified time period for the purpose of administering treatment. For example, an elder who is seriously depressed and suicidal and refusing hospitalization may be held for a time and be given antidepressant medications and therapy until she is no longer suicidal. The initial hold is temporary, generally 72 hours, but can be extended to a permanent conservatorship.

A permanent LPS conservatorship automatically terminates after one year, and further court proceedings must be initiated to reestablish it for another year. If the individual recovers, the conservatorship is removed. This type of conservatorship mandates that the individual be placed in the least-restrictive environment to receive mental health treatment. Depending on the individual's situation, an elder may be placed in a locked facility.

Federal law requires that all individuals residing in nursing homes be represented by nursing home ombudsmen. See Chapter 14, "Long-Term Care," for further information.

FACTORS LIMITING USE OF MENTAL HEALTH SERVICES

Just as other groups, some older people need mental health services. Despite elders have a great need for mental health services. And, because more people are living longer, the numbers of older people with mental disorders are going to increase substantially.

Despite the presence of mental health services in most communities, few people use them. This is true of all age groups, but elders, particularly ethnic elders, are least likely to use these services. Low utilization of mental health services by the older population can be attributed to their traditional beliefs about getting help for mental problems, to the attitudes of mental health providers, and to problems with the system itself.

Elder Beliefs

Consumer bias against the use of mental health services occurs among all age groups, but older persons are especially prone to resist psychiatric diagnoses, psychological explanations, and psychological help from a stranger. Many believe that anyone who needs a therapist is "crazy." Elders may believe that mental problems are not treatable or may not admit that they have a psychological problem. They may see the need for visiting a therapist as a weakness—an inability to solve their own problems. Further, older people may not be comfortable talking about their feelings and may believe that they should "tough it out" or "snap out of it" on their own.

Many older people mistakenly attribute their mental problems to physical ailments or to the aging process itself. These elders may be more likely to mention their psychological symptoms to their physicians than to seek out a mental health professional. On the other hand, some fear that if a mental disorder is found, they may be moved from their homes. Elders as a group are less likely to be aware of local mental health services. Since minority elders are particularly low users of services, cultural differences almost certainly influence elders' use of mental health services. When older people are educated about mental health services, they report an increased willingness to use them.[20]

With the aging of the baby boomers, some of these beliefs are likely to change. The baby boomers were adults during the time when mental illness came "out of the closet" and words like depression, stress, manic, anxiety and neurotic became household words. The new elders are more comfortable with psychoactive medications and nondrug therapies and are thought to be more "psychologically minded." Since they are more educated and more attuned to using mental health services than their predecessors, the demand for mental health services for elders will increase substantially in the next few years.

Provider Attitudes

The attitudes of those who work in the field of mental health can impact utilization. Some studies suggest that mental health practitioners have negative stereotypes about older adults, feeling they are less likely to change their behavior ("can't teach an old dog new tricks" mentality). The poor health status of some elders make it less likely for mental health practitioners to want to work with them. They may have belief that gains in treatment will be low because they have a limited life expectancy and poor health. Psychotherapists may not offer the type of counseling services that appeal to elder clients, especially those from different ethnic groups. And, some counselors believe that therapy is not useful for those with cognitive decline. Many therapists and mental health professionals lack training and experience in dealing with elderly clients and little research is available on the success of psychotherapy for elders.

Older people might exhibit symptoms of a mental disorder that differ from textbook definitions. Cognitive decline makes it difficult for a physician to get an accurate medical history in order to properly diagnose and treat a mental disorder. Physical disorders may mask mental disorders. Many symptoms of distress may be deemed irreversible or attributed to old age and may go untreated. And, most important, if an elder patient comes in with physical symptoms that need prompt attention, mental problems "take a back seat" to the more obvious physical complaints. For all these reasons, the rate of identification of mental disorders is low. But it has been suggested that the greatest obstacle to treatment is the failure of physicians to recognize mental illness in their older patients.

System Barriers

A lack of integration of the mental and medical systems is a major impediment to excellence in care. Historically, each system has acted independently with separate practitioners, reimbursement policies, programs, and staff. There is a trend toward integration (new federal laws to align reimbursement guidelines), but progress has been slow. Too often, mental health professionals know too little about medical problems that can aggravate mental illness, and medical health professionals are not comfortable caring for those with mental illnesses. As elders often have multiple medical diagnoses and complex medication regimens, there is risk of misdiagnosis, adverse medication effects, and aggravation of mental or physical condition without coordinated care.

For both physical and mental illnesses, elders are more likely to visit their physicians than to seek out mental health professionals. The physician is generally the "gatekeeper," being responsible to sort out the medical from the mental problems, and either initiate treatment or make a referral. Mental diagnoses are not easy in older people as they might exhibit symptoms that differ from textbook definitions. Cognitive decline makes it difficult for a physician to get an accurate medical

history in order to properly diagnose and treat a mental disorder. Physical disorders may mask mental disorders. Many symptoms of distress may be deemed irreversible or attributed to old age and may go untreated. And, most important, if an elder patient comes in with physical symptoms that need prompt attention, mental problems "take a back seat" to the more obvious physical complaints. For all these reasons, the rate of identification of mental disorders is low. But it has been suggested that the greatest obstacle to treatment is the failure of physicians to recognize mental disorders in their older patients.

Some primary care physicians are comfortable diagnosing and treating mental illness, but others feel ill equipped to manage mental illness and the behavioral complications of dementia. Dementia and cognitive impairment are classified somewhere in the middle between mental health and physical health in a kind of "no-man's land." Medical doctors are often not skilled in caring for individuals with psychiatric problems related to dementia. However, some mental health professionals see dementia as a hindrance to care: cognitive loss makes the elder less able to be treated or "rehabilitated" with individual and group psychotherapy. Many mental health programs exclude those with dementia or cognitive impairment. And, a good number of older people who are seriously ill develop cognitive loss and are left without a comprehensive system of care.

As mentioned before, historical differences in reimbursement with lower reimbursement for mental illness has contributed to the development of separate health care systems for medical and mental illnesses and lack of integration. Components of the Health Care Reform Act of 2010 will likely to increase the integration of mental and physical health systems. In addition, many demonstration projects have shown good outcomes when mental and medical services are linked. It will be interesting to see how reimbursement and federal policy affects the delivery of health care services as the health care reform plan is fully implemented.

The current supply of professionals trained in geriatric mental health is inadequate to meet the needs of the increasing numbers of elders in our country who are mentally ill. In many areas, there is a shortage of mental health services geared specifically to elders and offered by professionals skilled in working with older people. Further, many of the services that exist are physically inaccessible to older people, especially to those living in rural areas, because outreach is seldom provided for those who are unable to get to a facility on their own. In rural areas, these problems are exacerbated by the scarcity of mental health care facilities and professionals, especially psychiatrists. According to the U.S. Department of Health and Human Services, 60 percent of rural counties have inadequate numbers of psychologists, psychiatrists, and other mental health professionals who concentrate on treating elders.

Fragmented and complex, the mental health system too often stymies cooperation and coordination among private medical providers, community agencies, and institutions. Critics argue that there is no "system of care." Navigation through the available services and programs is almost impossible without a savvy advocate or case manager who is familiar with the various eligibility rules for programs. Because of these drawbacks, an interdisciplinary approach to meeting the multiple needs of mentally ill elders is not an option in most communities. Although some programs are available in some locations, what is available for a particular individual, given his or her income, insurance, geographic location and diagnosis, may be minimal.

FINANCING MENTAL HEALTH CARE

There are two major sources of payment for mental health services: *Medicare,* the federally funded insurance program for all individuals 65 and older, and *Medicaid,* the joint federal and state-funded program for the poor, blind, and disabled of all ages.

Medicare

Medicare provides health insurance to most elders aged 65 and older in the United States. The program operates as private insurance: Individuals enroll, pay premiums (a monthly fee), and co-payments (a small fee for each service), and deductibles (a certain out-of-pocket amount paid before the insurance kicks in). Medicare has three parts. Part A partially covers hospital services. Part B partially covers outpatient services. Part D partially covers prescription drugs. Expenses for mental health services for individuals who qualify are only a small fraction of the Medicare budget.

Medicare Part A partially reimburses the hospital for acute psychiatric hospitalization—an elder is so mentally ill that he or she must be hospitalized. Medicare reimburses a limit of 190 days in a lifetime for hospitalization in a *psychiatric* hospital. Individuals can stay up to 90 days at a time in *general* hospitals. Sixty days must elapse between 90-day hospitalizations before Medicare will pay again. For care in both psychiatric hospitals and general hospitals, the patient pays a deductible on first admission and a co-payment, depending on the length of stay. Mental health treatment in nursing homes is not covered under Medicare.

For mental health needs, Part B covers the services of physicians and mental health providers. This coverage includes 80 percent of Medicare-approved charges for physician services for *inpatient* mental health care (in a general hospital, a psychiatric hospital, or nursing home), including the monitoring of psychoactive medication. The reimbursement is capped at $1,100 per year. However, psychotherapy and treatment of patients with Alzheimer's disease have no cap on Medicare reimbursement. Regarding the amount reimbursed by Medicare for *outpatient* treatment, the Medicare Improvements for Patients and Providers Act of 2008 mandated that Medicare co-payment rates for outpatient psychiatric treatment be the same as for other medical services. Before 2011, Medicare paid 50 percent of outpatient psychiatric treatment while paying 80 percent of outpatient treatment for all other medical services. This copay difference (50 percent reimbursement for mental health and 80 percent reimbursement for medical services) was thought to be unfair and

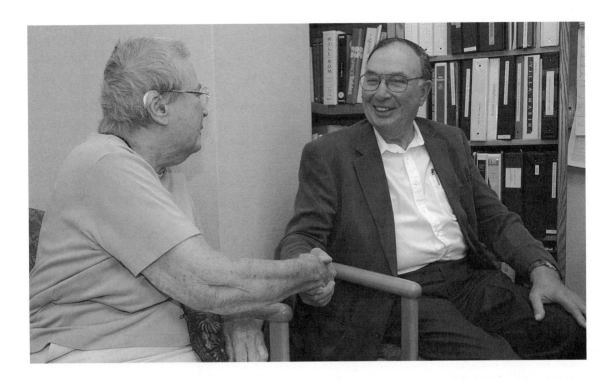

discouraged people from seeing mental health specialists. The Medicare reimbursement correction is being phased in gradually (2012, 60 percent; 2013, 65 percent; 2014, 80 percent). It is hoped that the reduced co-pay by Medicare recipients will encourage more individuals to seek needed psychiatric care. It is more likely that other steps beyond insurance parity will be needed before those elders seek the mental health care they need.

To use Part B, the person must pay the premiums, the yearly deductible, and the coinsurance for each service. Individuals who can afford them can purchase private insurance plans, called Medigap policies, which fill in the gaps of Medicare coverage by paying the deductibles and copays of Medicare (see Chapter 13, "Medical Care").

Medicare Part D helps Medicare beneficiaries pay for prescription drugs. It is a complicated program requiring elders to select the provider that best matches their present need for prescription drugs. Psychiatric drugs are included, but the list of Medicare-approved drugs is limited and varies with each insurance provider. In addition, due to

concern about over-prescribing psychiatric medications to elders, there are constraints on what is covered.

The next chapter will provide more detail on Part D. For current detailed guidelines for Medicare coverage, including mental health coverage, refer to the *Medicare and You* booklet, available at www. Medicare.gov

Government funding of mental health care and services is one important target of advocacy groups for the mentally ill who seek lower consumer costs. One important target of their advocacy work has been to address the difference in patient copay between mental health and physical health through Medicare because what Congress legislates for Medicare often becomes the norm for private insurance as well. Because of advocacy efforts, two important changes have been made to Medicare mental health coverage.

The Mental Health Parity and Addiction Equity Act of 2008 (MHPAEA) was passed by the federal government in response to pressure from advocates who wanted better insurance coverage for diagnosis and treatment of mental diorders. The act requires group health plans and health insurance issuers covering more than 50 people to ensure that financial requirements (such as co-pays, deductibles) and treatment limitations (such as visit limits) applicable to mental health or substance use disorder benefits are similar to the requirements for physical illness. This act does not require private insurers to offer mental health benefits, but stipulates that when they do, the services should be similar to physical health benefits.

Two years later, another law was passed as part of President Obama's "Health Reform Plan" of 2010 (H.R. 3590, the Patient Protection and Affordable Care Act) that includes language identifying mental health services as an "essential health benefit." Thus, insurance companies are now required to provide coverage, and that coverage must be equal to coverage provided for any other medical condition. Additionally, certain psychotropic medications are required to be covered under insurance company formularies. As part of that law, a new "high risk" pool allows those with preexisting mental conditions to obtain insurance. The law goes into effect in 2014.

Medicaid

Medicaid (*MediCal* in California) is the largest single payer of mental health services. States have some flexibility in the types of programs they offer to their residents, but federal guidelines set minimum standards for general hospital care, physician services, outpatient services in general hospitals, emergency room care, and nursing home care. Many clinicians and hospitals, however, do not accept individuals who qualify for Medicaid because the reimbursement is very low. Medicaid reimbursement rates to nursing homes are lower than the prevailing rates, with some states reimbursing the homes less than others. This practice discourages nursing homes from accepting Medicaid-eligible patients. Medicaid reimbursement for psychiatric care in nursing homes is even lower than for medical care.

You have read of the many ways in which the daily lives of those with mental disorders has improved in the last few years: effective drug treatments, a variety of formal and informal psychotherapies, laws that protect vulnerable elders, and other laws that respond to consumer issues regarding cost and access, and more. Nevertheless, significant problems remain regarding the care of the mentally ill. Funding and services have not matched needs. Those with serious mental illnesses are seldom able to negotiate a complex mental health system. New medications that improve care have been developed, but they are expensive, have multiple side effects, and, even when taken correctly, do not allow most seriously mentally ill people to live normal lives. Medications are expensive, and psychotherapy is out of reach for many elders who need it. Social services, housing, and jobs for the mentally ill are inadequate. Nursing homes, board and care homes, single-room-occupancy hotels, and the streets are ill equipped to deal with the myriad needs of this population. Funding for services has not matched the extensive needs. These ongoing problems and limited resources point the way for innovation in devising comprehensive, community-based services that address the unique needs of those who are mentally ill.

SUMMARY

Mental health in elders can be defined as the ability to adapt successfully to the transitions of old age. This ability is related to a number of physical, psychological, and situational factors, such as personality, physical health, financial situation, availability of social support, and coping strategies. Although most elders adjust readily to the stresses and transitions of old age, a few need outside assistance to deal with mental disorders.

In elders, mental disorders may appear for the first time during old age, but most appear years earlier. Several mental disorders are discussed in this chapter, particularly as they relate to elders: depression, anxiety, psychotic disorders, substance abuse disorders, sleep disorders, and two cognitive disorders—delirium and dementia. Some mental disorders are underdiagnosed in elders because their symptoms may be mistaken for age changes or chronic illness. Ongoing assessment is important to diagnose and treat mental illness in the older population. The common treatment for the majority of mental disorders is psychoactive medication, although some elders have access to psychotherapy and support groups.

Mental health services are available for elders in both community and institutional settings—public mental health hospitals, wards in general hospitals, nursing homes, community mental health centers, halfway houses, and individual and outpatient psychiatric services. These services are underutilized by elders for a number of reasons, including elder beliefs, professional biases, and system barriers. Governmental initiatives, supported by patient, provider, and family advocacy groups, are working toward improving the coordination, choice, availability, and delivery of mental health services in this country.

ACTIVITIES

1. Develop your own definition of mental health, taking age and cultural background into account. Identify some behaviors that are universally healthy or unhealthy. Ask several individuals to define mental health. Do their definitions work for older adults?

2. List the strategies that you use to cope with stress, both those that are effective and those that are not. Which strategies work best for you?

3. Review the transitions associated with aging (e.g., widowhood, changes in marital relationships, changes in relationships with adult children, retirement). Interview friends and family members at different stages of life, including those without children. What are their hopes and plans for these transitions? If they have already experienced them, what was the overall effect on their lives? How do the experiences of those without children or those who are not married differ from the experiences of those who are married with or without children?

4. Conduct a life review with an older person. Tape the conversation (audio or video) and write a summary for the class. Be sure to give a copy to the person interviewed.

5. Interview a representative from your local mental health department. Find out the percentage of clients who are aged 65 and older. Do they have any specialized mental health services for elders? Do they have a suicide prevention programs in place for the elder population?

6. Question elders about their attitudes toward mental illness and its causes and treatments, and compare their views with those of your classmates. How do the views of the two groups differ?

7. Make a list of the self-help groups in your community. If possible, talk with a group member to find out the percentage of participants over age 65. Attend a support group session, and describe your experience to the class.

8. Attend a meeting of Alcoholics Anonymous. Be sure to identify yourself as a guest. What proportion of attendees appear to be elderly? Question some of the participants about the impact of various services on their sobriety and the role of AA in their lives.

9. Find the resources in your community that offer programs to treat substance abuse (public, private, religious, AA, and medical-based programs). On what basis would you select one program rather than another? What is the cost of each? Which one would work best for an elder living in the community? Which one would work best for an institutionalized elder?

10. As people live longer, many younger elders will spend their retirement years caring for aging parents or spouses. How will this trend affect your plans for your old age?

11. Interview a nursing home administrator. What is the percentage of mentally ill elders residing in the facility? How are behavioral problems (e.g., wandering and disruptive behavior) managed?

What therapy is available? What is the educational background of the nursing home's therapist?

12. Explore the Web sites for NAMI and other family and patient advocacy groups. Compare their goals. What information is available on the Web sites? What do these groups propose as solutions to the problems of mental health and illness?

13. Visit a dementia unit in a hospital or nursing home and observe the patients. Interview the nurse's aides about the needs of the residents/patients. What kinds of behavioral problems do they observe? How do they manage these problems. Do they use medications or alternatives?

14. Call your local health department and inquire about services in your community for mental health and illness, eligibility requirements, and which services are appropriate for elders. Visit at least one site (e.g., a mental health clinic, a day care program, a board and care home, etc.). Observe the clientele and interview staff members about their program—their successes and their needs. Based on this needs assessment, design a staff or patient education module (video, PowerPoint, pamphlet, poster, handout, etc.) and provide it to the facility/site.

BIBLIOGRAPHY

1. Rowe, J.W., and Kahn, R.L. 1997. Successful aging. *The Gerontologist* 37:433–440.

2. Holstein, M.B, and Minkler, M. 2003. Self, society, and the "new gerontology." *The Gerontologist* 43(6):787–796.

3. Hansen-Kyle, L. 2005. A concept analysis of healthy aging. Nursing Forum 40(2):45–57.

4. Erikson, E.H. 1982. *The life cycle completed.* New York: Norton.

5. Carstensen, L.L., Gottman, J.M., and Levenson, R.W. 1995. Emotional behavior in long-term marriage. *Psychology and Aging* 10:140–149.

6. American Psychiatric Association. 2000. *Diagnostic and statistical manual of mental disorders: DSM-IV-TR.* Washington, DC: American Psychiatric Association.

7. Kessler, R.C., Berglund, P.A., Demler, O., Jin, R., Walters, E.E. 2005. Lifetime prevalence and age-of-onset distributions of DSM-IV disorders in the National Comorbidity Survey Replication (NCS-R). *Archives of General Psychiatry* 62(6):593–602.

8. Lyness, J.M. 2004. Treatment of depressive conditions in later life. *Journal of the American Medical Association* 291(13):1626–1628.

9. Centers for Disease Control and Prevention, National Center for Injury Prevention and Control. Web-based Injury Statistics Query and Reporting System (WISQARS): www.cdc.gov/ncipc/wisqars

10. Keller, M.B., McCullough, J.P., Klein, D.N., et al. 2000. A comparison of nefazodone, the cognitive behavioral-analysis system of psychotherapy, and their combination for the treatment of chronic depression. *New England Journal of Medicine* 342:1462–1470.

11. Pagnin, D., de Queiroz, V., Pini, S., and Cassano, G.B. 2004. Efficacy of ECT in depression: A meta-analytic review. *Journal of Electroconvulsive Therapy* 20(1):13–20.

12. Unutzer, J., Katon, W., Callahan, C.M., et al. 2002. Collaborative care management of late-life depression in the primary care setting. *Journal of the American Medical Association* 288(22): 2836–2835.

13. Substance Abuse and Mental Health Services Administration. 2011. *Results from the 2010 National Survey on Drug Use and Health: National findings.* NSDUH Series H-41. DHHS Publication No. SMA 11–4658. Rockville, MD: Substance Abuse and Mental Health Services Administration.

14 Ewing, J.A. 1984. Detecting alcoholism: The CAGE questionnaire. *Journal of the American Medical Association* 252:1905–1907.

The development of pharmaceuticals to prevent and treat a broad range of health problems is one of the many advances of modern medicine. Antibiotics to control bacterial infections, vaccines to prevent communicable diseases, and drugs to treat the symptoms of chronic illnesses have improved the lives of many people who otherwise would have suffered, even died, without them. Drugs also rid us of small irritants, such as headaches, itching, minor aches and pains, and constipation. Despite their many benefits, drugs may cause adverse effects—nausea, stomach ulcers, sometimes death. And prescription drugs are expensive, making them unaffordable for many who need them.

On the average, our nation's elders consume more medications than any other age group, mainly because they have the highest prevalence of chronic illness and age-related ailments. Although drug therapy provides significant benefits in managing chronic symptoms and minor conditions, drug use among elders comes with an increased risk of serious side effects due to age-related changes in physiology, deterioration from chronic diseases, and use of multiple drugs. In addition, the high proportion of adverse drug effects among the older population reflects the inadequacy of health professionals in assessing drug needs, prescribing appropriate drugs, supervising medication therapy, and educating elders to be active partners in their own health care.

Medication issues are of paramount importance to older people, their family members, and professionals who serve them. This chapter includes an overview of medication use among elders, the spiraling cost of prescription drugs, and Medicare Part D, the federal government drug insurance program. Pharmacokinetics, the way a drug works in the older body, is discussed. Problems associated with drug use and ways to counteract those problems are addressed. Finally, herbal medicine is explored. Specific medications used to treat chronic and acute illnesses are included in the chapters addressing those conditions (Chapters 4, 5, 6, and 7).

MEDICATION OVERVIEW

A *medication* is a substance that treats, prevents, or reduces the symptoms or the progression of a disease. Medications are chemicals that are taken into the body and interact within body cells, organs, and tissues to exert their effects. Medications can be classified in several ways: by the body system in which they act (e.g., cardiovascular drugs, gastrointestinal drugs), by their action in the body (what receptors they target, for example), by the diseases they treat (e.g., antihypertensive medications), or by their chemical structure (acetylsalicylic acid). Some medications treat symptoms (e.g., pain, nausea, or itchiness), but many more treat the underlying nature of the illness. For example, high blood pressure has no symptoms in many people, but the medication lowers blood pressure, which can be measured. Similarly, diabetes may have no symptoms, but the medications prescribed lower the blood sugar levels.

Medications are available in many forms. Most of us think of pills, capsules, or liquids, but medications can also be inhaled, applied to the skin, placed in the rectum, vagina, eye, or ear, placed under the tongue, injected under the skin or deep in the muscle, placed in the bloodstream directly, or even placed in the body cavity or in the cerebrospinal fluid that bathes the brain. Medication can be short-acting (exerting its effects for seconds, minutes, or a few hours) or longer-acting, with effects that last for many hours, days, or even longer. Some medications are "sustained release" which means that the medication is absorbed little by little, and the effects of the drug are sustained over a period of time. In general, short-acting drugs need to be taken more frequently than longer-acting and sustained-release medications.

Some medications are taken on a regular schedule; others are taken as needed. Some medications are prescribed for a short course; others may have to be taken for months, years, or a lifetime. Doctors use abbreviations, based on Latin phrases, to communicate about medications: For example *QD* means "every day," *QID* means "four times daily," and *PRN* means "as needed."

Unforeseen Problems with Miracle Drugs
"There's No Free Lunch"

They were miracles: Antidepressants without side effects, antipsychotics that did not cause tardive dyskinesia and turn patients into zombies, painkillers that reduced joint inflammation without damaging the stomach, and the female hormone that kept women young while protecting them against heart disease, osteoporosis, and Alzheimer's disease. Each of these drugs was introduced to the public with great fanfare and almost immediately was prescribed to millions. Over the years, however, large-scale studies began to turn up problems. Some miracle drugs had to be taken off the market.

The first miracle: Antidepressants without major side effects. Previous antidepressants caused problems with dry mouth and constipation and could be fatal if taken in overdose. The drugs were uncomfortable to take, and doctors did not like to prescribe them. Enter selective serotonin reuptake inhibitors, called SSRIs—a new class of antidepressants with fewer side effects and reduced dosing frequency. Millions of Americans flocked to their doctors and began taking them for depression as well as for a bevy of other conditions: anxiety, ennui, feeling a bit blue, sleeplessness. Then data began to emerge indicating that these drugs might increase the risk of suicide and were only marginally more effective than a placebo.

The second miracle: The new antipsychotic medications (e.g., risperidone, quetiapine, olanzapine) were first thought to be a miracle for those with bipolar disease, schizophrenia, and dementia because they did not cause tardive dyskinesia or excessive sedation. Over the years, however, they have been found to be related to diabetes, weight gain, possibly heart disease, and an increased rate of death among the older population.

The third miracle: Magical anti-arthritis drugs offered reduced pain and joint inflammation without any stomach problems. Doctors and their patients with arthritis were thrilled, as were a lot of other patients with pains of various types. Then data from a large-scale study revealed that these medications (called COX-II selective agents), including Vioxx, Celebrex, and Bextra, may be associated with an increased risk of heart attack and stroke, especially when they are used for long periods of time or in very high risk settings (immediately after heart surgery). The added blow: One of the older anti-inflammatory drugs (Naprosyn, Aleve) may also cause an increased risk of heart disease with long-term use.

The fourth miracle: Premarin and other estrogen replacement drugs were marketed for decades to post-menopausal women as the key to the fountain of youth. Early studies suggested that women who took these medications had fewer bone fractures, lived longer, had less heart disease, and had a lower risk of Alzheimer's disease. The large-scale Women's Health Initiative set out to prove these benefits in a randomized controlled trial and reported that Premarin, when combined with Provera or other progestins, caused increased rates of heart disease. Millions of stunned women flocked to their doctors for advice as to whether to continue these medications. The use of female hormones in the United States dropped precipitously.

And the list goes on: Weight loss and diabetes drugs that are associated with cardiopulmonary problems, breast implants that are linked to autoimmune diseases, allergy medications that interact with antibiotics to cause heart problems, cholesterol-lowering drugs that are linked to muscle degeneration. Some findings resulted in drugs being removed from the market (the manufacturer of Vioxx voluntarily recalled it). Other findings resulted in new warnings on package inserts or cautions.

The take-home lesson: Even though the clinical trials required by the FDA for drug approval are rigorous, the trials are not long enough and do not include enough people to identify side effects or risks that are rare or take a very long time to develop. Thus, every person who takes a new drug is a sort of guinea pig. Both physicians and consumers need to keep in mind that the perfect medication with excellent effectiveness and no side effects has not been invented and likely never will be! All drugs have risks, both known and unknown, that should be carefully balanced against any benefits.

A complete list of medical abbreviations is found at www.rxlist.com

The Food and Drug Administration (FDA) is responsible for ensuring that all medications sold in the United States are safe and effective. The FDA implements strict guidelines on which drugs are sold to the public, how they are packaged, and what information must be on their labels. The FDA Web site, www.fda.gov, provides information regarding the agency's role and the drug approval process.

Drugs may be sold in two ways: by prescription or over-the-counter. Prescription medications are those that have to be prescribed or ordered by a licensed professional (physician, dentist, and, in some states, nurse practitioner, physician assistant). Upon the legal signature of a licensed physician, the pharmacist can dispense the prescription medication to the patient. In contrast, nonprescription drugs do not require an evaluation by a physician or a prescription. They can be purchased over-the-counter from pharmacies, grocery stores, and other retail outlets by anyone. Nonprescription medications are carefully reviewed by the FDA to ensure they are safe for the majority of Americans. Examples of over-the-counter medications are cough and cold remedies, Tylenol, painkillers such as Aleve and ibuprofen, creams for athlete's foot, and wart treatments.

All medications have risks and benefits, and all have *side effects,* symptoms or problems that are not intended. For instance, a person may take a medication to reduce muscle pain, but its side effect is nausea or stomach pain. Sometimes side effects occur when the medication works "too well," such as daytime sleepiness that occurs after a sleeping pill is taken the night before or when the blood thinner causes bleeding gums with toothbrushing. The most common side effects of drugs are nausea, sedation, dizziness, and constipation. Stronger drugs generally produce more severe side effects. For example, the side effects of cancer chemotherapy are gastrointestinal bleeding, severe nausea and vomiting, loss of hair, and a reduced ability to fight off infections. Researchers who develop drugs find out about many of their side effects in the studies they conduct before drugs come to market. Based on their findings, manufacturers of drugs are required to list all known side effects of their products in the package insert.

We can often accept and tolerate short-term side effects. For example, if we have pneumonia and take an antibiotic and develop nausea or a reduced appetite, we deal with this side effect because we know we need the drug to get better. We tolerate the side effects because the drug is needed for only a short time, until we return to health. Side effects are more complex to deal with when a medication needs to be taken over a long period (perhaps for a lifetime), when the disease has no obvious symptoms, and when the side effects are significant. Imagine a blood pressure medication that you will need to take for the rest of your life even though it causes daily dizziness or sexual dysfunction. When side effects of a needed medication are severe, sometimes a second medication or a change in health behavior (exercise, healthy diet, stress reduction) may reduce side effects or reduce the need for the medication.

In addition to side effects, other important information is listed on package inserts. The package insert tells what symptoms or illnesses the drug can help, how the drug is broken down and excreted by the body, recommended dosage, and how long a dose lasts. The insert tells you for which populations the drug is approved and which populations have not been studied. Drugs may come with warnings or cautions. For example, the insert says that you should not drive or use heavy machinery after taking Valium or that a drug was not tested in people over age 75. Drugs also come with contraindications: The insert says the drug should not be taken by people who have a certain condition. Those with ulcers, for example, should not take Motrin, for it causes an increased risk of bleeding in the stomach. The package insert also lists potential interactions that occur when the drug is taken with other drugs or with certain foods. For example, some drugs cannot be taken with milk because the calcium in milk inactivates some of the drug, reducing its effectiveness.

Package inserts also list special information relevant to the elderly. In this chapter we discuss many of these topics in more detail.

ELDER MEDICATION USE AND COST

Part of growing older in American society means taking more prescription medications. Older adults are prescribed more drugs than any other age group. Even though they comprise only about 13 percent of the total population, they account for more than one-third of drug use.

The National Health and Nutrition Examination Survey reported that 90 percent of individuals 65 years of age and older used at least one prescription medication in the past month, and almost two-thirds of the elder population used at least three. Ethnicity affects drug use: Whites and blacks used more prescription drugs than those of Mexican descent.[1]

High drug use means high drug costs. The proportion of the health care dollar spent on prescription drugs continues to climb faster than inflation. Between 1990 and 2009, the nation's expenditure on prescription drugs increased from $40 billion to almost $250 billion.

Paying for Medication

Traditionally, Medicare, the federal health insurance program for individuals 65 years and older and other needy people, did not help to pay for prescription drugs unless an individual was in the hospital or in a managed care program. Consequently, many elders bought private supplemental insurance coverage that paid for a portion of their medications. A few were poor enough to qualify for Medicaid, and their prescriptions were paid for by the states in which they lived. Otherwise, elders used their income and savings to cover the costs of medications. They could reduce their costs if they bought in quantity by mail, purchased their drugs from Canada or Mexico, comparison-shopped in their communities, or even purchased large tablets and cut them in half. Some decided that the costs of the medications were too high and elected to go without.

Medicare Part D is a prescription insurance program offered by private insurers that is open to all Medicare beneficiaries. Individuals who are already in a Medicare managed care plan do not have to enroll in Medicare Part D because the cost of their drugs is included in the monthly premiums they pay for the managed care plan. The Medicare Part D program is mandatory only for those individuals who formerly had their drugs paid through Medicaid. Their premiums and deductibles will be paid by the Medicaid program (MediCal in California). Individuals in the Medicaid program are automatically enrolled in a prescription drug program. Chapter 13, "Medical Care," discusses Medicare and Medicaid in detail.

The U.S. government and private consumers spend a lot of money on prescription medications and the amount is growing. The share of U.S. health care spending accounted for by prescription drugs has steadily increased since the early 1980s, from 4.5 percent in 1982 to 5.6 percent in 1994, rapidly accelerating to 10 percent by 2005.[1]

These increases in government expenditures occurred even though most elders did not have Medicare coverage of prescription medications. Prior to 2006, Medicare, the federal health insurance program for those aged 65 and older and the disabled, did not pay for prescription drugs unless a beneficiary was in a hospital, had the drug administered in a physician's office (for example, chemotherapy), or was enrolled in a managed care plan. Some elders who qualified due to poverty had prescription medications paid for by Medicaid. Others purchased private insurance or paid out of pocket. Overall, more than 30 percent of the 44 million elderly and disabled beneficiaries of the program lacked insurance coverage for prescribed medications.[2]

The Medicare Prescription Drug, Improvement, and Modernization Act of 2003 established a voluntary outpatient prescription drug benefit known as Medicare Part D. This program took effect in 2006 and represented the largest expansion of an entitlement program since the start of Medicare itself. It was hoped that Medicare Part D would provide financial assistance to beneficiaries to take their medications, and by encouraging use of generics, competition among plans, and the anticipation of "financial deal making" between drug companies and insurance plans, would lower pharmaceutical costs. Some of these goals have been realized, but not all. As expected, offering coverage for prescription drugs actually increased use of these drugs— likely because those who previously couldn't afford the drugs didn't buy them, but now that the drugs are cheaper, they purchase them. However, these plans have not been sufficient to stem the rising costs of prescription drugs and are criticized for adding one more layer of complexity and one more player looking to make a profit into the system.

First, it is voluntary. Individuals have to sign up to participate. Individuals already in Medicare managed care do not enroll in Medicare Part D. Medicare managed care programs already offered a prescription drug coverage plan. Most elders do sign up (about 60 percent), with 30 percent having drug costs paid by Medicaid, employer coverage or other coverage. Ten percent lack prescription drug coverage.

Medicare Part D established a standard slate of benefits and then allowed the private health insurance market to develop plans and compete for enrollees. Medicare developed guidelines for standard coverage, which include the monthly premiums, yearly deductible, and a cap. A monthly premium is how much the person pays each month to continue the service. The deductible is how much the elder must pay out of pocket before the insurance kicks in. The cap is the maximum amount that an individual would have to pay for medications in a year. Currently there are scores of Medicare-approved plans offered by insurance companies across the country. Some plans offer more coverage or a lower premium. The Medicare Web site, www.medicare.gov, enables individuals to see which plans are offered in their geographical area and to compare plans. Information is also available by phone: 1-800-MEDICARE.

Upon reaching age 65, most individuals must decide whether or not to purchase prescription drug insurance through Medicare. Medicare prescription drug plans are not good for everyone, particularly those who use few medications or use prescription drugs that are not expensive. The monthly premiums and the yearly deductible are spent before any medicine is even purchased. Individuals who want a prescription drug plan need to weigh the benefits of the plans available in their area with regard to monthly premiums, deductibles, co-payments (the fixed percentages that participants pay for each prescription), the plan's formulary (list of drugs offered), and participating pharmacies. If individuals choose to enter the program at a later date, their monthly premium goes up at least 1 percent a month for every month they wait to join.

No plan offers payment on all drugs, so each person must research each plan to find the program that covers all or most of the drugs that he or she uses. Each drug plan offers a limited selection of drugs in each drug category. An elder may choose a particular plan because it covers the blood pressure medication he or she needs, even though it does not offer coverage for his or her cholesterol-lowering medication. Someone who is taking a drug that isn't covered by a specific plan can ask his or her physician to prescribe a drug that is covered. To hold down the cost of the monthly premiums, elders might choose plans that require them to change one or more of their medications. Doctors have to know about plan formularies so they can tailor their prescribing to the plan in which an elder is enrolled. If an individual changes plans, prescribed medications may also have to be changed.

Sounds complicated? It is. No plan pays for all drugs so individuals must research their present and possible future situation to find the program that is best for them.

There are multiple plans offering services in most zip codes and each has differences in what drugs it will cover, what percentage of each drug is paid for, the co-pays, deductibles, and the process for getting exceptions. Each plan must supply medications from each category (for example, beta blockers, antidepressants, anticoagulants), but they do not have to offer all the drugs in each category. These drugs may be similar but are made by different companies and have other differences—like how often a day they are taken, their side effects, and, of course, how much they cost.

For each category of drug, the insurance company develops a tier system. A "three-tier" system is the most common. The lowest tier is for inexpensive medications and generics. The next tier is for preferred brands—where the insurance company has made a deal with the pharmaceutical manufacturer to get a price break. These cost the insurer a bit more, and these costs are passed to the patient. The drugs in tier three are more expensive drugs that the insurance plan would rather not be used. To discourage use, they are more costly to the consumer with co-pays, and they involve more paperwork for the physician. For example, they may require "set therapy"—trying all the drugs that are on lower tiers and having these trials fail (for example, suffering serious side effects) before covering the more expensive drug. Or perhaps the drugs will require prior authorization, which is another kind of paperwork to discourage physicians from prescribing these more expensive drugs. Let's say we are talking about cholesterol-lowering drugs. The plan may have two drugs as the first choice (first tier), then three others as second choice/tier, and then others only for rare conditions. The plan decides which drug is on which tier based on the cost they pay (and the prices they negotiated) for the various drugs. If an individual is on a drug that is not first tier, the plan will not pay for the drug and will request the beneficiary and physician to switch to the drug that the company covers and gets the best price on. All plans can substitute generics and charge higher prices if brand-name drugs are chosen.

How do you find out what plan is best? First, individuals have to sign up. Medicare beneficiaries with private insurance that pays for medications or those not taking any may not need or want to sign up—but they must understand that every month they do not sign up adds 1 percent to their premium. There is a Web site that provides assistance. You enter your zip code and medications you are currently taking and can see a price comparison. Medicare consumers can compare the out-of-pocket costs they will pay under each plan, whether the drugs they are using are on the formulary or whether they would have to switch or get special authorization, convenience (where are the pharmacies, mail order?), and the reputation and satisfaction of the plan.

So here is how it works. Lisa turned 65, but was still working, so she didn't access Medicare Part D until she retired at 71 years old. She logged onto the Web site with her daughter to help her at the local library. She entered her zip code and the five medications she was currently taking. She found that no plan covers all the medications she is on as the first tier. One plan has her cholesterol and blood pressure medication as second tier, where she is responsible for a higher co-pay, but there is a requirement that she stop those medications and try the lower cost medications to see if they work before they will give her the medication she has been taking for the last decade. Plus, she noted that her doctor had told her he might have to add another blood pressure medication if her blood pressure isn't under control, but she doesn't know what that is. The monthly fees and co-pays differ between the two plans, and she isn't sure if she should change medications—would it be bad for her? She wants to call the doctor and talk about that before she decides.

Keep in mind that the average senior isn't adept at the computer and that these calculations involve many variables. Every time there is a change in medications, it is possible that a new plan is really "the best." There are co-pays, tiers, pharmacy locations, deductibles, generics, brand names, and "approvals" to be considered. It is not surprising that many seniors face difficulty and require assistance. Studies indicate that many are not on the optimal plan for them.

Currently there are scores of Medicare-approved plans offered by insurance companies across the country. Some plans offer more coverage or a lower premium. The Medicare Web site, www.medicare.gov, enables individuals to see which plans are offered in their geographical area and to compare plans. Information is also available by phone: 1-800-MEDICARE.

Despite its limitations, Medicare Part D still offers more coverage than in the past. However, this increased coverage comes at a cost. In 2010, Part D covered 29 million beneficiaries and cost the federal government $49 billion, for an average of close to $1700 per individual enrolled. Health care costs in general and drug costs in particular are increasing faster than the gross domestic product of the nation, and costs are ballooning as the baby boom generation enters its later years. It is no wonder that the entitlement programs like Medicare Part D continue to be in the public eye as costs increase.

Influences on Medication Cost

Medications are much more expensive in the United States than in other countries, and the price continues to rise much faster than inflation. There are a variety of reasons for this disparity.

High drug company profits

Pharmaceutical companies are one of the most profitable industries in the United States. Each year, CNN Money ranks the revenues of the 500 largest corporations in America, called the Fortune 500. In 2010, the six largest pharmaceutical companies earned almost $254 billion in revenues with an average profit of 19 percent. Eli Lilly led the pack at 41 percent profit, and Johnson & Johnson was second in line with close to 24 percent profit.

Change in population, change in prescribing habits

As the population expands, particularly those who are middle-aged and older, the need for drugs increase. Drugs are being developed for lifetime use and for conditions that might not have been recognized in the past or treated so agressively, such as elevated cholesterol, allergic rhinitis, overactive bladder, erectile dysfunction, chronic pain and some types of mental illness. Expert guidelines on diseases suggest the need for ongoing treatment with a combination of medications. For example, diabetics may need aspirin, lipid-lowering medications, ACE-inhibitors, oral hypoglycemics, a complex insulin regimen, and frequent monitoring to assure their blood pressure, glucose, and lipids are kept in a tight range.

Profit before the drug goes generic

When a pharmaceutical company first markets a drug, it takes out a patent that prohibits others from copying the drug until the patent expires (usually 20 years). Since other manufacturers can begin to make and sell generic versions of the drug that are significantly less expensive, profits need to be made within that time period.

Expense of research and development

Another reason for high drug prices is that the cost of developing and testing new drugs is expensive and risky. Pharmaceutical companies assert that research and development (R&D) yields only a few "success stories," so the price of drugs needs to be high in order for companies to recoup expenses related to each successful drug as well as expenses related to drugs that do not make it to market. Moreover, high profits need to be made quickly, before the patent on a successful drug expires. However, it is important to note that not all research and development costs are borne by the pharmaceutical companies. Many come from government grants or from researchers at universities and are then turned over to pharmaceutical companies to manufacture and market (and profit).

Marketing costs

To be effective, drug companies need to educate both the physician and the consumer so that the physicians prescribe them and consumers request them. The costs incurred to market drugs to the physician and consumers are added to the total drug costs. It is estimated that the drug industry spent more than $20,000 per physician in 2009 to market their products.[3] Further, the costs of direct to consumer advertising are about one fourth of the total marketing budget of pharmaceutical companies. Details on how marketing affects medication use is discussed in the next section.

What Is Your Opinion?
Taming Pharmaceutical Prices

Scientific research continues to uncover more and more about diseases and often these discoveries result in new and improved medications to treat them. However, the cost for health care in general, and medications specifically, continues to grow at a higher rate than inflation. We all want to have effective pharmaceutical medications, but we want them at a more reasonable price. How can we stem the continued cost increases?

One popular target is profits made by the pharmaceutical companies despite price-lowering deals and regulations. However, some suggest that if taking risks, studying, developing, testing, making and selling drugs wasn't profitable, nobody would do it. This can be shown when drugs go generic. They often lose their profit margin and so no company will make that drug. This can result in drug shortages. So, should we cap profits? Or leave the free market alone?

Liability issues also drive up the prices for pharmaceuticals. We see stories all the time about drug recalls or lawsuits due to a medication being contaminated, or found to be unsafe. Recalls, lawsuits, and adverse incidents can result in high costs for the pharmaceutical companies. Liability issues cost the drug makers billions of dollars from defending them, paying out claims, and paying high insurance premiums to cover this "expense." Maybe pharmaceutical companies should not be expected to "prove" that their drug is 100 percent safe or should not be subject to lawsuits. Should we limit drug liability—"buyer beware"—or continue to permit lawsuits when medications have negative side effects?

Another cost is research and development. Much research is still paid for by public sources: government laboratories, colleges and universities; but pharmaceutical companies also finance some of their own research and this can be very expensive. Many "good ideas" for drugs never work out, or never get tested. The FDA requires detailed studies on each drug, which are costly. These steps toward approval can be perceived as "irksome governmental regulations" that hinder growth and profit, or "necessary protections for consumers' health," depending on your point of view. Should we relax the testing regulations to make it cheaper to bring new drugs to market? Should public funds through the government and universities be funding research that results in profit for private companies as well as drugs for all? What is your opinion?

One way to bring costs down is to negotiate with drug companies. Large payers like big HMOs, Medicare Part D providers, or Medicaid, in some states, make financial deals with the pharmaceutical companies. These deals mean that the company may provide the members of one plan with a certain drug (e.g., one antidepressant) over the others *if* the pharmaceutical company gives the insurance company a "special price for volume and exclusivity." Some suggest that if there were national health insurance or if more states or large plans made these deals, consumers might pay a lower price for drugs. However, others feel that the government should not be in the position of negotiating prices. What is your opinion?

Good drugs gone bad

Many times after a drug is marketed, problems arise. Perhaps a user dies as a result of the drug, or new side effects are noted. The manufacturer may have to issue more warnings, or pay insurance claims, or even take the drug off the market. These costs are also added into the profit of medications. Liability costs are up as consumers sue drug companies when products have unanticipated side effects.

Companies have to factor into their bottom line the costs of product recalls or withdrawals and lawsuits.

Lobbying to protect their industry

Pharmaceutical companies have many lobbyists to protect their interests and their profits. Although lobbyists are expensive, they are effective at representing the interests of the pharmaceutical companies when new laws are considered. Both Medicare Part D and Medicare Advantage programs use government monies to fund private insurance and are run by insurance companies. The companies who sponsor Medicare part D and Medicare Advantage programs negotiate directly with the pharmaceutical companies to get "deals" on medications for their members, in exchange for exclusive contracts—for example, "we will only offer your cholesterol lowering drug to our plan members *if* you give us a 25% discount." These negotiations are why the formularies or medication coverage lists of the different plan differ. In contrast, Medicare itself does not negotiate directly with pharmaceutical companies to get lower prices for its millions of members and doesn't limit the drugs it pays for or insist that members use the lowest price choices. In other countries with government sponsored health plans, these plans *do* negotiate with pharmaceutical companies and this lowers the amount the government pays. It is believed that lobbying by the pharmaceutical companies has a strong influence on Congress and it is for this reason that the Medicare program does not request drug discounts from them.

Influences on Medication Use

Many individuals would not enjoy the quality of life they do today without drugs to cure some diseases, prevent others, and reduce the symptoms and progression of many chronic illnesses. And many people are alive today because of modern drug miracles—medications to control blood pressure, high cholesterol, diabetes, and congestive heart failure, to name a few.

However, in the United States there is an affinity for medication that goes beyond its effectiveness for some diseases. Americans tend to choose medications over making positive behavioral changes. Popping a pill is easier than changing unhealthy behaviors, and medication use is encouraged by physicians and pharmaceutical companies. In some cases, development of a medication defines a new "treatable disease,"

thus medication companies make their own new markets. This section will discuss these reasons in detail. Many people would rather take a pill to make them feel better than change negative health behaviors to prevent disease.

Many new and different drugs have been developed to successfully treat major diseases, and more people are taking these drugs. In the past, when an individual had an acid stomach, the solution was an inexpensive over-the-counter antacid. Today, many types of drugs work in multiple ways to protect the stomach. With the advent of safer drugs to treat elevated cholesterol, many people who would not even have known they had a condition to be treated are now taking "statins" every day for years. Another example is depression. There used to be few antidepressants on the market, and their side effects discouraged people from taking them unless they really needed them. Newer antidepressants have fewer side effects, and far more people are prescribed antidepressants than ever before. Further, in the past, only psychiatrists prescribed antidepressants. Now, general practitioners and family doctors commonly prescribe them not only for severe depression, but also to change mood, such as sadness, anxiety, and dissatisfaction. Also, within the last few years, several drugs have been developed and marketed, not to treat disease, but to enhance lifestyle, such as Viagra for increased sexual potency. The newly created market to improve men's sexual function with drugs has been a boon for the drug companies (and their stockholders). Most of the top-selling drugs are newly developed and cost more than older drugs because they are under patent and face no competition.

Some diseases (e.g., obesity and diabetes) are becoming more prevalent, so drugs that treat these conditions and their complications are more often prescribed. In addition, the standard of care is changing. For example, treatment of high cholesterol used to be recommended only for individuals who had experienced a heart attack. Now, the level of cholesterol to be treated with medication is falling, and treatment is deemed "appropriate" for more and more people.

As science reveals the complexity of many illnesses, the array of medications grows to treat them. For example, asthma is now treated with some medications to open the airways, some to reduce inflammation, some to provide long-term relief, and some to treat emergency flare-ups. Diabetics are routinely prescribed more than one medication—to lower blood sugar, to reduce blood pressure, to protect the kidney, and to thin the blood. After a heart attack, elders are encouraged to take beta blockers and ACE inhibitors to reduce the risk of further attacks, plus blood thinners, cholesterol-lowering medication, and often other heart medications as well. And to treat blood pressure, there are many classes of medications, each with different actions, side effects, and dosage profiles, and within each of these classes, there are various brands of drugs. Doctors have a dizzying array of medications to treat hypertension, and there are many individual differences among physicians in what drug is prescribed. Some doctors prefer to use one medication class and increase the dose if needed, while others prefer to keep doses low and add another drug.

Many factors influence the prescribing practices of physicians: where they trained, their past success with the medication, the medical journals they read, their perceptions of the severity of the problem, whether they believe the patient is likely to be nonadherent, their attitudes toward the elderly, and the pressure they receive from patients. Perhaps the most salient influence on physicians is their education and training in medicine. The prescribing practices of physicians with more recent training differ from those of physicians in practice for a long time. The doctor's choice of specialty also influences prescribing practices. For some diseases and conditions, standards guide prescribing. For example, the National Cholesterol Education Program specifies when elevated cholesterol should be treated and in which patients, and it even guides practitioners in medication use.

Pharmaceutical companies exert a significant influence on the prescribing practices of physicians. Because pharmaceutical companies must rely on physicians to sell their prescription products, they maximize their profits by encouraging physicians to write as many prescriptions as possible. They accomplish this goal in many ways. The companies advertise heavily in professional journals and send salespeople to inform physicians about their latest products and give them free samples. Once started with a "free sample," the patient and physician may not want to switch to a less expensive drug. Pharmaceutical companies promote product recognition by distributing items with the product name or company logo, such as prescription pads, coffee mugs, pens, and refrigerator magnets. Also, the companies sponsor medical conferences. They pay physicians as consultants to travel around the country to speak to their peers about a disease and the medications the company developed to treat it. Also, pharmaceutical companies pay physicians to participate in research on their products. And, they may fund physicians to conduct research and write scientific papers. The papers which are positive to the pharmaceutical industry are published in scientific journals, and the pharmaceutical companies help to market this "latest research" in the media. Not surprisingly, the studies which fail to find a result flattering to the company are not published. Studies show that although doctors feel they are not influenced, pharmaceutical companies are a major source of influence and education for practicing physicians.

Starting in the 1990s, pharmaceutical companies began to advertise directly to potential consumers of their drugs. They "educate" the public about particular health problems and advertise their drug solutions along with an admonition to "talk to your doctor." Full-page advertisements tout the benefits of medications to stop stomach acid, keep you dry when urinary urgency strikes, or improve your relationship through erectile drugs. Often the consumer is provided with research findings to support the use of these drugs for various common conditions, along with coupons and toll-free numbers for more information or referrals. These ads are regulated and often have a glossy first page, followed by detailed small print black and white pages (or detailed rapidly spoken sentences) about the risks of the medications. Ads are everywhere—magazines, newspapers, radio and on television, Companies have developed websites which market to consumers by providing "health information" and promoting their product at the same time. The companies get involved in disease-specific organizations where they can target those with the disease that their drug treats. In addition, the drug companies submit press releases about diseases and drugs to "educate" the public which serves as free advertising.

The ads encourage consumers to discuss these newer (often more expensive) medications with their physician, and the companies hope that the consumer will leave the office with a prescription for their brand. As a result, increasing numbers of consumers are going to their physicians with specific prescription requests. Advertisements can be helpful in encouraging individuals with treatable medical problems to see their physicians, but they are often misleading. Consumers rarely read the small print, which details the medication's indications, uses, and side effects.

Concern about the practices of pharmaceutical companies has prompted calls for increasing regulation, and the pharmaceutical companies are increasingly regulating themselves. Many physician organizations and specialty groups have developed ethical standards in regard to accepting gifts and financial compensation from pharmaceutical companies.

PHARMACOKINETICS

Pharmacokinetics is the study of what happens to a drug after it enters the body: how it is absorbed from the gut into the bloodstream, distributed throughout the body, metabolized (broken down), and finally excreted. An understanding of pharmacokinetics is necessary to determine why older people may respond differently to drugs than younger adults and to determine the drug dosage needed to maximize benefits and minimize side effects. For instance, how quickly a drug is absorbed and how long the active drug circulates in the blood before it is broken down determines how

often the drug must be taken. The effectiveness and toxicity of most medications are related to their concentration in the blood.

Drug Absorption

Most drugs taken by mouth are absorbed into the bloodstream from the stomach or small intestine. In contrast, injected drugs enter the bloodstream directly. Although a number of changes in the digestive system may accompany aging, experts in pharmacokinetics do not believe these significantly affect drug absorption. Digestive diseases or food and other drugs taken at the same time are more likely to affect drug absorption than age changes alone.

Drug Distribution

Medications taken by mouth usually dissolve in the stomach, then pass through the stomach lining into the bloodstream. The blood carries the medication throughout the body. Some drugs dissolve in the blood. Drugs may also be stored in fat or muscle to be released when the blood concentration of the drug declines. But most of the drugs entering the bloodstream "hitch a ride"—that is, they attach themselves to carrier proteins in the blood. Drugs are carried not only to the organ they affect but to all the organs of the body. For example, a medication for a headache does not go to the head specifically, nor does a heart medication concentrate in the heart.

How does a medication get to where it needs to be? Generally, the site of action of the drug has more "receptors" for that drug—places where the drug chemically binds and creates its intended therapeutic effect. The heart has a great number of "beta receptors," and that is why "beta blocker" drugs are so effective on the heart. However, the fact that drugs go everywhere is also a major cause of drug side effects. Anti-inflammatory drugs are taken to relieve pain or inflammation in the joints by blocking prostaglandins. However, prostaglandins in the stomach protect it from ulcers. So, anti-inflammatory drugs can reduce pain in the knees but cause a pain in the stomach or a bleeding ulcer. Likewise beta blockers, which reduce the heart rate, also affect the lungs (which also have beta receptors) and can aggravate asthma.

A number of age-related changes cause elders to distribute drugs differently. Elders generally weigh less than younger adults, so dosages appropriate for younger adults may be excessive for elders. Drugs distributed in body fluids are more concentrated in elders because they have less body fluid. Conversely, drugs stored in fatty tissues may last longer in elders because they have more fatty tissue.

Another influence on the distribution of medication within the body is the degree to which the drug attaches itself to a carrier protein (often albumin) in the bloodstream. When a drug is bound to albumin or another carrier protein, it is inactive. Only the unbound drug has a pharmacological effect so changes in the albumin levels will increase or decrease the effect of the drug. Albumin levels are lower in those who are ill or frail. Low albumin levels may result in a higher blood concentration of the active drug and more adverse drug reactions.

Even though the albumin level in the blood does not decline with age, it is reduced significantly in elders who have advanced illness or malnutrition. Low albumin levels may cause more of the drug to be distributed to where it needs to go, increasing its toxicity. Thus, a small decrease in albumin causes large increases in blood concentrations of an active drug. Furthermore, with age, each albumin molecule becomes less efficient at binding drugs. Thus, if an elder is taking many drugs that bind to albumin in the bloodstream, the active drug concentrations will increase. Low albumin levels are directly related to a number of adverse drug reactions in elders.

Drug Metabolism

Medications are metabolized (broken down) in the stomach, the liver, the kidneys, and in other sites as well. Generally, the process of metabolism breaks the drug down to a less active form, but sometimes the process can actually make the drug more potent. Metabolism is accomplished with enzymes, which work inside cells. There is great variability among individuals in the type and rate or speed by which they metabolize some medications. Some people may metabolize a particular drug quickly, needing a higher dose of the drug to have an effect, while others metabolize the drug slowly, needing a smaller dose. To add even more complexity, the foods we eat, our environment, and other medications we take also affect the rate of metabolism. Scientists are only beginning to understand drug metabolism. In general, elders tend to metabolize drugs more slowly than younger adults, likely due to a combination of age-associated changes, diseases, and the use of multiple medications.

Drug Excretion

Most drugs are eliminated from the body through the kidneys (urine) or the liver (stool). Some drugs leave the body unchanged . Others are metabolized by the liver and return to the stool or pass through the blood to the kidney.

The kidneys continuously filter the blood, capturing the circulating drugs, and eliminating them in the urine. Although kidney function varies considerably among older people, kidney blood flow and filtration ability decrease significantly with age. The consequent decrease in kidney function allows a drug to circulate longer in the body, thus increasing its effect.

Before medications that are excreted by the kidneys are prescribed to older people, their kidney function should be measured. Most dosages for elders are two-thirds to one-half the adult dose. The reduced dosage recommendations for many medications given to the elderly are based primarily on decreased kidney function.

Summary of Pharmacokinetics in Elders

The passage of a drug through the body is affected by many factors, such as kidney and liver function, amount of circulating blood, body weight, and body fat. Age-associated changes, chronic illnesses, dehydration, the presence of other drugs in the bloodstream, and immobility can also affect drug response. Genetic differences among individuals affect pharmacokinetics, and these, combined with environmental factors and aging, make prescribing and using drugs a risky business. We can never be exactly sure how an individual will react to a particular drug or drug combination, but we can take steps to reduce the chance of adverse events. One of the most effective strategies is "to start low and go slow," especially in those who are ill or elderly. Starting with low doses and increasing doses slowly will maximize improvement and minimize toxic effects.

The FDA requires labeling of all prescription drugs regarding their pharmacokinetics—factors affecting absorption, metabolism, and excretion, possible drug interactions, and special considerations for special populations. All prescription drugs must be labeled and include a package insert revealing information relating to the use by those age 65 and older. The insert summarizes the studies conducted on the use of the drug among elders and includes optimal dosages. However, the FDA does not require additional studies to be conducted on elders, and many drugs, especially the older drugs, have never been tested in this population. Likewise, most drugs have been tested on people who take only one or two drugs, not on people with multiple chronic illnesses who need to take many medications over a long period of time.

Because of the great variability among older people in the number and extent of health problems and the number of medications used, elders and their providers should educate themselves about their medications, "start low and go slow" with new medications, and be alert to possible adverse effects.

OVER-THE-COUNTER (OTC) DRUGS

Over-the-counter drugs play a vital role in America's health care system by enabling consumers to have easy access to safe and effective medications without having to go to the doctor for a prescription every time they have a minor symptom. Some of these drugs have always been available without a prescription. Others used to be dispensed by prescription and now are available without one. In any case, OTC drugs generally have these characteristics: (1) Their benefits outweigh their risks for most people. (2) The potential for misuse and abuse is low. (3) The consumer can use them for self-diagnosed conditions. (4) They can be adequately labeled. (5) Health practitioners are not needed for the safe and effective use of the product.

The U.S. Food and Drug Administration is the federal government agency that oversees OTC drugs to ensure that they are properly labeled, that they can safely be given to most Americans, and that their benefits outweigh their risks. By law, all information that is needed to use the drugs appropriately must be on the label and included in the package insert. The Food and Drug Administration estimates that there are more than 80 therapeutic categories of OTC drugs on the market today.

When consumers use OTC drugs, they take charge of reducing symptoms or curing a health problem themselves. The majority of all medical care in this country is self-care, especially among elders, and over-the-counter drugs play a major role. Almost everyone uses OTC drugs, either to supplement or substitute for medical care. Over-the-counter drugs should not be underrated. They are a quick and inexpensive drug therapy for temporary, minor conditions. Most OTCs are effective at reducing symptoms. In fact, some contain the same compounds as prescription drugs, differing only in dosage or packaging. Over-the-counter preparations save money and physician visits. These drugs can alleviate back pain, sore throat, gastrointestinal complaints, coughs, colds, constipation, and many other minor aches and pains. It is important to note, however, that many minor problems go away without any medication.

There is a downside to the use of OTCs. Some individuals are not able to accurately diagnose many of their own health problems and to choose an appropriate drug. Or they select a drug because of its packaging or advertising, not because of its suitability to treat their health problem. Some may not read labels and may use drugs improperly. As a result, the selected OTC drug may be ineffective, delaying needed care for a serious problem. For instance, what may be interpreted as heartburn may really be a heart attack. Use of over-the-counter medications may cause significant side effects—even death. For example, an older person might use Benadryl to reduce insomnia. However, she may experience urinary retention as a side effect, followed by confusion and life-threatening delirium. Self-prescribed medications might confuse a physician's diagnosis or may not be reported to the physician. Furthermore, because OTC drugs are mistakenly believed to be less potent than prescription drugs, consumers may overmedicate. Some over-the-counter remedies contain a mixture of ingredients, including sodium, sugar, alcohol, potassium, and magnesium, that can harm some individuals. Taking multiple remedies with combinations of ingredients can lead to a higher-than-recommended dose of some ingredients. Finally, there is a potential for drug interactions when some OTCs are taken with prescription drugs.

Despite the disadvantages, OTC drugs can contribute to good health if the right product is used for the right problem and label directions are followed. The FDA Web site (www.fda.gov) provides extensive information on over-the-counter drugs.

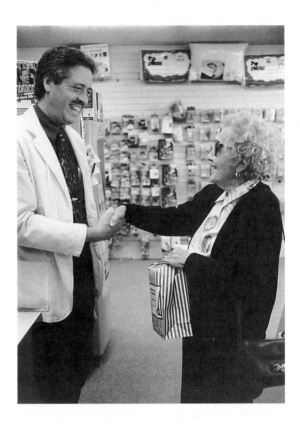

PRESCRIPTION DRUGS

Prescription medications can only be procured under the direction of a physician or other licensed professional with prescribing authority (e.g., physician, dentist, nurse practitioner, physician assistant) and dispensed by a pharmacist. They are usually used to treat more serious disease conditions and require monitoring to ensure they are safe and effective. Like nonprescription drugs, prescription drugs are monitored by the Food and Drug Administration, which sets strict guidelines on the information provided to patients and doctors, on doses, and on approved uses. However, physicians can and often do prescribe the drugs for conditions for which the FDA has not approved their use (a practice called off-label use). For example, some of the medications for seizures are used to treat pain. Some antidepressants are used to treat mood fluctuations that are not "major depression."

About 13,000 prescription drugs have been approved by the FDA and are grouped into major drug classes that share important chemical characteristics and intended effects. Each class has several medications marketed under different brand names, but all drugs within a class contain the same or similar basic drug ingredients.

Prescription drugs are as varied as the diseases and conditions they treat. For example, to treat diabetes, many types of insulin are available (long-acting, short-acting, very short acting). There are drugs that stimulate the release of insulin from the pancreas, others that help cells take up the glucose, and still others that work to decrease the rate at which sugars are absorbed from the intestine. An individual may take one or four of these medications for diabetes, plus separate medications to protect the kidney from diabetes, to lower cholesterol, and to lower blood pressure (the latter two are conditions related to diabetes and generally are treated together). Another example is the many classes of drugs to reduce high blood pressure. Some are diuretics that promote the excretion of water. Others work on the blood vessels or kidneys. Some work directly on the nerves that control the blood vessels. Others work to alter the hormones that affect blood pressure. Just as with diabetes, it is possible for one person to take one of three medications for blood pressure, each with a different action and side effect profile. A discussion of the many classes of drugs used by elders is beyond the scope of this text, although many classes of drugs are listed in the chapters that address treatments of various acute and chronic conditions (Chapters 4, 5, 6, and 7). Accurate and readable information on medications is available at www.nlm.nih.gov/ medlineplus and type "OTC medicines" in the search bar.

What drugs are most commonly used? In 2010, the number-one medication prescribed was hydrocodone/acetaminophen (Lorcet, Vicodin), an opioid pain reliever with over 131 million prescriptions dispensed. Simvastatin, a cholesterol-lowering drug (Zocor and generics) came in second with over 94 million prescriptions dispensed, and lisinopril, a medicine used for high blood pressure (Primivil, Zestril) was third with 87 million prescriptions dispensed.[4]

With regard to total spending for prescription drugs, the drug class that brought in the most revenue was cancer drugs, bringing in over $22 billion in 2010. The second class, which brought in more than $19 billion, was respiratory drugs (for example, asthma, allergies, COPD), and the third class, lipid regulators, had sales of close to $19 billion.[4]

GENERIC VERSUS BRAND-NAME DRUGS

When a pharmaceutical company develops a new drug, it is patented and sold only by that company under a single brand name. The patent expires after 20 years after which time any drug manufacturer can apply to the FDA to sell a generic form of the medication. More than half of all generic drugs are manufactured by the same company that makes the patented drug. The name of a generic drug is a simplified version of its chemical name. A generic drug has the same ingredients as the original patented version and must meet the same Federal Drug Administration standards for quality. The federal government conducts annual inspections on pharmaceutical companies to ensure that standards are met.

Generic drugs save consumers billions of dollars a year. Even more billions are saved when hospitals use generic drugs. Depending on the drug, generic drugs cost from 20 to 80 percent of the brand-name price. About three-fourths of the more than 13,000 approved prescription drugs on the market have approved generic equivalents. The rest are still under patent and cannot be sold generically. Of all prescription drugs filled, two-thirds are filled with generic drugs. According to data from the National Association of Chain Drug Stores, in 2010 the average price of a brand-name prescription was approximately $198, and the average price of a generic prescription was approximately $72— a savings of $126 per prescription.

Many people erroneously believe that brand-name drugs are better than generic drugs. This is at least partially due to marketing efforts by pharmaceutical companies and a belief that the more expensive "brand name" is better. There is evidence that pharmaceutical companies suppress publication of studies that show generics to be equivalent and also set up sham Web sites or organizations with "scientific" information about the benefits of brand names.

Even though the generic prescribing rates have increased in the last three decades, most physicians still prescribe brand names. Physicians may prescribe the brand-name medication because of name-brand recognition from ads in medical journals and from materials provided by the pharmaceutical company representatives who visit their offices. In contrast, generic drugs are not advertised or otherwise promoted by the drug companies. Physicians may also have more confidence with the brand-name drug they prescribe because it works for their patients, even though the generic drug would have the same outcome. Finally, a number of brand-name drugs do not yet have generic equivalents, so in some cases the physician must prescribe a specific brand.

Some people are hesitant to substitute a generic drug for another with a brand name. The patient may not trust a generic drug, believing it to be inferior because of its lower cost. Many elders have the attitude, "I want the best possible medication, and I'm willing to pay the price." Generic drugs may arouse suspicion because they differ in shape and color from the brand elders may have previously taken. However, Medicare Part D stipulates that generic drugs be prescribed when available, and this has been associated with increased use. Educating elders that generic drugs are safe, effective, and significantly less expensive than brand-name drugs would counteract negative attitudes toward generic drugs and save them a significant amount of money.

Consumers need to ask the physician to prescribe the generic equivalent, if available. Most states have passed legislation that permits the pharmacist to substitute a generic equivalent unless the physician specifically expresses that the substitution would not be in the patient's best interest. In addition, some HMOs and hospitals require generic substitution unless the physician specifically orders the brand-name drug. To find out whether there is a generic equivalent for a brand-name drug, search the Electronic Orange Book at www.accessdata.fda.gov/scripts/cder/ob/

POLYPHARMACY

Polypharmacy is the practice of prescribing multiple medications to a patient, particularly medications that are redundant, unnecessary, or excessive, or that interact with each other. Although the term is frequently used, it is defined in various ways. Defined most simply, polypharmacy is the taking of more than a certain number of medications—4 in some studies, 6 in others, and 10 in others. It is not always clear what is counted as a medication (eye drops? herbs? vitamins, over-the-counter medications?). However, some experts don't just count the number of medications, but are more interested

in whether they are indicated for that patient and whether the medications work well together. Combining drugs that interact with each other, giving unneeded medications (or not stopping medications when the need has passed), and giving drugs to elders that are potentially dangerous in this age group are all examples of "bad polypharmacy." Broadly defined, *medications* refers to all forms of drugs taken by whatever route—prescription drugs, over-the-counter drugs, and herbal medications—as well as to alcohol, smoking, and dietary influences on medications.

Polypharmacy may be initiated by the physician or the consumer. Some consumers visit two or more physicians and do not tell any of them about the drugs prescribed by the others. A consumer may use a number of OTC drugs in addition to a prescribed medication in order to deal with the symptoms of a health problem. Physicians who do not routinely ask patients what other drugs they are currently taking sometimes mistake a medication side effect for another illness. Polypharmacy places an individual at greater risk of adverse reactions, further health problems, increased expense of physician and hospital visits, and, in some cases, death.

Polypharmacy is common among elders because they are often prescribed several medications to treat multiple chronic diseases and conditions. Not all polypharmacy is bad: Many times multiple medications are recommended for treatment of a particular illness. However, polypharmacy always carries increased risk.

Patients can reduce the harmful effects of polypharmacy by losing weight, reducing stress, increasing exercise, stopping smoking, or initiating other positive health behaviors. Another way to reduce the harmful effects of polypharmacy is to bring all prescription and OTC medications, herbal and other supplements to each physician visit for assessment. Further, during every appointment, the physician should be asked whether any medications can be reduced or eliminated. When different doctors are seen, the patient should review his or her medications with each doctor. If a patient uses the same pharmacy for all prescriptions, the pharmacist is able to review the person's medication profile for interactions or alternatives and can call the doctor about worrisome findings. Patients may ask their physicians and pharmacists whether a drug is safe for elders and its side effects and interactions. The patient should ask the doctor whether it possible to take a medication less often or to lower the dose and under what conditions the drug could be discontinued.

DRUG INTERACTIONS

A drug interaction can be caused by a variety of adverse events that involve both prescription and over-the-counter medications. Drug interactions might be drug-drug, drug-alcohol, drug-food, and drug-herb interactions. Drug-drug interactions occur when a drug that is taken affects a chemical in the body that breaks down another drug, either raising or lowering the blood level of the second drug. Many hospital admissions of elderly patients for drug toxicity occur after administration of a drug that is known to cause drug-drug interactions, many of which could have been prevented. One of the most common drugs with multiple drug-drug interactions is the antiseizure medication Dilantin (phenytoin). Dilantin causes the liver to break down other drugs more rapidly, thereby reducing their effects. Another common example is Coumadin (warfarin), a blood thinner that has multiple interactions with other medications. Some medications make Coumadin much more potent; others render it less effective. To prevent or reduce drug-drug interactions, physicians need to be careful when prescribing and be able to recognize and act on medication-related symptoms. Further, patients should be educated about the drugs they are prescribed and know to inform the physician of unusual symptoms.

Alcohol interacts with many drugs and some disrupt the enzymes needed to break down the alcohol in the body. As a result, the effect of alcohol could be greater than usual, or the alcohol may increase or decrease the intended effect of the medication. Herbs also can interact with medications. For example, when *Gingko biloba* is used with warfarin, the combination can cause excessive blood thinning.

The intended drug action can also be reduced or enhanced by particular foods. Perhaps the most hazardous and well-documented case involves a type of antidepressant called monoamine oxidase inhibitors. When foods that are high in the amino acid tyramine (prominent in aged cheeses and red wine) are consumed with this type of antidepressant, the individual may suffer a very sudden rise in blood pressure. Another food-drug interaction may occur when the presence of food in the stomach impedes or enhances the absorption of a drug into the bloodstream. For example, acetaminophen (e.g., Tylenol) is absorbed faster on an empty stomach. In contrast, the absorption of griseofulvin, an antifungal drug, is enhanced when fatty foods are eaten before the drug is taken. Some drugs, such as antibiotics or anti-inflammatory medications, are taken with food to minimize gastrointestinal upset. But tetracycline is inactivated when taken with foods containing calcium, such as dairy products. Warfarin, described above, is rendered less effective if foods containing vitamin K are eaten. Grapefruit juice is known to interact with many drugs. For more information on drug-food interactions, see Chapter 10, "Nutrition."

ADVERSE DRUG REACTIONS

Any symptom in an elderly patient should be considered a drug side effect until proved otherwise.

Brown University Long-term Care Quality Letter, 1995

An undesirable or unexpected reaction produced by a medication is called an *adverse drug reaction* (ADR) or *adverse drug effect.* Adverse drug effects can occur because of drug interactions, incorrect prescribing or dosing, or individual reactions to the medication. One example of an adverse drug effect is an allergic reaction to a drug, such as a rash or swelling of the face or tongue. Another example occurs when a physician prescribes two medications that interact and the result is a toxic level of one drug.

Although some ADRs are not very serious, others cause the death, hospitalization, or serious injury of more than two million people in the

United States each year. Estimates vary depending on the population and the classification of adverse drug effects, but numerous studies show that adverse drug reactions result in preventable emergency room admissions, hospitalizations, and nursing home admissions and are endemic in both the community and within hospitals and nursing homes. Even in the hospital, adverse drug reactions occur, and these can result in longer lengths of stays, complications, and even, in some cases, death.

There are many different causes of adverse drug effects. Some adverse drug reactions are allergies, others are due to drug-drug interactions, and still others result from the way the drug is distributed, metabolized, or excreted. What does an adverse drug reaction look like? The symptoms of an adverse drug reaction vary, and most commonly affect the digestive system (e.g., upset stomach, diarrhea, constipation). Other symptoms might include confusion, depression, appetite loss, dehydration, unstoppable bleeding, fecal impaction, weakness, urinary incontinence or infection, falls, weight loss, postural hypotension, lethargy, unsteady gait, forgetfulness, hallucination, or tremors. It is interesting to note that many of the symptoms of adverse drug effects conform to the stereotypes of old age as well as diseases common to the elderly. Thus, adverse drug effects that would be diagnosed and treated in other age groups might be ignored by old people, their families, and health professionals.

Adverse drug reactions are also due to human error—prescribing the wrong drug or dose for the problem, administering the wrong dose, taking the drug at the wrong times, and taking a drug that interacts with another already prescribed. These errors can occur when the drug is prescribed by a physician, filled by a pharmacist, dispensed by a nurse in an institution or by a caretaker in the home, or taken on one's own.

Individuals over age 65 account for a higher percentage of hospitalizations and deaths from adverse drug effects than any other age group because of age-associated changes and a higher prevalence of chronic disease. Elders are more likely to experience side effects of medication than younger groups, particularly confusion, sleepiness, constipation, and changes in heart rate or blood pressure. The most serious side effects are from medication that causes sedation, confusion, dry mouth, inability to urinate, and delirium. The following characteristics increase the risk of many older people, particularly the very old and frail, for adverse drug effects:

- Weigh less: have less body water, less muscle, and more body fat
- Reduced ability of the liver to process some drugs
- Reduced ability of the kidneys to clear drugs out of the body
- More sensitive, because of dementia, to drugs that affect the brain
- Reduced ability to maintain blood pressure while on some drugs, predisposing elders to dizziness when rising too rapidly
- Reduced ability to adjust to external temperature by shivering or sweating
- More chronic diseases that affect drug absorption, metabolism, and level of drugs in the body
- More sensitive to medication side effects than younger population
- Take more drugs, increasing the risk of adverse drug reactions and drug interactions
- Less visual acuity, cognitive ability, and health literacy: reduced ability to read labels and take right pills at right dosage and right time
- Reduced short-term memory: forgetting to take medications

Looking at the above list, it is easy to understand why elders are at high risk for adverse drug reactions. Further, most medicines available today have not been specifically tested on older people who are using them, particularly those 75 and older. And, the medications are seldom tested upon individuals who are using other medications or have other chronic diseases, variables which become more common with advanced age.

Doctors and patients often assume that drugs are safe and that all adverse reactions are listed on package inserts. In fact, according to the FDA, most new drugs are approved with an average of only 1,500 patient exposures and usually for only relatively short periods of time. A drug that is tested in a few thousand people may have an excellent safety profile in those few thousand patients. However, soon after entering the market, the drug may be administered to several million patients. That means that some drugs that rarely cause toxicity are only detected after, not before, marketing, so any adverse drug reactions in that population are likely to occur after the drug has been approved. Seldane, Hismanol, Propulsid, and Vioxx are examples of wildly popular drugs that were removed from the market after approval due to adverse drug reactions and drug interactions in the general population. Other medications are still on the market but have new warnings based on postmarketing reports of adverse events. For example, cholesterol-lowering medications were found to induce acute problems with muscle weakness and breakdown, and now physicians and patients are cautioned to be aware of this reaction. Antipsychotics were found to be associated with increased risk of diabetes and stroke and premature death in the elderly demented patient, so now the packaging of these medications includes this warning.

The incidence of adverse effects has increased significantly over the last few years, in part because of better reporting but also because people are taking more drugs than ever before and are living longer and have more time to develop illnesses. Further, medical professionals keep reducing the range of symptoms considered normal, thereby increasing the proportion of the population taking drugs for conditions such as high cholesterol, hypertension, and obesity. For instance, blood pressure over 140/90 used to be considered hypertension, but now lower blood pressures are being diagnosed and treated. Likewise, more people are diagnosed with depression and prescribed antidepressants than in the past. Thirty years ago, no one treated high cholesterol, allergies, and impotence; therapies weren't available. It makes sense that increased drug use leads to more adverse reactions and subsequent illness.

Why do physicians persist in writing prescriptions for drugs that are listed as "dangerous" or "inappropriate"? Some do not know of these drugs' side effects or risks. Some physicians acknowledge that these drugs may be troublesome in this age group but believe them to be safe and effective for many elders. In some cases, there are few drug alternatives or the alternatives are expensive or are not covered by the elder's drug plan.

Under federal law, in nursing homes that are state licensed a pharmacist must complete a medication review for each patient at least every 30 days, and the pharmacist must note medications that are on the list of inappropriate medications and notify the physician with recommendations to review those medications.

Recently, various professional groups have devised lists of medications "not to be used" or which are "dangerous" or "inappropriate" for elders. Currently, the most rigorous tool is called the STOPP criteria (**S**creening **T**ool of **O**lder **P**ersons' potentially inappropriate **P**rescriptions). The criteria consist of 65 statements regarding specific medications that are potentially inappropriate for elders, divided according to body system (e.g., cardiovascular system, central nervous system). In addition to the name of the potentially inappropriate drug, a concise explanation of why the drug is not appropriate is listed. And some medications have additional risks listed, such as those with a particular disease or condition or inappropriate dosage level. Subsequent research on these criteria determined that they were significantly associated with avoidable adverse drug events that cause or contribute to hospitalization.[5,6]

The decision of how many drugs to prescribe or whether to prescribe drugs at all is complex because there are dangers in both overprescribing and underprescribing. The dangers of overprescribing medication to elders are clear: The more drugs, the more chance of side effects, and the more chance that drugs will interact with each other. Some drugs are highly associated with negative outcomes. However, it is important to note that there are also adverse consequences when drugs are underprescribed—that is, a drug that might have been beneficial was not prescribed or

Delirium Mistaken for Senility

When her regular physician was out of town, Mrs. M., an 89-year-old African American woman, became weak and fell. Her neighbors called an ambulance. Mrs. M. had a lot of tests done in the emergency room and was diagnosed with a urinary tract infection and dehydration. She was started on intravenous fluids and antibiotics and admitted to the hospital.

When she was seen the next day, she was confused and agitated, trying to get out of bed, insisting she had to use the bathroom. An indwelling catheter was placed, but Mrs. M. still felt she had to urinate and kept trying to get to the bathroom. She slipped through the hospital bed rails and fell and bruised herself all along one side. She pulled out her intravenous line, and it had to be replaced. She was given a benzodiazepine to calm her and help reduce her agitation. This resulted in brief periods of sleep, but when she was awake, she remained confused. She could recall her name but she did not know where she was, what day it was, or the phone number of any friends or family members. For her safety, she was put into a chair with an attached tray that did not allow her to stand up, and she was given doses of various medications for sedation. It was thought she might be depressed, so she was started on an antidepressant.

When the bladder infection was cleared, a decision was made to transfer Mrs. M. to a nursing home. Her primary physician returned to town. He was contacted to help with the plan to send her to a nursing home. He telephoned the patient's elderly sister, who lived in a nearby town, and they visited her. They were shocked at Mrs. M.'s appearance. They informed the medical team that she had been alert, highly functional, and able to care for her own needs at home, where she had lived alone for many years.

A review of her medical records revealed that Mrs. M. had been given at least six new medications. Unnecessary medications were discontinued. Over the next two weeks, her mental status improved. Mrs. M. underwent physical therapy to regain strength lost from being bed-bound. She had little memory of the hospitalization and was once again able to live independently in her own home.

the dosage prescribed was too small to have a therapeutic effect. Hypertension or high blood pressure, for example, will eventually result in kidney damage, heart damage, and death. Medications can keep blood pressure in the normal range and prevent these complications. Individuals with severe pain from cancer or another disease can live productive and fulfilled lives when their pain is managed. Underuse of beneficial drugs prescribed to older people is associated with increased illness, death, and decreased quality of life. The key issue for physicians is to prescribe the correct medication in the correct dose ("start low and go slow"), monitor the patient carefully for adverse events, and educate the patient to follow through with the drug treatment plan.

MEDICATION ERRORS

A *medication error,* as defined by the National Coordinating Council for Medication Error Reporting and Prevention, is any preventable event that may cause or lead to inappropriate medication use or patient harm while the medication is in the control of the health care professional, patient, or consumer. Put simply, medication errors are human mistakes in handling, preparing, or administering a drug that may be caused by the pharmaceutical company, pharmacist, physician, nurse, caregiver, or consumer.

Examples of medication errors are many and varied. Medication errors can be initiated by many people—the doctor, the pharmacist, the nurse, the patient, or the caregiver. The physician may not ask the patient about drug allergies, other drugs used, or look at lab results before prescribing a medication. The physician might prescribe the wrong drug or the wrong dose, or prescribe the correct medication but poor handwriting makes the prescription illegible and is misinterpreted by the pharmacist. For example, the doctor wrote QD (which is daily), but the pharmacist thought it said QID (four times a day), and the patient got too much. The pharmacist may also dispense the wrong drug or mislabel the drug. The caregiver may mistake one drug for another and administer the wrong drug, the wrong dose, give the drug too often, or not often enough. The nurse assistant in a hospital or nursing home might forget to administer the drug or give one patient's drug to another patient. The older person might forget to take the medicine, or take it too often. Or he or she might mistake one bottle of pills for another. As you can see, there are many individuals involved in medication use and many opportunities along the line for medication errors. Can you think of other examples?

Among the most important rules for nurses and others who are responsible for dispensing drugs to individuals at any age are the "5 Rights of Medication Administration": administering the *right* drug, in the *right* dose, through the *right* route, at the *right* time, to the *right* patient. Although this seems a straightforward task, data from a number of studies indicate that a significant number of medical errors are made in the home, physician's office, hospital, and nursing home.

Medication errors can have no impact at all, or they might cause pain, illness, hospitalization, or death. Medication errors are thought to be preventable and occur because of poor systems or systems breakdown, or individual errors. Even though only a few medication errors result in a bad outcome, far too many do. New studies are uncovering the alarming frequency with which medication errors occur in hospitals, nursing homes, and physician's offices.

Even though the frequency of medication errors are rough estimates, one thing is clear: Medication errors result in unnecessary deaths and excess injury and cost the nation billions of dollars a year in increased hospital stays and drug complications. It is estimated that close to 2 million drug-related injuries occur each year because of medical errors or adverse drug reactions. And about 40 percent of those are serious, life threatening, even fatal. Examples include falls with fractures, bleeding requiring transfusions, low blood sugar, and deterioration of kidney function. The drugs that most commonly cause errors are cardiovascular drugs, followed by diuretics, painkillers, antidiabetic medicines, and anticoagulants.

How can medication errors and adverse drug reactions be prevented? Multiple local, statewide, and national initiatives have been implemented to address this serious and growing problem. One of the first steps is to increase reporting of these errors to improve understanding of what is occurring, when, and why. Reporting is difficult, however, because health care organizations and professionals often are reluctant to report bad outcomes that may result in litigation. Organizations need to provide mechanisms for people to report errors without fear of retribution. Once errors are reported, there needs to be a system approach to investigation. Instead of blaming a particular doctor, nurse, or pharmacist, a broader perspective on the problem is needed. What went wrong? Why? What can be done to prevent future errors of this type? For example, if there are recurrent problems with physician handwriting, initiate a system of electronic orders.

There are other ways to reduce medical errors. One effective strategy is multiple checking: The physician writes a prescription for a medication, a nurse checks it, and a pharmacist checks it again. The hospital accrediting organization (JCAHO) has mandated many interventions to prevent medication errors, such as requiring hospitals to develop lists of drugs that are commonly confused: drugs that look alike and drugs whose names sound alike (e.g., Celexa is an antidepressant, and Celebrex is an arthritis drug). Another way to reduce medication errors is to mandate certain hospital procedures in dispensing medications. Increasing the involvement of pharmacists

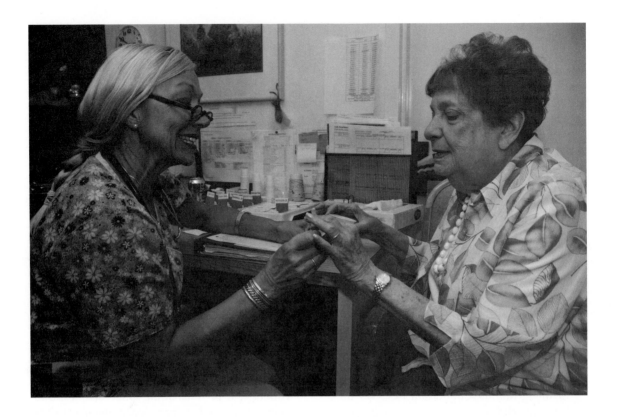

in the hospital and nursing home significantly reduces medical errors.[7]

Currently some medication errors are reported to the FDA, which has a division dedicated to medication error prevention. The Patient Safety Initiative, sponsored by the Agency for Healthcare Research and Quality, recommends a comprehensive interdisciplinary approach to reduce medication errors. For information about this initiative, see Chapter 13, "Medical Care."

PROMOTING EFFECTIVE DRUG USE

Generally, advancing age reduces the ability to manage and take medications while the number of prescribed medications increases. Some older people, especially those who are frail, may have other difficulties, such as poor vision, poor hearing, lack of education, dementia, poor health literacy, disability, and fewer social and financial resources, that complicate their ability to understand and comply with their medication regimen. Elderly patients often do not know the names, dosages, indications, or side effects of the medications they are taking.

Older people generally need more time to learn about the drugs they are prescribed. Often they cannot assimilate multiple facts at one time, or they may struggle to understand information presented to them after an exhausting physician visit. Many elders are hearing- or vision-impaired, and some are less educated or less fluent in English. To compensate for these difficulties, health professionals (including doctors, nurses, and pharmacists) should ensure that the patient not only understands the specifics of the drug therapy but also can carry out the instructions. Health literacy is discussed in Chapter 12, "Prevention and Health Promotion."

Adherence

Drugs don't work in patients who don't take them.

—C. Everett Koop, MD

Adherence, in the context of medication use, is the extent to which patients take medications as prescribed by their doctor or other health care professional. Even if the physician accurately diagnoses a disease or disorder and prescribes the appropriate drug, the health problem cannot be cured or controlled unless the patient takes the medication as directed. Estimates vary, but it is believed that from one-fourth to one-half of adults aged 60 or older are not following their medicine regimens. Although elders differ little from other populations in adherence rates, adherence is especially important for elders because they are prescribed more drugs and are more susceptible to drug interactions and adverse effects than other adult populations. On a national scale, nonadherence with prescribed medications results in a worsening of disease and, in some cases, death. Further, increased medical costs are incurred because of increased visits to physicians and hospitals.

Nonadherent Behaviors

A patient who does not adhere to a physician's instructions is said to be nonadherent or *noncompliant.* The word "noncompliant" has been used historically, but is being replaced with wording that sounds less paternalistic. Nonadherence may be unintentional (lack of knowledge or forgetfulness) or intentional (a deliberate choice not to comply). In either case, not taking prescribed medication as directed can result in a worsened condition, unnecessary hospitalization, even death. However, nonadherence does not always result in negative consequences. Nonadherence may occur because the patient has different care goals than the physician. For example, the patient may be less concerned about the long-term consequences of untreated hypertension as much as short-term consequences or side effects from the medications (such as dizziness, erectile dysfunction, or stomach upset). Some patients make drug dosage adjustments to minimize adverse effects or discontinue unnecessary medication without the physician's consent.

A number of behaviors can be classified as nonadherent. An individual may never get the prescription filled, may never take the prescribed medication (either intentionally or because of forgetfulness), or may take the drug improperly because of lack of knowledge. It is easy to forget the physician's explanation about one's illness, and even easier to forget detailed instructions on how to take the drug. In one elder population, as many as 90 percent of all nonadherence was the result of taking less than the prescribed dose of medication, whether from forgetfulness, intentional reduction to minimize adverse effects, or the desire to save money. Cost considerations may induce elders to not fill their prescriptions or to cut tablets in half or to skip doses in an attempt to make the bottle last longer. Some nonadherence is intentional: Elders may feel that they are "sensitive" to drugs or that the prescribed dosage is too high. They may lower the dose because of side effects or because they feel fine without the drug.

If an elder is not taking a medication as prescribed, it is important to find out why. Nonadherence lengthens recovery time, consequently increasing the costs of drugs, physicians, and hospitalization, and it raises the risk of medication errors and adverse effects. If an elder is not taking a medication because of a side effect, it is important to report the side effect to the physician so that another medication or a lower dose may be attempted. Patients must also report if they have discontinued a medication. If an elderly patient arrives in his physician's office with a blood pressure of 200/100 and the doctor previously prescribed a medication to lower blood pressure, the doctor is likely to increase the dosage. However, if the patient stopped taking the medication but then begins to take the new, higher dose, his blood pressure will be reduced too much, and he will be dizzy and again discontinue the medication because of the side effects! Elders and their providers may not always agree about medication type and dose, but it is critical to have open communication for good patient care.

It is tempting to place the blame for not adhering to a medication regime on the patient. However, the nature of the disease or therapy and the inadequacies of the physician may also be causes. Before the consumer health movement of the early 1970s, physicians and pharmacists withheld information about prescribed medications. Now, it is generally accepted that medical consumers have a right to know about their health status and all aspects of their medications—benefits, side effects, and alternatives. Providers and patients need to work as a team to promote rational drug use. Consumers have the right to decide whether or not to agree to a prescribed regimen. It is the physician's responsibility to give patients appropriate information so they can make these decisions. Table 8.1 describes common causes of nonadherence among elders.

Education to Increase Adherence

Although some adults are very educated about their medications, the overwhelming majority are not. Effective education increases the success of drug therapy; it does not guarantee adherence but is a necessary prerequisite. Patient education should include an understandable description of the disease and its progression, treatment goals, details about the drug therapy, and alternatives to drugs. Education may be accomplished by a physician, nurse, pharmacist, or health educator.

One important aspect of patient education is to determine whether the patient can administer the medication (e.g., swallow large pills, put drops in his or her own eyes). Some health professionals suggest "checking for understanding" by having the elder repeat information back to the health provider. It is likely that most elders require more time to ask questions about their health problem and treatment plan. The health provider must allow time to confirm that the information is understood. If possible, someone close to the patient should also listen to the discussion regarding the medication regimen, especially if she or he will monitor or administer it.

Child-resistant containers may be a barrier to adherence. The Federal Poison Prevention Act requires the use of child-resistant containers for

TABLE 8.1	Causes of Nonadherence Among Elders

PATIENT FACTORS
1. Never starts the drug therapy
2. Forgetfulness
3. Lack of knowledge
   a. Does not understand disease or importance of therapy
   b. Does not know how to take medication properly
   c. Visual or hearing decrements that preclude knowledge of medication use
4. Intentionally alters medication schedule
   a. Fear of dependence on medication
   b. Lack of trust in physician
   c. Dissatisfaction with results of medication
   d. Attempt to save money

NATURE OF DISEASE AND/OR THERAPY
1. High number of medications and dosage frequency
2. Long treatment time
3. Medication causes unacceptable side effects
4. High cost of medication
5. Disease has no symptoms
6. Unacceptable dosage forms (bad taste, can't swallow pills)
7. Low potential for therapy to cure disease or relieve symptoms

PHYSICIAN INADEQUACIES
1. Lack of explicit written and oral instructions
2. Poor relationship with patient
3. Physician's lack of confidence in treatment
4. Complicated drug regimen prescribed
5. Lack of specific instructions on medication label

both OTC and prescription medications to reduce the incidence of poisoning in children. However, child-resistant containers can pose a problem for some older people with impaired vision and reduced manual dexterity and strength. The most obvious consequence is that elders will not take the medication. Or they may break the container when trying to open it, causing injury. Or, once the cap is off, elders may not recap the container or may transfer the medication to another vial without identification or instructions for use. Uncapped medications may spoil or be ingested by grandchildren.

Some new cap models, mainly squeeze-and-turn designs, are child-resistant but can be opened by most older adults. Elders should request this type of cap and if possible try to open it in the pharmacy. With the consumer's permission, the pharmacist can place the prescription in a container with an easy-open cap. Such a container should be stored out of the reach of children.

One of the most important and neglected means of patient education to increase adherence is clear instructions on drug labels and educational information on handouts. The more information that is put on the drug label, the greater is the likelihood that the client will be able to understand and adhere with directions. Whenever possible, the medicine directions discussed in the physician's office should be supplemented with large-print, readable handouts that the client can refer to later. It is also important to assess whether the person's mental status, vision, coordination, and hand strength are adequate to take medication without supervision.

The following information should be discussed when any prescription is given:

- Name of medication (both generic and brand name)
- Amount of medication in each dose
- Appearance of the medication
- Why the drug is prescribed
- Major benefits and risks of medication
- Quantity to be taken
- Dosage frequency
- Method of administration
- Duration of therapy
- Precautions
- Special instructions
- What to do if a dose is missed
- Prescription refill information
- Storage requirements
- Adverse effects to report
- Interactions with food, other medications, or alcohol

- When effects of the medication should be noticed
- When to stop taking a drug
- How long the prescription should last
- What to expect if the medication is not taken
- Alternatives to medication

The package insert for each medication includes much of this information, but the small print size discourages reading. Ues www.medlineplus.gov to find information on a particular prescription drug.

Memory Aids to Increase Adherence

Because elders often take several drugs, keeping track of which medications to take at what time can be a major impediment to adherence. There are many techniques to help people remember medication schedules. The time to take medication may be matched with another daily activity, such as breakfast or bedtime. Medication can be placed in an obvious place (beside the coffee, toothbrush, or razor) to jog the memory. Elders can divide their week's medications into envelopes, pillboxes, or egg cartons labeled with the date and time of ingestion. The pharmacist can consolidate medications into labeled bubble-packs. Elders can use a medication calendar and check off boxes immediately after drugs are taken. The calendar can be shown to the physician to check compliance. Some individuals set a timer to remind themselves to take their medication. An electronic pill cap has been developed with a flashing red light and a loud bell that can be set to ring a number of times a day.

Probably the most elaborate medication reminder is the Monitored Automatic Pill Dispenser MD2, a dispensing system for tablets and capsules and a reminder system for medications not taken by mouth. The dispenser includes 60 cups for medications and is about the size of a coffeemaker. The system even has the capacity to call the caregiver if the medications are not taken on time. The downside is the cost: about $800.

Many other electronic gadgets have been developed to remind people to take their medications and even to record whether they took them on time. The problem with these is that the elder who is forgetful about medications is often not savvy enough to program or use the devices without assistance. When medication schedules change, it is imperative to update these tools. It is also important for the elder to be trained to use the tool and for there to be appropriate follow-up to ensure that he or she is using it.

Enhancing Oversight of Drug Therapy

A number of health professionals should be involved in effective drug therapy because each person has the potential to minimize adverse drug effects and provide helpful drug information to elders. In a team approach, the physician, pharmacist, nurse, social worker, and the older person cooperates to maximize benefits and minimize problems with drug therapy. The team approach, though effective, is rarely used in community settings.

The Physician's Responsibility

Physicians are primarily responsible for drug therapy. They must accurately diagnose the health problem, prescribe the correct type and dosage of medication, and supervise drug therapy. In addition, the physician must educate the patient about the disease and its treatment, including drug therapy. Since the majority of elders take prescription drugs for chronic diseases, it is imperative for the physician to allocate time to explain the drug regimen or to explicitly delegate that responsibility to a nurse, health educator, or pharmacist.

The following list indicates the many ways in which physicians may promote effective medication use. Failure in one or more areas may increase the risk of medication errors and adverse drug reactions:

- Obtain a complete drug, dietary supplement, and herbal medicine history, including drug allergies.
- Ask patients whether they think the drugs are working and if they noticed any side effects.
- Accurately diagnosis the health problem.
- Correctly calculate dosage or frequency of dosage appropriate for elders.
- Use correct drug name, dose, or abbreviation.

- Clearly write the prescription so there is no confusion about drug, dosage, and timing.
- Use generic drugs whenever possible.
- Consider food-drug, drug-drug, and drug-herb interactions.
- Suggest lifestyle changes.
- Give clear instructions regarding medication.
- Avoid duplication of drugs.
- Monitor side-effects of medications.
- Tell patients and those who care for them about the most common and most severe side effects.
- Tell patients and those who care for them what to do if the patient is sick, misses a dose, or experiences a side effect.
- Prescribe as few medications as possible and as low a dose as possible.
- Objectively evaluate whether the drug makes any difference.
- Assess the patient's kidney and liver function and prescribe accordingly.
- Consider the patient's lifestyle when recommending drug and dosage.
- Periodically review need for all medications.
- Consider nondrug alternatives.

The physician's lack of knowledge of the special medication considerations for older people can be attributed to an insufficient geriatric focus, insufficient pharmacology content in medical school, and limited opportunities for continuing geriatric and drug education for practicing physicians.

The Pharmacist's Responsibility

The traditional role of the pharmacist was to procure, store, prepare, and dispense drugs. Today, in addition, pharmacists in the hospital and community prevent, recognize, and intervene in drug-associated problems.

Pharmacists serve as a resource for both clients and physicians, providing information on proper drug use and on the adverse effects of both prescription and OTC drugs. Further, pharmacists provide a confidential record-keeping service for their customers. The records include drug history, drug allergies, and medical history. Pharmacists consult with the physician periodically to ensure the client is using the drug properly, and they alert the physician to potential drug interactions, adverse drug effects, and the negative impact of prescriptions ordered by other physicians. They can identify symptoms of serious diseases in their clients and refer them to their physicians when necessary. Pharmacists provide information on generic drugs and can assist the patient with medication scheduling and memory aids. In addition, they can instruct clients on the use of child-resistant containers and assess their need for easy-open containers. Many pharmacies also provide emergency service, delivery, and insurance billing service.

Many long-term care institutions and hospitals have instituted clinical pharmacy services to dispense and administer drugs, review drug utilization, and educate patients. When such services are implemented in an institutional setting, drug misuse drops significantly. Regulations from the Health Care Financing Administration have expanded the role of the pharmacist in long-term care institutions. Pharmacists now monitor drug regimens and dosages, eliminate unnecessary drugs, and ensure that patients understand and can administer their own medications when discharged. Medicare Part D recognizes the important role of the pharmacist on the health care team by providing reimbursement to the pharmacist for counseling and medical review services.

The Nurse's and Social Worker's Responsibility

The nurse's responsibility in drug therapy depends on the work setting. In a physician's office, nurses commonly provide drug education. In hospitals, nursing homes, or home health care, nurses carry out the plan of care devised by the physician; they administer medications, monitor drug reactions, and report problems to the physician. Nurses are in direct contact with the patient and are in a good position to determine if a new drug or change of dosage is needed. Nurses also play an important role in patient education. Nurses employed in nursing homes have a great deal of contact with patients over a long period of time, seeing patients

much more frequently than do physicians. Thus, their responsibility for monitoring drug regimens and side effects is crucial.

Social workers working with older people (e.g., in adult day health care or case management) should have a basic knowledge of medication-related problems and be able to refer clients with those problems to appropriate health care professionals. Some social workers are in a position to monitor medication consumption and adverse effects. Social workers might also discuss problems with adherence or medication complications with their clients' physicians. Unfortunately, few social workers are knowledgeable about the common health concerns of elders and associated medication issues.

An important role of social workers who work with older people is to serve as their health advocates by recognizing medication-related problems, helping to resolve them, and encouraging health practices that could reduce drug use. They are in a position to inform elders about generic drugs and assist in developing memory aids to increase adherence. They can encourage elders to keep medication records and to discuss all drugs with a pharmacist or physician. The social workers' advocacy role becomes especially important for

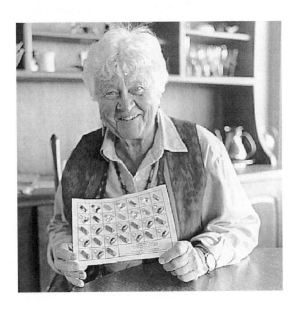

elders living alone because social workers may be the only professional with whom those older people have any contact.

The Elder's Responsibility

Consumers must take responsibility for their medication use. They need to actively seek drug information from their physicians and pharmacists, make decisions about treatment plans, and monitor their own drug therapy programs. Consumers can also decrease their chance of suffering adverse medication events by familiarizing themselves with their medications, reading labels and directions carefully, asking questions about all new medications, and reminding health care professionals about their allergies.

Everyone needs to keep a record of all over-the-counter and prescription medications they are currently taking. The record should list those taken daily and those taken only occasionally. The dosage, timing, and any adverse reactions should be noted. The reason the medication is taken should also be listed. The medication record should be brought to every physician visit and to every pharmacy visit that involves a new prescription. Unfortunately, most elders do not keep a list.

Individuals should use the same pharmacy for all prescriptions so that a complete medication history is on record at one location. Elders should also inform their pharmacists of the over-the-counter and herbal medications they use. Many physicians and pharmacists prefer that patients bring their medications to them for review. If any adverse reactions are noted, the physician should be called immediately so that the drug or dosage may be modified.

If the older person cannot manage his or her own medications, a caretaker or family member can help by accompanying the elder to the physician to get accurate information on the medication regimen, then properly administering the medication.

Be a Savvy Drug Consumer

- Tell the physician all physical complaints; lack of complete data can lead to inappropriate drug use. It might help to bring a written list to the doctor's office.
- Be aware that a physical problem may be caused by adverse drug effects or drug-drug/drug-food interaction. Report them to the physician.
- Keep a personal medication record, including both prescription and OTC drugs. Share this record when you visit each physician.
- Tell the physician of any allergic reactions experienced previously with drugs.
- Question the physician about alternatives to drug therapy.
- Know when, how, and with what to take drugs, as well as which foods to avoid. Read all drug inserts and consult your pharmacist or physician with unanswered questions.

- Follow medication instructions exactly. If in doubt, contact your physician or pharmacist.
- Don't mix medications without permission from your physician.
- If the drug schedule interferes with your lifestyle, tell your doctor immediately.
- Do not share prescription medication with others.
- Do not mix similar-looking medications in a pill box.
- Do not take medications in the dark or when not fully awake.
- Do not drink alcohol when taking drugs.
- Keep medications away from children.
- Destroy all outdated medication.
- Ask that childproof containers not be used if they are a problem for you.
- Ask for a generic substitution, if available.
- Ask for large-print prescription labels if you have vision problems.

A family member or friend can also monitor the elder's reaction to the drug, determine if symptom relief is sufficient, and keep drug intake records. In addition, the helper should be alert to potential adverse drug reactions and should contact the physician when they occur. An excellent fact sheet from the National Center on Caregiving at the Family Caregiver Alliance, called "Caregiver's Guide to Medications and Aging," offers guidelines for the safe and effective use of medications. It includes tips ranging from how to work with a pharmacist to how to recognize adverse drug reactions. It is available at www. caregiver.org

Medication Information Resources

Many people are surfing the Internet for medication information geared toward the layperson, and they are finding it everywhere. Web sites range from those offering low-cost medications without a doctor's prescriptions, to pharmaceutical company sites, to governmental and professional organization sites. The following lists provide a sampling of the reputable sites that offer excellent information regarding medication use and older people.

Government Sites

- The Food and Drug Administration, Center for Drug Education and Research, provides news on consumer drug information, warnings, recalls, and other drug information (www.fda.gov).
- The National Library of Medicine in cooperation with the National Institutes of Health offers current information on diseases and provides extensive resources and educational handouts for the layperson and the professional regarding medications and news alerts (www.nihseniorhealth.gov). Another project of the National Institutes of Health is a Web site specifically for older people. The site includes information about common diseases in large print and with audio (www.health.nih.gov/category/SeniorsHealth).

Professional Organizations

- The American Academy of Family Physicians has a senior section that includes a section on seniors and medicines and another on common conditions of older adults including treatments (www.familydoctor.org).
- The American Society of Health-System Pharmacists (ASHP) has a Web site that features information about why a medication is prescribed, how it should be used, potential side effects and warning signs of adverse drug reactions, special precautions and dietary instructions, information on what to do if a dose is missed, and storage directions. The site also provides breaking health and medication news and tips to help prevent medication errors and antibiotic resistance (www.SafeMedication.com).

The Physicians' Desk Reference

The *Physicians' Desk Reference (PDR)*, the "drug bible" of the medical profession, is a catalog of all prescription drugs available in a given year. Each year a new edition is compiled by the drug companies. The prescription drugs are listed in several ways to allow easy access—by generic name, brand name, and company selling the brand—and there are color illustrations of each pill (www.pdrhealth.com).

ALTERNATIVES TO DRUGS

Many alternatives to prescription and over-the-counter drugs are available to improve health and well-being. The most well-documented alternatives are exercise, weight loss, smoking cessation, and dietary changes, and they are discussed extensively in other chapters. We all know that such alternatives take work and that it is difficult to break long-standing habits. Instead, many people prefer the quick action and simplicity of medications. Some individuals prefer to augment their prescription drug use with herbal medications. A few use herbs exclusively for prevention and treatment.

Herbal remedies are the primary medical treatments for over three-fourths of the world's

A Skeptic's Guide to Medical "Breakthroughs"

Everyone is gratified by news of a major drug breakthrough, especially if it promises help for people who are seriously ill. And if you or a loved one has been praying for such a drug, the news may seem like a miracle.

But can you accept the good news at face value? All too often you can't, because many such reports are either exaggerated or are inaccurate interpretations of scientific findings. Significant advances in drugs and drug therapy don't happen nearly as often as magazines, television, or the Internet might lead you to believe. Sober skepticism is a good attitude to have when evaluating news about drug "breakthroughs." Here are a few guidelines:

- Where did the news report appear? Is it in a newspaper, magazine, or broadcast news service that regularly covers health and medical affairs and assigns specialized reporters to the subject? Or is it part of a publication or broadcast that emphasizes sensational stories that seem, and probably are, too good to be true? Is the reporter someone whose coverage of health and medicine you believe to be accurate and cautious? If you are doubtful about the news medium in which the report appears, it's probably best to take the story with a grain of salt.
- News stories about drugs producing complete cures and unscrupulous cyberspace marketers peddling "miracle" treatments especially for patients with cancer, AIDS, severe arthritis, or other grave illness, are likely to be cruelly wrong.
- What is being reported? The results of one study in a small number of patients are seldom, if ever, conclusive. This kind of preliminary information is presented at scientific meetings or published in scientific journals whose editors and readers know how to interpret such findings. News stories may place undue importance on these reports and jump to conclusions that the researchers themselves know are unjustified.
- Ask your health care provider what he or she knows about the story. While health care practitioners can't know everything, there's a good possibility that they will know about a truly important medical advance.

Most medical science writers and reporters try diligently to provide accurate and authoritative information. They avoid unfounded speculation, and they strive to put exciting discoveries in perspective. Their stories don't often grab front-page headlines or lead off the evening news, but they can be trusted to give you solid information. And that's a great deal better than false hope.

population. Many conventional medications come from plants (aspirin from willow bark, digitalis from foxglove, and warfarin from sweet clover). Even in industrialized nations, about one-quarter of all prescription medications contain ingredients derived from herbs. However, just like prescription and over-the-counter medications, herbs have benefits, risks, and side effects. Herbs are inexpensive, and many can be grown in the backyard. Herbal treatments do not require interaction with a health care provider. The movement in consumer advocacy toward being responsible for one's health and the high cost of prescription drugs make herbal therapy very appealing. On the other hand, some herbs can interact with some medications or foods, creating adverse effects. However, when compared with the adverse effects of drugs, herbal remedies almost never cause serious harm.

What are the differences between herbs and pharmaceutical drugs? Pharmaceuticals are standardized with fewer ingredients and components than herbs. An herb may contain multiple "types" of a single chemical, differing slightly; a medication is a purified version of just one of those chemicals. The FDA requires documentation of the effectiveness, safety, and potential of pharmaceutical drugs to interact with other medications. The FDA does not regulate herbs because it considers them food supplements. Because FDA approval is not required for herbal supplements, there is no guarantee of the safety, effectiveness, potency, or purity of the product bought in the store, and the product label may not accurately describe the potency or list all the ingredients.

Because herbal products are considered food supplements, their manufacturers cannot make health claims (e.g., suggesting that garlic may lower cholesterol) or place warnings about their products' use on the label. Although manufacturers are restricted from putting health claims on labels, their business depends on linking their products with health and vitality, so it is very common to see health claims and testimonials in their ads. An assessment of over 400 Web sites that provide information on the eight best-selling herbal products found that three-fourths of them were retail sites or were directly linked to another seller. Further, over 80 percent of those sites made at least one health claim. Besides being illegal, claims that herbal supplements treat, prevent, diagnose, or cure specific diseases are misleading.[8]

An incredible amount of material is available on the Internet and at local health food stores about herbal remedies, but most of it is testimonials—individuals telling about how the medication has worked for them. For accurate information on herbal medicine, see the following sources:

- The National Center for Complementary and Alternative Medicine conducts research on a variety of complementary and alternative medicines (including herbal medicine), trains researchers, and disseminates information to professionals and the public. Fact sheets are available for selected herbs with current research findings (www.nccam.nih.gov/health/herbsataglance.htm).
- The Office of Dietary Supplements, created at the National Institutes of Health under the Dietary Supplement Health and Education Act of 1994, has a lot of information on its Web site about herbal remedies and dietary supplements, including evidence-based reviews and fact sheets for many supplements (www.ods.od.nih.gov).
- *The Physicians' Desk Reference for Herbal Medicines* is the most complete reference on herbs available and is now in its fourth edition (2007). Information on the herbs in the book can be accessed on the Web at www.pdrhealth.com

Rigorous controlled clinical trials are needed to document the health claims of those who market herbal products, but at this time, no legislation requires them. Research regarding herbal supplements is beginning to appear in medical journals, though certainly not in proportion to their use. Drug companies seldom fund studies on herbs that are already available without a prescription because, even if these natural products are found to be effective, the companies will not realize a financial gain. Further, the dosages of herbs are very difficult to measure because the ingredients are not controlled by the FDA. To complicate matters even further, some herbal preparations use different parts of the plant (leaves, buds, roots), different forms of the herb, and different methods of extraction, and dosages are not standardized. Even when clinical studies are conducted, the size of the study and the research methodology make it very difficult to interpret the results.

The increase in interest and consumption of herbal remedies is paralleled by the consumption of vitamin and mineral supplements to enhance health, prevent disease, and even reduce the symptoms of common health problems. Their benefits and risks are discussed in Chapter 10, "Nutrition." Traditional healing practices in most of the world do not include most of the medicines to which we have become so accustomed. Instead, they depend on other theories of healing that have been used for hundreds, even thousands of years. Descriptions of the most common alternative healing approaches appear in Chapter 13.

Changing one's health behavior should be the first consideration in managing most chronic illnesses: In many cases, drug use may not be needed. For instance, weight loss, dietary change, and exercise can control adult-onset diabetes (type II diabetes), and increased fiber and fluid intake and daily exercise almost always help those who are constipated. However, for some diseases and disorders, drug therapy may be the most effective means to control symptoms and prevent the disease from worsening.

In addition to their benefits, almost every medication on the market is accompanied by unwanted side effects. The physician and the consumer must be aware of the long-term and short-term benefits of the medication and how it compares with nondrug alternatives. A cautionary note: Symptoms are a signal to the body that something is wrong. If self-care does not relieve the symptoms, seek a physician's advice.

The good news is that the human body has extraordinary healing powers and many health problems resolve themselves without a physician, a prescription, or a trip to the drug counter. As Dr. Lewis Thomas said, "The biggest secret of doctors is that most things get better by themselves; most things, in fact, are better in the morning."

SUMMARY

Elders use more medications than any other age group because of their high prevalence of chronic conditions. Advances in drug technology have revolutionized the management of symptoms of chronic illnesses in elders, but no medication can be considered fully safe. All have risks, benefits, and inadequate information available about long-term use, use in the elderly, use in combination, and how the drug will impact a particular individual. Elders are especially susceptible to adverse drug effects and drug interactions because of the high number of OTC and prescription drugs they take. Additionally, some age- and disease-related physiological states affect the drug dosages needed in elders. Adverse effects are more common among elders than among any other age group and can cause illness, hospitalization, or death.

Nonadherence with medication regimens is a prevalent, multifaceted problem. Effective patient education can increase adherence with drug regimens and reduce the risk of adverse drug effects. Nurses, pharmacists, physicians, social workers, and individual consumers can work together to maximize rational drug use. Finally, changes in lifestyle (losing weight, stopping smoking, exercising more) should be attempted before drug therapy is initiated because no drug is risk-free. When drugs are used, the lowest possible dose for the shortest possible time is recommended.

ACTIVITIES

1. Ask an older relative or friend to show you what OTC and prescription drugs he or she has at home. Find out how much this person understands about the medications' use, side effects, directions for administration, and shelf life. Ask which drugs the person is currently using. Remember to ask specifically about OTC medications such as laxatives, which are commonly used but infrequently reported. From your reading, do you note any drug misuse?

2. Go to the drugstore and examine the multitude of medications available for purchase. What are the most common symptoms being treated? Notice the differences between the package labeling of brand-name drugs and that of generic drugs, and compare prices. Notice how medications are clustered on the shelf and the varying dosage forms that are available. For a half-hour period, observe the individuals buying OTC drugs at the drugstore. How do they decide what to buy? Compare the purchases of elders and younger people. Keep a record and compare your results with those of other students in your class.

3. Collect child-resistant containers from pharmacists. Have a container-opening session in class, and assess which ones would be most difficult for elders with decreased visual and touch sensitivity and reduced physical strength to open. Interview five elders regarding their opinion of child-resistant containers. Are they aware that they can request an easy-open container?

4. Ask 10 people (any age) if they know what generic drugs are and if they request them. Be prepared to educate them on the difference between generic and brand-name drugs. Gather information regarding generic prescribing from a local pharmacy. Does your state have a law to encourage the use of generic drugs?

5. Collect all the OTC and prescription drugs in your home. Are the names and labels clear on the prescription drug containers? Do you know why each prescription was purchased? Is the medicine still usable (look at the expiration date)? Is it being properly stored? Do you have unfinished prescriptions that you are no longer taking? Why are you no longer taking them? Concerning the OTCs, are they really needed? Have you tried nondrug alternatives for headache, insomnia, constipation, and acid indigestion? How do you decide when to treat your symptoms with an OTC remedy?

6. Find 12 advertisements from 12 Web sites advertising drugs and analyze them. Is the information factual? What claims are being made? Compare the advertised prices to the prices at a local pharmacy. Where do the drugs cost less? Don't forget to include taxes and shipping costs in your calculations.

7. Compare the prices of five prescription drugs in the United States and Canada by using local pharmacies and Internet pharmacies. The drugs may be ones that you or family members commonly use. What is the savings?

8. The Canadian International Pharmacy Association site (www.cipa.com/patient-safety/) outlines steps for U.S. citizens to take when ordering from Canadian on-line pharmacies. Look up that document. Would you consider purchasing your prescription drugs from Canada? Why or why not? Would you feel differently if you were on a fixed income and couldn't afford the cost of the drug in the United States? See if you can find more recent information regarding the importation of prescription drugs from Canada by consumers in the United States.

9. Compare the prices of five prescription drugs that have both a brand name and a generic name. What is the savings?

10. Collect and analyze drug advertisements in medical journals and popular magazines. What types of medications are advertised in what type of publication? How many advertisements are geared to older people? How many purport to provide scientific information? How do advertisements marketed directly to consumers suggest that consumers obtain the product? Attempt to read all of the small print appearing with the advertisement. What new information do you garner from it? If a toll-free number is available, call for more information.

11. Bring an OTC medication to class. See what the members of the class, without reading the label information, believe the medication is used for. Then read the label. Any surprises? Discuss nondrug alternatives to each product.

12. Visit a health food store and examine the herbal remedies available. What can the store clerk tell you about each remedy? Are written materials available to guide you? Compare prices with other medications.

13. Interview adults about their compliance with prescribed medications. Do most people take all medications as prescribed, or is it more common to stop taking a medication after a while? Does adherence depend on particular factors that you can identify (for example, whether they can feel the medication effects, whether they are knowledgeable about the reason it was prescribed, whether the medication is for an acute or a chronic problem, or whether a physician explained the importance of finishing the prescription)? Are any of the interviewees intelligent noncompliers?

14. Develop patient information on nondrug alternatives to common health problems, such as insomnia, constipation, or cold symptoms. For example, insomnia: Use bed only for sleeping, eliminate daytime naps, drink warm milk before

bed, go to sleep at same time nightly, increase physical activity.

15. Find out what changes have been legislated since the initiation of Medicare Part D. What is the current status of Medicare Part D? Do elders save money? Are pharmaceutical companies increasing profits?

16. Generate a hypothetical list of medications (from four to eight medications) that you might be taking, and choose a pharmacy you prefer; then try to enter this list in the www.cms.gov Web site to see which preferred drug provider (PDP) would best meet your needs under Medicare Part D.

BIBLIOGRAPHY

1. Centers for Medicare and Medicaid Services. 2010. "National Health Expenditure Data." www.cms.hhs.gov/nationalhealthexpenddata

2. Neuman, P., Strollo, M.K.,Guterman, S., Rogers, et al. 2007. *Health Affairs* 26(5):630–643. Medicare prescription drug benefit progress report: Findings from a 2006 national survey of seniors. *Health Affairs* 26(5):w630–w643.

3. Weiss, J. 2010. Medical marketing in the United States. *The George Washington Law Review* 79: 260–292.

4. IMS Institute for Health Care Informatics. 2011. The use of medicines in the United States: Review of 2010. Parsippany, NJ: IMS Institute for Healthcare Informatics.

5. Gallagher, P., Ryan, C., Byrne, S.l., Kennedy, J., and O'Mahony, D. 2008. STOPP (Screening Tool of Older Person's Prescriptions) and START (Screening Tool to Alert doctors to Right Treatment). Consensus validation. *International Journal of Clinical Pharmacological Therapy* 46(2):72–83.

6. Hamilton, H., Gallagher, P., Ryan, C., Byrne, S., and O'Mahony, D. 2011. Potentially inappropriate medications defined by STOPP criteria and the risk of adverse drug events in older hospitalized patients. *Archives of Internal Medicine* 171(11):1013–1019.

7. Leape, L.L., Cullen, D.J., Clapp, M.D., Burdick, E., and Demonaco, H.J. 1999. Pharmacist participation on physician rounds and adverse drug events in the intensive care unit. *Journal of the American Medical Association* 282(3):267–270.

8. Morris, C.A., and Avorn, J. 2003. Internet marketing of herbal products. *Journal of the American Medical Association* 290(11):1519–1520.

Physical Activity

Those who think they have no time for bodily exercise will sooner or later have to find time for illness.

Earl of Derby

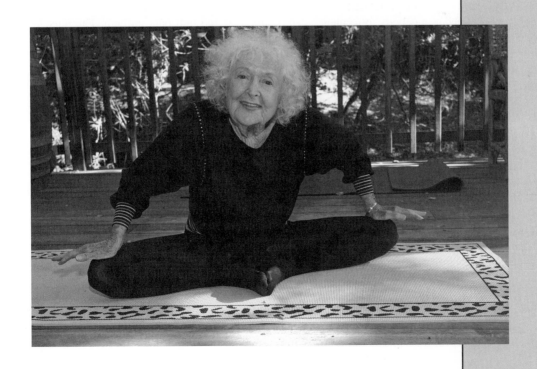

Before the Industrial Age, most people were not concerned about getting sufficient physical exercise because their active daily routine kept their muscles and hearts strong. As the workplace and home become more mechanized, fewer people get sufficient physical activity from their occupations and household chores. Most people must make an effort to become more active because it is easier to sit in front of the television or computer screen than to go for a walk or swim a few laps. Elderly people are even less likely to engage in physical activity than their younger counterparts, despite its proven value for all age groups. In this chapter we discuss components of physical fitness, the benefits of keeping active, the pitfalls of inactivity, and the role activity plays in the prevention and treatment of several chronic diseases. Patterns of physical activity in older adults, their attitudes toward exercise, and ways to promote a more active lifestyle in that group are addressed.

COMPONENTS OF PHYSICAL FITNESS

It is important to learn the difference between physical activity, exercise, and physical fitness. *Physical activity* is defined as any body movement that is produced by skeletal muscles and expends energy. *Exercise* is planned, structured, and repetitive body movement accomplished to maintain or improve one or more components of physical fitness. *Physical fitness* relates to the body's ability to perform physical activity—the higher the level of fitness, the greater the physical ability. At any age, being physically fit enhances quality of life, allowing individuals to meet ordinary and unexpected demands of daily life with ease. For elders, fitness may mean the ability to live independently, do household chores, shop for food, engage in active leisure pursuits, and withstand illness and injury. Physical fitness must be maintained. If an individual no longer strengthens his or her muscles or exercises aerobically, for example, the body rapidly loses fitness. The loss of fitness from inactivity occurs more rapidly among elders.

There are many components of physical fitness: cardiorespiratory endurance, muscular endurance and strength, joint flexibility, body composition, balance, and coordination. Some exercises are better than others for the type of fitness desired. For instance, jogging increases endurance and aerobic capacity, while dancing also increases balance and flexibility.

Cardiorespiratory endurance is the ability of the body's circulatory and respiratory systems to supply fuel during sustained physical activity. Keeping the heart rate above normal for an extended period of time strengthens it, whether these exercises are done at high, moderate, or low intensity. Exercises that increase cardiorespiratory endurance are called *aerobic,* meaning "with oxygen." These types of exercises maintain an elevated heart rate by repetitive or rhythmic motions of the two largest muscle groups, those that move the legs and arms. The heart pumps increased blood to these working muscles, and the lungs work harder to supply enough oxygen. The heart rate goes up, we breathe faster, and, with time, the muscles, heart, and lungs become more efficient. The force of each heartbeat gets stronger, and the heart pumps more blood with every beat. Small blood vessels develop in the muscles to bring more oxygen and nutrients to them. The muscles become larger. Any exercises that keep a person moving and raise the heart rate are aerobic: jogging, walking, aerobic dance, martial arts, shoveling, sweeping, swimming, bicycling, cross-country skiing, rowing. In the later years, a lower level of intensity of exercise may be aerobic, such as housecleaning or gardening.

The more intensely an individual exercises aerobically, the more oxygen must be inhaled and the harder the heart has to work. Thus, the most commonly accepted measurement of cardiovascular fitness is called *maximal oxygen consumption.* This is the amount of oxygen taken in and distributed to working muscles when a person is exercising at maximum rate. Fit individuals consume more oxygen than their sedentary counterparts.

As a person ages, cardiorespiratory endurance is *gradually reduced.* There is a steady decrease in maximal oxygen intake through middle age, and a more gradual decline in old age. This decline in cardiorespiratory endurance reduces peak exercise ability, lowers maximal heart rates, and lowers the efficiency of the heart. The reduction in maximal heart rate that occurs with age is universal—a loss of approximately one beat per minute per year—but the magnitude varies by fitness level, genetics, and disease state. Resting heart rate is much lower in those who are fit than in those who are not because a strong heart is able to pump more blood per beat. Athletes may have resting heart rates between 40 and 50 beats per minute, while those who are sedentary have heart rates around 80 beats per minute.

By age 80, the effects of gradual decline in cardiorespiratory endurance become noticeable, and it is harder to perform moderately strenuous housekeeping and gardening tasks or even to walk uphill: Rest periods may be needed while walking or working in order to reduce fatigue. Reduced oxygen intake can be lessened with aerobic exercise, but some decline occurs even in elite elderly athletes. Individuals who have exercised since midlife fare better than those who begin exercise after age 75, but exercise at any age helps increase oxygen intake.

Exercises that increase muscle strength and endurance but not cardiorespiratory fitness are called *anaerobic,* meaning "without oxygen." These exercises require so much muscle exertion that oxygen cannot be supplied to muscle tissues fast enough. Thus, the tissues begin to get their energy from a chemical pathway that does not require as much oxygen. Although these exercises may increase muscle strength and endurance, they do not strengthen the heart and lungs. Anaerobic exercises include sprinting, isometric or static exercises (e.g., grip squeezes), and some types of weight lifting.

Muscular endurance is the ability of a muscle to sustain work over a period of time, either to keep a muscle contracted or to alternately contract and relax the muscle. Muscular endurance is required to hold a heavy object for a long time or to continually repeat a motion, such as hammering, kneading bread, or sawing. Both aerobic exercises and anaerobic exercises increase muscular endurance.

Muscle strength is the ability to apply force by contractions of the muscles. Muscles get stronger when worked against resistance—the resistance of lifting, pulling, or pushing. Strength is important in a wide variety of daily activities, from opening a jar to carrying groceries. Strength training, also called resistance training, involves use of weights (free or in machines), balls, rubber bands, or gravity to provide resistance to various muscle groups. In addition to building muscle mass and strength, strength training also builds bone strength. Strengthening the muscles in the spine and abdomen improves posture and prevents backaches. Strong shoulders, arms, and legs are important in walking and activities of daily living. Strong muscles are needed to stay independent and active later in life.

Muscular strength peaks around 25 years of age, plateaus at 35 or 40 years of age, and then generally shows significant decline by the age of 65. *Muscle mass* also decreases, primarily due to a reduced number of muscle fibers. Changes are greater in the arms than in the legs. Loss of strength makes it more and more difficult to perform daily activities, such as carrying a 10-pound bag of groceries, walking to the mailbox, even getting up from a low chair. Men generally are stronger than women, but both lose their strength at the same rate. Thus, women are limited by a loss of strength at an earlier age than men. Muscle strength can be greatly improved with weight training, even in people who are very old and frail.

Flexibility is the ability to move the joints through a maximum range of motion without undue strain. Flexibility improves posture and physical performance, and it reduces the risk of joint injuries or strains. A person who is flexible can easily pick up an object from the floor, look behind, or reach a high cabinet. Flexibility in the neck and extremities prevents muscle strain; flexibility of the spine prevents low back pain and postural deformities. Inactivity, joint disease, and injuries to the joints and surrounding tissues can decrease flexibility. Flexibility is enhanced by exercising each joint separately with slow, regular, repeated stretching exercises. Ballet, modern dance, yoga, and aquatic exercises enhance flexibility.

The elasticity and flexibility of tendons, ligaments, and joints is reduced with advancing age.

In later life, adults lose flexibility in their hips and back and are less able to bend both forward and backward comfortably. As range of motion is reduced in major joints, elders may not be able to perform important tasks such as climbing into a car, getting in and out of a bathtub, squatting to plug in a cord, going up stairs or even combing hair. Elders can maintain or increase flexibility by gently moving joints through a full range of motion at least daily. These flexibility exercises can be done easier in warm water to reduce pain and the weight of the arms and legs.

Balance is an important component of physical fitness and is affected by many of the chronic diseases of old age. Problems with balance are a major reason for falls and other accidents among elders. Older people can improve their balance with practice. Dancing, yoga, martial arts, standing or hopping on one foot, and walking on a straight line improve balance.

Coordination is the ability to synchronize different actions of the body with each other and with vision. *Agility* is the ability to coordinate such movements and to change directions quickly and safely. Racquet sports, martial arts, aerobics, and dancing may provide the highest degree of training for coordination and agility.

Body composition refers to the proportion of fat, muscle, bone, and water that makes up the body. Ideally, one should have a high proportion of muscle and a low proportion of fat. In general, women have a higher percentage of body fat than men, and people who are fit have lower levels of body fat than people who are sedentary. Men generally have a higher proportion of muscle than women. Those of both genders who are fit have a higher lean body mass (more muscles) than their sedentary counterparts. Body composition cannot be measured solely by weight. Even though a person may have a constant weight over four decades, the body composition may be gradually changing as fat replaces muscle tissue. Body composition is an important consideration in measuring health and physical fitness.

Depending on a person's life stage, one type of exercise may be more important than another.

During adolescence, participating in physical activities that build bone and muscle is important. For middle-aged adults, aerobic exercises for cardiovascular fitness and weight loss are crucial. In the later years, weight-bearing exercises to increase muscle strength, flexibility, and balance are needed to maintain function and stay independent. At any age, the goal of developing a personal fitness plan is to seek a balance among different fitness components. Even individuals with significant physical limitations can find some form of activity that is enjoyable and beneficial.

BENEFITS OF PHYSICAL ACTIVITY

Regular participation in physical activity is one of the most effective ways for older adults, including those with disabilities, to help prevent chronic disease, promote independence, and increase quality of life in old age.

American College of Sports Medicine

No matter what our age, exercise is good for us. Regular physical activity slows, or even reverses, many of the age-related physical declines in the cardiorespiratory and musculoskeletal systems by improving the efficiency of the heart and lungs, increasing muscle strength and mass, improving elasticity and flexibility of tendons, ligaments, and joints, and reducing the level of bone loss. It also delays the onset or progression of several diseases and is believed to improve psychological well-being. In addition, exercise may be the best way to maintain independence in the later years. The report from the Department of Health and Human Services, called the 2008 Physical Activity Guidelines for Americans, developed by the Department of Health and Human Services, summarized the health benefits of exercise based on a review of scientific evidence and found:

Strong evidence that exercise is associated with

- Lower risk of early death, heart disease, stroke, type II diabetes, high blood pressure, adverse blood lipid profile, metabolic syndrome, colon and breast cancers

- Prevention of weight gain
- Weight loss when combined with diet
- Improved cardiorespiratory and muscular fitness
- Prevention of falls
- Reduced depression
- Better cognitive function in older adults

Moderate to strong evidence that exercise is associated with

- Better functional health in older adults—in other words, more ability to do daily activities
- Reduced abdominal obesity

Moderate evidence that exercise is associated with

- Weight maintenance after weight loss
- Lower risk of hip fracture
- Increased bone density
- Improved sleep quality
- Lower risk of lung and endometrial cancers[1]

Documentation of research findings for each benefit mentioned above can be accessed at www.health.gov/paguidelines

For people who want to reap the benefits of exercise, how much is enough? The answer changes as experts modify their recommendations based on new evidence. The 2008 Physical Activity Guidelines for Americans provides education and guidance for consumers and health professionals on the types and amount of education that provides substantial health benefits. The science-based document looks at the data supporting exercise, what type and how long in what populations, and issues "best practices" recommendations. The main idea behind the guidelines is that regular physical activity over months and years can produce long-term health benefits. This guideline was adopted by the American College of Sports Medicine and the American Heart Association, among others.

The 2008 Physical Activity Guidelines for Americans identified specific recommendations for different age groups in regard to exercise to promote health. In general, healthy older adults follow the guidelines for those 18–64 years old, but for those with chronic illness and disability, there are additional recommendations. The first four bullets below are guidelines for all adults, including elders.

- All older adults should avoid inactivity. Some physical activity is better than none, and older adults who participate in any amount of physical activity gain some health benefits.
- For substantial health benefits, older adults should do at least 150 minutes (2 hours and 30 minutes) a week of moderate-intensity, or 75 minutes (1 hour and 15 minutes) a week of vigorous-intensity aerobic physical activity, or an equivalent combination of moderate- and vigorous-intensity aerobic activity. Aerobic activity should be performed in episodes of at least 10 minutes, and preferably, it should be spread throughout the week.

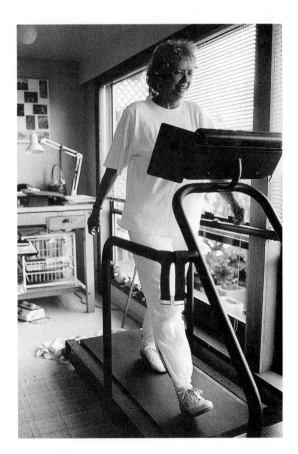

- For additional and more extensive health benefits, older adults should increase their aerobic physical activity to 300 minutes (5 hours) a week of moderate-intensity, or 150 minutes a week of vigorous-intensity aerobic physical activity, or an equivalent combination of moderate- and vigorous-intensity activity.
- Older adults should also do muscle-strengthening activities that are moderate or high intensity and involve all major muscle groups on 2 or more days a week, as these activities provide additional health benefits.

In addition to the above guidelines that apply to all adults, the following guidelines are just for older adults.

- When older adults cannot do 150 minutes of moderate- intensity aerobic activity a week because of chronic conditions, they should be as physically active as their abilities and conditions allow.
- Older adults should do exercises that maintain or improve balance if they are at risk of falling.
- Older adults should determine their level of effort for physical activity relative to their level of fitness.
- Older adults with chronic conditions should understand whether and how their conditions affect their ability to do regular physical activity safely.

(These recommendations are found at www .health.gov/paguidelines under Chapter 5, Active Older Adults.)[1]

Of note, the exercise program should be modified according to an individual's habitual physical activity, physical function, health status, exercise responses, and stated goals. Adults who are unable or unwilling to meet the exercise

---

It's Never Too Late

Maria Fiaterone, M.D.

Aging in modern society is in many respects an "exercise deficiency syndrome" which contributes to an excess rate of heart disease, diabetes, obesity, hypertension, high cholesterol, arthritis, osteoporosis, falls, and other chronic problems. Cumulatively, these diseases, as well as fatigue, muscle weakness, low endurance, stiffness, impaired balance, and low self-efficacy may result in a syndrome we call frailty.

Frailty, if difficult to define, is not hard to recognize. Ask a child to show you what an old person looks like. They will stoop over, pretend to have a cane in one hand, shakily grab furniture for support with the other, and slowly walk across the room. This mobility impairment, fear of falling, and weakness they so readily identify and mimic is at the center of frailty and is increasingly prevalent in our ever-graying society.

Is there a medical treatment for frailty? Is there a way to prevent it? Needless to say, if we could prevent all of the diseases which contribute to it we would minimize its impact. But much of it has nothing to do with a discreet disease. Instead it is an expression of poor exercise tolerance simply due to disuse or underuse of the muscles and heart.

Consider 80-year-old Jack LaLanne.* Is he frail? He is old, he has wrinkles, he has gray hair, but no one would call him frail. This is because exercise, particularly resistance training, or weight-lifting exercise, which he has advocated since his youth, has a remarkable preventive and restorative effect on the body. Exercise in the aged, even those up to 100 years of age, has now been shown to increase strength, muscle mass, aerobic capacity, bone density, flexibility, balance, neurological speed of movement, functional abilities, and overall activity level. Along with these physical changes, improvements

Continued

It's Never Too Late

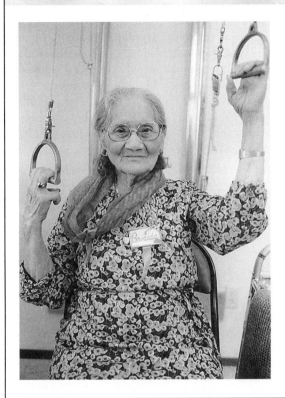

with respect to depression, morale, insomnia, and self-efficacy have been documented.

There is no pill that can perform even remotely as powerfully in this regard. Many older women who begin strength training are stronger than their daughters at the end of six months of weight lifting. Older men in their sixties and seventies who have lifted weights for many years have muscles that look and perform identically to those of 20-year-old men.

Obviously, exercise cannot prevent all age-related changes in physical functioning, nor can it avert all diseases, but we have become much too complacent at accepting as inevitable changes that are now clearly documented to be preventable or reversible even in extreme old age. Less frailty will mean more independence, fewer injurious falls, lower nursing home admission rates, decreased health care costs, and improved quality and perhaps quantity of life. "Life is short. Play hard" is a popular slogan, geared towards the competitiveness of youth. We would say, rather, "Life is long. Play well." The consequences of not playing are real and frightening. The rewards of a lifetime of healthful exercise, or of taking it up for the first time in your nineties, are enormous. Start now, and be fit for your life.

Excerpted from *Perspectives in Health Promotion and Aging* 1996; vol. II (4): p. 7. American Association of Retired Persons. Used with permission from Maria A. Fiaterone Singh, MD, FRACP.

*Author note: Jack LaLanne was 96 when he died in 2011. See his Web site: www.jacklalanne.com

targets outlined here still can benefit from engaging in amounts of exercise less than recommended as some activity is better than none. People without diagnosed chronic conditions (such as diabetes, heart disease, or osteoarthritis) and who do not have symptoms (e.g., chest pain or pressure, dizziness, or joint pain) do not need to consult with a health care provider about physical activity.[1] Details regarding each type of exercise outlined above will be discussed in the section, The Exercise Prescription.

HAZARDS OF INACTIVITY

Look at a patient lying in bed.
What a pathetic picture he makes.
The blood clotting in his veins,
the lime draining from his bones,
the scybala stacking up in his colon,
the flesh rotting from his sweat,
the urine leaking from his distended bladder,
and the spirit evaporating from his soul.

—Dr. R. A. Asher[2]

In the past, it was believed that prolonged bedrest promoted healing, and it was prescribed for many illnesses common in old age: low back pain, congestive heart failure, heart attacks. Now, bedrest is rarely prescribed because experts have documented that immobility does not promote healing.

Inactivity, especially if it is prolonged, is detrimental to individuals of any age. Currently, there is substantial evidence that prolonged inactivity delays recovery, reduces ability to function, and promotes deterioration of almost every body system (Table 9.1.) Also, immobility creates a cycle of further immobility, taking its toll on every body system, creating even more disability, and leading eventually to death.

Many people mistakenly attribute many signs and symptoms of inactivity to growing old when, in fact, they are related more to a sedentary lifestyle. Increased tiredness, decreased ability to tolerate physical exertion, reduced muscle strength, and joint stiffness are all factors associated with aging that can be dramatically improved with physical activity, no matter what the age or extent of initial ability. While it is true that there is some natural decline in ability to exercise, elders who are physically active are likely to stay well longer than those who are not.

TABLE 9.1	Effects of Immobility on the Body

CARDIOVASCULAR SYSTEM
Orthostatic hypotension causing dizziness when sitting or standing and perhaps falls
Heart works harder
Increased resting heart rate
Risk of blood clots in legs
Anemia
Decreased cardiac reserve
Decreased volume blood pumped per heartbeat

RESPIRATORY SYSTEM
Decreased lung function; shallow breathing so the bottoms of the lungs do not completely open and function, causing risk of pneumonia. It is more difficult to clear secretions from the lungs when lying flat and not moving; the cough is less forceful
Reduced coughing
Oxygen/carbon dioxide imbalance
Decreased aerobic capacity

GASTROINTESTINAL SYSTEM
Lack of appetite
Slowed digestion; food remains in the stomach longer, making a person feel full, and may reflux into the esophagus
Constipation

SKIN
Pressures on the skin can lead to skin breakdown and ulcers

MUSCULOSKELETAL SYSTEM
Bones begin to break down quickly, leading to more risk of fractures and osteoporosis
Decreased muscle strength and size
Reduced range of motion in joints

URINARY SYSTEM
Reduced bladder function
Increased calcium breakdown
Impaired bladder emptying
Urinary infection risk increases

METABOLISM
Increased triglycerides
Increased LDL cholesterol
Reduced metabolic rate
Altered drug metabolism
Tissue atrophy
Protein deficiency
Mineral imbalances

PSYCHOSOCIAL EFFECTS
Sensory deprivation
Anxiety and depression
Decreased learning capacity
Decreased problem-solving ability
Decreased motivation
Exaggerated or inappropriate emotions
Increased dependence
Disorientation

People who are sick, recovering from surgery, in pain, confused, or in hospitals or institutions are more likely to stay in bed, and this habit results in longer recovery times, increased risk of falls, and deconditioning. The routines in hospitals and nursing homes promote bedrest. Patients in hospitals and nursing homes are asked to call for help before trying to get up; staff are often busy and help is delayed. Staffing levels may be too low to take 10 minutes to transfer an elder to and from the bathroom, so there are delays and pressures to use catheters and stay in bed until staff are ready to help. Beds may have rails, which the elder cannot put down. Beds may not be at a height that makes it easy to get in and out. Elders may have intravenous tubes with pumps or catheters and other tubes that make it complicated to change locations without disrupting medical care. Elders may believe they "should" stay in bed, be fearful of falling or doing something wrong, or feel weak, tired, and unmotivated due to illness. They may be confused and disoriented or fearful. Institutions want to reduce falls and frail, ill, walking elders are at high risk for falls. There are few safe and supervised places to walk around in most hospitals and nursing homes.

To counteract the negative cycle of immobility, people of all ages should be encouraged to maximize activity to the extent possible while in the hospital and at home—even if they do no more than dangle their legs from the side of the bed or do range-of-motion exercises. If bedrest is absolutely needed (such as in the treatment of extensive pressure ulcers or some orthopedic problems), exercises can be done to maintain joint range of motion and strength. Those who do not need to be in bed need to be encouraged to get up and walk as much as possible. Muscle contraction exercises while in bed and appropriate positioning in bed can prevent muscle weakness. Other strategies to minimize the harmful effects of bedrest include use of bedside commodes, standing the patient briefly when transferring from bed to chair, encouraging the wearing of street clothes, and providing walkers and canes to patients to encourage walking.

Whenever possible, physical or occupational therapists should be utilized to improve the individual's physical tolerance for activity. A good axiom, taught to medical students over 50 years ago by Dr. R. A. Asher, still holds true today:

> Teach us that we may dread
> Unnecessary time in bed
> Get people up and we may save
> Our patient from an early grave.[2]

EXERCISE TO PREVENT AND TREAT DISEASE

If exercise could be packed into a pill, it would be the single most widely prescribed, and beneficial, medicine in the nation.

—Robert Butler

A physically active lifestyle is associated with a lower incidence of illness and death from a number of chronic diseases, particularly cardiovascular diseases, type II diabetes, some cancers, and osteoporosis. Besides reducing the risk of chronic disease, exercise is also prescribed to reduce the symptoms, progression, and complications of some diseases, such as osteoarthritis, obesity, and depression, allowing a person with a chronic illness to maximize function and stay independent as long as possible. General information on the diseases discussed below is presented in Chapters 4, 5, and 7.

Heart Disease

Heart disease is the primary cause of death and disability in the United States, and a main risk factor for the disease is a sedentary lifestyle. The role of exercise in the prevention of atherosclerosis and coronary heart disease is well documented: It controls weight, reduces blood pressure, increases the level of protective HDL cholesterol, reduces blood clotting, and lowers blood insulin levels. In addition to reducing the risk of coronary heart disease, regular and sustained physical activity is an important part of retarding the progression of the disease.

What is not yet clear is the exercise intensity needed to make a difference. Will walking do it? Or do we have to participate in more strenuous activities, such as jogging? Even light to moderate exercise intensity is associated with lower coronary heart disease rates among women. In one large study of almost 40,000 women, the minimum amount of exercise to have an effect was as little as one hour of walking a week, and the risk became lower with increased time spent walking. The walking pace did not seem to make a difference in this particular study. Interestingly, even women who were overweight, had high cholesterol levels, and smoked were able to reduce their risk with as little as one hour of walking a week.[3] Another study reported that both walking and vigorous exercise reaped similar benefits in reducing heart attack risk. Age, body mass, and ethnicity did not affect the results. The researchers also reported that prolonged sitting increased cardiovascular risk.[4]

Heart failure—a weakened enlarged heart that pumps inefficiently—can be improved with exercise. One study randomly assigned one group of elder men with heart failure 70 years of age and older to an exercise program that included 10 minutes of cycling on stationary bikes four to six times daily, followed by six months of cycling at home for 20 minutes a day. The other group did not exercise. The exercise group had more blood pumped with each heartbeat, better blood flow, and slightly reduced heart size.[5]

Exercise also has been documented to improve the pain of angina. Angina is a pain in the heart that is caused by exertion and occurs when the heart can't pump enough oxygenated blood through a narrowed coronary artery to nourish the heart cells. By reducing resting heart rate and the oxygen demand of the heart, exercise allows individuals with angina pain to do more work before feeling chest pain.

Those who suffer a heart attack benefit from a combination of strength and exercise training to reduce the risk of further attacks. These exercise programs are referred to as cardiac rehabilitation. One analysis of 48 studies (almost 9,000 patients)

regarding the effectiveness of exercise-based cardiac rehabilitation programs reported that those undergoing exercise-based cardiac rehabilitation programs after a heart attack had fewer future fatal heart attacks and fewer instances of death from other causes than those who did not participate. Further, participants experienced greater reductions in cholesterol, triglyceride levels, blood pressure, and smoking rates than nonparticipants.[6]

Cardiac rehabilitation programs offer other benefits, such as nutrition education and stress reduction, that improve participants' quality of life. The success rate of cardiac rehabilitation programs is comparable to that of other, far more invasive and expensive therapies. Further, participants may require less medication and are less likely to need further surgery than nonparticipants. However, elders are not always referred to cardiac rehabilitation programs. This may be because of other conditions that impair exercise ability, frailty, or biases in the health care system. The benefits for elders, especially elderly women and minorities, have not been well studied.[7]

Hypertension

Hypertension, or high blood pressure, is one of the most common disorders in the adult population. People with hypertension are more likely to die earlier from all causes and from cardiovascular disease. Exercise is a critical factor in prevention, treatment, and control of high blood pressure. Those who engage in regular vigorous exercise have a lower incidence of hypertension than those who do not, and this holds true even among those who are overweight. Regular aerobic exercise decreases blood pressure and reduces the increase in blood pressure that often accompanies aging.

Exercise is a cornerstone to treatment of high blood pressure, and its effect is most pronounced among those who exercise vigorously on a regular basis. Older people planning to initiate a vigorous exercise program need to be evaluated by a physician first. If they cannot participate in vigorous exercise, a moderate activity program is warranted.

Older individuals with hypertension need to know that they can safely exercise to reduce their blood pressure, and even if they cannot reduce their blood pressure to the normal range, they can reduce their chance of dying from hypertension-related complications.

At this time, the frequency, intensity, duration, and type of exercise that optimizes the blood-pressure lowering effect is not known. Endurance physical activity (walking, jogging, bike riding) and resistance exercise for at least 30 minutes a day on almost all days of the week are generally recommended.[8] High-intensity, anaerobic, or static exercises may be dangerous for those with hypertension and should be avoided because they cause a temporary increase in blood pressure.

Peripheral Vascular Disease

Peripheral vascular disease occurs when the arteries supplying blood to the legs are damaged or partially blocked. Not enough blood gets to the muscles, causing pain. When an individual tries to exercise, the blood vessels do not expand to supply more blood to the muscles. Consequently, the muscles cramp and hurt, causing the person to stop using the muscle. At rest, the muscle no longer needs so much blood, and the pain improves. This symptom is called intermittent claudication. Individuals with claudication are not able to walk easily and have a difficult time in carrying out their daily activities. Because inactivity causes further deterioration, they are at high risk of disability and dependence. The standard medical treatment is drug treatment and surgery. However, exercise is a recognized effective, inexpensive, and noninvasive alternative to reduce the symptoms and consequences of the disease.

People with claudication are instructed to walk to the point of moderate pain and limping, stop for a short rest, then continue to walk. The initial session should be at least 35 minutes of walking and resting. As the person's walking ability improves, the workout needs to increase in speed or intensity to ensure that leg pain always occurs. The goal is to exercise for 50 minutes from three to five training sessions a week. Exercising in this manner lengthens the time it takes before the symptoms appear.[9] Even though an individual will likely still experience the symptoms, exercise rehabilitation significantly improves pain-free walking time and distance and consequent ability to carry out daily activities.

Type 2 Diabetes

Diabetes is a chronic disease in which the body does not properly use insulin. Regular exercise plays a significant role in both the prevention and the treatment of type 2 diabetes (also called adult-onset diabetes). The relationship between exercise and diabetes is consistent among studies: The more individuals exercise, the lower is the disease risk, even among those who are obese. Exercise also reduces other risk factors common in diabetes, such as heart disease.

In addition to preventing diabetes, exercise (both endurance and strength training) is one of the cornerstones of nondrug therapy for adult-onset diabetes. Diabetics who exercise regularly need fewer oral medications and insulin because their body cells are more sensitive to their own insulin production.

The American College of Sports Medicine and the American Diabetes Association recommend that diabetics participate in mild to moderate aerobic exercise at least three nonconsecutive days a week, preferably five, at a level of 40 to 60 percent of an individual's maximum oxygen intake. The individual should exercise enough to burn 1,000 calories of energy per week. Duration of exercise should start at 15 minutes a day, building up to at least 30 minutes for each session. For most people with type 2 diabetes, brisk walking is a moderate-intensity exercise. Use of a pedometer is recommended. Further, it is recommended that resistance exercises be conducted at least twice a week, exercising 8 to 10 muscle groups each session, 10 to 15 repetitions for each group until the muscle is near fatigue.[10]

Unfortunately, older persons with diabetes who might benefit from exercise are often unable to participate at a high level of activity because of advanced heart disease, hypertension, or peripheral vascular disease. For this reason, people with diabetes should undergo exercise treadmill testing prior to beginning a moderately vigorous exercise program and be supervised by a qualified exercise trainer. In addition, because exercise can lower blood sugar and insulin needs, careful monitoring of blood sugar to prevent hypoglycemia (not enough sugar getting into the body cells) is warranted. For diabetics to continually reap the benefits of improved glucose tolerance and insulin sensitivity, exercise must be performed regularly, for gains are lost within 72 hours after the last bout of exercise.[10]

Obesity

Obesity and overweight are of epidemic proportions in our country: According to the results of the National Health Interview Survey in 2010, the percentage of obese adults in the United States has risen from 19 percent in 1997 to 28 percent in 2010. Among the 60+ population, the percentage is 27 percent.[11] Obesity is associated with a number of chronic health problems, including premature death, adult-onset diabetes, arthritis, hypertension, vascular disease, and respiratory problems. It is well known that a major contributor to obesity is physical inactivity.

Those who are only moderately obese can select from a wide variety of exercise activities, but generally fitness walking is recommended. Individuals who are more severely obese may suffer from other conditions that limit their ability to exercise (joint pains, reduced functional capacity, reduced range of motion) and may require even lower intensity exercise regimens (e.g., stationary bicycling or water aerobics).

The American College of Sports Medicine recommends that, in addition to reducing calories and fat, moderate weight loss occurs with 150–250 minutes of moderate-intensity exercise per week,

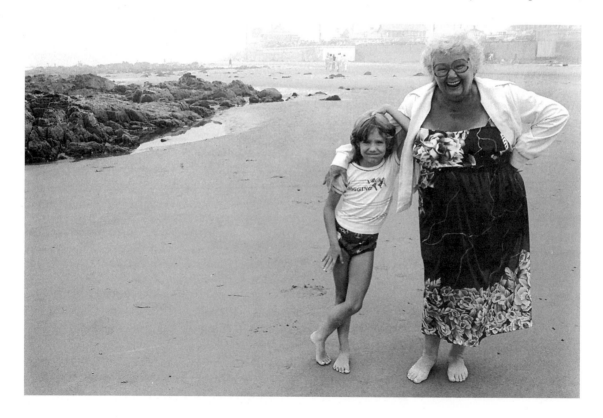

but for clinically significant weight loss and to prevent weight regain, more than 250 minutes per week is needed.[12]

One pound of body fat is lost for every 3,500 calories of energy expended. The primary goal of exercise for those who are overweight is to burn up 2,000 to 3,000 calories a week to lose weight. Refer to www.nutristrategy.com to find out the number of calories burned by various physical activities. In elders, generally lower-intensity and longer-duration exercises are recommended to reduce injuries. As weight is lost, individuals may shift to higher-intensity workouts to improve cardiovascular endurance.

Exercise recommendations for those who are overweight should be accompanied by dietary counseling. It is important not to begin a strict diet and an exercise program simultaneously. People on calorie-restricted diets with or without exercise often lose muscle tissue in addition to fat. However, when aerobic exercise is combined with a sensible diet, lean body mass is preserved and even increased but body fat is decreased.

Respiratory Diseases

Individuals with chronic obstructive pulmonary disease (COPD), which includes asthma, chronic bronchitis, and emphysema, have a difficult time just getting up in the morning and conducting their daily routines. Because individuals with pulmonary disease often lose additional lung capacity because exercising is hard, exercise is highly recommended to counteract the spiral of inactivity. It cannot repair damaged lung tissue, but it can improve lung function and prevent further deterioration caused by inactivity.

Exercise can increase the level of oxygen inhaled, improve breathing, reduce resting heart rate, and increase the tolerance for work. The exercises recommended for those with COPD are strength training two to three days a week and 20 to 30 minutes of supervised aerobic exercise at least three times a week, particularly exercises that strengthen the legs. Before beginning an exercise program, those with COPD should also undergo

an exercise treadmill test while oxygen intake is measured. If they have insufficient oxygen intake, supplementary oxygen may be required before or during exercise. Commonly, exercise causes shortness of breath and fatigue in individuals who have pulmonary disease, so a closely supervised program is recommended. These individuals are often more successful if they exercise after using bronchodilator inhalants.

Osteoporosis

A sedentary lifestyle is a major contributor to the rate and extent of bone loss, and consequent osteoporosis. A number of studies show a high correlation between level of physical activity and bone mass in older women. Weight-bearing exercises are recommended to prevent or at least reduce the decline in bone loss in both premenopausal and postmenopausal women. It can also significantly decrease the incidence of hip and leg fractures in both sexes. Results of randomized controlled trials confirm the positive effects of an exercise program on bone density, muscle mass, strength, and balance in older adults.[13]

Exercise has been shown to reduce the risk of hip fracture, and the degree of benefit is related both to the hours of walking a week and to the briskness of the walk. In one longitudinal study of over 61,000 middle-aged and older women, those who reported the longest duration and highest level of aerobic activity level (primarily walking) on a regular basis had the fewest hip fractures. Subjects who walked at least four hours a week had a significantly lower risk of hip fracture than those who walked for less than an hour a week. And the brisker the walk, the fewer were the fractures.[14]

Arthritis

Arthritis is the most commonly reported cause of activity limitation in elders, and limitations become more prevalent with advanced age. Patients with rheumatoid arthritis or osteoarthritis often suffer from physical deconditioning, which leads to a vicious cycle of joint pain, causing further reductions in movement. A two-year study of almost 6,000 older adults with arthritis reports that the biggest risk factor for decline in function over a two-year period was the lack of regular vigorous physical activity. Further, lack of regular activity doubled the odds of a decline in function. The authors assert that if all subjects of the study would engage in regular vigorous physical activity, the expected decline could be reduced by one-third.[15]

The joint pain and destruction of arthritis, the side effects of drug therapy, and fear of further injury or disability can reduce the desire to exercise. Although getting started may be difficult, evidence points to the role of exercise in reducing the pain and disability associated with arthritis.

Exercise relieves pain and improves joint function of people with both types of arthritis. Whether the person has rheumatoid arthritis or osteoarthritis, exercise must start gently and progress gradually. Because those with rheumatoid arthritis commonly have morning stiffness and those with osteoarthritis have more pain at the end of the day, exercise time needs to be adjusted.

Generally an exercise program for those with arthritis begins with passive range-of-motion exercises and progresses to aerobic exercise and weight training to increase cardiovascular endurance, flexibility, and muscle strength. Swimming or water exercises are particularly effective for elders with arthritis because they place less stress on joints.

Low Back Pain

Almost everyone experiences low back pain at some time. Physical inactivity is an important contributor to chronic back pain because a back with poor muscle tone is especially susceptible to fatigue, strain, injury, and tension. Most commonly, lower back pain occurs when muscles in the back and abdomen are too weak to keep the back in proper alignment. As a result, poor posture while lifting, sitting, standing, and walking increases the risk of back injury. Exercises that strengthen back and abdomen muscles can reduce the risk of back injury. Because the vast majority of back injuries are due to improper lifting, proper lifting techniques should be practiced as a preventive measure.

The goal of exercise for back pain is to strengthen muscles in the abdomen and back to improve posture, strengthen the leg muscles used in lifting, and improve flexibility and aerobic endurance. An exercise program that strengthens the abdomen and back muscles, in combination with a program of brisk walking, should be performed regularly for lasting improvement. Specialized exercises designed to strengthen the core muscles supporting the spine and pelvis and to maintain flexibility are among the most effective of all treatments for low back pain.

Cancer

Physical inactivity may play a role in the development of several types of cancer, particularly in cancers of the colon and breast. A number of epidemiological studies have proposed an inverse relationship between physical activity level and colon cancer risk: the higher the level of exercise, the lower the risk for colon cancer. It is believed that exercise works by increasing bowel activity, so that cancer-producing substances do not linger in the colon. Since obesity is also a strong risk factor for colon cancer, physical activity may also work indirectly to reduce colon cancer by weight loss.

Regarding breast cancer, there is evidence of a relationship between physical activity and a decreased risk of breast cancer among pre- and post-menopausal women. Exercise may lower breast cancer risk by reducing obesity and improving immune system function, or it may influence the levels of estrogen hormones in the blood.

Participation in moderate physical activity after a breast cancer diagnosis may decrease the rate of cancer recurrence. In one study, the greatest benefit occurred among women who walked from three to five hours a week. However, in that study, exercising longer than that did not increase survival. Exercise is an important component of cancer rehabilitation in general, improving both physiological factors such as energy, flexibility, and aerobic capacity as well as quality of life.[16]

Depression

The standard treatment for depression in older people is medication. However, some elders do not want to take drugs, others do not respond well to them, and still others cannot take them because of side effects. A body of research has indicated that aerobic and strength training exercises are a good alternative to medication for depression among older people, and high intensity is even more effective than low intensity.[17,18]

EXERCISE: A PRESCRIPTION FOR HEALTH

It is clear that a physical activity program for adults that includes cardiorespiratory, resistance, flexibility and balance training beyond activities of daily living is essential to maintain and improve physical fitness and health. For people who want to reap the benefits of exercise, take walks, go swimming, play sports, exercise at the gym, or clean their floors and dig in the garden. Elders may wish to engage in formal exercise programs in groups—joining a team or going to a class—or they may prefer solitary exercise programs. Many elders who did not exercise as younger adults will need to find physical activities that they enjoy, such as yoga, Pilates, tai chi, or a "prime of life" soccer team!

Exercise Goals

The amount and type of exercise recommended depends on the state of health of the individual, the reason for exercising, and the exercise goal. If physical fitness is the goal, a higher level of exertion is required. Likewise, if weight loss is a goal, a combination of vigorous exercise and longer duration (or more frequent) exercise is needed. However, for those who must participate in low-intensity exercise, those with diabetes, and those who want to lose weight, daily exercise is preferable. Several short sessions a day (at least 10 minutes each session) of low-intensity exercises may be easier than once-a-day exercises for older people with low endurance.

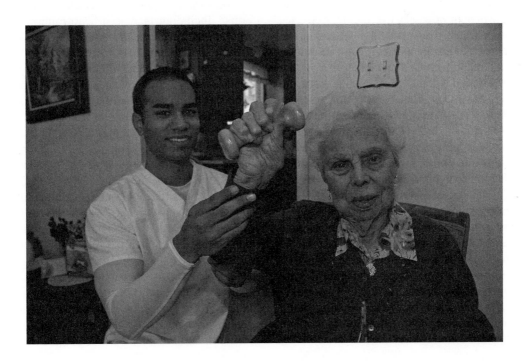

To promote cardiovascular fitness, activities that use large muscle groups should be emphasized. Expert recommendations do not specify a particular type of exercise because many different types can effectively promote health and fitness. Active elders may enjoy aerobic dance, bicycling, swimming, and brisk walking or jogging. More sedentary elders may enjoy walking or water aerobics. The first consideration is to select an activity that is enjoyable and can be accomplished reasonably. By far the most common exercise choice among elders is walking.

Walking is a form of aerobic activity that provides many benefits at any age and can be tailored to suit the individual's needs or preferences. For many people, walking with another person makes the exercise more enjoyable and provides social support to continue. A walking program is inexpensive: No special equipment is needed, no gym membership is required, and walking can be done almost anywhere. The Walking Site (www.thewalkingsite.com) is highly recommended for anyone interested in walking as exercise.

In addition to exercises to enhance cardiorespiratory fitness, a well-rounded exercise program includes strength or resistance training exercises. Free weights, hand weights, ankle weights, squeeze balls, elastic bands, and weight machines are used in strength training. For weight training among most older adults, at least one set (8 to 12 repetitions) that work on each of the major muscle groups (legs, hips, back, chest, abdomen, shoulders, and arms) is advised. The benefits are increased when two or three sets are accomplished for each muscle group.[1] To strengthen a muscle, it must be exercised to the point of fatigue. If desired, weight training can be accomplished more often if fewer muscle groups are exercised and the muscle group was not exercised on the previous day.

Resistance training has been shown to provide many benefits for older people, even the frail. This action builds and strengthens muscles, stimulates bone growth, and reduces the risk of falls. Most important, strong muscles allow an individual to stay independent and active, making it easier to go up stairs, get up from a chair, and carry groceries. In general, the older and more frail the individual is, the more important muscle-strengthening exercises and flexibility exercises become. See Box 9.1 for guidelines for strength training.

Measuring Physical Activity Intensity

How do you know how hard you are exercising? There are several ways to measure the intensity of aerobic exercise. The simplest method is to pay attention to how you feel and what you can do while exercising. The easiest way to measure exertion is the talk test. Can you talk while exercising? A person who is active at a light level of intensity should be able to sing while doing the activity. Someone who is active at a moderate level of intensity should be able to carry on a conversation comfortably while engaging in the activity. If a person becomes too out of breath to carry on a conversation, the activity can be considered vigorous. Another method is a scale of perceived exertion. One of the more well known is the Borg exercise intensity scale.[19] Perceived exertion is how hard you feel your body is working. It is based on the physical sensations a person experiences during exercise, including increased heart rate, increased respiration or breathing rate, increased sweating, and muscle fatigue. If you feel tired, your heart is racing, and you are breathing quickly, then you are likely in the moderate to strenuous range of exercising. Although this seems subjective, studies show that a person's own rating of his or her exertion is actually pretty well predictive of the actual level of exertion and heart rate.[19]

Monitoring the heart rate during exercise is another way to determine exercise intensity. Some activities are more strenuous than others, and intensities vary based on a person's age and physical fitness level. A 20-year-old in prime physical condition may find gardening relaxing whereas for a 70-year-old woman with flexibility restrictions gardening can be very difficult, or even impossible. One way to measure or monitor the level at which someone is active is to look at his or her heart rate.

For moderate-intensity physical activity, a person's heart rate should be between 50 and 70 percent

---

B O X 9 . 1

Guidelines for Strength Training

These guidelines can help you start resistance training and make exercising more enjoyable while reducing your risk of injury.

1. Set aside a specific time of day to exercise. Choose a time when you usually are not tired and not right after a meal.
2. Wear comfortable clothing. Encourage a friend to come with you.
3. Aim for 20- to 30-minute strength training sessions at least two times a week.
4. Start with a weight that is comfortable but challenging. It may weigh as little as a pound or two. Or start with resistance bands or with no weights at all. Exercises should not cause too much pain or stiffness or make you feel breathless or off balance.
5. Perform one set of 8–12 repetitions of each exercise slowly. When you can easily do 12 repetitions, add more weight. If you can, do two or three sets of exercises as the benefits will increase.
6. Slow lifting and lowering is more effective than quick repetitions. Swinging weights or using momentum is hard on the joints and does not build strength. Take at least 3 seconds (some say as much as 15 seconds) to lift, hold for 1 second, and release very slowly over 3 to 15 seconds.
7. How you breathe when lifting the weight is important. You should inhale before lifting, exhale while lifting, and inhale again while lowering the weight. Never hold your breath while lifting. If you have to hold your breath to lift, you are probably using too much weight.
8. Perform exercises that involve the major muscle groups (e.g., arms, shoulders, chest, abdomen, back, hips, and legs) and exercises that enhance grip strength.
9. Concentrate on a few muscle groups during each session. You may not want to use the same muscles every time you exercise. For instance, you might want to work your legs on Monday and your arms on Wednesday. You may want to mix a little strength training with some aerobic activity.
10. Rest a few seconds between sets.
11. Gradually increase the weight you are lifting, the number of times you can lift it, or even the slowness at which you lift it. Slow lifting allows you to focus on the muscle you are exercising.
12. It is normal to feel the muscle working and to feel it tiring, but if you feel pain, stop exercising.
13. Drink water to stay hydrated.
14. Take advantage of trainers available for free at most gyms to orient you to the program. A personal trainer can develop a program specific to your needs and goals and can provide motivation, but will be expensive.

---

of his or her maximum heart rate. Although maximum heart rate can vary, a good estimate is to subtract a person's age from 220. For example, for a 70-year-old person, the estimated maximum age-related heart rate would be calculated as 220 – 70 years = 150 beats per minute (bpm). The 50 percent and 70 percent levels would be:

- 50% level: 150 x 0.50 = 75 bpm
- 70% level: 150 x 0.70 = 105 bpm

Thus, a moderate-intensity physical activity for a 70-year-old person would mean that his or her heart rate remains between 75 and 105 bpm during the activity.

For vigorous-intensity physical activity, a person's heart rate should be between 70 and 85 percent of his or her maximum heart rate. For example, for a 70-year-old person, as in the example above, the estimated maximum age-related heart rate would be calculated as

220 – 70 years = 150 beats per minute (bpm). The 70 percent and 85 percent levels would be:

- 70% level: 150 x 0.70 = 105 bpm
- 85% level: 150 x 0.85 = 127.5 bpm

Thus, vigorous-intensity physical activity for a 70-year-old person will require that the heart rate remains between 105 and 127.5 bpm during physical activity.

Scientists have also determined which activities are generally more strenuous and require more effort than others. Of course there will be variation—some people can do ballroom dancing very slowly while others can make it more vigorous—but the following guides can be very helpful.

According to the Centers for Disease Control, examples of moderate intensity exercises are: brisk walking, water aerobics, bicycling slower than 10 mph, ballroom dancing, general gardening. Examples of vigorous intensity exercises are: race walking, jogging, running, swimming laps, and aerobic dancing.

Although intense exercise remains the ideal, significant benefits can be realized by exercising at a moderate intensity if conducted for at least 30 minutes.

It is important that intensity be tailored to the individual's state of activity and health. For most older people, a good initiation into regular exercise is brisk walking almost every day for at least 30 minutes. However, even this recommendation may be too much for some. Progression to a higher level of exercise intensity is often quite individual and is based on health status, physical capacity, personal goals, and motivation. Elders who have been sedentary should begin slowly, building up intensity and duration with time. Beginning an exercise program with vigorous exercise is associated with a high risk of injury and a high dropout rate. Many individuals who begin an exercise program expect a certain outcome. Perhaps they want to lose five pounds or have less back pain or be able to climb stairs without stopping to rest. Focusing on a realistic outcome can help them to maintain the program.

The Role of the Physician

Physicians are in an excellent position to influence their older patients to begin and continue an exercise program because older people are likely to have contact with physicians and are more likely than other age groups to follow their advice. Physicians are able to assess their patients' past and current physical activity level, discuss the health benefits, and work with the patient to develop and continue an appropriate physical activity program. The U.S. Preventive Services Task Force recommends that physicians advise all patients seen in primary care settings to increase physical activity.[20]

One manner in which physicians can formalize a recommendation to be more active is by prescribing exercise. An *exercise prescription* is a regimen of physical activity tailored to improve an individual's physical condition. It is agreed upon by both the physician and the patient and is designed to change the patient's current physical activity level by means of a reasonable strategy that will not be a burden and will likely continue. Just as a prescription for a medication includes the name of the medication, the frequency and duration of its use, and any special instructions, an exercise prescription provides a visible reminder of the physician's specific recommendations. A balanced exercise prescription includes aerobic activities for cardiovascular endurance, resistance exercises for strengthening the muscles, and exercises to improve joint flexibility. An exercise prescription should specify exercise type, frequency, intensity, and duration, and it should include directions on how to progress to higher exercise levels.

Exercise may be prescribed to maximize fitness, prevent illnesses and disorders due to inactivity, treat an existing illness or disorder, or rehabilitate after a crisis such as a heart attack or stroke. Depending on the goal, specific types of exercises may be suggested to improve muscular strength and endurance, increase joint flexibility, reduce bone loss, or improve cardiovascular endurance. For instance, weight lifting may be prescribed to increase muscular strength and

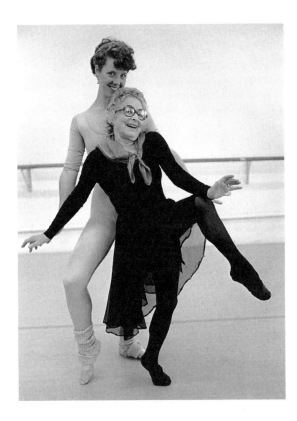

and programs still focus on physician education, the attention is moving toward community-based interventions and health promotion efforts to reach elders directly.

Risks and Complications of Exercise

The biggest risk of exercise is not starting.

American College of Sports Medicine

Although exercise is an excellent prescription to enhance health and reduce the onset or progression of disease, there are some risks: orthopedic injuries of the muscles or joints caused by injury or overuse, and cardiac problems caused by overexertion or dehydration. The most common risk is musculoskeletal problems related to too much physical activity: muscle soreness, shin splints, and joint pain.

The most serious complication is that an individual may suffer angina or even a heart attack while exercising. Warning signs of risk or complications include chest, arm, neck, or jaw pain; significant increase in shortness of breath, light-headedness, or fainting; irregular heartbeat; nausea or vomiting during or after exercise; prolonged fatigue after exercise; weakness or uncoordinated movements; and unexplained weight or exercise-tolerance changes. These warning signs could indicate an underlying disease or a need to alter the exercise. If any of them occur, the individual should be directed to stop exercising and contact a physician.

The fear that exercise will induce a heart attack inhibits many elders from exercising. This concern is overblown. There are reports of exercise inducing heart attacks but these are rare and overwhelmed by the evidence that exercise prevents heart attacks. If symptoms of a heart attack occur during exercise, such as shortness of breath and crushing chest pressure, the person should immediately stop and seek medical attention.

Certain individuals are at higher risk of cardiac complications during exercise. A few health conditions prohibit vigorous exercise: some types of angina, irregular heartbeat, congestive heart failure, and severe cases of hypertension, anemia, and obesity. Most individuals with these conditions

endurance, vigorous walking to enhance cardiovascular endurance and bone mass, and range-of-motion exercises to improve joint flexibility. Exercise may also be prescribed as part of a weight reduction plan. The exercise prescription for weight loss may be very different from a prescription for increasing muscle strength. The American College of Sports Medicine has developed exercise prescriptions for several chronic diseases, available in book form called *ACSM's Guidelines for Exercise Testing and Prescription.*[21]

More than a decade ago, intervention programs targeted physicians as the "best strategy" to improve fitness of adult and elder patients. Unfortunately, these campaigns did not succeed. There were too many physicians to reach, too much new information to give them, too much training needed, and too many other demands on physicians' time. Although the physician definitely has a role in the fitness of his or her patient have severe activity limitations that prohibit vigorous exercise; however, even among those with significant disability, being more active is associated with better outcomes.

Certain precautions can reduce exercise risks. The recommended dose of exercise should do no more than leave the participant pleasantly tired on the following day. Since exercise recovery takes time, vigorous training should occur every other day. Among individuals with preexisting joint disease, walking or swimming might be substituted for jogging or running to reduce falls and knee injury. If an elder has a history of falls, special care is needed in pursuing activities that increase balance ability and reduce fall risk. In older people who take medication to lower blood pressure, there is a danger of a sudden loss of consciousness upon getting up quickly or lowering the head below the heart. Some older people have a higher risk of hyperthermia (heat stress) and hypothermia (cold stress) and should dress appropriately for the

weather and not exercise in extremes of heat or cold. Elders should be encouraged to drink fluids before, during, and after exercising to prevent dehydration, instead of waiting to "feel thirsty." People with diabetes may fail to notice foot injuries because of reduced sensation; thus, they should regularly inspect their feet. No matter what a person's age or physical condition, shoes are important: They need to be lightweight, fit well, and provide adequate shock absorption and support.

A medical assessment can be used to prescribe an individualized exercise program consistent with the individual's current health status and ability. The assessment may also reveal health problems that may inhibit exercise or require special precautions. A medical assessment includes a medical history, a physical examination, laboratory work, and exercise testing. A medical history includes information concerning present and past levels of physical activity, physical symptoms suggesting conditions that would limit physical mobility, and

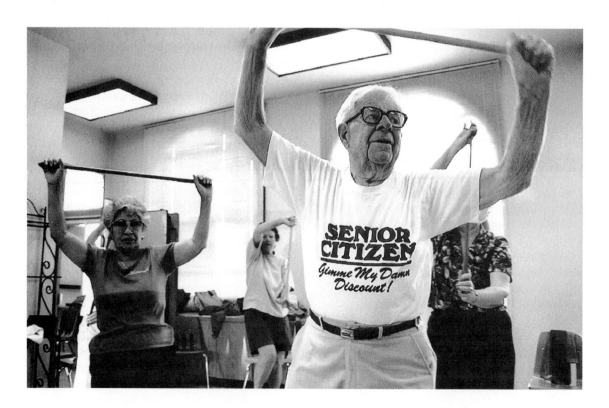

current medications used that impact on the ability and type of exercise to be prescribed.

The physical examination includes the measurement of resting heart rate, blood pressure, body weight, and evidence of cardiovascular disease. Laboratory studies might include blood count, urine analysis, tests for fasting blood sugar and blood lipids, and a resting electrocardiogram. An exercise stress test, in which an individual exercises on a treadmill or bicycle while his or her heart rate and function is evaluated, may be used as part of a medical assessment to determine a person's capacity for strenuous exercise.

Who should have a medical assessment before starting an exercise program? In general, those who develop pain or other symptoms while exercising or when increasing the intensity of exercise need to consult a physician. In addition, those with chronic conditions like diabetes and heart disease should already be under the care of a physician and should consult with their health care provider to develop the best exercise plan. Those who are inactive do not necessarily need to consult a doctor before exercising if they increase intensity gradually. Studies show that inactive people who gradually progress over time to relatively moderate-intensity activity have no known risk of sudden cardiac events and very low risk of bone, muscle, or joint injuries. Generally, moderate-intensity activity is safe and beneficial for individuals with chronic illnesses, but precautions may need to be taken. For example, people with diabetes need to pay special attention to blood sugar control and proper footwear during exercise activity.

ELDERS' ACTIVITY LEVEL

Despite the commonly known benefits of exercise on health and disease, a large proportion of the nation's population is sedentary, and the older we get, the more inactive we become.

The National Health Interview Survey conducted in 2010 gathered data on a representative sample of U.S. adults regarding leisure physical activity and whether or not the participants engaged in muscle strengthening exercises or aerobic exercises. The 2008 Physical Activity Guidelines for Americans was used to determine whether the level of exercise was sufficient. Regarding physical activity among people 65 and older, almost half engaged in no significant physical activity. Another 20 percent engaged in physical activity, but not sufficient to meet the guidelines, Thirty percent reported engaging in physical activity that met the federal guidelines. Regarding the two types of physical activity focused upon, almost two thirds of elder respondents reported no significant participation in either muscle-strengthening exercises or aerobic exercise. Twenty percent participated in aerobic exercise alone and 5 participated in muscle strengthening exercises only. Only 10 percent of individuals 65 and older reportedly engaged in both muscle strengthening and aerobic exercises that meet the federal guidelines for physical activity.[11] Given the many benefits of physical activity, why don't more elders exercise? Many factors influence their lack of physical activity.

Elders as a group are poorly educated about the importance of exercise for health and well-being. Physical education was not emphasized at home or in school when they were growing up, and much of what we know about the benefits of physical activity has been only recently understood. In the past, most people did not need to exercise for health. Instead, their daily routines were sufficient to maintain health and fitness. Most adults, particularly women, did not play sports. People did not swim laps or walk for fitness; they swam for recreation and walked to get places. Thus, they may have never participated in physical activity to enhance health and reduce disease.

Elders likely support the common belief that people should slow down in old age. Further, elders tend to exaggerate the risks involved in exercise after middle age and underrate their physical capabilities. Because of this, they might not exercise because they fear an accident or overexertion.

Elders may not exercise because of a lack of encouragement from physicians. Some physicians are poorly informed about the benefits of exercise or are unaware of the exercise capabilities of even the most disabled patients. Physicians may actually discourage exercise by advising their elder patients to "take it easy" or avoid stairs or overexertion, and they may overestimate the hazards of exercise in elders with chronic diseases.

Many older adults are likely to have symptoms of chronic illness that make it difficult for them to exercise. They may mistakenly believe that they cannot exercise vigorously enough to experience gains in their health. They may not realize that even a modest increase in activity improves physical and psychological health. Further, they may not know which exercises to perform to reduce their symptoms and improve their health.

Many older people do not care to be more physically active. It is far easier to take a pill to reduce disease symptoms than to perform daily, perhaps initially painful, exercises, especially when the benefits may not be immediate. Some people may even be dissatisfied when exercise is prescribed because they believe that doctors are trained and paid to prescribe modern drugs, not exercise that the patients must do themselves.

A shortage of exercise facilities and programs and transportation to them is a significant barrier to older people who do not drive. Even if they want to walk, the lack of safe walking and biking paths may contribute to low rates of exercise participation. Although walking is an excellent way to increase physical activity, extreme weather in some areas of the country prevents exercising outdoors year-round. Some elders may live in unsafe urban neighborhoods with sidewalks in disrepair or poorly lit at night. Or individuals might not feel safe walking in the neighborhood because of fear of crime.

EXERCISE PROMOTION

Given the low proportion of elders who regularly exercise, it is obvious that an important focus of health promotion should be to facilitate physical activity among the older population. Community efforts are needed. These would include education about the benefits of physical activity, effective exercise programming with supervision, ongoing support, transportation and exercise incentives, and availability and accessibility of safe physical activity and recreational facilities (e.g., recreational centers, parks, trails, public pools). Many

resources are available for organizations and agencies to promote physical activity programs among older people. An exercise program can be offered in many settings: multipurpose senior centers, fitness centers, parks, public pools, community colleges, rehabilitation facilities, assisted living facilities, nursing homes, and others.

Implementing Effective Exercise Programs

Ideally, individuals of all ages should be counseled to initiate and sustain a program of regular physical activity tailored to their health status and personal lifestyles. In this section we focus on factors to consider when developing and implementing effective exercise programs for older people.

Providing information to older people regarding the value of exercise and the types of exercises that improve health and reduce disease is a necessary first step in encouraging exercise. Information may be disseminated in national campaigns (e.g., billboards, radio spots, newspapers, books, or magazines), in a small group (e.g., senior center, church, assisted living facility), and in one-on-one interactions with professionals (e.g., physician, physical therapist, nurse, health educator).

Social support increases the success of an exercise program. After an extensive analysis of published studies, the national Task Force on Community Preventive Services reported strong evidence of the effectiveness of social support in both increasing physical activity and improving physical fitness among adults. They assert that social support networks (whether they be family and friends or new contacts in the program) provide supportive relationships that helped to increase physical activity and improve fitness. Examples of social support are using a buddy system, working towards group goals, or setting up groups to provide friendship and support while engaging in exercise (e.g. walking groups).[22]

Support from the health professional also motivates a client to continue an exercise regimen. Clients respond well to individual attention from the staff, and they adhere to an exercise program more readily when the professional and client mutually agree on an exercise contract, including objectives of the exercise program, specific instructions, time frame, and goal setting.

Psychological factors can influence participation in regular physical activity. A common characteristic of people who exercise is self-efficacy, the belief that they can be successful and accomplish their goals. Elders with high self-efficacy and self-confidence are more likely to start and maintain an exercise program. Those who have a desire to look better, who feel confident they can succeed, and who believe that exercise is healthful are more likely to be fit than those who do not accept the virtues of exercise or feel incapable of making a change in their lives. Another characteristic of people who are most likely to begin and maintain an exercise program is internal motivation: they gain enough pleasure and reinforcement from the physical activity itself. Others may need external reinforcement, such as support from their physician, noticeable physical changes, attention from staff, or socialization from peers to maintain their physical fitness program.

Cultural factors also play a role in exercise participation. Multiple surveys report that blacks and Latinos exercise less than their white counterparts. Studies are just beginning to identify barriers to physical activity for groups other than whites.

Participation in fitness programs is influenced by its location—whether it is in the home, in the neighborhood park, or in an exercise facility. Can the older person easily get to the exercise site? Is the location close to public transportation, are there crosswalks and traffic lights? Is the sidewalk repaired? Is there adequate lighting? Low crime rate in the neighborhood is another variable to consider in choosing the location. A shortage of appealing facilities and programs contribute to low rates of exercise participation among elders. The decor of a facility, type and volume of music, age of other participants, and type and level of difficulty of the exercise play a role in whether elders are attracted to the exercise program there.

Like younger people, not all older adults are alike. Some like to exercise in a group; others pursue solitary physical activity. Some prefer to exercise with others their own age; others prefer a facility with mixed ages. Some older people prefer same-sex facilities; others prefer to exercise with both men and women. If possible, financial costs should be minimal because many elders have limited funds for recreation. Ideally, a variety of free programs for older people would be available in a community, using effective marketing techniques so that elders are aware and are encouraged to participate in them.

To accommodate frail elders, a facility must be physically accessible (within easy walking distance, with adequate parking nearby, or serviced by public transportation) because transportation problems prohibit many from participating in programs. However, it is important to realize that the most widely recommended form of physical activity is walking. It can be done almost anywhere and has no equipment or dress requirements except a well-fitting pair of shoes. Supervised walking programs (at the local park or mall) reduce the fear of injury and crime.

Although most people might agree that exercise would be good for them, few are motivated to begin and continue a regular exercise program. Some experts feel that even the word "exercise" can serve as a barrier because it has negative connotations for some. Instead, use of the term "physical activity" may emphasize the lifelong, daily nature of fitness goals. Encouraging elders to become more active, rather than to exercise, may be more palatable. Many positive changes can occur with simple changes in daily habits, such as walking more, taking the stairs instead of the elevator, or routinely parking farther away from the intended destination.

Probably one of the most important considerations for health professionals is to find ways to motivate people to begin and sustain a regular program of physical activity in order to reap its benefits. Many studies have focused on the stages of change and are targeting their specific message of motivation to the stage of the elder adult. Some people have no interest in or intentions to increase their physical activity level; some are thinking about making a change; some are getting ready to make a change or are in the process of making a change. Others have made a change in their life to exercise more but want help to maintain the positive behavior.

Different strategies may be effective, depending on the stage of change the individual is in. For example, when people have not even considered exercising, the goal should be to educate them about the benefits of exercise so that they might consider the possibility of exercising in the future. However, for those who are in the process of making a change in their lives, hearing more about the benefits of exercise is less helpful than learning about ways to increase the amount of exercise in life or how to make exercise more interesting and fun.

Many times, individuals who haven't exercised before become motivated to exercise after they are diagnosed with a disease. For example, many people begin an exercise program after experiencing a heart attack. For others, in contrast, the illness and disability associated with chronic illness result in a reduced motivation to exercise. Individuals with chronic illnesses may fall into a cycle of reduced physical activity, resulting in poorer health and a vicious cycle of fatigue that further decreases the ability to engage in physical activity. Motivating individuals who are chronically ill to initiate an exercise program can be very difficult. They may believe their situation is hopeless, so they don't want to exercise. Or they have unrealistic expectations about what exercise can do for them. Also, exercise may temporarily worsen their discomfort by causing fatigue, pain, and breathlessness.

Even when an individual is successful in starting an exercise program, many factors influence whether the program is continued. Many individuals who begin a fitness program exercise sporadically and tire of the activity within a few days or weeks: Fewer than half of those who begin an exercise regimen are still participating after three or six months. Persistence in an exercise program often depends on whether the program and its health effects meet initial expectations. Studies show that exercisers are more likely to persist in their program if the goals they set and achieve are their own goals, rather than those of others. Additionally, those who initiate an exercise program of moderate intensity are more likely to continue with their program than those who train at high intensity. Elders are similar to younger individuals in offering a wide variety of reasons for terminating an exercise program: exercise is not enjoyable, they have difficulty in arriving to class on time, too expensive, inconvenient location, parking problems, insufficient staff attention, and belief that the exercise has little value.

Because exercise programs have a high dropout rate, every effort should be made to tailor the activities to fit the individual's motivation, ability, and lifestyle. Above all, the exercise program should be realistic, since too much exercise may cause discomfort, fatigue, and feelings of failure and too little may not produce results. Furthermore, the exercise regimen should be developed mutually by the individual and the health professional so it can become an integrated part of the person's daily routine. Finally, the person needs to be held accountable for meeting his or her exercise goals. Success at achieving exercise goals can be evaluated by use of an exercise diary or charts so that progress can be reinforced.

Helping individuals increase their activity level is more successful than just relying on health information or recommending an exercise prescription alone. The program CHAMPS II (Community Health Activities Model Program for Seniors) was developed to encourage and support long-term increases in physical activity of a group of sedentary older people with no serious health problems. The goal was 30 minutes of moderate intensity activity most days a week. Trained staff helped the participants to choose physical activities that could be continued over time, either individually or in a group. The staff was trained to motivate the clients to begin and continue a program tailored to their fitness level. They provided information on exercise and local programs, social support, and opportunities to build skills. Various motivational tools were used: skill-based workshops, telephone support, booklets, phone calls, exercise diaries, and monthly newsletters. At the end of the study, the group participating in the program increased caloric expenditure by almost 500 calories per week, equivalent to adding a mile a day of brisk walking five times a week.[23]

The National Physical Activity Plan

The National Physical Activity Plan is an ambitious document that contains a comprehensive set of policies, programs, and initiatives to increase physical activity of all Americans. Experts from many diverse fields and hundreds of organizations, both private and public, have spent years collaborating on the plan to determine ways to enable every American to live, work and play in environments that promote physical activity. The goal is not only to change individuals, but to change communities and the "national culture" in ways that promote health and fitness. The experts are divided into 8 sectors with each sector presenting strategies aimed at promoting physical activity. Each strategy also outlines specific tactics that communities, organizations and agencies, and individuals can use to address the strategy. Discussion of strategies from each group are beyond the scope of this text, but the list of sectors and one selected strategy from each sector is listed below.

Business: Develop legislation and policy agendas that promote employer-sponsored physical activity programs while protecting individual employees' and dependents' rights.

Education: Develop and implement state and school district policies requiring school accountability for the quality and quantity of physical education and physical activity programs.

Health care: Make physical activity a patient "vital sign" that all health care providers assess and discuss with their patients.

Mass media: Enact federal legislation to support a sustained physical activity mass media campaign. Parks, recreation, fitness and sports: Promote programs and facilities where people work, learn, live, play and worship (i.e., workplace, public, private, and non-profit recreational sites) to provide easy access to safe and affordable physical activity opportunities.

Public health: Develop and maintain an ethnically and culturally diverse public health workforce of both genders with competence and expertise in physical activity and health.

Transportation, land use and community design: Prioritize resources and provide incentives to increase active transportation and other physical activity through community design, infrastructure projects, systems, policies, and initiatives.

Volunteer and non-profit: Conduct outreach to non-profit groups' members, volunteers, and constituents to change their own behaviors and advocate for policy and system changes outlined in the National Physical Activity Plan. It is evident that professionals in almost every field can have a part in promoting physical activity in our nation. Recognizing that some strategies encompass multiple sectors, the Plan also has several overarching strategies:

STRATEGY 1 Launch a grassroots advocacy effort to mobilize public support for strategies and tactics included in the National Physical Activity Plan.

STRATEGY 2 Mount a national physical activity education program to educate Americans about effective behavioral strategies for increasing physical activity. Integrate the program's design with other national health promotion and disease prevention education campaigns.

STRATEGY 3 Disseminate best practice physical activity models, programs, and policies to the widest extend practicable to ensure Americans can access strategies that will enable them to meet federal physical activity guidelines.

STRATEGY 4 Create a national resource center to disseminate effective tools for promoting of physical activity.

STRATEGY 5 Establish a center for physical activity policy development and research across all sectors of the National Physical Activity Plan.

The National Coalition for Promoting Physical Activity (NCPPA) is spearheading implementation of The National Physical Activity Plan. They have defined priorities, measurable outcomes and annual objectives for advancing the plan and is looking for organizations interested in implementing the plan. For more information about the National Physical Activity Plan, check their Web site (www.physicalactivityplan.org).

SUMMARY

Regular physical activity has been documented to reduce many of the changes associated with the aging process. In addition, an active lifestyle contributes to good health and well-being, increases life expectancy, and reduces the risk of many chronic illnesses. Exercise is often prescribed to reduce the symptoms and delay the progression of several chronic diseases. Inactivity has many serious and debilitating effects on almost every body system.

Multiple professional groups have issued recommendations for physical activity to enhance health and well-being and to reduce the effects of chronic illness. The current recommendation is to participate in moderate exercise for 30 minutes on five or more days a week. A well-balanced exercise plan includes exercises to increase cardiorespiratory fitness, strength, and flexibility. The type, duration, and intensity of exercise depend on the individual's goals and state of health. Although exercise has some risk, for most elders there is little risk in gradually beginning a moderate exercise program such as walking. Studies point to a variety of individual, cultural, and institutional barriers to exercise. Multiple intervention trials have found ways to overcome these barriers. Many resources are available for the professional interested in developing and implementing exercise strategies that are appropriate for elders. Because of the wide range of benefits of an active life in the later years, several local, state, and national governmental and private organizations are working to improve fitness among our nation's elders.

ACTIVITIES

1. If you plan to work with elders, you will be a better role model if you yourself are physically fit and have a positive attitude about exercise. To better understand your own fitness level, monitor the amount and type of exercise you engage in for a week. Do you feel you get enough exercise per day? If not, what is keeping you from exercising more? What activities could you add to your schedule? What other activities might you omit to make room to exercise? Which exercise activities may you carry on through old age?

2. Interview five older people regarding their exercise beliefs and current practices. Also, ask them to compare the amount and type of physical activity they currently undergo with what they did 10, 20, and 30 years ago. Has their activity level changed? What are their reasons for changing their activity level? Ask if they want to increase their exercise level. If so, what activities might they initiate? Compare and contrast the responses of the individuals you interviewed.

3. Visit a local nursing home. What physical activity programs does it offer? Who attends? How might attendance be increased? Find out how much time is spent per day per resident in physical activity. You may wish to compare the activity programs in several nursing homes.

4. Design a 30-second television or radio spot to encourage elders to exercise. What approach do you take? Who might sponsor such an advertisement?

5. Discuss exercise concepts with five people of different ages: a child, a teenager, a young adult, a middle-aged adult, and an older adult. Compare their perceptions of how much exercise is enough, what exercises are effective, and how much exercising they do.

6. Create a 15-minute module to educate elders in a community setting about the value of exercise for older people. Develop objectives, an outline, and methodology.

7. Contact a local hospital that offers a postcoronary exercise/rehabilitation program. Interview staff about their patients' characteristics, exercises performed, ways in which professionals motivate clients to start and stay in a program, and dropout rates.

8. Ask a nurse or a physician in a local hospital or nursing home about the protocol for treatment and rehabilitation of bedridden patients. Outline a plan to improve their care, keeping in mind the resources available at the site.

9. A local fitness center has hired you to develop a fitness program for older adults. What type of

program will you design? How will you motivate elders to join and continue with the program? What types of advertisements will you use? What strategies could you use to motivate a chronically ill, postcoronary, bedridden, or sedentary elder to exercise?

10. What exercise programs does your community have for older adults? Compare the types of programs, the population utilizing them, and the cost. Talk to several individuals frequenting the programs.

11. Identify a local program to enhance the involvement of elders in physical activity. What

type of program is it? What components of health behavior change are targeted? Who is the audience? What is the evidence that the program is effective? How might the program be improved?

12. Follow the Recommended Guidelines for Exercise for one week. Document what you did to follow the recommendations. What barriers did you encounter? How did you overcome them? What did you find out about your preferences and habits? Monitor how well you feel—did you note any differences?

BIBLIOGRAPHY

1. U.S. Department of Health and Human Services. 2008. Physical activity guidelines for Americans. Washington DC: U.S. Department of Health and Human Services.

2. Asher, R.A. 1947. The dangers of going to bed. *British Medical Journal* 2:967–968.

3. Lee, I-M., Rexrode, K.M., Cook, N.R., Manson, J.A., and Buring, J.E. 2001. Physical activity and coronary heart disease in women. *Journal of the American Medical Association* 285(11): 1447–1454.

4. Manson, J.E., Greenland, P., LaCroix, A.Z., et al. 2002. Walking compared with vigorous exercise for the prevention of cardiovascular events in women. *New England Journal of Medicine* 347(10):716–725.

5. Hambrecht, R., Gielen, S., Linke, A., et al. 2000. Effects of exercise training on left ventricular function and peripheral resistance in patients with chronic heart failure. *Journal of the American Medical Association* 283(23):3095–3101.

6. Taylor, R.S., Brown, A., Ebrahim, S., et al. 2004. Exercise-based rehabilitation for patients with coronary heart disease: Systematic review and meta-analysis of randomized controlled trials. *American Journal of Medicine* 116(10):682–692.

7. Heran, B.S., Chen, J.M., Ebrahim, S.M., Moxham, T., Oldridge, N., et al. 2011. *Cochrane Database Review*. Issue 7.

8. Pescatello, L.S., Franklin, B.A., Fagard, R., et al; American College of Sports Medicine. 2004. American College of Sports Medicine position stand: Exercise and hypertension. *Medicine and Science in Sports and Exercise* 36(3):533–553.

9. Stewart, K.J., Hiatt, W.R., Regensteiner, J.G., and Hirsch, A.T. 2002. Exercise training for claudication. *New England Journal of Medicine* 347(24):1941–1951.

10. American College of Sports Medicine and the American Diabetes Association. 2010. Exercise and type 2 diabetes. *Medical Science in Sports and Exercise* 42(12):2282–2303.

11. U.S. Department of Health and Human Services. 2012. Summary Health Statistics for U.S. Adults: National Health Interview Survey, 2010. *Vital and Health Statistics* 10(252):1–80.

12. American College of Sports Medicine. 2009. Position Statement. Appropriate intervention strategies for weight loss and prevention of weight regain for adults. *Medicine and Science in Sports and Exercise* 41(2):459–471.

13. Kohrt, W.M., Bloomfield, S.A., Little, K.D., Nelson, M.E., and Yingling, V.R.; American College of Sports Medicine. 2004. American College of Sports Medicine position stand: Physical activity and bone health. *Medicine and Science in Sports and Exercise* 36(11):1985–1996.

14. Feskanich, D., Willett, W., and Colditz, G. 2002. Walking and leisure-time activity and risk of hip fracture in postmenopausal women. *Journal of the American Medical Association* 288(18): 2300–2306.

15. Dunlop, D.D., Semanik, P., Song, J., et al. 2005. Risk factors for functional decline in older adults with arthritis. *Arthritis and Rheumatism* 52(4): 1274–1282.

16. Burnham, T.R., and Wilcox, A. 2002. Effects of exercise on physiological and psychological variables in cancer survivors. *Medicine and Science in Sports and Exercise* 34(12):1863–1867.

17. Singh, N.A., Clements, K.M., and Fiatarone Singh, M.A. 2001. The efficacy of exercise as a long-term antidepressant in elderly subjects: A randomized, controlled trial. *Journal of Gerontology: Medical Sciences* 56A(8):497–504.

18. Singh, N.A., Stavrinos, T.M., Scarbek, Y., et al. 2005. A randomized controlled trial of high versus low intensity weight training versus general practitioner care for clinical depression in older adults. *Journals of Gerontology: Medical Sciences* 60A(6):M768–M776.

19. Borg, G.A.V. 1998. Borg's Rating of Perceived Exertion and Pain Scales. Champaign, IL: Human Kinetics.

20. U.S. Preventive Services Task Force. 2002. Recommendations and rationale: Behavioral counseling in primary care to promote physical activity. *Annals of Intern Medicine* 137(3): 205–207.

21. American College of Sports Medicine. 2010. *ACMS's Guidelines for exercise tests and prescription*. Baltimore, MD: American College of Sports Medicine.

22. Guide to Community Preventive Services: Promoting Physical Activity. www.thecommunityguide.org Accessed 12/20/2011.

23. Stewart, A.L., Verboncoeur, C.J., McLellan, B.Y., et al. 2001. Physical activity outcomes of CHAMPS II: A physical activity promotion program for older adults. *Journal of Gerontology: Medical Sciences* 56A(8):M465–M470.

Nutrition

Dietary habits of youth set the stage for health and disease in old age. The time to nourish your body for late life is now.

Alice Chenault

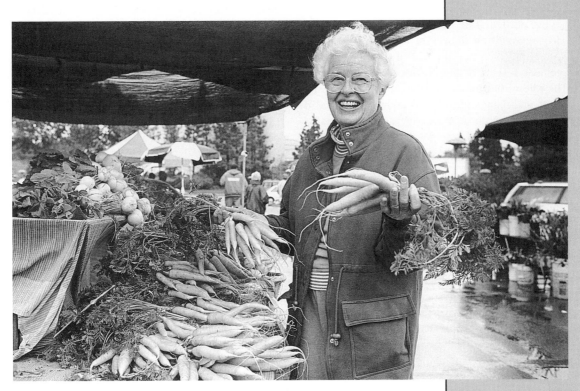

Our daily diet plays a significant role in our state of health and quality of life, no matter what our age. "You are what you eat" may not be literally true, but diet plays a clear role in health and well-being. Although the same nutrients are essential for individuals of any age, the changes that accompany aging may affect the amount of specific nutrients required by older people. Issues such as obesity, cholesterol, trans fats, and vitamin therapies are often in the news, raising public consciousness of the importance of eating well. Furthermore, new information regarding the importance of nutrition in health and disease underscores the need for nutritional counseling as an adjunct to medical therapy. Poor eating habits accelerate many age-related decrements and increase the likelihood of several chronic illnesses in later life.

In this chapter we examine the essential nutrients needed for all ages, and we outline a strategy for choosing a healthful diet. The challenges of nutrition research are discussed as well as research findings linking foods and food components to health. Obesity and malnutrition are addressed, paying particular attention to the importance of early recognition of weight loss among elders. Specialized diets and the role of diet in the management of selected chronic diseases are explored. The role of nutritional supplements in enhancing health and reducing disease is addressed. We also examine research regarding the nutritional status of older people and strategies to improve access to healthy meals among the older population.

ESSENTIAL DIETARY COMPONENTS

The human body requires a wide variety of nutrients to carry out its essential functions, to provide energy for metabolism and action, to build and repair tissues, and to reproduce. In this section we discuss the essential components of a nutritious diet and common food sources for each nutrient.

More than 40 nutrients have been identified as playing a role in health. The metabolism of protein, carbohydrates, and fat supplies the body with energy for growth and maintenance. Vitamins and minerals are needed to manufacture enzymes that are needed for cell growth and maintenance. Water is perhaps the most essential element in the body. A person can live for over a month without food but for only a few days without water. Even though dietary fiber is not a nutrient (because it travels through the digestive system unchanged), it too plays an important role in physical health.

Each individual requires a different quantity of various nutrients that depends on activity level, response to stress, drug use, age, gender, body size, and health condition. Over the years, attempts have been made to standardize nutritional requirements to assist individuals to make good food choices. Perhaps the best-known standards are the Recommended Dietary Allowances (RDA) developed by the Food and Nutrition Board. The Food and Nutrition Board is a working group within the Institute of Medicine, which is a part of the umbrella organization, the National Academy of Sciences. As the relationship of diet and disease becomes clear, the RDA is continually modified. Whereas the RDA used to be simply the amount of nutrient necessary to prevent deficiency disease, it now focuses on levels sufficient to achieve health benefits. The *RDA* is the nutrient intake level that meets the requirement for nearly all individuals of a specified age range and gender. In contrast, the *AI* (Adequate Intake) is the nutrient intake level of healthy people assumed to be adequate, and it is based on current research. The *UL* (Upper Limit) is the highest daily nutrient intake likely to pose no risk of adverse health effects to almost all of the general population. It is not a recommended level, and there are no established benefits of a higher level. In fact, there may be increased health risks of consuming above the UL.

The Dietary Reference Intakes in this section are from the Food and Nutrition Information Center of the United States Department of Agriculture. If the reader desires more detail than is provided in the text regarding nutrient requirements, refer to their Web site (www.fnic.nal.usda.gov) and click on "Dietary Guidelines for Americans."

Calories

The body is fueled by food, which provides energy for us to function. With the exception of diet sodas, black coffee, and tea, almost all food contains some usable energy in the form of protein, carbohydrates, or fat. The amount of energy contained in foods is measured in kilocalories (commonly referred to as calories) and represents the amount of energy required to heat 1,000 grams (about a quart) of water by 1 degree Celsius. Thus, if you burned the energy in a 10-calorie piece of candy, you could heat 1,000 grams of water 10 degrees Celsius. Calories in food do more than warm the body, they provide fuel for our organs, brains, and muscles to function. The usable energy of calories of food can be in the form of fat, protein, or carbohydrates. Most foods contain a combination of these substances. By weight, fat contains the most calories (9 calories in every gram), while carbohydrates and proteins contain about 4 calories per gram.

Because fat is so concentrated, a relatively small portion contains more than twice as many calories as the same-size portion of a food that is predominantly carbohydrate or protein. Some high-energy foods release as much energy as explosives. For instance, a two-inch square of fudge (185 calories) releases as much energy as a small stick of dynamite, and a double-dip ice cream cone (334 calories) releases energy equivalent to one-half cubic foot of natural gas. Although we consume huge amounts of energy, we do not explode because it is released gradually by the enzyme-coordinated process of metabolism.[1]

Everyone needs calories to survive, but the amount needed differs and depends on a person's gender, size, rate of metabolism, and activity level. To put it simply, bigger, taller, more active, and younger men need more calories than smaller, shorter, less active, and elderly women. There are many reasons why caloric requirements diminish with age. The proportion of body fat increases, and muscle mass decreases. Further, there is a gradual reduction in resting metabolic rate after maturity. Finally, as a group, elders are generally less physically active than younger adults and need fewer calories. Although caloric need tends to decline with age, there is a significant calorie variation among what individuals of the same age require:

Table 10.1	**How Many Calories Each Day Are Needed for People over Age 50?**
A woman	1,600 calories if her physical activity level is low
	1,800 calories if she is moderately active
	2,000–2,200 calories if she has an active lifestyle
A man	2,000 calories if his physical activity level is low
	2,200–2,400 calories if he is moderately active
	2,400–2,800 calories if he has an active lifestyle

Source: http://www.niapublications.org/agepages/nutrition.asp

For instance, elders who are very physically active need more calories than those who are bedridden. No matter what our age, when we eat more food than our body needs, the excess calories are stored as fat to be used in times of increased need. Although there is a general decrease in the amount of calories needed as we age, the need for vitamins and minerals and other micronutrients does not decline. This presents a quandary for elders: how to get the same amount of vitamins and minerals into fewer calories per day. This challenge means that elders cannot "waste" any calories on foods that are not rich in nutrients.

Water

Water is needed for almost every body process, including getting food through the body, circulation of blood, eliminating waste, and regulating body temperature. All chemical reactions within the body need water; even small changes in water balance can lead to metabolic problems. In addition, water, especially hard water, provides the body with needed minerals such as zinc, magnesium, calcium, and copper.

According to the Food and Nutrition Board of the Institute of Medicine, older men require about

16 cups of liquid a day, with about 13 cups from water and beverages. Older women require about 11 cups of liquid a day, 9 from water or other beverages. Elders have less body water than younger groups and are more susceptible to dehydration. Healthy older people are not as likely as younger people to complain of thirst, and they tend to drink less than younger people, suggesting that elders cannot rely totally on their thirst mechanism to determine needed water intake. Symptoms of mild dehydration include weakness, confusion, dry mouth, and flushed skin. Symptoms of more severe dehydration include sunken eyes, dry loose skin, and low urinary output. On the other hand, excessive water consumption can aggravate some diseases, such as congestive heart failure, by making the heart and kidneys work too hard. It also can dilute the important salts in the body. Thus, some elders are prescribed diets with fluid restriction.

Proteins

Foods rich in protein are required for almost every aspect of the body's functions. Proteins are broken down into building blocks called amino acids. We eat proteins, and our body breaks them down into amino acids, then reassembles them again into new proteins in our body organs and cells. Imagine proteins as structures built with Legos—we eat them in one form—multicolored structures with various sizes and shapes of blocks. In digestion, the body breaks them apart and send them around to where they are needed, and then within cells, these blocks are reassembled in different configurations to make cells, organs, enzymes, and nearly everything else in the body. They are reassembled according to instructions in our genes. Some amino acids (called *nonessential* amino acids) are manufactured within the body; other amino acids (called *essential* amino acids) must come from the food we eat. Proteins may come from vegetable or animal sources. Once ingested, proteins are broken down into amino acids in the intestines and are absorbed so they can be used to build and repair body tissues or be burned for energy. The body requires more protein during periods of rapid growth, illness,

and recovery from surgery or injury. Although older people may need less protein to maintain their declining muscle mass, they often have increased needs due to illness.

Many people from developing nations do not get sufficient protein in their diets. However, in the United States, many people consume an excessive amount of protein. The metabolism of excess protein, especially animal protein, can put a strain on the liver and kidneys and can deplete the bones of needed calcium. The Food and Nutrition Board recommends that individuals over age 50 get 46 grams (women) to 56 grams (men) of protein a day. Because protein needs are increased in times of stress or during recovery from a wound, those who are chronically ill or bedridden, or who have pressure ulcers, are at high risk of protein deficiency and should increase their protein consumption to twice the Recommended Daily Allowance (RDA).

Major dietary sources of protein are nuts, legumes, fish, meat, eggs, and dairy products.

Carbohydrates

Carbohydrates provide the major source of calories because they are inexpensive and easy to prepare, store, chew, and digest. Carbohydrates are easily broken down and provide an immediate source of energy. Foods classified as carbohydrates vary widely. *Simple carbohydrates* are sugars such as sucrose, fructose (found in fruits), and lactose (found in dairy products). Sugars include sweets such as table sugar, honey, jelly, and candy. Milk and fruits also contain simple natural sugars. *Complex carbohydrates* are starches that take longer to digest but provide energy over a longer period of time. Starches include legumes and starchy vegetables, such as potatoes, and whole grains. Simple sugars enter the bloodstream immediately. Complex carbohydrates must be broken down into sugar by saliva and stomach enzymes before they enter the bloodstream. When sugars are ingested, they enter the bloodstream quickly, creating a burst of sugar energy, followed by a drop in sugar energy. When complex carbohydrates are eaten, digestion is slower and thus the sugars are released into the body over a longer period of time. This process of digestion releases the sugars more gradually and consistently into the bloodstream. Insulin, a hormone produced by the pancreas, facilitates entry of sugar into each body cell to produce energy.

There is a new focus on carbohydrates these days. Many of the modern "diets" focus on reducing carbohydrates, attributing symptoms of fatigue, irritability, pain, and obesity to the ingestion of carbohydrates. However, nutritionists continue to recommend carbohydrates, particularly whole grains and fresh fruits and vegetables, as an integral part of a healthy eating plan.

Most carbohydrates come from plants—fruits, vegetables, grains. Carbohydrates vary by the amount of processing of the natural product. If a whole grain is processed to create white flour and white bread, this product has fewer naturally occurring vitamins and minerals and less fiber than a wheat berry ingested whole and unprocessed. Carbohydrates also vary by the ease in which they are digested and converted to sugar. Foods that easily convert to sugar (e.g., white bread and simple sugar) are said to have a *higher glycemic index,* and those that take longer to convert to sugar (e.g., whole-grain barley) have a *lower glycemic index.* Speaking generally, foods with a lower glycemic index are more healthful, higher in fiber, lower in calories, and higher in nutrients and are associated with an increased sense of fullness after eating.

Since complex and simple carbohydrates vary in their effects, currently the emphasis is to increase the amount of complex carbohydrates in the diet and to reduce simple carbohydrates. This recommendation adds fiber to the diet, reduces total calorie consumption, and provides important vitamins and minerals. The Food and Nutrition Board recommends that individuals 51 years and older consume 130 grams of digestible carbohydrates a day. According to the board, the acceptable range of carbohydrates is 45 to 65 percent of total calories, with no more than 25 percent of calories coming from sugars added to food during production and processing. No deficiency disease of carbohydrates is known because complex carbohydrates are the most available and inexpensive of all the food groups.

The main sources of carbohydrates are whole-grain breads and cereals, rice, beans, pastas, fruits, and starchy vegetables. Less healthy sources include cakes, cookies, white flour, and candy.

Fats

Despite their negative press, fats are important because they are a major energy source. They also help to absorb fat-soluble vitamins, insulate and cushion the body, and are needed to make new cells. Fats also provide flavor to food and a feeling of fullness. All animal and plant foods contain fats. Foods high in fats include dairy products, vegetable oils, and red meat. Fats can be made by the liver or may be ingested in the diet.

There is little danger of insufficient fat intake in the United States. Even if someone ingests no visible fat, about 10 percent of all calories would still be derived from fat. On the average, Americans consume an average of 40 percent of their calories as fats. Recommendations vary, but most experts suggest that fats should comprise only 30 percent of dietary calories and some suggest 15–20 percent. Excess fat intake can be particularly harmful for elders because it provides calories in a concentrated form with few vitamins, minerals, fiber, or other nutrients. In addition, some elders have a reduced tolerance for fat due to digestive problems.

There are many different types and subtypes of fats. Two major types are triglycerides and cholesterol. The main role of triglycerides is to produce energy. Triglycerides are made of two- or three-long chains of molecules called fatty acids connected to a short carbohydrate backbone. Triglycerides may be polyunsaturated, saturated, or monounsaturated, depending on the way the molecules are chained together.

Saturated fats are generally found in animal products such as meat and butter and are solid at room temperature. A diet high in saturated fats is strongly associated with an increased risk of atherosclerosis, elevated cholesterol, and heart disease. Hydrogenated and partially hydrogenated vegetable fats (also called trans fats) are manufactured counterparts to saturated fats that are produced by bubbling hydrogen atoms through liquid oils. The use of trans fats enhances the taste, texture, and appearance of food. Trans fats are commonly found in store-bought crackers, cookies, and cakes, and in solid margarines and deep-fried foods. Because of known risks to health, the FDA requires that all food labels list the grams of trans fats in the food product.

Unsaturated fats are generally liquid at room temperature, although they may solidify in the refrigerator. *Polyunsaturated* fats, such as margarine and most vegetable oils, protect against heart disease, but they may be associated with an increased risk of cancer. *Monounsaturated* fats, such as olive oil and fats found in avocados and nuts, are thought to be the healthiest type of fat. Most foods contain combinations of more than one type of fat. It is recommended that the majority of fat intake come from foods containing monounsaturated and polyunsaturated fats. Food labels are the most reliable guides to the amount of various types of fat in foods.

Cholesterol is perhaps the most commonly discussed fat these days. Cholesterol is a very complex molecule that looks different from other fats. It is needed to maintain cell membranes and to manufacture vitamin D. Cholesterol is found only in animal products. Even nuts and avocados have no cholesterol.

The body does not require cholesterol from food because the liver can make what it needs. In most people, the liver responds to high-cholesterol diets by making less cholesterol and getting rid of it faster. Many people can eat very high-cholesterol meals and not have elevated blood cholesterol levels. However, the bodies of some people do not compensate for high-cholesterol intake, and unless the cholesterol they ingest is kept low, an excess of cholesterol will appear in the bloodstream. For more on blood cholesterol levels, see Chapter 4.

Omega-3 fatty acids and alpha linoleic acids are considered "good fats," and experts recommend we eat more of these. Omega-3 fatty acids are found in fatty fish (e.g., albacore tuna, salmon, sardines), and eating a high level of these fats is associated with a reduced risk of heart disease, lower blood fats, decreased blood clotting, and other benefits. Alpha linoleic acids (e.g., soybeans, tofu, canola, walnuts) are converted to omega-3 fatty acids in the body and may also be healthful.

Major sources of fat are animal and vegetable oils, meat, fried foods, cheese, butter, ice cream, and whole milk.

Fiber

What used to be called "roughage" is now called "fiber," and health experts are encouraging people to eat more of it. Fiber is the undigestible parts of plants. *Soluble* fiber (which gets sticky when in contact with water) is found in oats, beans, barley, fruits, and vegetables. It is known to lower cholesterol levels and stabilize blood glucose levels. Fiber can add volume to foods, helping you to feel fuller after eating fewer calories. *Insoluble* fiber is especially important to prevent constipation, for fiber absorbs water as it passes through the colon. This makes the stools larger but softer and easier to pass.

There are other benefits to adding fiber to the diet. A high-fiber diet is associated with low serum cholesterol and a decrease in blood pressure. Individuals who consume a diet high in fiber have lower risks of cancer (especially of the colon), diverticulosis, diabetes, and heart disease. Since high-fiber diets are associated with a high consumption of fruits, vegetables, and grains, the effect may also be due to the vitamins and minerals found in those foods, which are known to enhance health.

The Food and Nutrition Board recommends that individuals over age 50 consume 21 grams (women) to 30 grams (men) of fiber a day. High-fiber foods such as oat bran and barley have received approval by the Food and Drug Administration to be labeled with statements about their protective abilities for heart disease. In the United States, the average adult consumes about half the recommended amount of fiber. Some older people may eat even less fiber, because foods rich in fiber are often hard to chew. For some, a fiber supplement such as Metamucil is recommended to relieve constipation or lower cholesterol. People should increase their dietary fiber slowly because a rapid increase can cause gas, diarrhea, and abdominal cramping.

Foods rich in insoluble fiber include corn, wheat bran, fruit and vegetable skins, and leafy green vegetables.

Vitamins

Vitamins are a diverse group of chemicals needed in small amounts to enable the body to complete a variety of chemical reactions: energy production, growth, maintenance, and repair of body cells. Some vitamins are considered to be nonessential—they are needed but our bodies can produce them. Nonessential vitamins will not be discussed here. Other vitamins are essential, and, since they cannot be made in the body in sufficient amounts, they must be included in the diet. Fat-soluble vitamins (A, E, D, and K) are stored in body fat and the liver to be used as needed. Excessive levels of these vitamins can be toxic. Water-soluble vitamins (carotenoids, vitamin C, and the B-complex vitamins) do not build up to toxic levels because they are regularly excreted in the urine. However, they need to be ingested more often and are more easily destroyed by cooking than are the fat-soluble vitamins.

This section discusses each vitamin, its role in health, signs of deficiency, and common dietary sources. The role of specific vitamins in preventing and treating chronic diseases and disorders of elders is discussed in a later section.

Vitamin A

Vitamin A (retinol) can be ingested directly, or it can be made by ingesting food containing carotenoids (the most prominent is beta-carotene) that are then converted to vitamin A by the liver. High doses of retinol are toxic, but carotenoids are safe even in high quantities. Carotenoids are actually pigments and can cause the skin to turn orange if an individual eats a large amount of carrots or takes edible "tanning pills."

Vitamin A is essential for vision, skin, and mucous membrane function. It is also an antioxidant (see Chapter 2, "Biologic Aging Theories and Longevity"). Vitamin A deficiency may be due to inadequate intake or to an impaired ability to absorb or store the vitamin. Causes of impairment might be liver disease, reduced bile production, and antibiotics and laxatives. A severe deficiency of this vitamin is first evident with reduced night vision and dry eyes, which can lead to blindness. Vitamin A deficiency may also cause rough and reddened skin, increasing the susceptibility to infections. The RDA for women over age 50 years is 700 micrograms; for men over age 50, 900 units. The upper limit for vitamin A consumption is established at 3,000 micrograms.

Observational studies have found that people who eat a diet high in vitamin A, or those who have higher blood levels of this vitamin, have increased immune cell function and reduced risk of several chronic diseases. It was hoped that dietary supplements of vitamin A or carotenoids might confer the same benefits. However, studies on supplements have not supported a beneficial effect. Perhaps the most famous study is a large randomized trial that reported an increase in lung cancer among elder smokers who took beta-carotene supplements.[2] Other research has revealed another negative effect of too much vitamin A: its tendency to weaken bones and increase fracture rates.[3]

Vitamin A derivatives (e.g., Retin-A and Accutane) are used to treat dermatological conditions, including acne, facial wrinkling from sun damage, and precancerous lesions.

Animal products are a major dietary source of vitamin A. Major dietary sources of carotenoids are orange and yellow fruits and vegetables, especially apricots, cantaloupe, sweet potatoes, and carrots.

Vitamin B Complex

The vitamin B complex was originally thought to be one vitamin, but as more B vitamins were discovered, subscripts were added. More than 20 B vitamins have been identified, but only 8 are essential for humans. All B vitamins are water-soluble, that is, they are not stored in the body. Each B vitamin is known by a number and a chemical name. All play a role in cell reproduction or the breakdown of protein, fat, and carbohydrates.

Thiamine (B$_1$) enrichment of foods in our country has largely eliminated the dreaded disease beriberi, which leads to paralysis, heart failure, and death. However, between one-third and one-half of all Americans, particularly the poor and alcoholics, suffer from mild thiamine deficiency. Symptoms are appetite loss, nausea, depression, and mental confusion. Alcoholics are often deficient in thiamine, probably because of inadequate intake, insufficient absorption, and heightened need. Because of the prevalence of thiamine deficiency among alcoholics, it has been suggested that alcoholic beverages be enriched with the vitamin. The RDA for thiamine is 1.2 milligrams for adult men and 1.1 milligrams for adult women.

Major dietary sources of thiamine are whole and enriched grains, legumes, organ meats, and green leafy vegetables.

Riboflavin (B$_2$) is essential for the action of other B vitamins. Deficiency is characterized by visual problems, cracking of the corners of the mouth, and scaly skin rashes. Strict vegetarians, alcoholics, and individuals who take estrogen supplements are at higher risk for riboflavin deficiency. Some experts believe riboflavin to be the most common marginal deficiency among elders and the poor. The RDA for riboflavin is 1.3 milligrams for adult men and 1.1 milligrams for adult women.

Major dietary sources of riboflavin are liver, dairy products, and whole or enriched grain products.

Niacin (B$_3$) deficiency causes pellagra, characterized by the "four D's": dermatitis, diarrhea, dementia, and death. Pellagra used to be a widespread disease, but now that refined carbohydrates are enriched, this deficiency is uncommon except among alcoholics. Mild deficiencies may appear as depression and mental confusion. High doses of niacin are successfully used to treat high cholesterol levels and are much less expensive than the other cholesterol-lowering drugs. Excessive

intakes of niacin are associated with liver damage. The body is able to make its own niacin if the amino acid tryptophan is ingested. The RDA for niacin is 16 milligrams for adult men and 14 milligrams for adult women.

Major dietary sources of niacin are meat, poultry, and legumes.

Pantothenic acid (B$_5$) is found in a wide variety of foods and is manufactured by intestinal bacteria. Because of this, a deficiency state does not exist. However, marginal deficiencies may contribute to disease states. The RDA for pantothenic acid has not been determined but the AI (adequate intake) is 5 micrograms for all adults.

Major dietary sources of pantothenic acid are vegetables, fruits, and meats.

Pyridoxine (B$_6$) is essential for antibody production and brain and nerve function. Deficiency of pyridoxine is rare. The need for pyridoxine increases for individuals who ingest high levels of alcohol or protein, use prescription medications such as levodopa, are heavy smokers, or use estrogen supplements. The RDA for pyroxidine is 1.7 milligrams for men over 50 and 1.5 milligrams for women over 50.

Major dietary sources of pyridoxine are bananas, vegetables, meat, liver, whole grains, and egg yolks.

Biotin (B$_7$) is present in all foods; however, it is lost in food processing and refrigeration and is not added back during enrichment. Though not common, symptoms of deficiency are gastrointestinal distress, fatigue, and depression. Persistent diarrhea or long-term therapy with antibiotics or sulfa drugs can create a deficiency state. The RDA for biotin has not been determined but the AI is 30 micrograms for adults.

Major dietary sources of biotin are organ meats, legumes, egg yolks, nuts, and whole grains.

Folate (B$_9$) is a plant-based vitamin that has received increased attention because of its role in prevention of neural tube defects when taken by pregnant women and its possible role in reducing risk of cardiovascular disease. Folic acid is a synthetic form of folate used in vitamin supplements and used to fortify foods such as cereals and breads.

Folic acid is about twice as potent as folate. Because of this confusion, the newest RDA refers to "dietary folate equivalents." The RDA for folate is 400 micrograms for adults. Thus, to meet the RDA of 400 micrograms of "dietary folate equivalents," a person must consume 200 micrograms of folic acid.

Because folate is known to prevent certain birth defects, and campaigns in the late 1990s to increase dietary intake among women were ineffective, the Food and Drug Administration now requires food manufacturers to add folic acid to foods containing enriched white flour. This has reduced birth defects. Low folate intake is relatively common in the population. Heavy alcohol consumption, estrogen therapy, chemotherapy, and some other drugs can reduce folate levels. Although folate is plentiful in foods, it is inactivated when cooked for even five minutes. Intestinal bacteria also synthesize this vitamin, but taking antibiotics can reduce the synthesis. Deficiency is most common among institutionalized elders and alcoholics. Anemia is the first sign of folate deficiency.

Major dietary sources of folate are cereals, lentils, beans, spinach, and pasta.

Cobalamin (B$_{12}$) is synthesized by bacteria found in the digestive tract. Other sources are meat, poultry, fish, and dairy products. Strict vegetarians may become deficient unless their intestinal bacteria produce sufficient quantities. Rarely, however, does anyone manifest vitamin B$_{12}$ deficiency due to inadequate intake. A deficiency is more likely due to inadequate absorption from reduced stomach acid. This condition, called pernicious anemia, is most common in those over age 50. Those at highest risk are individuals who had surgery on their intestines, who take antacids or seizure drugs, or who consume a lot of alcohol.

It is estimated that as many as 20 percent of the elderly have low vitamin B$_{12}$ levels.[4] The synthetic form of B$_{12}$, available in vitamin pills and in fortified grains and cereals, is recommended for elders because their bodies may not fully absorb the natural form of the vitamin. Injections of the vitamin can rapidly correct the deficiency, and these may be followed by monthly B$_{12}$ shots, weekly inhalation from a nasal spray, or daily pills to keep levels in normal range. The RDA for vitamin B$_{12}$ is 2.4 micrograms for all adults.

Major dietary sources of vitamin B$_{12}$ are meat, liver, kidneys, fish, yogurt, cottage cheese, and eggs.

Vitamin C

Vitamin C (ascorbic acid) is an important component of the cell structure (e.g., collagen and elastin) that hold the body together. Additionally, it plays a role as an antioxidant and enhances the absorption of iron and calcium from the small intestine. Severe vitamin C deficiency causes scurvy, characterized by a loss of appetite, irritability, and depression, followed by sore bones and joints and excessive bleeding from gums. The disease was first noticed in sailors on long voyages without fresh fruits and vegetables. Although scurvy is now very rare, some experts believe that a mild deficiency can cause increased susceptibility to illness. Marginal deficiencies of vitamin C or the B vitamins may aggravate neurologic symptoms. Use of certain drugs increase the need for vitamin C, particularly persons who take estrogen supplements or high doses of aspirin, and those who smoke cigarettes or who drink alcohol heavily.

The amount of vitamin C needed for optimal health is highly debated. Although only minimal levels are needed to prevent scurvy, some experts believe that higher levels of vitamin C in the diet prevent illness and enhance recovery. Studies show that vitamin C levels are reduced during infection, surgery, or stress. Elders with wounds, particularly pressure ulcers, are often prescribed vitamin C to speed wound healing, although there is no scientific evidence to support this practice. Some people use vitamin C products to forestall the development of colds, and there is some evidence to support its effectiveness. Any vitamin C not used is excreted in the urine. Large doses may interfere with some diagnostic laboratory tests and cause diarrhea. The RDA for vitamin C is 90 milligrams for adult men and 75 milligrams for adult women. The tolerable upper intake level of Vitamin C is 2,000 milligrams.

Major dietary sources of vitamin C are citrus fruits, cantaloupe, watermelon, strawberries, Brussels sprouts, and broccoli.

Vitamin D

Technically, vitamin D (calciferol) is not a vitamin but a hormone because it is manufactured in one part of the body and affects another part. When skin is exposed to sunlight, vitamin D is activated in a complex chain of events that also involves the kidneys and liver. The end product, calciferol, increases the amount of calcium absorbed from the intestines; without it, calcium is poorly absorbed. In other words, without enough vitamin D, the body cannot absorb the calcium that is in food. Consequently, the needed calcium must be taken from the bones.

The vitamin D requirement can be met by sunlight exposure and food supplements. Exposing the hands, face, and arms to sunlight for 15 to 20 minutes two or three times a week will suffice. Sun exposure must be longer in the winter months, when vitamin D production is less efficient. Since blacks average lower serum levels of vitamin D than whites, they need a longer sun exposure than do whites. Sunscreen products prevent absorption of UV rays.

In addition to the production of vitamin D from the sun, vitamin D is also present in foods, particularly in oily fish. Just a teaspoon of cod liver oil has more than 3 times the RDA. Because of widespread vitamin D deficiency in children that resulted in weakened bones, called rickets, milk and some cereals are now fortified with a form of vitamin D. However, the level is often not sufficient for many adults as one cup of fortified milk provides one-fourth of the daily vitamin D requirement. The RDA for vitamin D is 600 international units (IUs) for adults aged 51–70 and 800 IUs for those older than 70. Recommendations are based on minimal sun exposure. The tolerable upper intake level of vitamin D is 4,000 IUs.[5]

A deficiency in vitamin D causes rickets in children and osteoporosis in adults—both diseases severely weaken the bones and increase susceptibility to fractures. The link between vitamin D deficiency and increased risk of fractures is compelling.

In addition, studies support a role for vitamin D deficiency in the development of skin, breast, prostate, and colon cancers, type II diabetes, and cardiovascular disorders including hypertension. Researchers estimate that as many as one-half of all elders have a marginal deficiency of vitamin D. Elders who are bedridden, ill, and institutionalized are at highest risk.

Individuals with kidney and liver disease are more likely to exhibit a vitamin D deficiency, as are people who take bulk laxatives, antacids containing aluminum, cholesterol-lowering drugs, mineral oil laxatives, and drugs for epilepsy.

Even elders with an adequate intake can exhibit a vitamin D deficiency. Elders may be at higher risk of vitamin D deficiency for several reasons: reduced ability of the skin to make the vitamin, insufficient sunlight exposure, reduced intake of milk, and decreased absorption. Vitamin D levels may vary seasonally, with levels lower in the winter and higher in the summer. In the Northeast, many people do not get enough vitamin D from the sun; they must rely on fortified milk or vitamin supplements.

Major dietary sources of vitamin D are cod liver oil, salmon, mackerel, tuna, sardines, and fortified milk.

Vitamin E

Vitamin E is another antioxidant that prevents and repairs free radical damage to the cell caused by normal cell metabolism. Multiple studies show an association between high blood levels of vitamin E from food and reduced risks of many diseases, including cardiovascular disease, cancer, cataracts, diabetes, and Alzheimer's disease. Unfortunately, multiple studies of vitamin E supplementation in individuals without vitamin E deficiency have not revealed a consistent benefit. Perhaps this finding indicates that other components of foods containing vitamin E are important. Or perhaps alpha tocopherol, the type of vitamin E that supplements generally use, may be the "wrong" tocopherol or form of vitamin E. An analysis of several studies revealed that high-dose vitamin E supplementation (over 150 international units per day) was associated with an increase in mortality.[6] Vitamin E can cause increased blood clotting when taken in high amounts. The RDA for vitamin E is 15 milligrams for all adults and the tolerable upper intake level is 1,000 milligrams.

Vitamin E deficiency can result from inadequate intake. Even with sufficient intake, individuals who are tube-fed or who cannot properly absorb fat can show symptoms of vitamin E deficiency. Symptoms are serious and obvious and include anemia and nervous system abnormalities.

Major dietary sources of vitamin E are vegetable oils.

Vitamin K

Vitamin K is manufactured by bacteria in the large intestine. The main function of vitamin K is to promote blood clotting. Vitamin K deficiency is very rare in adults, but it can occur in individuals on long-term antibiotic therapy because the antibiotics kill the bacteria in the colon. Additionally, people who have difficulty in absorbing fats or who take mineral oil are at higher risk of deficiency. Symptoms of deficiency include anemia, prolonged bleeding, and easy bruising. The RDA for vitamin K has not been determined but the AI is 120 micrograms for adult men and 90 micrograms for adult women.

Major dietary sources of vitamin K are leafy green vegetables.

Minerals

Minerals are inorganic substances needed in relatively small amounts for proper body function. Some are a necessary part of cell structure, body fluids, and tissues; others have very specific functions (e.g., iodine needed to make thyroxin, iron to produce hemoglobin). Some minerals, such as calcium, magnesium, phosphorus, sodium, potassium, and chlorine, are needed in amounts greater than 100 milligrams per day (macronutrients). Other minerals, such as iron, iodine, copper, manganese, zinc, chromium, fluorine, and selenium, are needed in trace amounts (micronutrients). In addition, trace elements, such as tin, vanadium, silicon,

arsenic, nickel, and cadmium, may be important, but recommended doses have not been established. The quantity of each mineral needed is no measure of the mineral's relative importance in the body.

Mineral deficiencies are more common than vitamin deficiencies. Although vitamins are usually present in foods in similar amounts throughout the world, some areas are very poor in specific minerals and trace elements, predisposing residents of these areas to deficiencies. In elders, mineral deficiencies may be related to decreased absorption, marginal diets, medications, and disease states. This section discusses the role of selected minerals in health and disease, signs of deficiency, and common food sources.

Calcium

Calcium is the mineral needed in the highest quantity by the body. It is crucial to bone formation, blood clotting, heartbeat regulation, muscle contraction, and neuron function. Dietary calcium is absorbed through the small intestine with the help of vitamin D. Blood calcium levels must remain constant. Both high calcium intake and physical activity stimulate calcium to deposit in the bones. Conversely, low intake gradually depletes calcium from the bones to maintain a constant blood level of calcium.

The RDA for calcium intake for men between 51 and 70 years of age is 1,000 milligrams, 1,200 milligrams for men over 70. For women beginning at age 50, the RDA is 1,200 milligrams.[5] Multiple studies document that the average daily calcium intake for older men and women is much lower than the RDA. Low calcium levels in older people can be due to low calcium intake, reduced absorption in the intestine, or low levels of physical activity. Marginal calcium deficiency may be aggravated by low-cholesterol diets prescribed to manage hypertension, which discourage intake of calcium-rich dairy products. Furthermore, a high-protein diet, soft drinks containing phosphoric acid, and some drugs reduce blood calcium levels. Low consumption of calcium has been associated with reduced bone density in normal men and women and increased susceptibility to fracture. Calcium deficiency has also been linked to hypertension.

Calcium supplements have been shown to increase bone mass and to reduce the risk of hip fractures among the elderly. However, the gains quickly disappear when the supplement is stopped.

Dairy products are by far the most effective dietary source of calcium. Further, milk is fortified with vitamin D to facilitate calcium absorption. Also, cereals and orange juice are increasingly being fortified with calcium. Even though some green vegetables have calcium, many contain substances that reduce calcium absorption (e.g., the oxalic acid in spinach). A high-fiber diet is known to reduce calcium absorption, so vegetarians may need to increase overall calcium intake.

Since it can be difficult to get enough calcium each day, supplements are suggested, particularly calcium carbonate (e.g., Tums), because they offer a high proportion of usable calcium. For some people, calcium supplements cause constipation. There is little danger of *eating* too much calcium because the excess is excreted, but the Food and Nutrition Board recommends that no more than 2,000 milligrams of calcium be ingested a day. There is some evidence that taking too many calcium supplements can result in kidney stones.

Calcium is found in dairy products— yogurt, milk, and cheese, some brands of tofu (check label)—sardines, and collard greens.

Chlorine

Chlorine works with sodium to maintain the acid-base and fluid balance of the body and is a component of the hydrochloric acid secreted by the stomach. Almost all chlorine is consumed in the form of sodium chloride (salt). Because salt is ubiquitous in our food, no dietary deficiency is known. However, chlorine is commonly added in small quantities to community drinking water to reduce the growth of bacteria. Research suggests that the chlorine in drinking water may be carcinogenic, leading to an increase in bladder cancer, particularly in men.[7] Although the health benefits of germ-free water outweigh the possible cancer risk, potential exposure to chlorinated water over a lifetime is significant. Other methods to purify community water are available and should be considered. The

RDA for chloride has not been established but the AI is 2 grams for adults between 51 and 70 years and 1.8 grams for adults over 70 years.

Major sources of chlorine are salt and animal products.

Chromium

Chromium enables body cells to use the glucose from the bloodstream when insulin is present. Long-standing chromium deficiencies may promote adult-onset diabetes. Chromium supplements have been reported to increase uptake of glucose into the cells from the blood. Food processing drastically decreases the amount of chromium available in foods, and this mineral is not replaced by the enrichment process. The RDA for chromium has not been established but the AI is 30 micrograms for men over 50 and 20 micrograms for women over 50.

Chromium-rich foods include brewer's yeast, blackstrap molasses, potatoes, wheat germ, whole grains, and mushrooms.

Copper

Copper helps transport oxygen from the lungs to the body tissues. This mineral is also important in producing the structural fibers collagen and elastin. Symptoms of copper deficiency include anemia, reduced immunity, loss of color in the skin and hair, and damage to the brain and spinal cord. The RDA for copper is 900 micrograms for all adults.

Major dietary sources of copper include shellfish, nuts, cocoa, dried beans, mushrooms, and whole grains.

Iodine

Iodine is needed to make thyroxine, the thyroid hormone which regulates metabolic rate. Iodine deficiencies result in hypothyroidism due to inadequate production of thyroid hormone that can result in an enlarged thyroid (goiter). Radioactive iodine is used therapeutically to treat thyroid disease. Iodine deficiency is rare in the United States because iodine is routinely added to salt. The RDA for iodine is 150 micrograms for all adults.

Major dietary sources of iodine, besides fortified salt, are saltwater fish, clams, oysters, and seaweed.

Iron

Iron is the key component of hemoglobin, which transports oxygen from the lungs to peripheral tissues, and of myoglobin, which transports oxygen to working muscles. Iron is needed to make several enzymes that convert nutrients into energy. It is also needed to produce elastin and collagen, maintain the immune system, and assist in nerve transmission.

Iron is continuously recycled by the body and is depleted only through blood loss. Iron-deficiency anemia is common among elders and may result from impaired iron absorption or from blood loss due to disease or injury. A common cause of blood loss is irritation of the stomach causing bleeding from medications such as aspirin. Insufficient iron causes a shortage of red blood cells, consequently reducing the amount of oxygen available to the tissues.

Symptoms of iron-deficiency anemia are weakness, headache, and heart palpitations. Anemia can lead to congestive heart failure (see Chapter 4, "Chronic Illnesses: The Top Five Killers"). Those who have a vitamin C deficiency may also be more susceptible to iron deficiencies because vitamin C enhances absorption of dietary iron. It is important to realize that anemia is caused by many things besides iron deficiency; only iron-deficiency anemia is treated with iron. Iron levels in the blood are easily tested, and an iron supplement should not be used unless it is needed. Iron supplements commonly cause constipation.

Excess iron can be unhealthy. A disease called hemochromatosis prevents the normal excretion of iron, and iron builds up in the liver, causing cirrhosis. Individuals with this disease should eat a low-iron diet and have periodic blood draws to reduce their iron level. The RDA for iron is 8 milligrams for all adults over 50 years old.

Major dietary sources of iron are liver, dried beans, raisins, prunes, shellfish, and some meats.

Magnesium

Magnesium is required for every major biological process, including the metabolism of glucose for energy, DNA and RNA synthesis, nerve cell function, and muscle relaxation. Magnesium also lowers blood lipid concentrations, stabilizes the heartbeat, and decreases blood clotting.

Marginal magnesium deficiency is extremely common in the U.S. population. This deficiency is particularly common among elders. It may be caused by a low-calorie diet, diabetes, alcohol use, heavy exercise, excessive diarrhea and vomiting, and use of diuretics or digitalis (blood thinner).

Symptoms of magnesium deficiency are nausea, diarrhea, tremors, and loss of appetite or coordination. Magnesium deficiency is the result of a long-term dietary deficiency and occurs when the body has used up its stored magnesium. Occasionally blood tests are normal even though the body is dangerously low in the magnesium stored inside the bones and cells. Detecting a magnesium deficiency requires sophisticated tests of blood and urine.

Studies show a possible link between low magnesium intake and development of diseases as diverse as diabetes, osteoporosis, hypertension, atherosclerosis, cardiac diseases, and asthma. However, it remains unclear whether magnesium supplements benefit persons without a deficiency disease. The RDA for magnesium for men over 30 is 420 milligrams and 320 milligrams for women over 30.

Dietary sources of magnesium include whole-grain cereals, black, navy, lima, and pinto beans, lentils, almonds, and spinach.

Phosphorus

Phosphorus is crucial for every cell reaction that releases or uses energy. This mineral is also an important part of DNA and RNA molecules, cell membranes, and bones, and it helps balance blood acidity. Vitamin D regulates the levels of phosphorus in the blood by controlling the rate at which it is absorbed and excreted. A deficiency is rare because phosphorus is abundant in all proteins and is used as an additive in processed foods such as soft drinks. However, excessive phosphorus intake (soft drinks and meat contain high quantities) may predispose an individual to osteoporosis by increasing the rate of bone demineralization and increasing calcium excretion. The RDA for phosphorus is 700 milligrams for all adults.

Dietary sources of phosphorus are red meats and many soft drinks.

Potassium

Potassium is involved in nerve conduction, muscle contraction, regulation of heartbeat, and body fluid balance. Studies suggest a role for potassium in reducing the excretion of calcium, in stroke prevention, and in preventing abnormal heart rhythms. Diarrhea, the use of diuretics, excessive sweating, and fasting can cause potassium deficiencies. Symptoms of deficiency are rapid heartbeat, muscle weakness, nausea, and vomiting.

High potassium intake has been associated with a decreased risk of hypertension and cardiovascular disease, and the effects may be even more important in blacks.[8] Thus, those who eat diets rich in fruits and vegetables containing potassium have lower blood pressure. Some diuretic drugs used for hypertension deplete potassium, so supplemental potassium is prescribed to maintain blood potassium in the normal range.

Potassium supplementation can have side effects. It can be dangerous for individuals with kidney disease or those on potassium-sparing diuretics. A potassium overdose at only five times the RDA can be fatal. The best way to increase potassium intake is through increased dietary consumption of foods high in potassium. The RDA for potassium has not been established but the AI is 4.7 grams for all adults.

Major dietary sources of potassium are potatoes, raisins, bananas, avocados, cantaloupe, orange juice, sardines, and skim milk.

Selenium

A trace mineral that was once believed to be poisonous, selenium is now known to be a strong antioxidant. It works with vitamin E to protect the immune system by preventing the formation of free radicals and producing antibodies. The pancreas needs selenium to function, and selenium is important to maintain tissue elasticity. The RDA for selenium is 55 micrograms for all adults.

Dietary sources of selenium vary, depending on where the foodstuff is grown. Meat and grains are a good source, as is brewer's yeast.

Sodium

Sodium is needed for nerve transmission and muscle contraction, and it helps maintain the acid-base balance of the blood. It also works with potassium and chloride to affect how much water the body retains and eliminates. Sodium deficiencies are rare because the body needs only about 200 milligrams per day (the amount in one-tenth of a teaspoon of salt). In our country, sodium excesses are common because most processed foods are high in sodium. The RDA for salt consumption is 1,300 milligrams per day for those aged 50 to 70 and 1,200 milligrams per day for those over age 70. The recommended maximum daily consumption is 2,300 milligrams. Excess sodium intake is eliminated in the urine.

The greatest danger of a high-sodium intake is high blood pressure. About half of the people with hypertension cannot effectively eliminate sodium and are said to be "salt-sensitive." Elders are more likely to be salt-sensitive than younger individuals because sensitivity to sodium increases with age. Consuming too much salt further raises the blood pressure of those who are salt-sensitive. The excess sodium in the blood pulls water into the bloodstream from the tissues—water that ordinarily would have been excreted. This excess volume in the blood causes blood pressure to rise. If the arteries are not flexible enough to accommodate the increase, a stroke, congestive heart failure, buildup of fluid in the lungs, or kidney disease can occur. Those with congestive heart failure are also sensitive to salt intake because sodium causes fluid retention, which leads to more stress on the heart. A salt-restricted diet often reduces hypertension.

There is no easy way to determine who is salt-sensitive except by long-term monitoring. Salt-sensitive people need a restricted-salt diet. Cutting back on sodium reduces high blood pressure.

Dietary Supplements: How Can You Spot False Claims?

Be savvy! Although the benefits of some dietary supplements have been documented, the claims of others may be unproven. If something sounds too good to be true, it usually is. Here are some signs of a false claim:

- Statements that the product is a quick and effective "cure-all." For example: "Extremely beneficial in treatment of rheumatism, arthritis, infections, prostate problems, ulcers, cancer, heart trouble, hardening of the arteries, and more."
- Statements that suggest the product can treat or cure diseases. For example: "shrinks tumors" or "cures impotency." Actually, these are drug claims and should not be made for dietary supplements.
- Statements that claim the product is "totally safe," "all natural," or has "definitely no side effects."
- Promotions that use words like "scientific breakthrough," "miraculous cure," "exclusive product," "secret ingredient," or "ancient remedy." For example: "A scientific breakthrough formulated by using proven principles of natural health-based medical science."
- Text that uses overly impressive-sounding terms, like those for a weight-loss product: "hunger stimulation point" and "thermogenesis."
- Personal testimonials by consumers or doctors claiming amazing results. For example: "My husband has Alzheimer's. He began eating a teaspoonful of this product each day. And now in just 22 days, he mowed the grass, cleaned out the garage, and weeded the flower beds; we take our morning walk together again."
- Limited availability and advance payment required. For example: "Hurry. This offer will not last. Send us a check now to reserve your supply."
- Promises of no-risk "money-back guarantees." For example: "If after 30 days you have not lost at least 4 pounds each week, your uncashed check will be returned to you."

Source: www.ods.od.nih.gov

A low salt diet reduces blood pressure levels, enabling some people to stop blood pressure medication.

In 2008, Congress requested that the Institute of Medicine recommend ways to reduce sodium intake in the general population. Subsequently, the Institute of Medicine recommended that this change would need to occur with legislation directed at restaurants and manufacturers mandating that they slowly reduce salt content of prepared food to enable the population to adjust.

Foods high in sodium include sausages, cured hams, hot dogs, fast foods, canned soups, salad dressing, ketchup, mustard, pickles, cheese, chips, and pretzels.

Zinc

Zinc is present in more than 300 enzymes needed for a variety of chemical reactions in the body. It plays an important role in the synthesis of DNA and in proteins involved in immunity. It is also essential for night vision. Zinc deficiency is characterized by a reduced sense of smell, delayed wound healing, and increased susceptibility to infection. Although severe zinc deficiency is rare, marginal zinc deficiencies may be common among elders, especially the poor and hospitalized. Progressive zinc deficiency may play a role in the gradual, age-related decrease in immune response. Zinc lozenges, taken within 24 hours of onset of symptoms, reduces the duration and severity of the common cold in healthy people.[9] The RDA for zinc is 11 milligrams for adult men and 8 milligrams for adult women.

Major dietary sources of zinc include oysters, other seafood, and red meat. Nuts and legumes contain high levels of zinc but also high levels of compounds that reduce its absorption in the body.

DIETARY GUIDELINES FOR AMERICANS

Are you old enough to remember the "Basic Four" food groups? Most middle-aged and older adults recall this effort by the U.S. Department of Agriculture (USDA) to help Americans plan meals and eat more healthfully. Although "Basic Four" is forever a part of our lexicon, these groups are now out of vogue.

The "Food Guide Pyramid," released in 2000, provided a simple visual representation of a recommended diet, heavy on whole grains, fruits, and vegetables, and light on fats, oils, and sweets. Some dietary experts found fault with the Food Guide Pyramid, saying that it recommended too many servings of food daily, didn't take into account physical activity levels, and wasn't balanced, allowing for "good fats" like those found in nuts and olive oil. Researchers were unable to find significant reductions in chronic diseases among people who followed the Food Guide Pyramid.[10] These complaints led to the revision of the guidelines called "My Pyramid." The new food pyramid had more specific advice than its predecessor regarding portion sizes and calories to be consumed daily. Physical activity was added as a new element, and people with access to the Internet could input data about themselves in order to customize

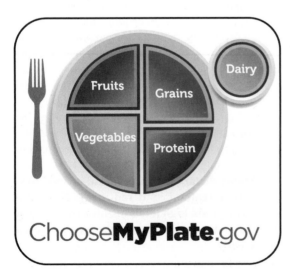

their pyramid. However, many professionals said that the pyramid allowed for too much reliance on refined grains, meat, and dairy products and that it wasn't fair to those without Internet access.

In 2011, the government released a new recommendation that stepped completely away from the pyramid graphic. The new model is called "My Plate." My Plate is a graphic representation of a balanced plate, with half the plate taken up with a combination of fruits and vegetables and the other half with grains and protein. It also includes a small circle for dairy, suggesting a glass of milk or a cup of yogurt. In addition, My Plate has suggestions like "enjoy your food, but eat less," "switch to fat-free or low-fat (1%) milk," and "drink water instead of sugary drinks." The graphic is a simpler, prettier, and more straightforward way to look at eating. However, it does not differentiate between different kinds of food groups (for example, the protein from beans or processed meats) and doesn't include an exercise component. Nonetheless, for the most part it has been met with appreciation. Online, people can get healthy recipes and daily tips or create a customized eating plan. The plan also has a social media component (daily updates via Twitter, for example). Check out the Web page at www.choosemyplate.gov

THE STUDY OF DIET AND NUTRITION

Most people are interested in what they can eat to stay healthy and reduce their risk of disease, and many experts offer advice about foods that we need to eat more of and foods that we should avoid. It is very difficult, however, to answer questions about what foods to eat and how much to eat, for most research is suggestive.

Why is it so difficult to find out what kind of diet is healthy? Most Americans have access to a tremendously varied diet. We can eat a variety of foods year-round. Some are grown locally, but most are grown and packaged in different parts of the United States or in other countries. Further, many people do not eat the same foods regularly. They eat different foods at home, in others' homes, and in restaurants. Most people eat both prepackaged and fresh foods. The foods we eat vary tremendously based on how they are prepared, where they are from, and what micro-ingredients they contain. Foods grown in one place may contain different nutrients than foods grown in another. For example, all apples are not the same. One is flavorful and juicy and has a thick skin; another is mushy and sour. One is a week old; another is a month old. One is small; another is large. It is difficult to measure the nutrients found in a single apple (or any other food) accurately, and this difficulty is compounded when various kinds of apples (or other types of food) from different locations are consumed. Further, food contains many components. Some we understand—minerals, calories, water content—but we do not understand many others that occur in tiny and variable amounts.

In addition to differences within food categories, there are differences among individuals, and it is not clear that the same diet is good for all people. We know that some people can tolerate a high-salt diet without problems while others develop high blood pressure, and some individuals can eat higher-fat diets than others. There are likely differences in how individual bodies digest and utilize foods and nutrients. Particular foods cause gas, heartburn, intestinal distress, and even allergic reactions in some individuals.

Scientists studying the effect of nutrition on health and disease find it very difficult to determine the "average" diet of a person or a population. Researchers attempt in various ways to accurately determine what and how much elders are eating. Each method has its strengths and weaknesses. Surveys are conducted to find out what people are eating and compare their food intake to their risk of disease or to the levels of certain vitamins in their blood. The most common survey is a 24-hour *dietary recall*. Individuals list the types and amounts of foods they ate in the last 24 hours. Sometimes the period is extended beyond 24 hours. A *food record* is usually used to record the types and quantities of all foods eaten over a specified period, usually three days. In a *dietary history,* individuals answer questions regarding the foods they generally eat, the portion

sizes, the frequency, and the food preparation methods used. Individuals might be asked to estimate whether they consume a certain portion size of yams, hamburger, corn oil, or eggs once daily, more than once daily, five to seven times weekly, two to four times weekly, or less than once a week. They also might be asked how long they cook their vegetables and how often they salt their food. Trained dietitians/nutritionists review the results of these surveys, calculate the amounts of various nutrients, vitamins, and minerals consumed, and then estimate the degree of nutrient deficiency or excess.

Surveys rely on self-reports: Individuals are asked to remember or record foods eaten over a specified time period or to estimate how often they consume certain foodstuffs. What is the average number of daily servings of fruits and grain that you ate last week, or so far this month or this year, or over your lifetime? If you don't know, you are not alone. Most people are notoriously poor at remembering what they ate, and those responding to food surveys may not tell the truth—underestimating the number of potato chips and overestimating the amount of broccoli. Poor recall, lack of consistency in filling out the forms, overreporting of nutritious foods and underreporting of junk foods to please the interviewer, and inadequate information about portion size and method of preparation are only a few of the limitations of data from surveys. Studies based on surveys may be biased against different racial or ethnic groups who eat traditional foods that are likely not included on standard questionnaires. It may be difficult to estimate serving sizes or food composition when meals are delivered by Meals on Wheels or served in a restaurant or nutrition site. Also, diet may change over time or vary by cohort or age.

Population studies of community elders may underestimate nutritional deficiencies because they exclude some groups at high nutritional risk: the bedridden, isolated, cognitively impaired, and homeless. And, the information gathered may be less accurate than with younger groups. Those with cognitive or memory impairment are less likely to be able to remember what they ate and to record their dietary intake. Additionally, population data tell little about individual variation. For instance, a study may show that, on the average, elders get enough protein, but, in fact, some may get too much and others too little.

Nationwide surveys, the most widely respected measures of adult nutrition, are periodically conducted to assess whether adults in the population are receiving adequate nutrition. These surveys use some of the methodologies discussed above, including 24-hour dietary recall and dietary history. Three examples are the National Health and Nutrition Examination Survey (NHANES), the Nationwide Food Consumption Survey (NFCS), and the U.S. Department of Agriculture's Continuing Survey of Food Intake by Individuals (CSFI). These and smaller studies provide information about the nutritional status of elders in community and institutional settings.

The National Health and Nutrition Examination Survey (NHANES), conducted periodically since 1971 by the National Center for Health Statistics of the Centers for Disease Control and Prevention, is one of the largest and most-cited studies on nutritional intake. It utilizes a nationally representative sample of 5,000 individuals of all ages each year. The survey includes both an interview and a physical examination. Participants are asked demographic, socioeconomic, dietary, and health-related questions. The physical examination includes medical and dental examinations, physiological measurements, and laboratory tests by medical personnel to gather health and nutrition information such as blood levels of vitamins and minerals, body fat and body composition, height, weight, and blood pressure.

Findings from the survey are used to determine the prevalence of major diseases and their risk factors. They also serve as the national standards for height, weight, and blood pressure. Numerous researchers use the data for research and epidemiological studies. Information on the NHANES is available at http://www.cdc.gov/nchs/nhanes.htm

The overwhelming majority of studies on nutrition measure the nutritional status of a group of individuals at one point in time to see whether there is a relationship between blood levels of nutrients or dietary habits and the subsequent development of disease. Studies may compare persons who have a particular disease with those who do not on some indicator. For example, researchers interested in possible relationships between melanoma and vitamin D may take a group of patients recently diagnosed with melanoma and ask them about their intake of fortified milk and compare their answers to those of a group of patients who do not have a diagnosis of cancer. Then the researchers may draw blood from all the patients and compare vitamin D levels.

Such studies can provide valuable insights into possible relationships between diet and disease, but they are flawed. People who have been diagnosed with a disease differ from those who have not. They are more concerned about their health and in finding out what they might have done differently to keep themselves from getting sick. Thus they may misreport the past—saying that they were either more or less "healthy" than they actually were. Also, the research findings do not indicate whether the nutrient affected the development of the disease or the disease affected the nutrient.

Other studies follow a group of individuals over time and monitor what they eat and measure weight, body mass index, and blood levels of vitamins, minerals, and other nutrients. As individuals develop diseases, the researchers can look at the measures taken earlier on them to see whether the disease may have a nutritional correlation. For example, a study might find that those who ate a lot of blueberries were less likely to develop heart disease. Although studies of this type are preferable to cross-sectional studies, they also face problems. For example, those who eat blueberries may also have other positive lifestyle factors (such as consumption of a lot of other fruits, high levels of physical activity, or even being able to afford to eat blueberries), any one of which might be the actual reason why blueberry eaters are less likely to develop heart disease.

The gold standard for determining the benefits of various nutrients or nutrient supplements is randomized controlled double-blind trials. In these studies, researchers randomly assign individuals (called subjects) to receive either a placebo (a pill that looks real but contains no active ingredient) or a nutritional supplement. "Double-blind" means that neither the subjects nor the researchers know who receives which pill. At the end of the study period, the subjects are evaluated for outcome (for example, the number who had heart attacks). Statistical calculations are done to determine whether there is any association between the nutrient and the subsequent outcome. These studies allow researchers to "control" for all the other things that might cloud the true association between nutrition and disease. These studies are expensive because they can measure only one thing at a time, they involve a lot of people, and they often must continue for years to see whether there is any benefit. Not surprisingly, there are very few randomized controlled trials on nutrition or nutritional supplements.

Despite the challenges of nutritional research, the results of many nutrition studies are reported as fact daily in the media. Headlines proclaim: "Beta-carotene linked to lower bladder cancer rates!" "Blueberries breakthrough for cancer patients" "Omega-3 Fatty Acids Reduce Alzheimer's Disease by 30%!" "South Beach Dieters Lose More Weight." We must be thoughtful as we read press reports about the effect of a particular nutrient on disease. Understanding the types of nutritional studies conducted and their strengths and weaknesses can help us to look at the latest fads and breakthroughs with a critical eye.

NUTRITIONAL STATUS OF ELDERS

Major changes have occurred in the average American diet during the lifetime of the current elder population. The current cohort of elders is likely the first to experience radical changes in diet and food choice in American culture. When they were growing up, everything was made from scratch and foods were eaten fresh and in-season locally. They are now growing old amid microwave ovens, fast-food restaurants, prepackaged dinners, frozen foods, and a dizzying array of produce, ethnic food, and other choices unheard of in the past.

Today, there is increased reliance on prepackaged foods and eating out. Consequently, as a nation, we are consuming more fat, salt, and sugar and fewer whole grains. Within the past few years, there has been a small reduction in fat consumption, particularly animal fat, likely due to research linking dietary fat and heart disease. Consumption of fresh vegetables has been increasing over the last quarter century, but Americans still eat far too little produce and whole grains. Consumption of sugar is rising annually, and the consumption of sodas has been skyrocketing, often taking the place of milk and juices.

Americans consume more than enough calories to keep them overweight but still suffer from deficiencies in many nutrients—including calcium and vitamin D. This trend is even more widely noted among elders. The combination of their increased nutrient requirements due to age and disease and their diminished caloric intakes threatens to increase their risk of nutritional deficiencies. The NHANES reported that over the 30-year period from 1971 to 2000, the number of calories people consumed increased, portion sizes became larger, more meals were eaten outside the home, snacking increased, and there was an increased consumption of supersized sodas. The number of adults taking a multivitamin or using "vitamin"-enriched foods or beverages also increased over the last three decades.[10]

COMMON NUTRITIONAL PROBLEMS

In this section we explore the two most common nutritional problems of American elders: overnutrition and undernutrition. Overnutrition includes obesity and the challenges of dieting, and undernutrition includes unintended weight loss.

Obesity

Obesity and overweight have reached epidemic proportions in America and affect individuals of all ages. According to measurements of body

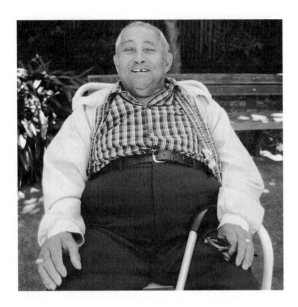

mass index (a ratio of height to weight), more than one of three individuals 60 years of age and older who participated in a national study reported height/weight combinations that placed them in the obese category (BMI over 30).[11] Check the body mass index calculator at www.nhlbisupport.com/bmi to determine your body mass index. Studies show that individuals with body mass index values between 19 and 22 have the best health and the lowest mortality. Health risks begin to accrue at about a BMI of 27 to 28 and increase after a BMI above 30. These risks include chronic illness, surgical complications, sleep apnea, cancers, musculoskeletal disorders, and psychological problems.

Excess weight as measured by BMI is not the only risk to your health. It also matters where the excess fat is stored. If you carry fat mainly around your waist, you are more likely to develop health problems than if you carry fat mainly in your hips and thighs. This is true even if your BMI falls within the normal range. Women with a waist measurement of more than 35 inches or men with a waist measurement of more than 40 inches may have a higher disease risk than people with smaller waist measurements because of where their fat lies.

To measure your waist circumference, place a tape measure around your bare abdomen just above your hip bone. Be sure that the tape is snug (but does not compress your skin) and that it is parallel to the floor. Relax, exhale, and measure your waist. Increased waist size is associated with cardiovascular disease, high cholesterol, high blood pressure, and diabetes.

What is it about excess weight that is associated with health problems? Obese people are also, in general, less active. This promotes further weight gain, of course, but in addition, these individuals lack the protective and health-promoting effects of exercise. Because of decreased mobility and more weight, obese elders are more susceptible to accidents and injuries from falls, painful joints, and overuse. It is more difficult to examine an obese person, so they are more likely to suffer skin problems related to their folds, as well as surgical complications related to poor healing. In addition, obesity is associated with a lower socioeconomic status, which is also associated with poor health outcomes. One of the less obvious reasons is that the obese are often malnourished. Individuals gain weight because they eat too many foods that are high in sugars and fats and low in vitamins and other nutrients. In other words, eating too many calories that are "empty" of nutrition leads to weight gain but not to health. Many of those who are overweight are actually deficient in body proteins and critical nutrients, which means they are in poor health. Some suggest that the obese are more likely to have psychological problems related to stress, guilt, self-hatred, and anxiety due to the American bias and discrimination against overweight individuals. Because these factors all interrelate, it is difficult to tell whether being obese is unhealthy, or whether the lack of health is more related to lack of exercise, poor intake of nutrients, being poor, and being stressed.

It is important to note that the relationship between poor health and being overweight is not as clear-cut or well studied in the elderly, especially those of very advanced age. Some studies suggest that being a little overweight is actually healthful

The Obese Resident
Individual Problems, Staff Problems

Ms. M. is a morbidly obese 65-year-old woman who is 5′1″ tall and weighs close to 400 pounds. She has been obese most of her adult life but was able to live independently. A few months ago, she fell and suffered a hip fracture and was admitted to a nursing home for recovery.

Despite physical therapy, she has been unable to recover her ability to walk and unable even to assist the staff to help her get out of bed. Four staff members are needed to move her from her bed, and they have to use a mechanical lift with special capacity. She feels badly that she is so heavy and they have to work so hard. Moving Ms. M. to a specialized extra-wide wheelchair takes about 40 minutes. In order to place a canvas sling under her, staff must roll her from side to side. The ends of the sling are fastened to hooks on the lift, which hauls Ms. M. from bed and lowers her into the wheelchair, where she sits with the sling underneath her because her weight prevents its easy removal.

Since Ms. M. spends most of her time in bed, she has to have a special air mattress to prevent pressure sores. Her showers routinely take more than two hours to accomplish twice weekly. Despite her weight, blood tests indicate that she is malnourished, and the dietitian works hard to provide her with a diet that is low in calories and fat but high in protein. She takes great pleasure in eating and has difficulty following a calorie-restricted diet. She frequently develops fungal rashes in her skin folds and under her breasts. Although she is continent, she is unable to get up to go to the bathroom quickly enough (the lift is required), so she uses disposable briefs, which aggravate the problems of excess moisture. Staff caring for her suffer a high rate of work-related injuries while trying to move her.

in the later years. It is difficult to determine whether this is because the heaviest unhealthy people have died. Maybe it is because some of the thinnest elders may be the most ill or may be smokers or ex-smokers. Perhaps overweight people have stronger bones and muscles. It has been suggested that those who eat a balanced diet may have to be a little overweight when caloric needs are so low in old age. Some suggest that because elders lose height with age and a natural "expansion of the waistline" occurs, perhaps the waist circumference and the BMI index are not the best measure of ideal weight. It may be that there is a benefit of a little fat "reserve" to be used in case of illness or padding in the case of a fall. Fat produces the female hormone estrone, so it may be that fat reserves somehow protect the bones. Although being lighter is associated with improved health, there is less evidence that weight loss and dieting are as effective as never gaining the weight in the first place.

The problems associated with overweight and obese people are clear. It is easy to say that these people should just "lose weight" or "get healthy." However, this is both an individual problem and a societal one. What contributes to obesity in our country? Many factors have been identified. One is that food is marketed like never before with advertisements that promote snacking and overeating while linking food with pleasure, fun, and status. There are many advertisements about food, but rarely are the advertised foods healthful. Unhealthy foods rich in fat and sugar are often less expensive and more convenient than healthful foods. For many reasons, including subsidies, it is cheaper to buy a soda, a hotdog, and a bag of chips for lunch than it is to purchase a sprout and hummus sandwich on whole grain bread paired with carrot sticks and an apple. In addition, food manufacturers are adding increasing amounts of fats, salts, and sugars to food that might otherwise be healthier in an effort to tempt the American palate. It is not uncommon to add sugar, fat, and salt to a single item, both as part of the cooking process and then as a topping (think nachos—tortilla chips soaked and cooked in oil, then topped with pure fat in the form of cheese). In the United States, sugar and other sweeteners are added to food that in other countries contains no sweeteners, such as salad dressings, sauces, buns, frozen dinners, stews, beans, and meats. Many foods also have very high levels of salt, and many mix all three: sugar, salt, and fat. Prepared foods are much higher in salt, sugar, and fat content in this decade than they were 20 years ago. Portion sizes have exploded as well—the size of a drink or hamburger or what is served in a restaurant or advertised as "normal" is growing. There is a rise in the use of sweetened caloric beverages, such as soda, which provide no nutrition, but which are often ingested throughout the day. There is an increased tendency toward fast, premade, or convenience foods, which are generally of lower nutritional value. Food is more available, and social gatherings are often based around eating, with unhealthy foods always on the menu.

Because obesity is an individual problem and a societal issue, to address obesity, efforts need to focus both on individual behavior and public policy. However, public policy efforts can be controversial—as some ask, what should be the role of the government in the promotion of healthful eating? We saw earlier how the government funds research on nutrition and issues guidelines to promote healthful habits. Other community-based projects to promote healthful eating have included:

- Establishing farmer's markets and community gardens in low-income neighborhoods to increase access to fresh fruits and vegetables
- Regulating vending machines in schools and changing the composition of school lunches
- Subsidies for farms and producers of healthful food to reduce the costs of these foods
- Mandating more information be provided on food labels or how "low nutrition foods" can be packaged, sold, or advertised
- Regulating the fat content of foods sold in restaurants, requiring labeling and offerings of healthful foods

- Adding a tax on "junk foods" to fund nutrition programs
- Linking nutrition education to other services provided to the poor or ill

An individualized approach generally involves identifying who is at risk or is already obese or overweight, assessing the situation, and then developing a plan for the person to lose weight and maintain a lower, healthier weight. The American Dietetic Association reviewed the literature in weight management and concluded that the overall trend is associated with reduced calorie needs as we age combined with less exercise. They have a series of recommendations about how to lower and maintain weight based on evidence. Some of their recommendations are the following:

- Assessment of overweight/obesity should include body mass index (BMI) and waist circumference and evaluation of metabolic rate to better identify the calories a person needs.
- An individualized diet low in calories is recommended. Calories can be reduced by eating less fat or less carbohydrates or both. Weight loss should include portion control—reducing the size of meals and only eating until one is 80 percent full. Calories should be spread throughout the day in 4–5 meals and snacks including breakfast. It may be better to eat more in the morning compared to the evening. Very low calories diets work quicker than reduced calorie diets, but there may be problems with weight regain.
- For some people who cannot control the food they eat, the use of meal replacements— drinking a can of a supplement or eating a prepacked item—can replace 1–2 meals a day. Low-glycemic diets are not recommended.
- Eating 3–4 servings of low-fat dairy foods daily is recommended to get enough calcium.

The best strategy is likely different for each person, but it should be comprehensive. Looking at the psychology of weight (monitoring oneself, managing stress, reducing access to tempting foods, problem solving, making plans for contingencies, social support, and cognitive therapy) can help lead to more weight loss and keeping it off.[12]

In managing obesity in elders, it is critical to remember that even obese elders may be malnourished and have nutrient deficiencies. Because older people have higher nutrient needs due to aging and chronic disease, it can be challenging to meet these needs on reduced-calorie diets. Nevertheless, older people likely realize many health benefits from gradual weight loss, just as younger adults do. Even a small amount of weight loss can reduce disease, particularly knee pain from arthritis, improved blood sugar management for diabetes, and reduced blood pressure and cholesterol level.

Any weight loss plan should focus on reducing calories and maximizing fruits, vegetables, whole grains, and regular exercise. The proposed diet should take food preferences, lifestyle, and income into account. Although many approaches to weight loss have been promulgated, none is as effective or as inexpensive as a combination of reduced calorie intake and increased calorie expenditure (eat less, exercise more). Giving elders skills to change their eating and exercise habits is an important step in achieving weight loss. It is important that regular support and monitoring of food intake and exercise occur. In extreme cases of obesity, medications or even surgery may be effective.

Malnutrition

Malnutrition occurs when a person has an inadequate intake of energy-rich foods. Malnutrition may occur among individuals no matter what their weight. American elders who are malnourished generally have protein-calorie malnutrition. Malnourished individuals undergo complex changes in metabolism that enable them to break down body tissues for energy. At first, expendable tissues, such as fat stores, are mobilized. However, after prolonged malnutrition, muscle and even organ tissue must be utilized. Individuals who are malnourished also reduce their metabolic rate since they are trying to conserve energy. Further, both

the function of the immune system and healing processes are reduced.

People who are malnourished may display symptoms of mental illness. One classic study placed a group of healthy young men on a calorie-deficient diet for six months. The subjects lost weight and reported feeling insecure, irritable, moody, and depressed. They also had no emotional control and no interest in others, and they were unable to make decisions.[13] Because these symptoms are similar to those of people with mental illness, it is important that nutritional inadequacies be ruled out before a diagnosis of disease is made. Malnutrition is not limited to the less-developed parts of the world. Even obese individuals may be malnourished.

Surveys reveal that a significant proportion of American elders suffer from insufficient calorie intake and other nutrient deficiencies. In general, data from national surveys indicate that at least 10 percent of older people interviewed did not consume sufficient calories to meet energy and nutrient recommendations. Further, a substantial proportion of older people had vitamin and mineral intakes below two-thirds of their nutritional requirements. Although the United States produces more than enough food to feed its people, studies continually show that food insufficiency (an inadequate intake of nutrients) is found in the U.S. population, including the elderly.

Analysts of the National Health and Nutritional Examination Survey compared the nutritional status of elders who had enough to eat with the nutritional status of those who did not and reported that those who did not eat enough consumed fewer calories, less protein, less fat, and fewer carbohydrates and had lower intakes of vitamins and minerals. Further, they ate fewer servings of meat and vegetables and had less variety in their diet. Not only did they eat less, but blood levels of nutrients were lower and those who did not eat enough food were more likely to be underweight. They also were more likely to report that their health was fair or poor than did others in their age group. As to be expected, the majority of individuals who did not get enough food were poor.[14] Malnourishment among older people in our country is likely due to a combination of factors: poor food choices, lack of appetite, inability to shop and prepare food, social isolation, and poverty.

Because older people in nursing homes and hospitals are very ill and frail, it is not surprising that many studies report a high rate of malnutrition among that population. Hospitalization exposes elders to the stresses of disease, surgery, and diagnostic and treatment procedures that further deplete their nutritional stores. Many elders lose weight while in the hospital, especially those who require surgery and those who stay in bed. The following list shows the many reasons for malnourishment among institutionalized elders:

Multiple chronic and acute illnesses

Reduced appetite

More need for help in eating, which may not be recognized

Gastrointestinal complaints (nausea, vomiting, diarrhea, constipation)

Medications that affect digestive system, appetite, alertness, taste, and smell

Illnesses that require altered diets that are not appealing

Unfamiliar foods (especially among ethnic elders)

Impaired cognition, confusion, and mood changes

Impaired ability to communicate

Decreased thirst response

Intentional fluid restriction because of fear of incontinence or choking

Psychosocial factors such as isolation and depression

Monotony of diet/quality of "hospital food"

When those considerations are combined with their higher nutrient requirements and increased demands of disease, it is no wonder that the rate of malnourishment is so high. If these factors are not recognized and corrected, there is a tendency toward a downhill spiral of weight loss, reduced immune function, dehydration, development of pressure ulcers and other complications, further dependence, and continued institutionalization. Older people who are malnourished heal more slowly, are more frequently readmitted to the hospital, and exhibit higher rates of infection, accidents, and death.

Many experts suggest that all elders admitted to the hospital have a dietary consultation immediately and then on an ongoing basis with frequent assessments of weight and quantity of food eaten to determine the extent of weight loss. In skilled nursing homes, regulations mandate initial and ongoing nutrition assessments and intervention. Physicians and personnel working in institutions are able to reduce barriers to eating so that malnutrition does not occur there. Medications should be minimized, teeth and mouth problems should be addressed, mealtimes should not be rushed, and nutrient supplements should be provided when needed. In addition, personnel may encourage the patient's family and friends to provide favorite foods to increase appetite. Former food restrictions may be liberalized to increase calorie consumption (e.g. fatty foods, high sugar snacks, and desserts).

Unintentional Weight Loss

Unintentional weight loss has many causes. Weight loss may be related to an acute illness: a cold, a bladder infection, or diarrhea. Alternatively, weight loss may indicate a psychological or psychiatric illness such as depression, anxiety, or loneliness. Weight loss without dieting may be due to an undiagnosed cancer, thyroid disease, or heart or lung disease progression. Weight loss, especially if accompanied by anorexia or lack of appetite, may be due to dementia, cancer, swallowing problems, or the end stages of a terminal illness. Oral health problems—pain in the mouth, ill-fitting dentures, gingivitis, or poor teeth—may cause involuntary weight loss, especially among the frail. Being in the hospital or nursing home is associated with a higher rate of weight loss for the reasons stated above. Any significant weight loss that occurs without dieting in an elder should be quickly investigated.

A Case of Malnourishment
Problems and Solutions

Peter S. is an 89-year-old Italian American man weighing only 100 pounds at 5'5" tall. He is moderately demented. His family reports that he has always been thin and active, and even today he is in constant motion, walking with his walker around the halls of the nursing home. He is often anxious, looking for something. He is served frequent small meals, but he picks at his food and has to be reminded and encouraged to stay in the dining room and eat. Sometimes the nursing home staff feed him. He takes his medications with Boost, a liquid nutritional drink. When he developed a urinary tract infection and had to take antibiotics, he ate even less and spent some days in bed. He lost three pounds over a week and now has a small pressure ulcer on his upper buttock that is very slow to heal. When members of his family bring in food that he is familiar with and share a meal with him, his eating improves.

The interdisciplinary team—the dietitian, the nursing staff, the physician, the physical and recreational therapists, and the social worker—meets with Peter S. and his family. It is decided that because Peter S. eats more with others present, he will be placed in a dining program in which he will eat with a consistent group of residents and staff every day in a location outside his regular unit. He is also participating in a restorative exercise program that allows him to walk outside, which reduces his anxiety and seems to stimulate his appetite. He is given a low dose of Tylenol for his arthritis pain. His family is encouraged to come in as much as possible and to bring him food and encourage him to eat.

The social worker begins to meet with Peter S. briefly on a daily basis to reassure him about issues he is anxious about. Traditional music that he has always loved is provided in his room, and he now lies down for a time in the morning and afternoon to listen to it. Over the next four weeks, Peter S. gains weight and now weighs 107 pounds. He appears calmer and happier.

An investigation into weight loss needs to begin with a thorough medical history and physical examination, with particular attention to symptoms of illness, bowel concerns (constipation, diarrhea, nausea, or heartburn), availability of food, psychological issues, appetite, food preferences, eating habits, and any associated life changes. Because elders who are losing weight are at a high risk of developing pressure sores, a thorough examination of the skin should be conducted. A rectal exam can rule out fecal impaction or retained stool. Laboratory tests can look at the cholesterol, salts, and protein in the blood and check for anemia and signs of vitamin and mineral deficiencies. The services of a speech therapist may be sought to screen for swallowing difficulties. Other tests may be indicated. A dietitian should be consulted to review the diet and weight patterns and to develop a nutritional plan of care (see Box 10.1).

When unintentional weight loss is identified, the first course of action is to support the individual nutritionally while investigating the cause. Nutritional interventions to promote weight gain are legion but work best if individualized. Ways to promote weight gain include offering high-calorie and nutrient-rich foods and "comfort foods," encouraging eating with friends and families, assisting in shopping and meal planning, increasing the visual appeal of foods, and offering fewer and smaller meals on a schedule. For individuals with swallowing problems, alternative food textures may be offered. Often, a medical problem is found that needs to be treated (e.g., dental care, antibiotics for an infection, or relief of constipation). A moderate exercise program may be recommended to improve appetite and health.

For some individuals who don't want to eat or cannot eat sufficient calories, liquid nutritional supplements may be helpful. These may include

---

BOX 10.1

The Dietitian's Role

A dietitian is a trained professional who is an expert in nutrition and food choices as they relate to health. A dietitian is able to consult with your physician to review your medical diagnosis and your prescribed medications and is able to assess your dietary intake. Dietitians analyze the amount of calories, protein, fat, water, fiber, vitamins, and minerals that you need to be healthy, based on your individual characteristics and needs. A dietitian develops nutritional care plans and counsels and educates individuals and their families regarding many aspects of diet and nutrition. Dietitians are commonly involved in the care of people who need special diets, such as those with kidney disease, food allergies,

eating disorders, or diabetes. They also supervise care of people who, because of illness, injury, or surgery, need liquid food given through a tube or an IV line. Dietitions work in hospitals, nursing homes, physicians' offices, and independent office practices.

Registered dietitians have a bachelor's degree and supervised experience, and they have passed a national exam. They operate under referrals from physicians. In some states, they can order laboratory tests. Many people who call themselves nutritional experts or nutritionists lack the license and training of a registered dietitian. To find a registered dietitian, check the American Dietetic Association's referral service (1-800-877-1600) or www.eatright.org

---

vitamin or mineral supplements, concentrated oral nutrition, intravenous nutrition, or feeding through a tube inserted into the nose or directly into the stomach. Many times supplements such as Ensure and Boost are prescribed to increase the ingestion of nutrients—particularly vitamins and minerals, calories, and proteins. Products such as bars and puddings offer concentrated nutrition in small volumes of food.

Although these nutritional supplements are widely used, there is limited evidence as to whether they offer much benefit to elders, particularly those who are healthy.[15] There seems, however, to be some benefit for the frail and for those at high risk (such as those in the hospital, after surgery, or with pressure ulcers).[16]

When weight loss is associated with anorexia or lack of appetite, patients may be prescribed medications to stimulate appetite. Preparing visually appealing meals and offering foods that are enjoyable to eat are important. Sometimes a small amount of alcohol is prescribed to be taken with the meal to improve appetite.

Because unintentional weight loss can be serious among sick older people, all should undergo a thorough physical examination and a complete

nutritional history when admitted to a hospital or nursing home. In addition, elders in hospitals and nursing homes need ongoing monitoring, because reduced appetites, weight loss, and nutrient deficiencies are common. Ongoing monitoring of weight and dietary intake and correction of factors contributing to weight loss are necessary.

DIETARY CONSIDERATIONS FOR SELECTED DISEASES AND CONDITIONS

Poor nutrition is known to contribute to a number of chronic diseases and disorders common to older people. Some diseases (e.g., diabetes) are worsened when particular types of foods are eaten. In these cases, dietary modification reduces the symptoms. Other diseases respond to particular vitamin or mineral supplements. Multiple explanations have been proposed for this phenomenon. A nutrient deficiency may have predisposed the patient to illness in the first place. Or the disease process may have created an increased need for some nutrients. Furthermore, some diseases associated with old age may actually be caused by nutrient deficiencies.

Good eating habits have the potential to prevent or reduce the progress of many chronic diseases.

The exact role that proper nutrition or dietary supplementation can play in the prevention and treatment of chronic conditions is the subject of many research studies and is still poorly understood. The role of diet in several selected diseases and conditions is examined in this section.

Osteoporosis

Osteoporosis, a disease associated with weakened bones and an increased risk of fractures, is highly associated with low dietary intakes of calcium and vitamin D.

Elders can meet the RDA for calcium and vitamin D with a diet high in fruits and vegetables, low-fat dairy products, and calcium-fortified foods. Foods are preferable to supplements because there are many other nutrients in food. However, if dietary intake is low, then supplements should be used. Calcium supplements are inexpensive and generally are well tolerated and well absorbed if taken properly.

Cancer

It is estimated that about one out of three cancer deaths is due to diet, and much research is focusing on the food-cancer connection. Several nutrients are hypothesized to play a role in the prevention of cancer. Multiple large studies have suggested that diets rich in fruits and vegetables, high in fiber, and low in fat are associated with reduced risk of many cancers, including colon, breast, and prostate. These studies suggest that both whole foods and particular nutrients may play a role in the development of cancer.

Whereas some nutrients (e.g., beta-carotene, vitamin C, and calcium) are thought to protect against the development of cancer, others (e.g., food additives and fat) may actually promote cancer. Many of the cancers common in the Western world, including colon, prostate, and breast cancers, are thought to relate to dietary habits. Cooked meat compounds (nitrates) and fungal toxins present in some foods are known to increase cancer risk. Further, high consumption of meats and saturated fats, high alcohol consumption, and obesity are associated with the development of cancer. Deficiencies of several vitamins have been associated with cancer. Low levels of antioxidant vitamins (vitamin E, vitamin C, beta-carotene) in the diet or the bloodstream are associated with increased risks for many cancers, including gastrointestinal cancers, lung cancer, breast cancer, and prostate cancer. Intake of many minerals (e.g., selenium and calcium) and vitamins (particularly antioxidants) and plant components is associated with reduced risk of some cancers.[17,18]

How might diet affect cancer risk? There are many types of cancers, and each type has its own biology, risk factors, treatments, and patterns of development, making it hard to make associations. However, all cancers are abnormal cells that grow and spread unchecked by the body's immune system. It is thought that dietary components may work in the body to prevent cancer by reducing the chance for genetic mutations, modifying hormones, or improving the function of the immune system.

Unfortunately, vitamin and mineral supplements do not seem to work consistently to protect against cancer, and some studies even show increased cancer rates among people taking supplements.[19,20] These studies show the complexity of the relationship between cancer and vitamins and minerals, and they point to the need for further study and careful consideration of supplementation.

Eating a lot of fruits and vegetables is associated with a reduced risk of many cancers. Cruciferous vegetables (broccoli, cabbage, and Brussels sprouts) may protect against tumor formation by releasing a chemical that helps to rid the body of cancer-promoting toxins. These vegetables are more effective if eaten raw. Also, compounds found in garlic, chili peppers, and onions may protect against cancers. Consumption of green and black teas that contain antioxidants is also associated with reduced cancer risk. Consumption of cooked tomatoes in pasta or pizza sauces has been linked to lower rates of prostate cancer. In addition, there is strong evidence that a high-fiber diet is associated with a reduced risk of colorectal cancer.[21]

A high-fat diet is associated with breast, prostate, and colon cancers in animal and large-scale epidemiological studies. However, the association is not strong and not consistent because it is unclear if a high-fat diet predisposes one to develop cancer or accelerates the growth of an existing cancer. It also is not clear which types of fats are the most harmful, although animal fats, trans fats, and polyunsaturated fats have been implicated.

Some additives and preservatives are converted to carcinogens during digestion. For instance, sodium nitrate, used to preserve meats, is converted into nitrosamine, a cancer-causing agent. Vitamin C can neutralize nitrosamines in the body and is sometimes added to foods containing nitrates to prevent toxin formation. Some preservatives (e.g., BHT) act as antioxidants and may be protective against cancers. Saccharin, an artificial sweetener, is known to cause cancer in laboratory animals. Salted and pickled foods are related to the development of stomach cancer.

Cancer increases the need for certain nutrients, but the disease and its treatment often diminish the ability or desire to eat. Lack of appetite occurs in many cancer patients at the time of diagnosis and during advanced illness. *Cachexia,* characterized by a loss of appetite, weight loss, and weakness, is common in advanced cancer victims and is caused by the diversion of nutrients to support growing cancer tissue. Cancer therapies can also reduce food intake or absorption. Radiation therapy can irritate the small intestine and cause diarrhea, reducing the absorption of nutrients into the bloodstream. Those undergoing chemotherapy may experience nausea, vomiting, a full feeling, and changes in smell and taste perception. Both radiation and chemotherapy are associated with pain inside the mouth, which further reduces nutrient intake.

Diabetes

Diet plays a powerful role in the prevention and treatment of diabetes. Both what you eat and how much you eat (and weigh) affects your chance of developing diabetes, how well the diabetes is managed, and whether complications develop. About one in five elders over age 60 has diabetes, so the effects of diet are potentially significant for many.

One of the greatest contributors to type 2 diabetes (adult-onset) is obesity. Most adult-onset diabetics in the United States are obese, and persons who are overweight have an increased risk of developing the disease, especially those who have a large waist. Studies show that people at high risk for type 2 diabetes can prevent or delay the onset of the disease by losing as little as 5 to 7 percent of their body weight.

The top priority for diabetic diets is weight control. In overweight or obese people, the body cells do not respond well to circulating insulin, so blood sugar levels rise. Thus, weight loss is critical to improve diabetic control and reduce complications. For the vast majority of diabetics who are overweight, weight loss is the only treatment necessary. Weight loss is accomplished through (no surprise here!) increased exercise and reduced calorie intake. It is important, however, not just to lower calories but to look carefully at the balance of nutrients in the diet.

Obesity is not the only contributor to diabetes. The amount, timing, and quality of foods eaten also affect the illness. Another important area is consistency in when and how much food is eaten, particularly for individuals who take pills or inject insulin. Diabetics need routine in their diet so that a constant blood sugar level can be maintained and they do not suffer from hypoglycemia (low blood sugar) from skipping meals or from hyperglycemia (high blood sugar) from eating a high-sugar meal. Diabetics must have a high-fiber diet, because fiber slows the rate of digestion and the rate at which sugars are absorbed into the bloodstream. Because diabetes is often associated with high blood pressure and high cholesterol and cardiovascular disease, the DASH eating plan is recommended (see below).

Heart Disease

Many studies have linked the incidence of heart disease with a high intake of saturated fat. Even though most experts agree that saturated fats should be reduced in the diet, there is a controversy about whether polyunsaturated fats or monounsaturated fats are safer substitutes. Current recommendations are to reduce all dietary fat to below 30 percent, with less than 10 percent of all fat to be derived from saturated fats. A decrease in dietary fat reduces both illness and death from atherosclerosis and heart disease. Obesity also plays a major role in increasing the risk of heart disease, and weight loss is known to reduce that risk.[22]

Numerous observational studies report the association of many vitamins, minerals, and dietary components with the development of cardiovascular risk factors, atherosclerosis, hypertension, and cardiovascular disease. Low serum levels of the antioxidant vitamins (A, C, and E), minerals (magnesium and selenium), B vitamins, soy proteins, coenzyme Q, and other nutritional components have been implicated in the development of heart disease. However, interventional studies (in which subjects are provided with supplements of vitamins, minerals, or dietary components and later tested) have reported inconsistent results. Some studies show benefits, others show higher risks, and still others show no effect at all unless the individual had a deficiency at the start of the study. There are two exceptions: Niacin supplementation in high doses is an effective treatment for elevated cholesterol, and omega-3 fatty acid supplementation may be helpful for cardiovascular disease.

It is clear that diet plays an important role in cardiovascular health. Those who already have heart disease or are at high risk of it (those with hypertension, obesity, a sedentary lifestyle, smokers, high cholesterol levels, or a strong family history) are recommended to follow the DASH eating plan (Dietary Approaches to Stop Hypertension), which is based on a diet high in protein, complex carbohydrates, and monounsaturated fats, and low in saturated fats, trans fats, and simple sugars. The DASH eating plan focuses on educating people how to cook using less fat and how to prepare and eat more fruits, vegetables, low-fat dairy products, whole grains, fish, poultry, and nuts. The diet is low in red meat, sweets, and sugar containing beverages and rich in vitamins and minerals (particularly magnesium, potassium, and calcium), protein, and fiber. Studies on the DASH eating plan among those with heart disease showed rapid and sustained reductions in blood pressure, particularly if it includes a low sodium diet. Details on the DASH eating plan can be found at www.nhlbi.nih.gov and type DASH Eating Plan in the search bar.

Dysphagia

Dysphagia, difficulty swallowing, is a common diagnosis among elders. Alzheimer's disease, strokes, and other cognitive and physical impairments can create problems in the coordination of biting, chewing, and swallowing food. Signs of possible swallowing problems include weight loss, eating more slowly, food "pocketing" (the presence of unswallowed food in a person's mouth an hour after a meal), drooling, and coughing or choking while eating. Swallowing problems can lead to aspiration, which occurs when food or liquid meant for the stomach is mistakenly taken into the lungs, possibly causing aspiration pneumonia, a very serious condition.

Swallowing problems can be diagnosed by a speech therapist or through tests in which a person is asked to swallow a radio-opaque liquid or food and X-rays are taken of the swallowing process. Depending on the type of swallowing problem, exercises or changing the way a person eats sometimes can help. Alternating bites of food with liquid, tucking one's chin while swallowing, or using a straw may help.

Individuals with dysphagia need special diets and food preparation. Their food may be pureed in a blender or chopped up or minced. Sometimes, liquids must be thickened to reduce the risk of aspirating fluid into the lungs. Some people cannot tolerate even water—it makes them choke. They need water to be thickened to a nectar or even a pudding-like consistency so they can safely drink it. Many foods—such as those that are fibrous or of mixed textures (e.g., salad)—should be avoided. Making the food palatable is often a challenge, and individuals with dysphagia have difficulty ingesting enough fiber to prevent constipation. Specific information about dysphagia diets, foods to use and avoid, and how to prepare meals for those suffering from dysphagia is found at www.asha .org and type Dysphagia in the search bar.

Artificial Feeding

Persons no longer able to take food in by mouth—perhaps they have a cancer growing in the mouth or esophagus, their intestines are not working, or a severe stroke has left them no longer able to swallow safely—must be fed artificially. Artificial feeding may be accomplished by inserting a tube into a vein or directly into the stomach or intestines. To decide which kind of artificial feeding is best, the first consideration is whether the feeding will be needed for a short time or long-term. In addition, it must be determined whether the stomach and intestines are functioning to move food through and appropriately absorb nutrients. Short-term artificial feeding may be used for elders who are malnourished to increase their stamina, for those who are undergoing cancer chemotherapy, or for those who are unable to eat after surgery. Elders with cancer of the throat or stomach and those with severe bowel problems often must be fed through tubes (intravenous or into the intestine) for prolonged periods of time because they are unable to take oral nutrition. Likewise, those with neurological illnesses, such as strokes or end-stage dementia, are often unable to swallow and may be maintained by tube feeding for months or years.

If the intestines are working and a short-term solution is needed, a nasogastric tube is often the first step. The tube is inserted through the nostril, down the back of the throat, through the esophagus, and into the stomach. This procedure can be done by a nurse at the bedside. The tube is left in place and taped to the nose, and fluids and liquid foods (such as a liquid nutritional supplement) are inserted through the tube with a syringe. This is a temporary measure. The tube can cause a lot of irritation of the nose and throat and is unsightly and uncomfortable.

If long-term feeding is necessary, then a hole is punctured into the skin of the abdomen and a tube is threaded into the stomach or jejunum. If the tube is placed in the stomach, it is called a G-tube (G for gastric), and if it is placed in the jejunum (the small intestine), it is a J-tube. If there is one tube in each, it is called a G/J tube. The tubes make it possible to bypass the mouth and provide water, food, and medications directly into the stomach or intestines. A person can still eat with a J or a G tube, and most people do not find the tube painful. However, the tubes can dislodge, cause skin irritation around the opening, or leak, and elders who are confused may pull them out.

If the digestive system is not functioning temporarily (perhaps because a portion of the intestines was removed or, after surgery, the intestines have not yet started functioning again), the best option is to initiate intravenous (IV) or parenteral nutrition. In this case, a solution of sugars, fats, proteins, vitamins, and minerals are introduced directly into the bloodstream through a vein through a long tube. This is a high-risk procedure that requires a large IV line that is usually inserted into a central or major vein in the chest.

Because there is a risk of infection, deficiency diseases, and problems with the balance of nutrients in the bloodstream, IV feeding requires careful monitoring in a hospital or nursing home. Individuals receiving intravenous nutrition often receive insulin and frequent blood tests to ensure the balance of nutrients is correct. Artificial feeding of any type may cause nutrient imbalances, fluid overload, or agitation related to being "hooked up" to tubes and should be supervised carefully by a physician and a dietitian. IV nutrition has a high rate of complications, including nutritional deficiencies and imbalances and infection. For these reasons, IV feeding is often recommended for short-term nutrition (for example, in the case of a bowel obstruction) to reduce severe nutritional deficiencies.

Long-term use of artificial feeding must be carefully considered. Artificial feeding is a medical procedure that is associated with risks and benefits. It is important that elders or those deciding for them fully understand the risks and benefits when making these decisions. Most patients and families do not consider artificial feeding unless there is a good chance that the patient's condition will improve. On the other hand, some

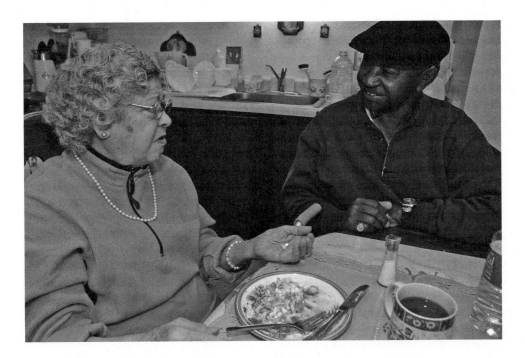

believe that withholding artificial feeding is like starving a loved one to death; they may not want to prolong life artificially but are concerned that death by starvation or dehydration is inhumane. The decision is especially challenging because it must be made quickly, and because many individuals needing artificial feeding never expressed their wishes about it. Many physicians no longer routinely recommend tube feeding of patients with neurological problems such as strokes or with end-stage dementia because there is little evidence that it brings significant improvements in length or quality of life.

The general consensus in the medical field is that dehydration is not uncomfortable and that measures can be taken to ease any discomforts related to terminal illness. Many times, a compromise is sought. For instance, if an elder suffers a massive stroke that affects swallowing, artificial feeding may be used during rehabilitation. However, if the elder remains unconscious, artificial feeding may be discontinued to allow the individual to die. To provide a more natural end of life, the dying individual may be fed small amounts of

liquid or food even though he or she is not able to swallow very well and risks aspirating the food.

EFFECT OF DRUG USE ON NUTRITIONAL STATUS

Many prescription and over-the-counter drugs affect nutritional status. Some irritate the stomach, cause nausea, vomiting, diarrhea, or alter the absorption or excretion of nutrients. Others alter electrolyte balance, carbohydrate or fat metabolism, or levels of healthful bacteria in the digestive tract. Drugs that alter taste perception can drive people either to overeat in search of satisfaction or to lose their appetite. Appetite may be increased directly by some drugs or indirectly by improving mental status. Grapefruit juice is a powerful inhibitor of one of the enzymes that break down many medications. Current diet, other drugs taken concurrently, and presence of chronic illness must be taken into account when analyzing the effect of drug intake on nutritional status. Table 10.2 illustrates a few of the more common food-drug interactions.

TABLE 10.2	Selected Nutrient-Drug Interactions

Antacids: Magnesium salts can cause diarrhea, which can impair intestinal absorption. Reduce acidity of stomach, perhaps altering protein digestion.

Antibiotics: Tetracycline can block absorption of iron, magnesium, and calcium salts. Other antibiotics can impair folic acid action in the body.

Anticoagulants: Can cause vitamin K deficiency. When taken with vitamin E supplements, may cause excessive blood thinning.

Anticonvulsants: Can induce folate and vitamin D deficiencies.

Antidepressants: Can accelerate breakdown of vitamin D.

Antidiabetics agents: Some inhibit absorption of B_{12}.

Aspirin: High doses may cause gastrointestinal bleeding, which can result in anemia. Can increase requirements for vitamin C, K, and folic acid. Can cause nausea and vomiting. When taken with vitamin E supplements, may cause excessive blood thinning.

Barbiturates: Can speed breakdown of vitamin D. Excessive sedation may cause missed meals. Can impair absorption of folic acid.

Cancer chemotherapy: Causes nausea and vomiting. Impairs appetite and absorption.

Colchicine: Can inhibit secretion of enzymes needed to break down complex sugars.

Corticosteroids: Can decrease pancreatic enzymes and cause stomach irritation. Can impair absorption of vitamins C, A, and D, folic acid, and potassium.

Digoxin: Can cause nausea and vomiting.

Diuretics: Can cause loss of potassium in the urine. Low levels of potassium in the blood can cause mental confusion and high blood pressure. Long-term use may cause calcium and magnesium deficiency.

Estrogen: Extended therapy can result in deficiencies of folic acid and vitamin B_6.

Ibuprofen: Can cause stomach irritation.

Laxatives: Can cause diarrhea-like effects whereby food passes through the intestines too quickly to be totally absorbed. Mineral oil binds fat-soluble vitamins, impairing their absorption.

MAO inhibitors: Cannot eat foods containing tyramine (wine, hard cheeses, chocolate, beef, or chicken livers).

Opioids: Can cause nausea and vomiting unless taken with food.

Alcohol causes many nutrient deficiencies. First, we have to remember that alcohol has calories. They have been called empty calories because although they provide energy, they do not provide other nutrients, vitamins, minerals, fat, or protein. Individuals who drink heavily tend to eat less because they have reduced appetite. When those who drink heavily do not eat or eat poorly, weight loss and nutritional deficiencies develop. In addition, alcohol affects food absorption and utilization by damaging the stomach, liver, and pancreas. Excessive alcohol consumption can lead to deficiencies in proteins, water-soluble vitamins, magnesium, potassium, and zinc. Zinc absorption is decreased, and its excretion is increased. Magnesium is excreted in abnormal amounts in alcoholics and excessive iron is absorbed, causing liver damage.

Heavy drinkers often have inadequate vitamin D production, resulting in calcium deficiency and osteoporosis. Some vitamins and minerals are needed in higher amounts in alcoholics to repair the damage caused by alcohol. Thiamine, and to a lesser degree other B-complex vitamins, are particularly subject to depletion since they are needed to metabolize alcohol.

Cigarette smoking also increases the need for particular nutrients. The Food and Nutrition Board recommends that smokers get more vitamin C. In addition, deficiency of B-complex vitamins, especially B_{12} and folate, may act synergistically with cigarette smoking in the development of lung cancer. For smokers, as for other adults, it is best to increase consumption of nutritious foods to raise levels and supplement only if deficient. Although cigarette smoking is traditionally associated with weight loss, it may actually result in weight redistribution, with more fat concentrated in the midsection, a weight pattern associated with increased mortality.

To reduce the chance of food-drug interactions, elders need to be directed to read prescription inserts carefully and talk to their physician or pharmacist about food-drug interactions. The package insert has a section on nutrient-drug interactions— the print is small, but the information is important. Also, some medications should be taken with food, and others should be taken on an empty stomach. If that information is not on the label, it is important to search it out in order to maximize the effect of the drug. No matter whether a new drug is prescribed or a drug has been taken for a long time, it is important to ask the physician or pharmacist whether the drug increases any vitamin or mineral deficiencies.

VITAMIN AND MINERAL SUPPLEMENTS

Vitamin and mineral supplements are usually ingested in pill form, though sometimes as liquids or powders. They provide varying amounts of single vitamins or minerals or combinations of vitamins and minerals (called multivitamins) intended to supplement food intake "just in case" a person's nutritional needs are not being met by food. Multivitamin supplements are intended to supply at least 100 percent of the Recommended Daily Allowances of vitamins and minerals. There are many brands of multivitamins on the shelves, some of them specifically formulated for older people. The majority of older people take some type of vitamin and mineral supplement to promote health.

One of the most controversial issues in nutrition is whether supplements of particular vitamins and minerals or a multivitamin supplement should be recommended to older people. A search through the medical literature or on the Internet brings up thousands of articles and studies suggesting that Supplement A is healthful or that Supplement B prevents disease, boosts the immune system, improves vision or energy, or reduces risk of cancer. It

seems obvious that supplements are good. Many doctors recommend them. What can be the problem?

Although most people believe that taking vitamins promotes good health, there is no scientific consensus as to whether they are effective. While it appears that many studies show a benefit of vitamins ingested as supplements, the researchers who review those studies report that no benefits are evident, and they criticize the studies for their weak research methodology.[23,24] Studies seem to indicate that, with a few exceptions, vitamin and mineral supplements do not seem to improve health unless the person taking them has a deficiency.

How can it be that high vitamin intake from foods and high blood levels of vitamins are so beneficial while vitamin supplements do not offer the same benefits? Aren't vitamins like a kind of insurance, giving us what our bodies need in case we don't follow a good diet every day? The only studies that can answer the question about whether vitamin or mineral supplements (either alone or in combination) have beneficial health effects are randomized controlled trials. As you recall, these trials involve giving vitamins to one group of people, giving a placebo to another group of people, and not telling participants of either group which pill they are getting. After varying lengths of time, depending on the study and assuming both groups continue to take the pills, the two groups are compared to see whether the group receiving the supplement performed better than the group without supplementation on one or more health measures.

One area where researchers hoped to find a benefit of supplementation was antioxidants. Three antioxidants—vitamin C, vitamin E, and beta-carotene—have received much media attention for their possible role in preventing heart disease, cancer, and other illnesses. These nutrients are believed to help the body protect itself from damage caused by free radicals (see Chapter 2, "Biologic Aging Theories and Longevity").

Many population-based studies have documented that people who eat a diet high in antioxidant vitamins, or those with high blood levels of these vitamins, have lower rates of cancer, hypertension, stroke, heart disease, and other conditions—and even greater longevity. Studies also show that those who choose to take antioxidant supplements have a lower rate of many types of cancers. Controlled trials of antioxidant supplementation, however, found them not to be as helpful as first believed and, in some cases, harmful.

Antioxidant supplements are not a substitute for eating healthfully. Why not? It may be that what reduces the risk of cancer and heart disease is not the specific vitamin but rather the habit of eating a variety of fruits, vegetables, and whole grains that happen to be high in antioxidants. While fruits and vegetables are rich in vitamins C, E, and beta-carotene, they also contain literally hundreds of other compounds, many of them not fully characterized, that may be the "real" health-protective molecules. Beta-carotene, for example, may not by itself be healthful, but may instead serve as merely an "indicator" for a host of other beneficial chemical substances found in fruits and vegetables. Further research is attempting to isolate other helpful compounds that may influence the positive health effects. For instance, compounds called flavenoids, found in many fruits and vegetables, are associated with reduced cancer risk. The few antioxidants that have been isolated and packaged into pills are likely a very small component of the benefits from eating whole foods.

What could possibly be wrong with taking supplements? We do know that several good studies report increased risk of disease and death from taking some types of supplements (vitamin E and beta-carotene), and this finding is concerning. Maybe the chemical form of the vitamin supplement is not what the body needs, or perhaps the supplement inhibits the body from absorbing other important nutrients in food. Supplements may be contaminated and have unhealthful ingredients in them. Supplements may interfere with medications that are taken or possibly even interfere with appetite and food intake. Or individuals may be taking the "wrong supplement."

What about the purported benefits of supplements on other areas of health: immune system, cognitive function, eye health? A meta-analysis of studies on vitamin supplementation and immune function found little support for supplementation.[23] Likewise, a meta-analysis of several randomized placebo-controlled trials of supplements believed to counteract cognitive decline found no consistent benefit.[25] Finally, studies on supplements for eye health support the role of vitamins and a mineral supplement for some elders who already have certain forms of age-related macular degeneration, but research does not support the use of supplements to prevent eye disease or treat diabetic eye disease or cataracts.[26]

So, should all elders take a multivitamin? About one-third of the population already does and these are often the healthier people—so, should we all take a multivitamin to be healthy? Although it sounds good that a multivitamin promotes health by "filling in any gaps" from poor diet, the scientific research does not support the health benefits of taking a multivitamin. A study published in 2009 from the Women's Health Initiative found no association between multivitamins and cancer or cardiovascular disease risk or total mortality in postmenopausal women.[27] In 2006, a National Institutes of Health State-of-the-Science Panel reviewed the randomized controlled trials and determined the evidence was insufficient to make recommendations to prevent chronic disease in healthy people.[28] The U.S. Preventive Services Task Force (www.ahrq.gov) does not recommend a multivitamin in healthy adults for disease prevention.

So, if the experts do not think healthy adults need multivitamins (or there is not enough evidence to suggest they help anyway), then who should take supplements at all? Those who should take supplements are those whose intakes are insufficient to supply the basic recommended amounts through food. This may include those on very low calorie diets, those with diseases that deplete vitamins or minerals, those who are ill (with increased requirements), or those who have difficulties absorbing these essential elements. The American Dietetic Association position paper on vitamin supplementation provides some guidance on when vitamin supplementation should be considered.[29]

The most likely vitamins recommended may include vitamin D and calcium for those with low

FDA Oversight of Dietary Supplements

Because dietary supplements are considered to be food, not drugs, the FDA regulates dietary supplements under a set of regulations different from those covering foodstuffs and prescription and over-the-counter drugs. Although drug manufacturers must prove their products are both safe and effective prior to obtaining FDA approval for distribution, manufacturers of dietary supplements do not. No regulations ensure the purity, strength, or even the presence of the ingredients listed on the labels of dietary supplements. Further, their safety or effectiveness is not guaranteed. Why does the FDA have less oversight over supplements than over food or drugs? Both the companies that make supplements and the

consumers who use them do not want to have to visit a physician to purchase them.

If the FDA receives complaints from consumers that a supplement is dangerous after it is on the market, the agency investigates. In general, multiple serious complaints must be received before the FDA acts. The FDA does monitor the labeling and package inserts of products to ensure they meet the law and do not make false claims. The Federal Trade Commission regulates the advertising of dietary supplements. The label information must not mislead the public. For instance, no statement of prevention or treatment of particular disease may be made if scientific evidence does not support it.

intakes and inadequate sun exposure, B vitamins for those with absorption problems, and omega-3 fatty acids for those with diets low in fish. If supplements are taken, it is important to inform the doctors about their use because they can interfere with some medications.

The Office of Dietary Supplements, part of the National Institutes of Health, aims to improve knowledge about supplements by evaluating scientific information, stimulating and supporting research, disseminating research results, and educating the public. The agency provides up-to-date supplement fact sheets with recommendations on daily intakes together with information on nutrient consumption and health status, risks of excessive intakes, groups at risk for inadequate intakes, and related topics. See www.ods.od.nih.gov

FACTORS AFFECTING NUTRITIONAL STATUS

A number of variables affect food selection and consequent nutritional status. This section surveys some of the many factors influencing food selection and nutritional status among elders.

Physiological Factors

Disability from chronic illness can severely affect mobility, energy level, and visual acuity and thus decrease interest in eating and ability to shop for and prepare food. Visual decrements can make it difficult for elders to read labels, comparison-shop, and cook. Reduced mobility may force an elder to shop only at nearby stores, which may be expensive or offer little selection. Disabled elders may overuse prepackaged foods. Medication-related problems (reduced ability to taste or smell, lack of appetite, dry mouth, and nausea) affect the ability and motivation to eat. Further, dental problems, such as ill-fitting dentures, lack of teeth, and poor oral hygiene, can make chewing difficult and reduce motivation to eat. Food intolerances and the necessity of following a prescribed diet can also affect interest in food and narrow food choices. Alcohol misuse is a very common cause of lack of interest in food and subsequent malnutrition.

Psychological Factors

Emotional state can have profound consequences on an individual's motivation to shop for and prepare nutritious meals. Anxiety and depression can cause either a diminished appetite or overeating. Elders who are lonely or grieving may be less likely to cook for themselves and may depend on toast and tea or processed snack foods. Those who are depressed or who have low self-esteem may not want to leave the house to shop or may be too lethargic to cook. Medications affecting alertness can impact diet as well.

Educational Factors

Level of education and knowledge about nutrition affect food choices and methods of meal preparation. Elders with a high educational level generally have fewer nutrient deficiencies than those with less education. For instance, elders with a low educational level may fry foods, whereas those with more education may steam or broil their foods. Elders who are illiterate, who have minimal nutrition education, or who speak English poorly may be unable to read and understand product labels. Also, elders who are less educated may select foods based on advertisements or coupons. Items available by coupons are often those that are highly processed and low in nutrients. Those with severe cognitive deficits may be incapable of shopping or preparing meals for themselves.

Economic Factors

Financial status influences the quality and quantity of food purchased. Income is related to diet quality. Go to a poor area and look to see if there are health food stores, produce markets, or grocery stores. Many times there are not, and instead there are convenience stores that sell processed items with a long shelf life that are full of sugar, simple carbohydrates, and fat. Poor-quality food is cheaper than high-quality food. It may take more time to purchase and prepare higher quality foods, which can be difficult for those who are disabled or need to work long hours. Elders who are poor are less likely to have an adequate diet because many high-nutrient foods are expensive. Elders who rely on economic assistance programs are more likely to have poor nutritional intake. Those with higher incomes can afford to spend more on food. However, a high income does not ensure nutritional adequacy.

Living Arrangements

Social interaction patterns affect food intake and nutritional status. People living alone have the poorest diets. Social isolation can also affect the motivation to shop, prepare meals, or eat well. Many elders do not like to prepare and eat a meal alone or go out to eat alone. Older men living alone have poorer diets than those living with a spouse; however, this same trend is not noted among older women. Elder women tend to eat a greater variety of foods than men and are more likely to choose fresh fruit, vegetables, and milk products, while men eat more meat. Also, older people who live alone may have physical or mental problems that make food preparation difficult. Other variables might reduce the ability to shop for food: living in a high-crime area, inability to drive a car, and lack of access to public transportation.

Cultural Attitudes and Behaviors

Differences in eating patterns among age groups are common because each generation grew up in a different cultural milieu. For instance, many elders associate white bread with wealth and beans with poverty. Elders from varied ethnic backgrounds may limit food choices to traditional foods that are available locally. Food consumption habits established early in life may be hard to break. However, numerous studies show that elders are open to trying new foods and that eating patterns may change dramatically with age.

Environmental Factors

The availability of community nutrition programs, distance from shopping facilities, transportation availability, and geographical location can also affect food choices and nutritional status. Elders in the inner city may have reduced access to supermarkets, and often small grocery stores close to home are expensive. Inner-city elders, especially women and those who have a hard time walking, may be reluctant to shop because they are afraid of being crime victims. Fresh fruits and vegetables are more available and less expensive in some areas than in others. Climate may affect food choices. Winter snows and excessive heat may confine some older people to their homes. Additionally, elders in rented rooms or hotels have limited access to cooking or refrigeration facilities.

NUTRITION ASSESSMENT

Health professionals need to be alert to signs and symptoms in elders suggesting poor nutrition. Malnutrition and dietary inadequacies generally develop gradually, and manifestations are subtle. Nonspecific symptoms may be attributed to age changes or chronic illnesses and be ignored by both the elder and the physician. Nutritional status is notoriously difficult to evaluate and may not be seen as a priority for elders or their physicians.

Assessment of dietary practices is an important part of medical care. Federal regulations now specify that nutritional screening be included when elders are provided with home health services and in hospitals and nursing homes. Assessment should include measures of weight taken over time to document weight gains or losses that may have been missed by the elder or family. In addition, assessing dietary intake (including level of appetite, number of meals per day consumed, and the person's recall of foods eaten) is important. Accounts from family members are very helpful. Physical complaints that may be related to food should be followed up: constipation, stomach upset, anorexia (lack of appetite), and functional status (particularly ability to shop and prepare meals) are important. Important components of the nutritional assessment include an evaluation for alcoholism, as well as information about alterations in psychosocial status (e.g., recent bereavement), depression, and medications used.

A physical examination can give important information about dietary practices. Many oral and dental problems, for example, are associated with poor nutrition. During a physical exam, it is important to evaluate whether an elderly patient can swallow well. Coughing after taking in liquids, for example, may signify that the elder is aspirating food into the lungs. Muscle wasting, reduced cognitive skills, and clinical signs of dehydration are important clues that malnutrition may be present. Blood tests can detect the consequences of a poor diet such as low levels of protein in the blood, anemia, low levels of vitamins, abnormal cholesterol measurements, and imbalances in salts.

Tools and resources developed by the Nutrition Screening Initiative can be helpful. The Nutrition Screening Initiative (NSI) was a collaborative project of more than 25 professional organizations committed to identifying and getting services to people with the greatest nutrition risk.

The National Screening Initiative includes a brief 10-item checklist that is easily scored and can accurately identify noninstitutionalized older persons at risk for low nutrient intake and dietary health problems. To educate elders and those who care for them, the group also identified several warning signs of poor nutrition to accompany the questionnaire. Although the project ended in 2006, the questionnaire and warning signs of poor nutrition are useful and can be downloaded at www.cdaaa.org

NUTRITION EDUCATION AND COUNSELING

Nutritional education and counseling can prevent or reduce the progression of disease and improve general health and well-being. Although physicians may provide dietary counseling, they are inadequately trained in this area, and nutritional counseling can be time-consuming. Therefore, it is often preferable for a trained nutritional counselor to provide counseling and education to elders—assessing dietary deficiencies, setting goals to improve diet, and monitoring progress.

Individual sessions with elders and their families may discuss nutritional problems and develop acceptable solutions. Nutrition education can be effective in a group setting. Lectures, cooking demonstrations, and discussions regarding a variety of interesting nutrition topics can be accomplished at senior centers, nutrition sites, assisted living complexes, and churches. Cooking classes, potlucks, and community gardens provide elders with opportunities to socialize while learning about healthy eating. Pamphlets, large print nutrition newsletters in simple language, nutrition columns in local newspapers, and television–based cooking programs are only a few of the ways to sensitize older people about the importance of diet and health. In some places, elders are trained as peer nutrition counselors to reach out to the homebound.

Nutrition education and counseling should not be a one-shot educational session; it is most effective if continued over a long period of time. The counselors and clients can regularly review and adapt the diet regimen to the clients' changing needs or wants. Success is increased if spouses or friends attend the counseling sessions to give support to the clients. These individuals may be counseled on ways to ensure that elders under their care are receiving adequate nutrition.

To be effective, nutritional counselors must consider the multiple factors that affect nutritional status—food preferences, cultural issues, educational level, economic status, and health condition—when advising clients on dietary practices. Special efforts should be directed toward low-income, uneducated, isolated, and minority elders. It is also important that counselors are trained not only in providing information but in facilitating behavior change.

Perhaps one of the most critical aspects of working with older people to improve their nutrition is to understand their cultural backgrounds. Each year, the older population of the United States becomes increasingly ethnically and racially diverse. It is imperative for individuals preparing to work in the field of health and human services to have the knowledge, attitudes, and skill to be able to communicate with and meet the varied needs of this diverse group. In the field of nutrition counseling and education in particular, learning about traditional foods and ways of food preparation, and becoming sensitive to the meaning of food in another's culture, are pivotal before any education and counseling occur. Just as food in our culture has many layers of meaning, so it is with other population groups. Influences such as religion, views of the family, levels of income, social meanings of food, and traditional foods and their preparation have a tremendous impact on individuals' lives.

Materials directing health messages to a particular ethnic or racial group should be thoughtfully produced. Not only must they be provided in the languages of target populations, but also they should take cultural differences and literacy levels into consideration. Further, diagrams and photographs should be culturally specific, relevant, and effective. It is imperative that the materials be pilot-tested on the target population before distribution.

Encouraging older people to attend nutritional education and counseling programs involves reeducating professionals who work with older people about such programs' importance. A major component of the Nutrition Screening Initiative is the education of physicians and other professionals about the importance of good nutrition, strategies to screen for nutritional risk, techniques to ascertain etiology of risk, and methods to improve patients' nutritional status through education and counseling.

NUTRITION PROGRAMS

The federal Administration on Aging allocates funds for the Elderly Nutrition Program to each state, which then allocates funds to each local Area Agency on Aging to provide a daily meal to elders. In addition, volunteers provide nutrition screening, nutrition education, and meal-planning counseling to participants. Two types of nutrition programs are offered. *Congregate meal programs* are community-based and are directed to elders who are able to leave home. Transportation is generally provided to

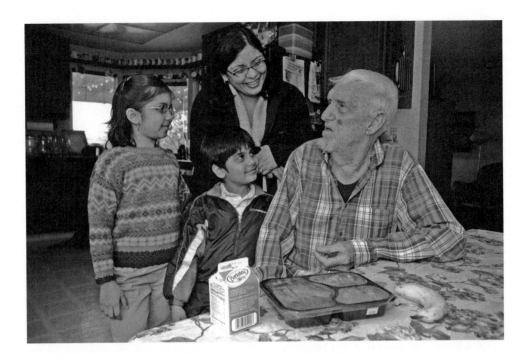

the site. The community feeding programs may be offered at churches, senior centers, congregate living facilities, or schools. Besides the meal, the program provides the opportunity to socialize. In contrast, *in-home programs* (usually called "Meals on Wheels") deliver meals to the homebound. During the meal delivery, the volunteers monitor the health of the homebound and make sure they are getting the help they need. An older person who is no longer homebound becomes ineligible for home-delivered meals.

Both programs are offered at no cost to individuals 60 years and older. They are mandated to provide at least one-third of an individual's daily nutritional needs, and they are geared to deal with individuals with special dietary requirements. Because federal funding is not sufficient to meet the needs of the community to serve all elders, state, county, or city resources, donations, private foundations, the United Way, volunteer support, and contributions from older adults generally augment the federal money. Even with augmented funds, many communities have waiting lists as the number of individuals who want to participate

surpasses the amount of money available for meals. Some communities do not offer nutrition programs for older people.

Elders served by congregate and in-home programs often are at high risk for nutritional deficiencies. They are likely to be either over- or underweight, have physical impairments, be poor, or live alone. New federal guidelines require states to screen potential clients for congregate meal and in-home nutritional programs with the National Screening Initiative questionnaire, mentioned above. An evaluation revealed that both programs were quite successful in providing high-quality nutrition-rich food to many individuals who otherwise couldn't afford it. Participants had lower rates of nutritional deficiency for many vitamins and minerals in comparison with elders not participating. These programs have been found to be effective at serving isolated, poor, and minority elders referred through physicians, hospitals, or nursing homes.

According to the Administration on Aging, in 2009 the congregate meal program served almost 1.7 million elders and the home-based program served almost 900,000 elders (www.aoa.gov).

However, many eligible elders remain on waiting lists, particularly those who need meals at home. Many social service experts are frustrated by the limitations of these feeding programs and by the number of elders who still go hungry. Most programs offer only one meal a day, and many serve only on weekdays. The people served, and those waiting for food, are often very ill, very poor, and very old.

The U.S. Department of Agriculture revealed that close to 8 percent of elders did not have enough of the right types of food needed to maintain their health or simply did not have enough to eat. Despite the lack of funds to purchase food, most elders who are eligible for the federal Supplemental Nutrition Assistance Program (SNAP, formerly called the Food Stamp Program) do not sign up for it. Only about one-third of eligible elders participate, with an average award of about $75/month. The reasons for nonparticipation include lack of information about how the program works and who can qualify, the stigma of receiving public benefits, and the complicated application process. Federal and state modifications of the Food Stamp Program have included providing online applications and changing from food stamp coupons to debit cards to purchase groceries. Some include dietary education or restrictions on the types of foods that can be purchased. Innovative programs allow use of SNAP funds at farmer's markets to promote the consumption of fresh fruits and vegetables. A prescreening tool to determine qualification for SNAP can be found online at http://www.snap-step1.usda.gov Applications and further information are available at all Social Security offices and online at www.ssa.gov and type Food Stamps in the search bar.

The types of nutrition programs and the ways in which communities fund them vary tremendously. They may be financed locally by churches, United Way funds, private organizations, local taxes, or other means. Free dinners, soup kitchens, and home-delivered meals for the homebound are available in many communities. Many restaurants and cooperative grocery stores offer discounts to older people. The expansion of current programs and the development of new programs are needed to provide quality nutrition to special groups of elders, especially those who live in rural areas and the inner-city and those who are minorities, socially isolated, homebound, and poor.

SUMMARY

Good nutrition is an essential component of health throughout life. The science of nutrition is fascinating and provides insight into how water, carbohydrates, proteins, fats, vitamins, and minerals interact to allow us to live. As we age, many factors can alter our nutritional status: the medications we take, the diseases we develop, our level of exercise, and age-associated changes in metabolic rate, sense of taste and smell, and cognitive decline. In general, elders' reduced metabolic rate means they need to eat fewer calories than younger people. This makes it all the more important that elders eat foods high in nutritional value to assure a healthy diet. The My Plate model for Americans stresses the importance of a varied diet, the type of food ingested, and exercise. Specific recommendations are made for elders. The Institute of Medicine specifies recommended daily intakes of nutrients for health, as well as adequate intakes to prevent deficiency and upper limits for various nutrients.

Old age is associated with many diseases that affect nutritional status: osteoporosis, anemia, heart disease, elevated cholesterol, hypertension, and diabetes, to name a few. Diet therapy is an important component of the management of these illnesses. In addition, elders have trouble with both obesity and malnutrition, which require careful assessment and treatment. Elders are more likely than younger people to have diseases that affect their ability to swallow safely, and they may need modified diets or feeding through a tube or a vein. Elders are at higher risk of nutritional deficiency and are more likely to need a multivitamin supplement. Decisions about supplements are challenging because the research and recommendations of experts are complex and contradictory.

Sexuality is central to human existence. In addition to its obvious importance for the continuation of the species, it is responsible for the organization of our society. On a personal level, sexuality plays a central role in our view of ourselves and how we relate to others. Sexuality encompasses a wide range of sensual or erotic feelings or behaviors, including sexual fantasy, affectionate hugs among friends, flirtatious glances, and genital intercourse among lovers. Attitudes and behaviors regarding sexuality are an integral part of one's personality. Early sexual attitudes and experiences significantly affect our expression of sexuality at all ages. The views of families, peers, and culture also tremendously influence sexuality by defining acceptable and unacceptable behaviors.

In this chapter we explore the diversity of sexual behavior in the later years, with special attention to women living alone, lesbian and gay elders, and frail elders who live in nursing homes. The effects of several chronic diseases, medications, and surgery on sexuality are discussed. Sexual dysfunction—its causes, diagnosis, and treatment—are addressed. Individuals working in health and human services need to be sensitive to the range of sexual needs and concerns of their older clients in order to better serve them. Accurate information about sexuality in later life helps professionals to foster an accepting atmosphere. Such knowledge also facilitates a realistic view of sexuality in our own later years.

Misconceptions of Elder Sexuality

The topic of elder sexuality is fraught with misinformation and bias, which, in turn, affect our attitudes toward older people and ultimately our own sexual feelings and behavior in later life. Americans live in a youth-oriented, consumer-based society. Images of sexy young men and women are used to sell anything from lawn mowers to nightwear. Consequently, we have a narrow view of sexual attractiveness that is associated with the physical characteristics of youth: beautiful young women with firm and shapely bodies and handsome, muscular, slim-hipped men. To a much larger extent than we may realize, images on television, in motion pictures, and in magazines both shape and reflect our impressions of what is beautiful or sexy.

Because older persons (and most of the younger population) do not conform to popular culture's image of sex appeal, nobody wants to look old. The cosmetic industry takes advantage of this fear of growing old by turning our trepidation into its profit. Products such as wrinkle creams, age spot removers, and hair dyes to cover the gray reinforce our fear of aging and consequent loss of sexual attractiveness. Botox injections, face-lifts, and dermapeels compete for the business of fighting against looking our age. Cosmetic surgery is at its peak. More people than ever are paying to be nipped and tucked, augmented and reduced, and sculpted with scalpels to seek unreachable standards of beauty—or at least look "better."

The belief that only the young are sexually appealing damages young and old alike. The prejudices of the young against growing old will continue as the young age, eventually making them victims of their own negative attitudes. Older women seem to be especially affected by society's narrow image of female sexuality. What if we were to define sexuality and sensuality more broadly to include realistic traits that can be valued throughout the life course: grace, competence, good humor, sexual energy, and playfulness? How might we contribute to that change?

Laypersons and health professionals alike may not see the sexual needs and concerns of older persons as important. Elder lovers expressing affection in public are often described as "cute" and commented on as if they were children—amusing but not to be taken seriously. Physicians may consider elder sexuality inconsequential; few take a sexual history or discuss sexual concerns with older patients. They may brush off patients' concerns about sexual dysfunction, saying that sex is not that important at their age or that a dysfunction is just part of growing old. However, because sexual dysfunction may be a symptom or a consequence of disease or of a medication side effect, the discussion of sexual issues is critical to accurate diagnosis and treatment.

SEXUAL ACTIVITY IN LATER LIFE

Most elders maintain an interest in sex. Studies consistently show that sexual activity not only is possible but is practiced by elders into their 80s and 90s. Although the majority of men and women retain the capacity to become sexually excited and orgasmic, studies consistently report a gradual decline in the frequency of intercourse with advancing age. In general, sexually active couples have intercourse less frequently, and the proportion of sexually active couples diminishes.[1] The most recent national survey on sexuality of older adults included in-home interviews of more than 3,000 men and women between 57 and 85 years of age living in the community. Overall, the prevalence of sexual activity declined with advancing age. However, even in the older age group, more than half of those who were sexually active participated in sexual intercourse at least two to three times per month and almost one-fourth reported the activity at least once a week.[2]

Even though the frequency of intercourse diminishes somewhat with advancing age, its quality may remain as good or even improve for many. A mail survey of more than 1,400 men and women aged 45 and older was conducted by the American Association of Retired Persons (AARP). Reduced sexual activity was reported with advancing age: About 60 percent of men and women aged 45 to 59 years said they had sex at least once a week, but by 75 years and older about 25 percent engaged in sexual intercourse at least once a week. The good news is that two-thirds of the individuals responding said they were extremely or somewhat satisfied with their sex lives.[3]

Multiple factors besides age influence intercourse frequency in the later years. The most obvious is the availability of a partner, especially for women. In the national study mentioned above, older women were significantly less likely to report sexual activity than older men, primarily because of the lack of a partner, and the difference increased dramatically with advancing age. And, among women without a spouse or other intimate relationship, only 4 percent reported being sexually active

Come to Me

by Sue Saniel Elkind

Come to me looking
as you did 50 years ago
arms outstretched
and I will be waiting
virgin again
in white that changes to splashes of roses
as we lie together
Come to me smiling again
with your mortar and pestle
and vitamin pills
because I am given to colds
and coughs that wrack us both
Oh come to me again
and I will be there
waiting with withered hands
gnarled fingers
that will leave their marks
of passion on your back.

From *When I Am Old I Shall Wear Purple: An Anthology of Short Stories and Poetry.* Edited by S. Martz. Manhattan Beach, CA: Papier-Mâché Press.

within the previous year. For men without a spouse or consistent partner, only 22 percent were sexually active. Health problems play a significant role in the frequency of sexual intercourse. In that same study, both women and men who reported fair or poor health were significantly less likely to engage in sexual activity than those reporting very good or excellent health. Finally, the same psychological factors affecting intercourse frequency among younger populations are also important in the elderly: boredom with partner, preoccupation with career or economic pursuits, mental or physical fatigue, overindulgence in food or drink, physical and mental infirmities of individual or partner, and fear of impotence.[2]

Another sexual behavior practiced by older people is masturbation. Although the vast majority of men and women have masturbated at some time in their lives, there remains a reticence to discuss the topic among both men and women of all ages. Masturbation has been considered a sin throughout Christian history, and many religious groups still believe it to be immoral. Because it is such a sensitive topic, it is difficult to obtain accurate information about elders' masturbatory practices. Although scientists and health care professionals consider masturbation to be normal and even beneficial, personal masturbation frequency is rarely discussed openly.

Few studies on sexual practices include questions on masturbation. In the national study mentioned above, about half of the men and one-fourth of the women reported that they engaged in masturbation within the previous year. The percentage of those engaging in the practice decreased with advancing age. Interestingly, the percentages were similar between those who were in a current relationship and those who were not. The study also included questions regarding oral sex. This practice also decreased with advancing age. Almost 60 percent of those who were in the 57–64 age group who were sexually active reported engaging in oral sex within the past year and about 30 percent of those who were sexually active in the 75–85 age group reported engaging in it. The prevalence of the practice was similar among both men and women.[2]

Masturbation is beneficial both physiologically and psychologically. It maintains the elasticity and lubrication of the vagina for women and preserves the ability to have an erection in men. Orgasms, with or without a partner, are known to reduce stress and induce sleep. Masturbation gives individuals control over their own sexuality, stimulates sexual appetite, and is a way to enjoy sexuality without relying on a partner. On the flip side, when openly practiced in public by institutionalized elders with dementia who have decreased social inhibitions, it may cause distress among those who share living quarters or staff who care for them.

Although sexual behaviors encompass more than intercourse and masturbation, these behaviors capture researchers' attention because they are more easily measured. Data from surveys are relatively easy to collect. However, survey results regarding elder sexuality are difficult to interpret for a number of reasons. Studies may be hindered by a "cohort effect." For instance, if elders report less frequent intercourse than middle-aged adults, there are several ways to interpret the information. Perhaps the elders who responded may have not declined in frequency but never were as sexually active as those who are now middle-aged. Or those who are now old are less comfortable with reporting their sexual practices. In order to get around the comparison between age groups, the same group of individuals can be followed over a long time period (longitudinal study).

Another drawback to surveys regarding sexual practices among elders is the "volunteer bias." People who are willing to participate in studies about their sex lives may not be representative of others in their age group. They may be more open to talking about sexuality, may engage in more frequent sexual activity, or may have a higher interest in sex than the general population. And there is the cultural bias: Men may be more inclined to overestimate their sexual activity to show they are more virile, and women may underestimate sexual activity for fear of being judged as "unladylike." Whether elders are truthful in answering questions on a survey about their sexuality is unknown. Further, numerical data on frequency of sexual intercourse and masturbation present a limited view of sexuality.

CHANGES IN SEXUAL RESPONSE WITH AGE

In the late 1960s, sex researchers Drs. William Masters and Virginia Johnson were the first to document the physiological sexual response of both men and women by carefully measuring physiological responses during intercourse of 694 adult men and women in a laboratory setting.[4] As a result of that study, Masters and Johnson identified four distinct phases of sexual response in both males and females: (1) excitement—the development and increase of sexual tension in response to stimulation, (2) plateau—the intensifying of sexual tension until it reaches the extreme level, (3) orgasm—those few seconds of sexual release with primary focus on the pelvic area, and (4) resolution—the move from the height of orgasmic stimulation to the resting state.

Unfortunately, that study did not tell us much about age differences in sexual response because only 20 men and 11 women aged 60 or over were included. Among the 20 men over age 60 who were observed, sexual excitement developed more slowly, the intensity of penile sensation was lessened, and increased time and more direct stimulation were needed to achieve an erection when compared to younger men. The plateau period was longer in older men, allowing them to maintain an erection longer before the need to ejaculate. Often a full erection was not achieved until ejaculation was imminent. Ejaculatory force was reduced and orgasm intensity and length were shorter in older men. During orgasm, elder men also had fewer pelvic muscle contractions, diminished sexual flush, and less nipple and testes engorgement with arousal than younger subjects. After ejaculation, the erection subsided more rapidly, and a longer time was needed to achieve another erection. Older men also frequently went from the plateau phase to the resolution phase without ejaculation.

Among the 11 older women observed, Masters and Johnson reported a reduction in vaginal lubrication and greater expansion of the vagina with stimuli when compared to the younger women. Nipple erection and clitoral response to stimulation were no different than in younger women. Both the orgasmic and the resolution phases were shorter in older women. However, the capacity to achieve orgasm, even multiple orgasms, did not change with age. Among the women in the sample who had intercourse at least twice weekly, little to no age-associated changes in sexual response were noted. Just as in other body systems, the "use it or lose it" phenomenon seems to play a role in sexual functioning.

Although the classic work of Masters and Johnson greatly expanded knowledge of human sexual response, their work on describing changes in sexual response in older men and women cannot be considered conclusive because of small sample size, scarcity of other corroborative research, effects of a laboratory setting on normal sexual response, and the unknown health status of the participants. In the mid-1960s, Masters and Johnson admitted that more studies needed to be conducted on elders. And a half century later, we know little more than we did then, because little subsequent research has expanded or replicated their preliminary impressions of the human sexual response among elders. Until collaborating studies are reported, age-associated changes in sexual response remain unknown.

"Aging makes sex less imperative. You can take it or leave it, and that uncovers something that is precious. I can report that women look better to me now than they did when I was young because when I was young, sex was demanding. It was ego; I could be attracted to a woman that I despised, and then not feel good about myself. Now it seems possible to admire only women whom I like, which feels good. It feels cleaner and purer."

—Abraham Maslow

SEXUALITY IN SPECIAL ELDER POPULATIONS

This section focuses on the sexual concerns and issues of three special groups: older unmarried women, lesbian and gay elders, and elders living in nursing homes.

Older Unmarried Women

Women without spouses comprise a large proportion of the elder population and include the never-married, the divorced, and the widowed. Older women are less likely to have a male partner than women of other age groups. Women outnumber men at all ages, and the gap widens with advancing age. Overall, within the 65 and older group, there are 100 men for every 140 women. By age 85, there are 100 men for every 216 women (more than twice as many women as men). Because women live longer than men and usually marry older men, the probability of widowhood is high. In 2009, older men

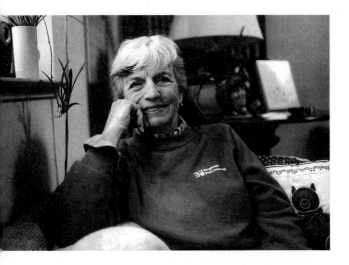

were much more likely to be married than older women (72 percent vs. 42 percent), and there were more than four times as many older widows (8.9 million) as widowers (2.1 million).[5]

Societal attitudes play a role in the lack of male partners for older women. Older men are more likely to seek relationships with younger women than with women their age or older. This preference has been attributed largely to the cultural attitude that says a man's value is determined by career or financial success and a woman's value is determined by how young she looks rather than by what she does. Although there are many advantages to older women–younger men relationships, the trend in that direction is not significant and is unlikely to affect those already in their later years. Because of the unbalanced sex ratio, a heterosexual relationship may not be a viable alternative for many older women, whether by choice or circumstance. Instead, they may explore other alternatives for sexual satisfaction: expanding affectionate relationships with men and women, exploring sexual fantasy, erotic books and films, and masturbation.

Lesbian and Gay Elders

Elders today grew up during a time when many people believed that homosexuality was a mental illness and homosexual practices were immoral. Consequently, many who are sexually attracted to the same gender have kept their feelings hidden from their family and friends, and it is difficult to determine their numbers. The National Gay and Lesbian Task Force estimates that there are 3 million elder gays and lesbians in the United States.

Lesbian and gays, no matter what their age, experience discrimination by both the personnel and the policies of health and social services organizations. In the past, homosexuals were considered mentally ill, and efforts were made to change their unhealthy same-sex attractions and behaviors. Even though the American Psychiatric Association eliminated homosexuality as a mental disorder from its classifications of mental disorders in 1973, many people in health and social service settings still believe that homosexual behavior is abnormal. This attitude is considered *homophobic* (fearful of people who are homosexual). The behavioral responses of health and social service personnel may range from subtle (embarrassment and excessive curiosity) to blatant (hostility, harassment, and avoidance of physical contact).[6] Such behaviors are not surprising because physicians receive little or no information about sexual orientation in medical school. Past discrimination makes elder gays and lesbians cautious or suspicious of health care, and they are consequently less likely to use health care services or to trust health personnel.

There is concern that discrimination and bias toward lesbians and gays may impact the care they receive. *Heterosexism* is the prejudice that heterosexuality is the only appropriate way to express love and sexuality. Asking "Are you married?" may be awkward for those who do not have the legal right to marry. Asking instead, "Do you have one significant person in your life or a partner?" may elicit more information.

Perhaps the most important issue for gays and lesbians who become ill is how "family" is defined as it relates to support, caregiving, visitation rights, and participation in health care decisions. The heterosexual view of what constitutes a family

Older Lesbians and Gay Men
An American History Lesson

The historical context in which older lesbians and gay men formed their sexual identity is important to understand. "Coming out"—acknowledging one's sexual orientation—has only recently been brought into public discourse by younger lesbians and gay men as a part of their need to identify and define their true selves. The Gay Rights Movement, or post "Stonewall Period," is not part of the life experience of today's older lesbians and gay men. As young adults, these elders tended to acknowledge their sexual orientation only to themselves—if at all. Hiding their sexual identity was often a survival strategy in a homophobic society whose laws and policies labeled homosexuality as immoral, pathological, and illegal.

Churches forbade membership to gays and lesbians who were open and honest about their identity. States had laws that criminalized romantic sexual expressions by two consenting adults of the same gender. A lesbian or a gay man brave enough to acknowledge her or his sexual identity to a family physician or psychiatrist could be institutionalized as chronically mentally ill.

During the McCarthy era, the hunt for Communists in government, in the armed forces, and in the entertainment world linked homosexuality to subversive activity. It was considered not possible to be both a good citizen of the United States and a homosexual.

This age cohort has been so bound by social pressure and by fears of disclosure, immediate discharge from employment, and humiliation that it created a hidden life. Consequently, many older lesbians and gay men have never disclosed their homosexuality. Two older, single women living together were likely to be dismissed as "just two old spinsters" or as "old retired teachers living together." Gays in later life were labeled as "confirmed bachelors" or were said to have not found the right person to marry. Some gay men found safety in marriage while having sexual relations with men. Lesbian women often married, had children, and lived their emotional lives with a significant woman friend (Claes and Moore, 2000, pp. 185–186).[7]

does not conform to the family structure of gay and lesbian elders. Although some individuals

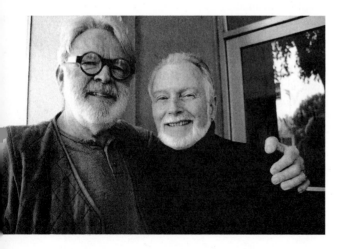

may rely on their biological family, others may be alienated from their children. Some rely predominantly on an informal network of gays and lesbians including a partner and close friends.

Unfortunately, gay and lesbian couples commonly encounter legal obstacles that prohibit their visiting and participating in health care decisions for an ill partner. It can be tragic to be excluded from a bedside vigil because "only immediate family" are permitted or to have an estranged family member be the one called to make decisions in place of a person who appears to be "just a friend," but in fact is a long-term companion. Health professionals should be proactive in asking people whom they wish to make decisions for them in the event they are unable and who can share information about a person's condition.

HIV/AIDS and the Older Adult

The Centers for Disease Control and Prevention estimate that the number of Americans aged 50 and older who were living with diagnosed cases of HIV/AIDS in 2007 was over 155,000, accounting for almost 30 percent of all cases.[8] Treatments have extended the life of those who contracted HIV+ and AIDS before their later years, so more individuals are growing old with the disease. But some contract the disease after mid-life, primarily because of anal intercourse between men. Heterosexual transmission is increasing in the over-50 age group, although the proportion is small.

AIDS is caused by the human immunodeficiency virus (HIV), transmitted from person to person in blood and semen. Over time, the virus disables the immune system. After the virus infects the body, the person may have no symptoms for years, then may manifest only vague symptoms such as fatigue, loss of appetite, night sweats, diarrhea, or increased susceptibility to colds. Later, the person becomes more disabled, loses weight, and becomes very susceptible to opportunistic infections (that is, infections that usually do not affect individuals with normal immunity). When people with HIV+ antibodies in their blood develop a major opportunistic infection or manifest other severe signs of infection, they have AIDS.

Researchers have discovered that older adults with HIV/AIDS do not fare as well as younger victims. The aging process is more compressed: They are more likely to get other illnesses and become frail. Further, treatment may not be as effective and/or they are more likely to experience adverse effects to medications.[9] The three major mechanisms to contract AIDS for any age group are intercourse (anal and vaginal) without a condom, sharing needles among intravenous drug users, and receiving a blood transfusion before 1985.

Those who are older or heterosexual may not believe themselves to be at risk and so may not use condoms or request testing. Physicians are less likely to think of HIV in an older population.

Later diagnosis means a delay in initiating therapy to prevent the progression of the disease. Managing AIDS cases in older patients is particularly difficult. Physicians must manage the opportunistic infections, chronic diseases, and polypharmacy (taking many medications) in the face of their patients' diminishing physical reserves, as well as the multiple problems inherent in treating persons with AIDS. Little is known about the interaction of HIV medications with other chronic illnesses, or about HIV medication regimens commonly prescribed to elders. The stigma still attached to AIDS may affect the care that elder AIDS patients receive, whether at home or in a nursing home.

The National Association of HIV over Fifty is a forum to exchange information and share concerns and issues about HIV and the older adult (www.hivoverfifty. org). Although most AIDS patients are cared for in the home by informal caregivers, many also rely on home health services and hospice care. Nursing homes are often used in the latter stages of the disease. SAGE (Senior Action in a Gay Environment) provides social support and education services to older gay men and lesbian women who are dealing with HIV/AIDS—both to those infected and to their caregivers, friends, or relatives. For more information, contact SAGE at www.sageusa.org

These preferences should be codified into advance directives and durable power of attorney for health care or finances, conservatorships, or other legal arrangements. The book *A Legal Guide for Lesbian and Gay Couples* is helpful.[10]

Educating professionals who work with elders can raise awareness and improve the responsiveness of agencies to the needs of the gay and lesbian population. Training should be broad to sensitize both the administration and the staff to the presence of unconscious heterosexism and homophobia in the organization. Using the acronym RESPECT, one health professional describes ways in which an organization can become more available to the gay, transgender, and lesbian population:

R   Review existing practices and policies in the agency.

E   Educate administration, staff, and residents about a range of taboo topics regarding sexuality and human relationships.

S   Share ideas to unlearn homophobia and heterosexism.

P   Promote diversity and the prevention of homophobic practices.

E   Explore and evaluate areas for continued learning and teaching.

C   Change beliefs and attitudes by getting all involved.

T   Transition to a diversity-friendly facility and practice with continued support by administrators.

The same professional provides awareness exercises that may be utilized in organizational training.[11]

Community resources for lesbian and gay elders are more likely to be available in large cities. They include services to homebound elderly gays, hospice programs, housing programs, information and referral services, and support services for caregivers. Some agencies have initiated services specifically for elder gays and lesbians and others (e.g., YMCA and senior multipurpose centers) have expanded their services to meet their needs. The Lesbian and Gay Aging Issues Network works nationally to raise awareness about the concerns of gay, lesbian, bisexual, and transgender elders and the unique barriers they encounter when trying to gain access to housing, medical care, long-term care, and other needed services. For a very extensive links page and a monthly newsletter, go to www.asaging.org and click on "diversity issues."

Senior Action in a Gay Environment, at www.sageusa.org, is the oldest and largest social service and advocacy organization dedicated to lesbian, gay, bisexual, and transgender individuals.

The Web page has links to other related organizations. The Gay and Lesbian Association of Retiring Persons, at www.gaylesbianretiring.org, is a niche market provider of benefits and services and is working toward building retirement communities (from independent living to skilled nursing homes) for members.

Elders in Institutions

Many institutionalized elders do not have an interest in or capacity for genital sexuality because most are there because of severe mental and/or physical problems. Serious disabling illnesses and treatments impact their sexual thoughts and ability to function. They may be more concerned with day-to-day living, eating, and body care than with sexual intercourse. It is important to remember, however, that sexual expression encompasses more than intercourse: It is a basic human need. Young or old, lucid or demented, strong or frail, the need for touch, companionship, love, and intimacy does not disappear when a person walks through the doors to live in an institution. Some individuals are there to recuperate and will return to their own homes. Others, even those who are very frail, might participate in a broader range of sexual activity in a supportive environment. Although a few institutionalized elders report an interest in intercourse, a larger proportion are interested in other types of sexual expression, such as touch, affection, companionship, and keeping up their appearance.

The institutional setting presents many barriers to a resident who desires intimate sexual activity. A big drawback is the lack of a willing and able partner. The majority of nursing home residents are single women. Even if a woman were interested in a sexual relationship, the opportunity for a willing and able male partner is slim.

The lack of privacy is common in a nursing home. The structure of the facility is designed to easily track its residents. Nurses' stations are placed so that the comings and goings of residents can be easily monitored, and the doors to the rooms are usually open. Residents' rooms are small, usually with two or more beds per room. When rooms are shared, usually a curtain provides the only separation between the beds.

There are various ways in which institutions can promote privacy. Married couples can room together. Or a room can be held in reserve for couples who wish to be intimate without fear of interruption. A system of "signs" such as "Do not disturb" can be set up after frank discussions with staff about how frequently elders need to be observed. Integration of men and women on the same wing or floor increases the amount and type of sexual expression among residents.

The attitudes of nursing home staff toward elder sexuality strongly influence sexual expression among the residents. Nurses and other long-term care staff are likely to have negative or patronizing attitudes toward sexual expression of older people under their care. Even though the residents enjoy touch, hugs and kisses, even eroticism, some staff may not be comfortable with all types of sexual behavior. Staff may voice their acceptance of elder sexual expression, but their actions may not be as supportive.

The sexual needs and concerns of patients are often overlooked by staff members who care for the residents. And, administrators seldom have the motivation to modify the living environment to better meet the sexual needs of the residents. Thus, the sexual needs of those elders residing in institutions are commonly ignored, overlooked, ridiculed, perhaps even regarded with disgust by staff who only vaguely understand the sexual needs of older people. Expressions of sexuality are likely to be seen as behavioral problems to be solved instead of expressions of a basic human need for love and intimacy.

Fostering elder sexuality and developing guidelines for sexuality in the nursing home is very challenging for administrators and staff. How can sexuality be supported among the residents with limited privacy? What about overnight visits with the spouse living at home? Usually the facility cannot accommodate overnight guests, especially if the individual does not have a private room. Other, more complex issues are not uncommon. Should staff intervene when two residents are sexual with one another when one is cognitively impaired? How can the staff be sure that the sexual activity is consensual if one partner cannot make her wishes known? And what if a resident who has a spouse outside the institution is sexually involved with another resident? How should the negative responses of the family regarding the sexual interest and activity of their institutionalized family member be addressed? Might there be legal ramifications? With the above scenarios, there is a delicate balance between the mandated resident's right to privacy and the staff's need to provide the resident with safety and supervision.

Another important concern for personnel is how to handle inappropriate sexual behavior. Those with dementia can be disinhibited and have sexual conversations, public displays of sexual behavior such as disrobing or masturbating, and inappropriate advances or touching of others. Those with dementia can get confused—when staff are bathing them or cleaning their genitals, they may think this is a sexual encounter. They may become frightened and resistive or alternatively may try to engage in sexual acts with staff, even putting staff at risk of harm. Staff need to monitor to ensure that all sexual encounters between residents are consensual, that no one is being taken advantage of, and that sexual behaviors are private so as not to disturb others. It can be a delicate balance to ensure privacy and safety at all times. Inappropriate sexual behavior of a resident toward a staff member or another resident can be very burdensome to the staff and disruptive to other residents and their families.

How can administrators sensitize staff to the residents' sexual needs when a staff member has conservative values regarding sexuality? A variety of educational programs have been designed to assist nursing home staff to recognize and support the many expressions of sexuality, sensuality, and affection among residents and to redirect any inappropriate sexual activity, especially among those with dementia. Inservice programs can increase staff knowledge and encourage a more tolerant attitude toward elder sexuality.

They'd Never Tell

Laura Goodwin, RN

He came to her every Wednesday,
after he had his tub bath, with his best black
suit on that the nurse's aides had helped him with,
his hair all slicked back (the few strands he had left
which encircled his head like a halo),
he shuffled over to her room in his oversized thick-
soled shoes,
a big smile on his face.

She, in turn, was waiting for him in her room,
her hair all freshly done in a beehive by the beauty
parlor,
with her best pink dress on,
sitting in her easy chair with a smile on her face, too.

She was allowed to have a bit of whiskey at bedtime,
which, after the nurse gave it to her, she kept on her
bedside table,
waiting for their meeting.

She had asked the administrator of our nursing home
for a double bed,
when he refused, we nurses pushed both of the twin
beds together in her room,
after he went home for the day.

He would look back and forth before he knocked on
her door,
and she would make him wait for a few seconds
before she said,
"Who is it?,"
As if she didn't know.
When he replied, she let him in.

The nurses always placed an invisible "Do not
disturb" sign on the door.
He always left at seven a.m.,
blew a kiss to her, and said, "I love you."
She always said, "I love you too."

The nurses then would all hurry up to rearrange the
room,
before the administrator got in for the day,
giggling with excitement the whole time at our
deception.
None of us would ever tell.

Now they are both just memories I carry with me,
happy memories that make me smile,
and I wonder if someday I'll be living in a nursing
home,
and need someone not to tell.

Used with permission from Laura Goodwin RN.

THE EFFECT OF CHRONIC ILLNESS ON SEXUALITY

It is well documented that relationships and sexual satisfaction enhance the quality of life. Even when one member of a couple has a chronic illness that restricts many other areas of life, sex is a significant source of comfort, pleasure, and intimacy. Further, a satisfying sexual relationship provides the opportunity for one who is chronically ill to feel normal—to be affirmed as a man or woman—despite restrictions in other aspects of daily living.

Sexuality may be compromised by physical and emotional problems that accompany chronic disease. The illness may cause an individual to feel tired, depressed, and uninterested in sexual activity. Furthermore, some chronic illnesses, or surgeries associated with them, alter personal appearance, thereby affecting body image, self-esteem, and sexual interest and performance. However, intercourse can provide intimacy and relaxation, reduce isolation and depression, divert attention from physical problems, and help the person to feel "normal." The degree to which chronic illness affects sexual capacity and interest is highly dependent on the extent of disability, and on the elder's coping skills, attitude toward sexuality, and motivation for sexual activity. In cases in which intercourse is not an option, it is important for the health provider to discuss alternate ways to foster intimacy.

Couples vary in their support for one another during periods of illness and disability. The degree that they accept changes in sexual activity is related to the strength and previous communication patterns of the marriage. The well partner may lose sexual interest because of concern of causing more pain or because the ill partner is no longer interested. Chronic illness also changes the dynamics of a relationship. For instance, the ill person may have difficulty with being dependent or "waited on," or the caregiver may be too overworked and exhausted to enjoy sexual intercourse.

Health care professionals who work with older people need to be aware of the effects of various diseases on sexuality. Unfortunately, sexual dysfunction and dissatisfaction are often undetected and undertreated because of communication barriers between physicians and their chronically ill patients and lack of training in human sexuality. Despite multiple magazine advertisements in which popular politicians and movie stars discuss erectile dysfunction and promote Viagra and other medications, most patients and health care providers are reluctant to discuss issues surrounding sexual function.

Certain general guidelines are helpful to maximize sexual satisfaction among elders with chronic illness. Changing medications or reducing the dosages of medicines that affect sexual performance should be considered. Further, medications can be prescribed to reduce symptoms associated with sexual activity (e.g., medications for joint pain in a patient with arthritis or nitroglycerine in a patient with chest pain). Elders can be counseled on alternative sexual positions or alternative means of sexual expression. And, if erectile dysfunction is a problem, drugs, devices, and surgery can be offered. Unfortunately, even though broaching the issue of sexual problems by the physician is critical, it is seldom done, especially with older patients.

Selected chronic illnesses that significantly impact elders' sexuality are surveyed in the remainder of this section. Though not discussed here, sexual problems commonly accompany other diseases and conditions such as obesity, dementia, and low back pain.

Heart Disease

Individuals who have had a heart attack are often cautious about resuming intercourse because they have the misconception that sexual activity will bring on another attack. A number of studies report that the majority of couples decrease or eliminate intercourse after the husband experiences a heart attack. The most commonly reported reason for reduced sexual activity is decreased ability and lowered satisfaction. It is not clear whether the decrease in performance and interest is due to drugs, organic problems, or psychosocial considerations. If the person who has a heart attack is also a smoker, the likelihood of impotence increases significantly. In studies of women, heart attacks cause a similarly reduced level of sexual activity and fear of resuming sexual activity.

Despite the fears of those who have had a heart attack, the physical demands of intercourse are minimal, and sexual activity may be both physically and psychologically beneficial: It reduces tension, aids sleep, increases self-esteem and self-image, and is an enjoyable, low-level physical activity that serves to normalize their lives. The physical demands of intercourse are no greater than walking around the block or up a staircase. Generally, physicians recommend that intercourse may be resumed 8 to 12 weeks after a heart attack. Intercourse can be assumed to be safe if the individual passes an exercise treadmill test. Although it is true that sexual activity can trigger a heart attack, the risk is extremely low and is reduced further in those who exercise regularly. If chest pain usually occurs during intercourse, physicians generally prescribe nitroglycerine to be taken immediately before sexual intercourse.

Cardiac rehabilitation programs, commonly prescribed after a heart attack, provide a good opportunity for the health professional to discuss impaired sexual function with the cardiac patient. Discussions might include what to expect after a heart attack, concerns regarding erectile dysfunction, the safety of engaging in sexual activity, the effect of heart medications on sexual function, and the emotional impact of heart disease on the sexual relationship.

Hypertension

Hypertension can accelerate atherosclerosis of the arteries supplying the penis and increase the incidence of erectile dysfunction (another word for impotence). Many elders who have hypertension have some degree of sexual dysfunction, both from the disease and from the medications used in treatment. Thiazide diuretics are commonly prescribed drugs used to treat high blood pressure because they are inexpensive, safe, and cause few side effects. However, complaints of decreased desire, difficulty in maintaining an erection, and difficulty with ejaculation are common among those who take diuretics. Another class of blood pressure drugs, beta blockers, often reduces sexual performance; newer drugs or lower dosages are less likely to cause problems. One study of hypertensive women reported a high proportion of women who reported sexual dysfunction of more than five years. Further, those women reported a low frequency of sexual activity despite the availability of a partner.[12]

Stroke

Individuals who have experienced a stroke—particularly those who are older and became the most disabled from the stroke—report a significant decline in sexual activity.[13] A stroke is likely to decrease satisfaction with sexual function in both men and women.

Cancer

The effect of cancer on sexual interest and function depends on the location and extent of the cancer and the type of treatment. Sexual interest and activity may be impaired because of the patient's physiological reactions to the cancer or treatment, such as nausea from chemotherapy, incision pain, and fatigue, or because of psychological factors, such as depression, fear of death or disfigurement, or fear of losing one's spouse.

The importance of sex in a person's life should be considered in the decision regarding the type of cancer therapy to be prescribed. For instance, radiation treatment for prostate cancer for a sexually active man may be more desirable than a prostatectomy (surgical removal of the prostate), not because of its success rate but because the surgery may significantly reduce the ability to perform sexually.

Although being able to be sexual after cancer treatment is an important part of the recovery process, partners of individuals with cancer may worry about whether they are well enough for sexual activity, or a lover's altered appearance may make his or her partner uncomfortable. Furthermore, the well partner may feel guilty about having sexual interest when the ill partner feels sick or depressed. Also, couples may not have privacy for sexual expression when one partner is hospitalized. Although sexual activity may have to be put on hold temporarily, restoring a sex life is a key part to feeling healthy and normal again.

Both those with cancer and their partners need support and education to understand the effect of the disease and its treatment on sexuality. Physicians rarely discuss sexual performance with their cancer patients, either before or after surgery. It is important that a physician discuss the effects of radiation and chemotherapy on sexual desire and performance, and how to deal with the feelings stirred by seeing a partner with a surgically altered body. Self-help groups are effective for those with cancer to share information and gain support. The American Cancer Society has initiated self-help groups for individuals who have undergone a mastectomy (breast removal), an ileostomy (bladder removal), or a colostomy (colon removal). Cancer treatments have a significant effect on elder sexuality and are discussed under "Surgery" later in this chapter. The American Cancer Society has many good resources regarding cancer and sexuality (www.cancer.org)

Dementia

The sexuality of individuals with dementia can be problematic. Although they may retain sexual interest and physical capability, their cognitive state is impaired. They may no longer be able to make decisions regarding the social consequences of their behavior, control their sexual impulses, or even recognize their loved ones. These deficits are not generally important in early dementia, but as dementia progresses, difficulties arise. Individuals may become less inhibited—a formerly conservative woman may undress in public, masturbate excessively or in plain view of others, or make advances to another man. There are no effective treatments to deal with hypersexual impulsive behavior in those with dementia. Individuals with these tendencies require redirection and supervision when in public or high-risk situations to ensure they are safe. Families may have to deal with uncomfortable situations, both within the home and in the nursing home. As an example, a woman placed her husband who was diagnosed with dementia in a nursing home. During his time there, he had a series of romantic and sometimes sexually intimate relationships with other residents and no longer recognized his wife when she visited.

This was bittersweet for his wife, who noted that even though the relationships made him happy, she personally felt the loss of her husband and his affection for her. An elderly woman with dementia was noted to be screaming when her husband attempted sexual relations with her in the nursing home. The staff were unsure whether she was able to understand or consent, but the husband stated this was the way it always was. These and other examples bring up many ethical and moral dilemmas, both for the family and for the nursing home staff.

Diabetes

Diabetes is the most common cause of impotence, and the proportion of affected men increases with advancing age. Studies report as many as three-fourths of men who have type 1 (juvenile-onset) diabetes become impotent as their disease progresses. Impotence can also occur in those with type 2 (adult-onset) diabetes. In both cases, erectile dysfunction occurs 10 to 20 years from the

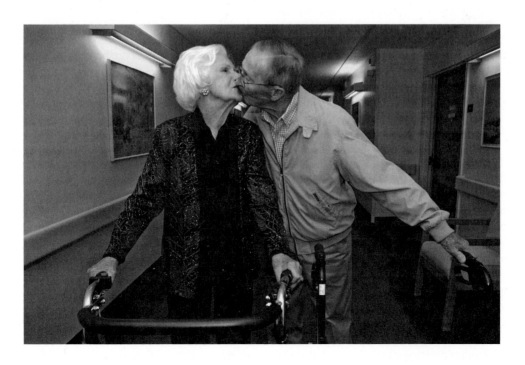

Sexuality and Parkinson's: A Spouse's View

In any relationship between a man and a woman, whether there is a disability or perfect health, there is a need for loving, caring, and sharing, and what more perfect way is there than through our sexuality?

As in all aspects of our life together, I have learned to accommodate Sid's parkinsonism, just as he has, and to make the necessary adjustments. But I have never given up on showing my love for him, either by voice, touch, or in our sexual relationship.

When Sid and I first started dating, his parkinsonism was already well advanced, but somehow it didn't prevent our love for one another from growing and ripening into a lifetime commitment to one another. From the very beginning, I realized that there would have to be careful timing and flexibility on my part to respond to the moment. I learned to adjust to sexual experiences at any hour of the day and in any part of the house. Instead of making it awkward and embarrassing, it made it more exciting. I learned that sometimes I would need to be the aggressor. I found it fun to dress in very feminine attire and to make myself as attractive as possible with makeup and scent. Sid's appreciation makes it worth the effort.

Each of us brings to a relationship all of the feelings and attitudes we have developed over the years of our lives. Sometimes these include some myths and misconceptions. Included is the myth that sexuality and feelings of love are for the young and beautiful people as portrayed by the mass media.

Another misconception is that disabled people can't and shouldn't have a full and satisfying sexual life. Neither of these wrong ideas should be perpetuated by the parkinsonian or the spouse.

In coping with a chronic illness, there is a delicate balancing act of adequate rest, exercise, diet, positive emotions, controlling of stress, and, most important of all, giving and accepting love. I have found that there is no more satisfying way of giving and accepting love than through sexual expression. This doesn't necessarily mean that you have to experience a mutual orgasm. It can be cuddling and fondling as a daily routine. One of my favorite times of the day is our afternoon rest period when cuddling is an important part. Sometimes it leads to a relaxed nap, and other times it can result in a fuller sexual expression.

Even when the sex act can't be completed, we both gain a sense of being loved and secure in the knowledge that the next time will be better. I have found it elating to realize that sex doesn't have to cease to exist as one grows older and has to deal with health problems. In fact, it can be the best time of your life. You certainly have more freedom when you are older, and there are fewer distractions and interruptions.

If you have the right attitude, the sexual relationship with your Parkinson partner can become one of the most rewarding in your life.

Reprinted from *Patient Perspectives on Parkinson's* by Sid and Donna Dorras, 1997. National Parkinson Foundation.

onset of the disease. Researchers generally agree that impotence is caused by the destruction of the nerves that open the penile arteries to permit the blood to enter. Although the ability to experience an erection is lost, sensation, orgasm, and ejaculation may remain unaffected.

Tight diet and drug control can reduce the risk of impotence in men with either type of diabetes. Careful screening is necessary to determine whether the erectile dysfunction is drug induced or caused by other physiological or psychological factors. If impotence occurs even when diabetes is controlled, the chance of recovery is unlikely, and penile implants may be considered.

Arthritis

Arthritis is a very common condition among older people and can impact sexuality in many ways. Those with arthritis may be less interested in sex because of chronic pain, and they may be less able to engage in sexual activity because of pain, joint stiffness, and reduced flexibility. Like elders with other chronic conditions, elders with arthritis need education and counseling to cope with the sexual consequences of their disease. Education should include a discussion of alternative sexual positions to reduce pain, varied forms of lovemaking, the value of a warm bath and analgesics before sexual activity, and planning for sexual activity during times when pain levels are low. Those with hip replacements need special advice regarding when intercourse can be resumed and which positions minimize the danger of dislocation.

OTHER FACTORS INFLUENCING SEXUAL FUNCTION

Sexual function can be influenced by factors other than chronic illness: medication, alcohol and tobacco use, surgery, and psychosocial variables. In this section we discuss the effects of these variables on sexual interest and activity in the later years.

Medications

Some common prescription drugs can cause or aggravate sexual difficulties. Many medications reduce sexual desire and increase the difficulty in achieving orgasm, particularly those used to reduce high blood pressure and alter mood. Some over-the-counter medications also affect sexual drive or performance among both men and women (e.g., Benadryl, used for allergies).

The adverse reaction of a drug on sexuality depends on the dose, duration of therapy, other drugs taken at the same time, psychological factors, and the state of the circulatory, hormonal, and nervous systems. The patient should be made aware that the prescribed medication may impact sexual function, and if the side effects are unacceptable, alternative drugs or other treatments should be considered. If the physician does not address the sexual side effects of a particular medication, frustration with reduced sexual function may cause an individual to stop taking a necessary medication, sometimes without the physician's knowledge. Because patients are reluctant to initiate a conversation with their physicians about the side effects of medications upon sex interest and performance, taking a sexual history can provide an avenue for the individual to discuss sexual concerns.

Alcohol and Tobacco

Alcohol has a negative effect on sexual potency in both men and women. The validity of Shakespeare's words, "[alcohol] provokes the desire, but takes away the performance," is well documented. Although low blood levels of alcohol may accelerate sexual arousal by reducing inhibitions, increased blood alcohol levels diminish performance. The use of alcohol over the long term can cause a reduced blood supply to the organs. This has a significant effect on the ability to achieve and maintain an erection. Chronic alcohol use is known to cause reduced testosterone levels and reduced testicular size. There is also reduced nerve sensitivity in the penis, which varies among individuals. Excessive alcohol use can cause temporary erectile difficulties, and long-term abuse causes irreversible loss of erectile function, even if drinking is stopped. About three-fourths of alcoholic men are impotent: Alcoholism is the most common cause of erectile dysfunction among men in their middle years. Women alcoholics also suffer from decreased libido and have difficulty achieving orgasm.

Cigarette smoking reduces blood flow to the organs, primarily because of the development of atherosclerosis in the vessels, including those in the penis. Smoking increases the rate of erectile dysfunction, and the longer a man smokes, the greater the risk.

Surgery

Surgery has the potential to interfere with sexual interest and ability, particularly prostatectomy (removal of prostate), hysterectomy (removal of the uterus), mastectomy (breast removal), knee and hip surgery, and stomas (artificial openings in the abdomen for urine or feces). Whether or not surgery causes sexual problems depends on the extent of nerve and blood vessel destruction in the genital area. Although all pelvic surgery is associated with an increased risk of impotence or other sexual dysfunction, some operations are more destructive than others. Additionally, there is a psychological component to sexual problems arising after surgery. Individuals may feel they or their partners are too fragile for lovemaking, or the changes in the body caused by surgery are perceived as unattractive. In couples for whom communication is an issue, difficulties may arise. One partner may not initiate sexual activity for fear of "pressuring" the partner who has had surgery. At the same time, the individual who had surgery may feel unattractive and may think the partner feels the same way.

Perhaps the most dramatic impact on sexual functioning for men occurs with surgery on the prostate gland, generally due to cancer. Prostate cancer surgery is the most common pelvic surgery affecting erectile function. Many of the treatments of prostate cancer (e.g., radiation, testosterone-blocking medications, removal of the prostate) carry a high risk of sexual dysfunction. Radical prostatectomy, the removal of the prostate gland through the abdomen, almost always causes erectile problems, although newer strategies may spare the nerves. Many men can experience an orgasm, but can no longer obtain an erection. Procedures that are less dramatic still result in erectile dysfunction and men with these procedures often have psychological changes related to their sexual function as well as physical ones.

Being older, having an enlarged prostate, and suffering from erectile difficulties before surgery increase the risk of erectile difficulties after surgery.[14] It is important to note that even if the capacity for an erection is lost, penile sensation and ability to reach orgasm will usually be unimpaired. Nevertheless, men who have had prostate cancer surgery report that their resultant erectile dysfunction goes beyond the sex act and affects the quality of sexual intimacy, everyday interactions with women, sexual imagining and fantasy life, and their perceptions of masculinity.[15]

Some prostate procedures can cause retrograde ejaculation, where the ejaculate flows into the bladder to be excreted during urination (called retrograde ejaculation) instead of outside the body. Although this condition has no effect on erection or orgasm, it seems to have a significant negative effect on sexual satisfaction. Educating men and their partners about the impact of surgery on their sexual behavior may help.

Pelvic surgery can also affect sexual function among women. A hysterectomy, or removal of the uterus, is the second most common operation performed on women in our country (cesareans are first). Evidence is conflicting regarding whether one type of surgery for hysterectomy affects sexual function more than another. In general, most women who have had a hysterectomy report no difference in sexual function, but a few report a great improvement and just as many report a decline. Since a hysterectomy is frequently performed to reduce disease or discomfort, it is easy to understand why sexual interest would increase when the medical problem is resolved. Alterations in sexual function are more likely when the ovaries are removed because the decrease in estrogen may result in thinning of the vaginal wall and decreased lubrication. Bladder surgery may also affect the nerves in the pelvic area.

Women's perceptions of their sexual attractiveness may be affected by a mastectomy (breast removal). A woman's breast is a symbol of female sexuality in our culture and is a significant part of most women's sexual identity. Breast cancer surgery has been shown to alter a woman's sexuality: body image, feelings of attractiveness, and sexual interest and activity. Older women, however, generally rate their sexual adjustment after mastectomy more positively than younger women.

Knee and hip surgery have an effect on sexual activity, at least among males. One study of elderly males who had recently undergone hip or knee surgery concluded that both sexual activity and erectile function declined, especially among the men who had impaired function before the surgery. And the older the man at surgery, the higher was the risk of sexual problems.[16]

Both sexual interest and frequency of intercourse can be affected by the surgery that creates an artificial opening (stoma) in the abdominal wall. In general, these openings are created to reroute the excretion of urine or feces because of obstruction, inflammation, or cancer. Multiple types of stomas are possible. Adjustment to a stoma can cause embarrassment regarding the stoma, alteration in body image, and anxiety about leakage or odor, each of which can impact sexual interest and desire in the patient or partner. Specialized nurses can assist in stoma management, and support groups are available to help individuals adjust.

Psychosocial Considerations

At any age sexual difficulties are likely combinations of biologic, attitudinal, and situational problems. The sexuality of elder men and women, like sexuality in other age groups, is highly influenced by individuals' psychosocial

---

Sexual Satisfaction in the Later Years

Jerry Phelps, Ph.D.
Psychologist, University of California, San Diego

Despite common stereotypes, sexual relations can be quite satisfying and enjoyable for older adults, and in some cases can even be more fulfilling. A good sexual relationship for adults of any age includes positive and open communication, flexibility in sexual behaviors, willingness to overcome new barriers, and curiosity.

The key to sexual enjoyment at any age is mutual satisfaction with the relationship. The qualities of a good relationship—trust; the ability to communicate sexual needs, limits, and concerns; learning to accommodate to the partner's needs; and a caring and solution-oriented mindset—can help to overcome the physical challenges that come with growing older.

The biggest challenge to sexual satisfaction in the later years is coping with physical changes that accompany age and dealing with the effects of chronic illness: pain, decreased libido, erectile dysfunction, lower energy, vaginal dryness and sensitivity, and a slowed arousal and orgasmic response. Older people who report sexual satisfaction say that they continue to learn to adapt to these changes. They are motivated to embrace a variety of sexual practices, such as oral sex, mutual or self-masturbation, and use of vibrators or other sexual aids. These practices add variety and are often more sexually satisfying for female partners than intercourse. Other practical tips help couples to cope with changes that accompany age and illness. Use a lubricant to reduce vaginal pain from intercourse or use manual and oral stimulation instead of intercourse. Schedule sex for early in the morning, when energy and libido are highest. Pay attention to skeletal pain and use positions that limit pain's impact.

One somewhat surprising finding in older adults is that many report increased sexual satisfaction. Since it takes a longer time to achieve an erection and ejaculation in men, couples choose oral and manual stimulation to satisfy their partners. Women frequently increase sexual satisfaction when their partners engage in longer foreplay, stimulate them to orgasm manually or orally, and engage in intercourse less often. When partners focus less on intercourse, men with erectile difficulties also find that they can be manually or orally stimulated to orgasm with a flaccid or semi-erect penis.

Often, growing older brings an appreciation of life's simple pleasures. Without the duties of regular childcare or work, older couples have more time to explore their sexuality. They have the opportunity to appreciate more fully all of the moments of the sexual experience—courtship, flirtation, arousal, the pleasure of giving pleasure, and the closeness and warmth of a sexual satisfaction. One does not go to a symphony to hear the final note, however "climactic." Similarly, focus less on the climax of sex, instead enjoying each note, the ups and downs of the experience, the person you are with, and the time you can spend together.

Used with permission of Jerry Phelps, Ph.D.

adjustment and health. The quality of the relationship is an important component in maintaining sexual interest and satisfaction. Many long-term couples have unresolved resentments, anger, and stereotypical patterns of communication or sexual intimacy that impact their ability to adjust their sexual routine to changing physical or emotional circumstances.

Although the media are full of advice about how to improve communication and achieve fulfillment in marriage and relationships, today's elders grew up in a time when there was no such advice. They tended to believe that marriage was "for life" whether the couple was compatible or not, and sex roles back then were more rigid than they are today. It is likely that men and women focused more on the day-to-day tasks of raising a family and earning a living than on improving their communication or maximizing their sexual inventiveness. Despite a lifetime of marriage and sexual activity, some elders may not have the communication skills needed to adjust to the changes that accompany aging.

Just like members of other age groups, elders are influenced by the societal attitude that older people are sexless. But, as we grow older, if we are not recognized, and do not recognize ourselves, as masculine or feminine, a degree of self-identity is lost. An older woman who accepts the widely held belief that a youthful and firm body is necessary for sexual attractiveness may hesitate to initiate or encourage sexual interaction, feeling that she doesn't measure up. Similarly, older men are victimized by the emphasis on physical performance. They may focus on the act of ejaculation itself rather than on a range of sexual expression. They may judge their sexual adequacy by comparing the frequency of intercourse, the rapidity in attaining an erection, and the firmness of their erection with their performance in their younger years. Such thinking is likely to set up a vicious cycle of sexual problems and strained relationships. With the aging of the population and new attitudes about sexuality, it is hoped that more positive views of aging and sexuality will be the norm.

SEXUAL DYSFUNCTION

Sexual dysfunction is a physiological impairment in sexual response that prevents sexual arousal or orgasm. The national study of over 3,000 mature adults between 57 and 85 included several questions regarding their extent of sexual dysfunction.[2]

Of those participants who were sexually active, about half the men and women reported having at least one bothersome sexual problem and a third reported at least two problems. Among the men, the most prevalent problems reported included difficulty in attaining or achieving an erection, lack of interest in sex, climaxing too quickly, anxiety about performance, and an inability to climax. The most bothersome problem reported was the difficulty in achieving or maintaining an erection. For women, the most common problems were lack of interest in sex, difficulty with lubrication, inability to climax, finding sex not pleasurable, and pain. The most bothersome problems encountered by women were pain, difficulty with lubrication, and finding sex not pleasurable. The respondents who rated their health as fair or poor were more likely to report sexual problems than those with very good or excellent health. The study questioned the respondents who had been sexually inactive for at least three months. The most commonly reported reason among women was the partner's physical health, although women were twice as likely as men were to report a lack of interest as a reason for sexual inactivity.[2]

There are many causes of sexual dysfunction among men. Because healthy men have the interest and capacity for sexual activity into very advanced years, the primary cause of erectile dysfunction, or impotence, in older men is not the aging process but damage to the nerves and blood vessels in the penis from diabetes and high blood pressure. Further, several of the drugs used to treat chronic illnesses affect sexual performance. Erectile dysfunction is more common among older people because they use more prescription drugs and have more illnesses that affect desire and performance. It must be noted, however, that reduced erectile function is considered dysfunctional only if one or both partners are concerned with the reduced sexual interest or ability.

Four factors are needed for male potency: (1) normal male sexual organs, (2) normal levels of testosterone and other hormones, (3) an adequate nerve and blood supply to the penis, and (4) a healthy psyche. Any one missing factor may result in partial or complete erectile dysfunction. *Erectile dysfunction* is the persistent inability to achieve or maintain an erection sufficient for satisfactory sexual performance. It is the most common sexual dysfunction among men. Occasional failure to achieve or sustain an erection is normal for men of all ages and does not qualify as erectile dysfunction. Even men who have erectile dysfunction may maintain sexual desire and even the capacity to reach orgasm.

Studies vary widely in their findings about the extent of erectile problems in the population. It is common for men to report more difficulty with erections with advancing age. One longitudinal study mailed a questionnaire to almost 32,000 male health professionals between the ages of 53 and 90. One-third reported erectile problems within the last three months. The proportion of men who experienced sexual desire, ability, and orgasm decreased sharply with age. Physical activity and leanness were associated with fewer erectile problems; chronic illness, obesity, smoking, alcohol consumption, and television viewing time were associated with more erectile problems.[17] In another study, regular intercourse was associated with less erectile dysfunction.[18]

Erectile dysfunction negatively affects sexual relationships and overall quality of life. Fears about erectile dysfunction can be debilitating to both partners, and fear itself can impede sexual satisfaction. In some cases, a vicious cycle is initiated whereby the couple is trapped in a pattern of fearing erectile difficulties, which decreases the quality of the sexual interaction, which results in higher rates of erectile dysfunction, which can cause irritability, insecurity, blaming, and more fear, further decreasing sexual interaction and satisfaction. Studies document that men who are successfully treated for erectile dysfunction experience improved satisfaction with their sex life, their relationship, and their general mental health.[19] The American Foundation for Urologic Disease has a toll-free hotline to dispense free information on erectile difficulties (1-800-473-0616) and a Web site (www.impotence.org)

Women also suffer from sexual problems. The term *female sexual dysfunction (FSD)* was recently defined by a consensus committee within the American Foundation for Urologic Disease. The definition includes both physiological and psychological symptoms. FSD includes pain during intercourse (dyspareunia), involuntary vaginal spasms that interfere with penetration (vaginismus), and genital pain following stimulation during foreplay (noncoital sexual pain). In addition, the following are considered to be dysfunctions only if the symptom causes the woman distress: chronic lack of interest in sexual activity (hypoactive sexual desire disorder), persistent or recurrent phobic avoidance of sexual contact with a partner (sexual aversion disorder), persistent or recurrent inability to attain or maintain sexual excitement (sexual arousal disorder), and chronic difficulty in attaining, or inability to attain, orgasm following sufficient arousal (orgasmic disorder).[20]

Little research has been conducted on the prevalence and cause of sexual dysfunctions among older women. It is evident that women's sexuality is tied to physical, psychological, and social factors. A prominent researcher at the Kinsey Institute urges caution in approaching female sexual dysfunction as a purely physiological phenomenon because female sexuality is less under hormonal control than male sexuality. This researcher and others suggest that hormone replacement or other drugs may be ineffective in solving problems with female sexuality, and they propose that more attention be placed on complex relationship issues.[21] For more information regarding both male and female sexual dysfunction, refer to the American Foundation of Urologic Disease Web site, www.afud.org

Diagnosis of Sexual Dysfunction

Elders are often reluctant to volunteer information about sexual behavior to a physician, but they are more likely to need help than younger clients. They may consider their problems to be due to the normal aging process, or they may minimize the importance of their sexual needs and desires, or they may be embarrassed to broach the topic. To make matters worse, health professionals may lack training in taking a sexual history or may feel they do not have time. They may be uncomfortable initiating discussions with a person who is older than they, or they may have inadequate knowledge of the sexual needs of older people. Health care providers may consider elder sexuality inconsequential; few take a sexual history or discuss sexual concerns with older patients. They may brush off patients' concerns about sexual dysfunction, saying that sex is not that important at their age or that the dysfunction is just part of growing old.

Sexual dysfunction, however, may be a symptom or a consequence of disease or a medication side effect, so the discussion of sexual issues is critical to accurate diagnosis and treatment. The high incidence of erectile dysfunction and female sexual dysfunction in the elder population makes discussions about sexual concerns imperative, despite the reluctance of both elders and physicians. Many chronic illnesses, medications, and surgeries have an impact on sexual function, and this impact should be discussed at the same time the disease and drugs are discussed. Because of the high rate of sexual problems among women, inquiry about female sexual health concerns should be a part of routine gynecological visits, no matter what the woman's age.

Diagnosis of sexual dysfunction, like other diagnoses, requires a thorough medical history (including psychosocial factors), a physical examination, and laboratory testing to pinpoint the cause of the problem and to determine an effective treatment. The medical history should include a thorough listing of current and past diseases and their treatment, family disease history, alcohol, tobacco, drug intake, and a sexual history.

A sexual history provides information to aid in diagnosis and serves as a vehicle for patient education. Often when conducting the sexual history, the practitioner can uncover misconceptions or misinformation about sexuality that serve as the basis for sexual dissatisfaction. Additionally, the practitioner can use this opportunity to discuss the impact of drugs or illness on sexual function. A sexual history should include the following topics:

- available partner(s), number and gender
- history of present relationship with partner
- if not mutually monogamous, safe-sex practices
- satisfaction with relationship with partner
- frequency and types of sexual activity
- satisfaction with frequency of sexual activity
- level of communication with partner about sexual matters
- current social situation, including life stressors
- illnesses that affect sexuality (desire, attitude, and activity)
- presence of pain during sexual activity (genital or other)
- frequency and turgidity of erections
- quality of ejaculation and orgasm
- use of medications and noticed effect on sexual interest and performance
- use of alcohol, tobacco, or other recreational drugs and noticed effect on sexual interest and performance

Information obtained from the sexual history can be combined with physical examination findings and diagnostic tests to determine the cause of erectile dysfunction or other sexual difficulties. A physical examination is important to uncover possible contributors to sexual problems. For instance, a pelvic examination can uncover the presence of vaginal infections or atrophic vaginitis (a condition resulting from low levels of estrogen). Laboratory evaluations, including measurement of hormones, cholesterol level, blood pressure, and liver function, are also important in identifying contributing causes for sexual dysfunction. If the doctor suspects problems in the blood supply to the penis, the blood vessels in the penis can be evaluated by ultrasound or arteriography techniques (dye is injected into blood vessels and an X-ray is taken). Taking a penile blood pressure can help evaluate erectile difficulties; a low penile blood pressure is associated with vascular disease and increased risk of heart attack or stroke.

Treatment of Sexual Dysfunction

Depending on its origin, sexual dysfunction can be treated in a variety of ways. Many medical conditions and prescription drugs can cause sexual dysfunction, and treating the medical problem or changing the medication type or dosage may be all that is needed to remedy the problem. When a sexual dysfunction is psychological in origin, the patient and partner might be referred to a sex therapist. If the problem is due to chronic illness or to a hormone deficiency, drugs, injections, or implants might be prescribed. If a problem with the veins or arteries in the penis leads to erectile dysfunction, surgery can be performed. The health professional should understand that not all elders want their sexual problems treated. A sexual dysfunction needs to be addressed only if it is considered to be a problem by the individual or the partner.

The overwhelming majority of treatments for sexual dysfunction focus on restoring male erectile function, even though a significant proportion of women cannot reach orgasm. What accounts for this discrepancy? Does it exist because most researchers are men, and impotence is of greater interest to them? Or does it exist because women can participate in the sex act and satisfy men without excitement and orgasm? Are data on women more difficult to gather than data on men? Medical treatments to restore sexual functioning are discussed in the following paragraphs. Sex education and counseling, mentioned later in the chapter, are also appropriate treatments.

Medications and Hormones

The search for a substance to enhance sexual function is probably as old as civilization itself. Oysters, chocolate, rhino horns, and Spanish fly are only a few of the many potions claiming to increase sexual desire and performance. However, some are risky. Spanish fly, made from a species of European beetle, is perhaps the most dangerous. It irritates the urinary tract as it leaves the body, causing blood to rush to the sex organs. It is a poison that can burn, leading to scarring, infections, and even death.

By far the most talked about medication to help men with erectile dysfunction is Viagra (generic name, sildenafil), the pill that entered the market in 1998. The little blue pill has become one of the most profitable medications in history: Millions of men have taken the drug for erectile dysfunction. It must be stressed that Viagra is not an aphrodisiac. It does not increase sexual desire; it enhances the ability to have and maintain an erection.

In order to understand how Viagra works, it is necessary to know the mechanism of a normal erection. An erection begins in the brain when a stimulus (vision, touch, smell, even a thought) stimulates a particular set of nerves that send messages down the spinal cord, around the prostate gland, and into the penis, where they direct cells to produce a chemical called cyclic GMP. The chemical relaxes muscles in two spongy cylinders of the penis, allowing them to fill with blood, ultimately stiffening the penis. The expanding spongy tissue then squeezes veins that normally drain blood from the penis, trapping the blood inside. Viagra works by blocking the enzyme that breaks down the cyclic GMP. As a result, the cyclic GMP accumulates in the penis and gradually results in an erection. Viagra is taken in pill form about an hour before sexual activity. The drug should not be taken more than once a day.

Although Viagra doesn't work for everyone, research confirms it is an effective treatment for many men with erectile dysfunction. Men with medical problems and elders may benefit as well. However, with prolonged use higher doses may be needed. Viagra is used for women as well at times, although it is not as well studied.

The side effects of Viagra may be significant: headaches, upset stomach, and vision abnormalities. Further, the drug is incompatible with nitrate drugs commonly used for heart problems. Both Viagra and nitrate drugs lower blood pressure. Combining the two drugs causes blood pressure to drop dangerously low. Finally, it is expensive, costing about $10 a pill. There have been very interesting debates regarding the number of pills for which health insurance companies should reimburse the insured per month. Over the years, Viagra has brought in billions of dollars to Pfizer stockholders, and Pfizer has spent millions of dollars marketing it. It is hard to escape the advertising for this product.

The FDA has since approved two drugs from other drug companies that work in the same way: Levitra and Cialis. These newer drugs are reported to have reduced side effects, rapid onset of effect, and longer duration of action.

Another way to increase sexual performance for men is to inject a drug into the penis prior to intercourse to produce an erection. Several drugs can be used in this way: paraverine, phentolamine, and alprostadil (prostaglandin E). All are effective and widely used. These medications produce an erection within 5 to 10 minutes of the injection and last 30 minutes to an hour even in the absence of stimulation. Injections cost about $2 to $4 apiece. Their use is restricted to no more than three times weekly, and they must be spaced at least 24 hours apart. The most common side effect of the medications is penile pain, occurring in about one in ten men. Prostaglandin E, a hormone that naturally occurs in semen, seems to cause the fewest side effects. It may also be prescribed as a suppository that can be inserted into the urethra by means of a slender plastic tube.

Natural therapies have been suggested to help with erectile dysfunction including acupuncture, red ginseng, yohimbe, horny goat weed, DHEA supplements, and gingko biloba.

Hormonal therapy has been reported to increase sexual desire in both men and women.

Testosterone replacement enhances erectile function and libido in men if they have a low testosterone level. Testosterone may be injected (usually every other week), a patch may be placed on the skin, or a gel may be rubbed into the skin. A testosterone pill is available in Europe but is not yet approved by the FDA to be sold in this country. Testosterone supplementation does not appear to increase sexual desire if testosterone levels are in the normal range. Long-term use can be associated with significant complications, particularly prostate cancer and blood clots. Because long-term safety remains uncertain, it is recommend that testosterone replacement not extend more than three years.

Several hormones are utilized to treat women with sexual dysfunction. Physicians prescribe estrogen replacement therapy for menopausal and postmenopausal women. Estrogen is combined with progesterone in women who have a uterus. Dehydroepiandrosterone (DHEA), an androgen produced naturally by the body that declines drastically in early adulthood, seems to increase testosterone production in older women, resulting in increased libido.

Testosterone supplements may be prescribed with estrogen for older women to enhance sexual drive and increase energy and sense of well-being. However, more study is needed to determine who should be treated with testosterone, what dose is ideal, and whether there are short- or long-term side effects. Women on this therapy should be carefully monitored because the drug can increase facial hair and cholesterol.

Mechanical Aids

Penile implants are useful for men with impotence caused by an irreversible physical problem. They have high rates of patient satisfaction. Two major types of permanent implants are commonly used to make the penis rigid enough for intercourse. One type consists of bendable plastic rods implanted into the penile shaft. In this case, the penis is in a permanent state of erection. When an erection is desired, the penis is positioned. Athletic supporters may be worn so the erection is not detectable in street clothes. The second major type is an inflatable implant that creates an erection when fluid is pumped from an implanted reservoir into two cylindrical chambers implanted in the penile shaft. The fluid pump is activated when a bulb in the scrotum is squeezed, causing the cylinders to expand. When the need for an erection is over, a valve is pressed, allowing the fluid to flow from the cylinder back into the reservoir. The advantage of the inflatable implant is a natural appearance of the penis. However, neither type of implant will restore arousal or orgasm if these capacities are lost. The cost of the surgical procedure for a penile implant is between $10,000 and $15,000. Most insurance plans, including Medicare, cover the procedure with some level of patient copay.

Another mechanical aid for impotence is the external vacuum device, which uses suction to draw blood into the penis; backflow of blood is prevented with a tight band at the base of the penis. A clear plastic tubular device is placed over the penis and pressed firmly against the pelvic area, and a hand pump creates suction that draws blood into the penis. An erection occurs in 3 to 5 minutes and lasts up to 30 minutes. Men using this device achieve orgasm but do not ejaculate. The band should not be worn for longer than 30 minutes. Men who can achieve but not sustain an erection may benefit from the tight band alone. A splinted condom worn on the outside of the penis, after an erection is achieved by vacuum, may also be used. The vacuum device is economical (from $100 to $450), does not require surgery, and no prescription is needed.

Sex Therapy

Most models of sex therapy have developed from the classic work of Masters and Johnson[22] and are based on the assumption that sexual problems arise because normal sexual response

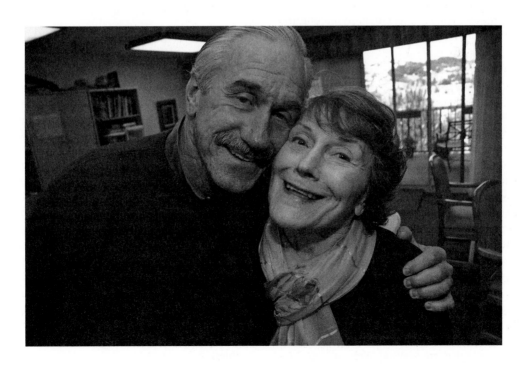

is blocked by anxiety or fear of failure. Masters and Johnson assert that both partners are responsible for the sexual dysfunction. Generally, a male-female cotherapist team provides education, counseling, and daily assignments for the couple, usually progressive exercises in mutual pleasure along with verbal feedback. The goal of the mutual pleasure-giving exercises is to learn that sexual contact should not be goal oriented (orgasm), but lovemaking should be pleasurable in itself. The therapists request that the clients refrain from intercourse for a time to reduce performance anxiety. This type of therapy is the most effective in cases of psychological impotence and premature ejaculation.

A different counseling approach may be used when the problem extends to other aspects of the relationship. Long-standing dissatisfaction with both sexual and nonsexual aspects of the relationship or lack of communication skills indicates a need for more general counseling. Other counseling approaches may also be needed by individuals seeking help with sexual problems created by chronic illness. There is little information regarding the use or success of sex therapy among the older population.

SEX EDUCATION

Ignorance is probably the greatest deterrent to sexual function for all ages, especially older people. Elders are likely to be less knowledgeable about sexuality than any other age group because they had little or no sex education in their earlier years. Studies show a high rate of sexual misinformation among elders, which may adversely impact their sexual satisfaction.

There is almost no information in the literature regarding sex education for elders. This lack may be due to the belief by some health educators that elders are neither sexually active nor interested in learning about sexuality.

The advent of the Internet has opened up many new opportunities for sex education. It is well known that pornographic Web sites are the most commonly accessed "sex education" on the Internet, but other less provocative resources are also available. Elders can ask questions anonymously, read blogs, watch videos, and access educational materials for free 24/7 in the privacy of their own homes with the click of a mouse. Education can be written or visual, directed toward men and women, and there is plenty there for all ages. However, the elders of tomorrow may have completely different issues, having grown up in the 1960s and 1970s, when sexuality became more open. The following list is only a sample of sexual issues that might be addressed in sex education classes for older people:

- The physiological changes with age that affect sexual interest and activity
- The effects of illness and surgery on sexual interest and activity
- Modes of alternative sexual expression
- Ways to maintain a healthy sexual identity
- The effects of medication and alcohol on sexuality
- HIV and the older adult
- Learning to communicate with a partner about sexual needs
- How to discuss sexual problems with your doctor

Family members and those who work with elders also benefit from education about elder sexuality, especially those who work in institutional settings. The attitude of the health professional is an important variable in the educational process for any age group. An older person's willingness to discuss sexual concerns depends on the professional's openness and comfort with the topic. Just as professionals should not be judgmental of sexually active elders, neither should they pressure an older person to conform to sexual norms of younger adults. Health professionals need to take elders' educational levels and cognitive abilities into account when developing programs. Just like other types of health education, sex education is more successful if elders are involved in the planning, topic selection, publicity, and group facilitation.

SUMMARY

Studies clearly show that sexual interest and activity continue into old age. However, many people still have misperceptions of elder sexuality. Studies on elder sexuality are sparse and generally have small sample sizes and other methodological problems. Although sexuality encompasses a number of behaviors, most studies have concentrated on intercourse and masturbation. Preliminary work shows that these behaviors tend to decrease slightly with age. However, intercourse frequency is highly dependent on the presence of a partner. Evidence seems to indicate that individuals who continue sexual activity throughout life have little alteration in sexual response.

It is difficult to make generalizations about elder sexuality because there are a number of elders with different characteristics and needs regarding sexuality, such as unmarried women, older gays and lesbians, and older people who are institutionalized. Furthermore, some chronic illnesses, including arthritis, heart disease, cancer, and diabetes, are likely to affect elders' sexual interest and ability. Other factors that influence sexual interest and activity are testosterone deficiency, prescription drugs, overuse of alcohol, and psychological factors.

Sexual dysfunction, an impaired ability or interest in sexual activity, can occur among men and women. Sexual problems may be due to drug reactions, psychological concerns, or physiological factors. Sex therapy, drugs, penile implants, and hormones are available to treat sexual dysfunctions. Although education about elder sexuality is uncommon, it has the potential to increase knowledge and change attitudes—for elders, their families, and the professionals who work with them.

ACTIVITIES

1. Ask 10 individuals of different ages these three questions:
   a. What is your age?
   b. At what age do you think sexual activity ceases?
   c. At what age do you think sexual interest ceases?

   Compare your responses with those of other students in class. How do the results differ among age groups? What informal conversations did your questions stimulate?

2. Interview five students about their estimates of the frequency of sexual activity by their parents and by their grandparents. How do the responses compare to average frequencies discussed in the chapter?

3. Visit a local skilled nursing facility and interview both an administrator and an aide about the sexual life of the residents. Ask the administrator to describe regulations pertaining to sexual activity in the nursing home. Does the right to privacy extend to sexual activity? Notice the physical layout of the nursing home. How does it discourage or encourage sexual intimacy?

4. Develop model guidelines for expressions of sexuality in a nursing home. Include guidelines for gay, unmarried, and married couples; the severely demented; privacy for masturbation; sex education; and maintaining personal appearance.

5. Collect cartoons and greeting cards that address sexuality in the later years. What images do they project about older people?

6. Develop an educational campaign to educate older adults about safe-sex practices.

7. Choose at least one Web site mentioned in the chapter, browse the site, and write about what interested you and what you learned.

8. Choose a topic regarding elder sexuality that might be presented at the local senior center. Develop a lesson plan that includes objectives and content to be discussed. List the resources you used in developing your presentation.

9. Develop an in-service educational program for nurse's aides regarding sexuality among institutionalized older people, including objectives and major content areas. Provide at least three educational resources for the instructor.

10. Do a Web search on sexuality and elders. What kinds of educational materials can you find? How would you categorize them?

BIBLIOGRAPHY

1. Starr, B.D., and Weiner, M.B. 1981. *The Starr-Weiner Report on sex and sexuality in the mature years*. San Francisco: McGraw-Hill.

2. Lindau, S.T., Schumm, L.P, Laumann, E.O., Levinson, W., O'Muircheartaigh, C.A., and Waite, L.J. 2007. A study of sexuality and health among older adults in the United States. *New England Journal of Medicine* 357(8):762–774.

3. AARP. 1999. AARP/Modern Maturity Sexuality Survey—summary of findings. Research.aarp.org/health/mmsexsurvey_1.html

4. Masters, W.H., and Johnson, V.E. 1966. *Human sexual response*. Boston: Little, Brown.

5. Administration on Aging. 2011. A profile of older Americans. U.S. Department of Health and Human Services. www.aoa.gov

6. Brotman, S., Ryan, B., and Cormier, R. 2003. The health and social service needs of gay and lesbian elders and their families in Canada. *The Gerontologist* 43(2):192–202.

7. Claes, J. and Moore, W. 2000. Issues confronting lesbian and gay elders: The challenge for health and human service providers. *Journal of Health and Human Service Administration.* Fall: 181–202.

8. Centers for Disease Control and Prevention. 2007. HIV/AIDS Surveillance Report 19, Table 12. Atlanta: U.S. Department of Health and Human Services.

9. Population Reference Bureau. 2009. HIV/AIDS and older adults in the United States. *Today's Research on Aging* 18:1–7.

10. Hayden, C., Clifford, D., and Hertz, F. 2010. *A legal guide for lesbian and gay couples*. Berkeley, CA: Nolo Press.

11. Metz, P. 1997. Staff development for working with lesbian and gay elders. *Journal of Gay and Lesbian Social Services* 6(1):35–45.

12. Burchardt, M., Burchardt, T., Anastasiadis, et al. 2002. Sexual dysfunction is common and overlooked in female patients with hypertension. *Journal of Sex and Marital Therapy* 28(1): 17–26.

13. Giaquinto, S., Buzelli, S., DiFrancesco, L., and Nolfe, G. 2003. Evaluation of sexual changes after stroke. *Journal of Clinical Psychiatry* 64(3):302–307.

14. Hollenbeck, B.K., Dunn, R.L., Wei, J.T. Montie, J.E., and Sanda, M.G. 2003. Determinants of long-term sexual health outcome after radical prostatectomy measured by a validated instrument. *Journal of Urology* 169(4):1453–1457.

15. Bokhour, B.G., Clark, J.Q., Inui, T.S., Silliman, R.A., and Talcott, J.A. 2001. Sexuality after treatment for early prostate cancer: Exploring the meanings of "erectile dysfunction." *Journal of General Internal Medicine* 16(10):649–655.

16. Nordentoft, T., Schou, J., and Carstensen, J. 2000. Changes in sexual behavior after orthopedic replacement of hip or knee in elderly males— a prospective study. *International Journal of Impotence Research* 12(3):143–146.

17. Bacon, C.G., Mittleman, M.A., Kawachi, I., et al. 2003. Sexual function in men older than 50 years of age: Results from the health professionals follow-up study. *Annals of Internal Medicine* 139(3):161–168.

18. Koskimäki, J., Shiri, R., Tammela, T., Häkkinen, J., Hakama, M., and Auvinen, A. 2008. Regular intercourse protects against erectile dysfunction: A Tampere Aging male urologic study. *American Journal of Medicine* 121(7):592–596.

19. Giuliano, F., Pena, B.M., Mishra, A., and Smith, M.D. 2001. Efficacy results and quality-of-life measures in men receiving sildenafil citrate for the treatment of erectile dysfunction. *Quality of Life Research* 10(4):359–369.

20. Basson, R., Berman, J., Burnett, A., et al. 2000. Report of the international consensus development conference of female sexual dysfunction: Definitions and classifications. *Journal of Urology* 163(3):888–893.

21. Bancroft, J. 2002. The medicalization of female sexual dysfunction: The need for caution. *Archives of Sexual Behavior* 31(5):451–455.

22. Masters, W.H., and Johnson, V.E. 1970. *Human sexual inadequacy*. Boston: Little, Brown.

CHAPTER 12

Prevention and Health Promotion

Our fascination with the more glamorous "pound of cure" has tended to dazzle us into ignoring the more effective "ounce of prevention."

Jimmy Carter

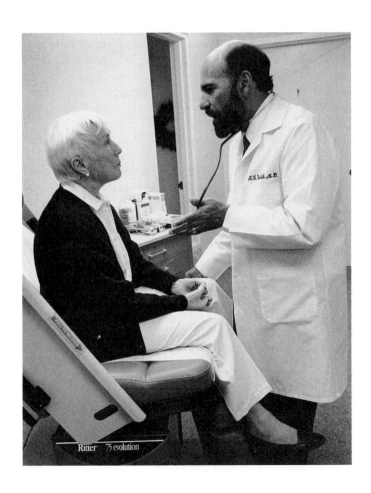

Health behaviors and lifestyle play an important part in the development and severity of many illnesses. Unlike genetic factors, which are beyond our control, our lifestyle—what we eat, our exercise habits, whether we smoke cigarettes or drink alcohol, even our reactions to stress—can be modified to reduce the risk of disease. And abundant information about ways to enhance our health is available. But even though most of us know what a healthy lifestyle is, and its importance in preventing disease, improved health behaviors do not necessarily follow. For example, even though there is ample evidence of the harmful consequences of cigarette smoking, about one-fourth of all American adults smoke. And even though most people are aware that obesity reduces the quality and length of life, more than half the adults in the United States are overweight or obese, and few people exercise regularly. Similarly, the benefits of some screening tests in reducing illness and death have been documented, but relatively few Americans undergo these procedures.

Historically, physicians placed little emphasis on encouraging older people to engage in health promoting activities to prevent or reduce disease and disability in later life. It was believed that it was too late for change or that elders would be unwilling to alter long-standing habits. However, it is now known that older people are at least as likely to change health habits as younger groups. And changing poor health habits, even late in life, can forestall disease, disability, and death.

In this chapter we discuss the three major types of prevention that improve the health of older people: *primary prevention,* practicing good health habits and getting vaccinated to prevent an illness; *secondary prevention,* engaging in particular health screenings to detect disease at an early, treatable stage; and *tertiary prevention,* properly caring for an already established disease to stay as well as possible, minimize its negative effects, and prevent complications. The Healthy People Initiative—the national public health effort to reduce illness, disability, and death in the United States—is explored.

Health promotion is an important activity for health professionals. Health promotion is defined, and attention is given to ways to help older people change negative health habits. We explore health behavioral interventions that have been shown to reduce the rate of illness and death and increase the quality of life for older people. Behaviors that keep individuals from choosing and maintaining healthy lifestyles are addressed. We also examine the importance of public policy in promoting health for the greater good.

PREVENTION: AN OVERVIEW

In the health field, *prevention* refers to any activity that reduces the incidence and severity of disease, disability, and premature death. A prevention activity may be self-initiated: Brushing one's teeth, eating fruits and vegetables, participating in physical exercise, and getting a flu shot are just a few examples of the many choices individuals make every day that impact their health status. A prevention activity may be initiated by a professional for individuals—for example, prescribing a screening test, assessing a client's home for accident hazards, and educating a patient about how to take medication. A professional may also work with groups—implementing exercise classes, conducting stop smoking classes, or facilitating self-help groups for individuals with a particular disease.

Prevention activities can also be designed by a health organization or agency to reach a broader audience: public service ads on television, health fairs, health department flu clinics, and billboards. Probably the prevention efforts that benefit the greatest number of people are health advocacy efforts by groups of individuals that culminate in new laws and regulations at the state and national levels: reducing toxic waste, strengthening worker safety, bans on smoking indoors, mandatory seat belt use, and many other health-affirming actions.

There are three major types of prevention activities: primary, secondary, and tertiary. *Primary* prevention is what most people think of as prevention: eating well, getting sufficient exercise, wearing a seat belt, getting sufficient sleep. Another example of primary prevention is being vaccinated to prevent an illness.

Secondary prevention activities, also geared toward those who appear healthy, are designed to detect a condition that otherwise would not be discovered. For example, Ann feels healthy, but laboratory tests indicate diabetes, and a blood pressure reading indicates high blood pressure. These diagnostic tests (also called screening tests) are administered to individuals who have no observable sign of disease in order to detect illnesses at an early, treatable stage. Screening tests are available to detect many types of diseases. Some can be accomplished by the individual at home; others require a physician or other health professional. The most common screening tests used by older people are discussed later in the chapter.

Tertiary prevention activities include the many types of treatments for individuals with existing illnesses. Tertiary prevention is designed to prevent further disability, complications, or death. One example of tertiary prevention is reducing blood pressure and cholesterol to reduce the incidence of heart attack. Another example is monitoring and treating high levels of blood glucose to prevent a diabetic person from developing kidney failure, blindness, or nonhealing wounds. Tertiary prevention that is specific to particular diseases is not discussed in this chapter. For coverage of treatment for the major diseases and conditions, see Chapters 4, 5, 6, and 7.

When most of us think of prevention, we relate it to the choices we make daily to maintain or improve our health. Or we might think of the education we receive at the physician's office. Although we do not usually think of prevention as involving whole communities, community-based health promotion programs may be very successful at reducing disease and disability. These programs may target a particular health problem (e.g., accident prevention, smoking cessation, disease screening) or offer a comprehensive wellness program. They may occur through health maintenance organizations or in community settings such as senior centers, assisted living facilities, and nutrition sites. In addition, many prevention activities focus on populations, or groups of people who share some characteristics in common.

THE HEALTHY PEOPLE INITIATIVE

We can all think of many ways to improve the health of individuals and the community, but where do we start? How do we decide what health issue to focus on, whom to target, what program to implement? And how will we know if we are successful?

One of the largest government-sponsored programs to establish priorities and set goals to improve the health of Americans is the Healthy People Initiative. The federal Department of Health and Human Services and more than 650 local, state, and federal agencies (both governmental and private) have come together to identify the top priorities to improve the health of Americans and to set health goals for various subgroups (e.g., elders, children, minorities).

The Initiative provides specific health objectives and outlines ways to meet those objectives in a format that diverse groups working together can use. The plan is based on the best scientific knowledge and is used for decision making and action. It can be envisioned as a road map to better health for all that can be used by many different people. Individuals can use the document to set their own health goals, and community leaders can use it to assess their community, prioritize health concerns, and implement needed programs. At the state level, the objectives can serve as a blueprint for determining where health funds should be spent. The goals can be implemented by states, counties, communities, professional organizations, groups whose concern is a particular health problem, or a particular population group.

The Healthy People concept was first developed in 1979 upon release of the report *Healthy People: The Surgeon General's Report on Health Promotion and Disease Prevention*. Among the goals of the report were the reduction of mortality among four different age groups (infants, children, adolescents, young adults, and adults) and an increase in independence among older adults. Specific numbers were targeted for each group, to be achieved by 1990. Many of the goals were met for infants and children. Goals for adolescents were not achieved, and there were insufficient data to assess whether goals for older adults were achieved.

Healthy People 2000 built on the lessons of the Surgeon General's 1979 report, with even more collaboration and more advanced science. Many of the *Healthy People 2000* objectives specified improving the health of groups of people who bear a disproportionate burden of poor health—including the poor, minorities, and those without health insurance. The framework of *Healthy People 2000* consisted of three broad goals: to increase the span of healthy life for Americans, to reduce health disparities among Americans, and to achieve access to preventive services for all Americans. Under these goals were more than 300 national objectives focused on health promotion, health protection, and preventive services.

The goals of *Healthy People 2010* were to increase individuals' responsibility for their health and the health of their communities, to encourage communities at the state and local levels to develop activities that promote health and healthy environments, and to increase all Americans' access to high-quality health care.

The document set forth two broad goals: to increase the length and quality of healthy life and to eliminate health disparities among ethnic and racial subgroups. The two broad goals were grouped into 10 leading health indicators: physical activity, overweight and obesity, tobacco use, substance abuse, responsible sexual behavior, mental health, injury and violence, environmental quality, immunization, and access to health care. The leading health indicators were intended to educate the population about the most important changes we could make to improve our health and reduce disability. Measurable objectives within each indicator were tracked, measured, and reported throughout the 10-year period.

The latest initiative is Healthy People 2020. The stated goals of Healthy People 2020 are to attain high-quality, longer lives free of preventable disease, disability, injury, and premature death; achieve health equity, eliminate disparities, and improve the health of all groups; create social and physical environments that promote good health for all; and promote quality of life, healthy development, and healthy behaviors across all life stages. There are four foundation health measures that will indicate progress toward these goals: General health status, health-related quality of life and well-being, determinants of health, and disparities. For a more in-depth look at these indices and goals, please refer to www.healthypeople.gov

The Healthy People initiatives and goals establish priorities for health for all Americans. But which of the many objectives are the most important to individuals? What should you, your parents, your grandparents, and your clients do to stay healthy and prevent illness? To answer this question, multiple expert panels and professional associations have reviewed the literature and recommended primary and secondary prevention activities shown in many studies to have value.

Perhaps the best-known set of recommendations for prevention activities is published by the U.S. Preventive Services Task Force (USPSTF). The Public Health Service directs the USPSTF to rigorously evaluate clinical research in order to assess the merits of preventive measures, including screening tests, counseling, immunizations, and preventive medications. Members of the USPSTF review the clinical evidence supporting various preventive activities, the recommendations of experts, and the risks and benefits of each activity, and they make recommendations based on the strength of the supporting evidence. The group's recommendations are considered the gold standard for preventive services delivered in the clinical setting. The pioneering efforts of the task force culminated in the *Guide to Clinical Preventive Services,* first published in 1989 and now available and continually updated on the Web at www.ahrq.gov USPSTF research and recommendations and periodic updates regarding each disease are beyond the scope of this chapter. To see the most current recommendations, go to the Agency for Healthcare Research and Quality's Web site: www.uspreventiveservicestaskforc.org/adultrec.htm

The How of Prevention: Principal Findings of the U.S. Preventive Services Task Force

1. **Interventions that address personal health practices are vitally important.** Those who provide health care services need to understand that people's personal health habits—what they eat, whether they exercise, and what behaviors they engage in, such as wearing seat belts, driving habits, avoiding smoking, and attitude—can have more to do with health than any blood test or physical exam at the doctor's office. Clinicians must encourage those seeking services to take responsibility for their own health and change their behaviors to extend their life and improve their health.

2. **The clinician and patient should share decision making.** Different people look at risks and benefits differently. Some are willing to go through a lot of pain and discomfort to find something that might be wrong, others prefer to "not know" unless there is a curative treatment.

3. **Clinicians should be selective in ordering tests and providing preventive services.** Although there are some screening tests, such as mammograms for older women, that have been shown to reduce deaths, most tests offered have not been proven to extend life, and many have side effects or can harm the patient. To choose the right screening test, a clinician must consider age, gender, health status, and patient preferences and know the evidence supporting the use of that test.

4. **Clinicians must take every opportunity to deliver preventive services, especially to those with limited access to care.** Many people at the highest risk of disease are those least likely to seek care. So when they do come to the doctor for something (perhaps they need a physical exam for work or have a skin infection), it might be a good time to talk to them about health behaviors or give them immunizations and/or screening.

5. **For some health problems, community-level interventions may be more effective than personal ones.** It is far easier to make a law requiring people to wear seat belts or to put air bags in cars than it is to constantly remind and/or check up on people.

Adapted from the *Report of the U.S. Preventive Services Task Force, Guide to Clinical Preventive Services,* 2nd ed. (Williams and Wilkins, 1996), pp. xxviii–xxxii.

PRIMARY PREVENTION: VACCINES AND PILLS

The most effective way to prevent disease involves positive health behaviors—activities that we do every day to stay healthy. Wearing seat belts, eating healthfully, cleaning the teeth and gums, preventing excess sun exposure, not smoking, being physically active, maintaining relationships and social ties, and maintaining a positive mental outlook are examples of positive health behaviors that are considered primary prevention activities. Many chapters in this book pay particular attention to several positive health behaviors in promoting good health and will not be discussed here. This section will highlight two other types of primary prevention activities that apply to older people: adult immunizations and daily aspirin to prevent heart disease and stroke. The CDC calculates statistics for immunization rates and updates their Web site frequently about the vaccine recommendations, new strains of flu, and other preventive strategies for elders. Refer to www.cdc.gov for more information.

Influenza is a debilitating but generally self-limiting viral infection that causes incapacitating weakness, fevers, chills, and body aches. In elders, particularly the chronically ill, an influenza infection may be life threatening. The vast majority of deaths attributed to influenza occur among people over age 65, particularly those who are frail. Affected individuals are at high risk of developing pneumonia. See Chapter 6 for details on the disease.

An annual flu shot, given in the fall before flu season starts, provides the best protection against influenza and its complications. Because the virus mutates quickly, the influenza vaccine is reformulated by the Centers for Disease Control and Prevention each year to target the strains that are most likely to cause an infection in the upcoming winter. The individual is injected with just enough of the inactivated virus to enable the immune system to set up a defense against it. A yearly vaccination is required because the immunity lasts only a few months. The vaccine is likely more effective at preventing illness among healthier elders (who are likely to recover without the vaccine) than among the very old or frail (who are at higher risk of death from influenza). There are two ways to receive the influenza vaccine: the shot (containing killed virus) and the nasal spray (live, weakened virus). Only the shot is recommended for those 50 years of age and older.

People 50 years of age and older, particularly those who are frail or who have chronic medical problems, the institutionalized, and those who have significant contact with elders, are advised to be vaccinated each year in October or November before flu season starts. The vaccination has been shown to reduce the risk of flu, its complications, and subsequent hospitalization and death from all causes during flu seasons.[1] Medicare covers yearly influenza immunizations for individuals 65 and older.

Pneumococcal pneumonia is an inflammation of the lungs caused by the pneumococcus bacteria (see Chapter 6). It is a significant cause of illness, hospitalization, and death among those 65 and older. The vaccine is made from several strains of the inactivated pneumococcal bacteria. The vaccine reduces the risk of contracting pneumococcal pneumonia in all ages, but it is most effective in healthy adults who are able to mount an adequate immune response. A single vaccination is recommended at age 65 for healthy elders. Boosters are recommended for some groups at

particularly high risk of infection—for example, those with kidney failure. The vaccine lasts about five years, and it is hoped that immunizing elders while they are healthy will protect them later when they are less able to fight off infection. The cost of the pneumococcal vaccine is covered by Medicare.

Shingles is a painful, blistering skin rash caused by the chickenpox (varicella-zoster) virus. According to the Centers for Disease Control and Prevention, all adults aged 60 and older should get the shingles vaccine (Zostavax), regardless of whether or not they have had shingles (or chickenpox as a child). Although the symptoms go away, the virus stays latent in the body and can be reactivated, even years later. The vaccine is a live vaccine given as a single injection to the upper arm. It isn't fail-safe, but it can reduce the severity and duration of the disease. The shingles vaccination will only be covered if you have a Medicare Part D Prescription Drug Plan. The amount of copayment for the vaccination varies, depending on the plan.

Tetanus is rare in the United States, but when it does occur, most individuals contracting the disease are over age 50 because many older people do not have up-to-date tetanus immunizations. The tetanus vaccine is mixed with a vaccine for diphtheria (Td) and should be given as a primary series in childhood with boosters every 10 years in adulthood. Refer to Chapter 6 for more information on immunizations and the diseases they prevent. Medicare will pay for a tetanus vaccination only if exposed to the disease or condition.

Heart disease risk is reduced in some populations when aspirin is taken every day or every other day. Aspirin has a long, successful history of reducing fever, headaches, and muscular pain. Aspirin also can decrease the stickiness of blood platelets, reducing the risk of blood clots. The U.S. Preventive Services Task Force strongly recommends that physicians talk to their patients who are at risk for coronary heart disease, addressing the benefits and harms of aspirin therapy. The USPSTF declared that for men aged 45–79 and women aged 55–79 years, the potential benefit of a reduction in myocardial infarctions and ischemic strokes, respectively, outweighs potential harm due to an increase in gastrointestinal hemorrhage. Others at high risk who could benefit from a daily baby aspirin include postmenopausal women, smokers, and individuals with abnormal cholesterol levels, high blood pressure, a family history of cardiovascular disease, or diabetes.[2]

Aspirin therapy has some undesirable side effects, including stomach upset, gastrointestinal bleeding, and hemorrhagic stroke. A valuable online tool at www.med-decisions.com is helpful as a guide. The final decision on such long-term therapy should be made after consultation with a physician.

SECONDARY PREVENTION: SCREENING

A screening test is a tool used to find disease in people without symptoms, hopefully in an early, treatable stage. The tools used to identify a disease are many and varied. A blood test can screen for diabetes, high cholesterol, or kidney damage. A scale can screen for obesity. An eye chart can screen for vision problems. A rectal examination or mole-check can screen for cancer. An X-ray (mammography) can screen for breast cancer. A questionnaire can screen for alcoholism, dementia, or depression.

Screening may be offered to the general population, but it is usually best targeted to those at risk of the disease. Mammograms, for example, are not routinely done on younger women because their risk of developing breast cancer is very low and their breast density is high, making the results difficult to interpret. In some cases, screening tests are offered only to individuals at high risk. Only diabetics, for example, would require screening for problems that affect diabetics, such as diabetic kidney disease.

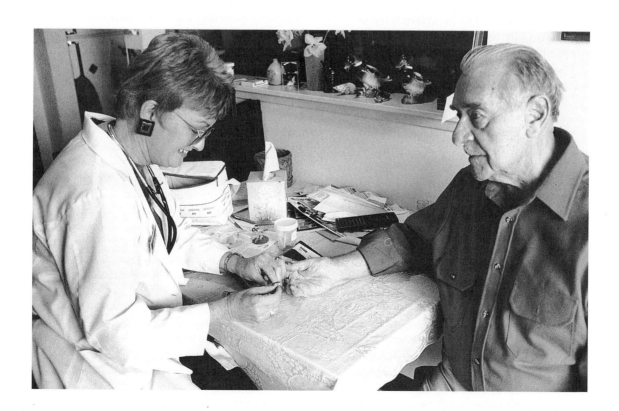

Certain characteristics must be met before screening is recommended on a wide scale:

1. **The test must be able to detect the illness before any signs or symptoms of the disease are evident to the patient or the health care provider.** Once symptoms are present, the individual should participate in the necessary diagnostic tests, and treatment should proceed.

2. **The test must be accurate with a minimum of false positives or false negatives.** *False positive results* occur when the test is positive (indicates that the individual has the disease) but the individual does not have the disease. *False negative results* occur when the test is read as negative (no disease is detected) but the individual does have the disease. Although no test is perfectly accurate, false positive results can cause mental distress and subject healthy people to unnecessary tests or procedures. For example, some of the screening tests for ovarian cancer have high rates of false positives, and women with these results may need to have surgery to find out if cancer is present. In contrast, false negative results can delay treatment and provide a false sense of security. For example, mammography in younger women has a high rate of false negatives so a woman is told her mammogram is normal but she is really harboring a cancer. Because of this reassurance, she may ignore other warning signs of cancer.

3. **Screening and early treatment of disease should improve the health of the patient.** Although it seems intuitive that early detection is a good practice, this is not always the case. For example, some illnesses are almost always fatal (such as some cancers and neurological diseases), and discovering them earlier does not change the end result but merely gives the individual more time to live with (and worry about) the diagnosis. For example, prostate cancer often grows slowly and may be present in many men who die of something else.

Detecting it earlier and subjecting men to treatment (which may be harmful) may not make any difference in their life expectancy, especially if they die of heart disease before the prostate cancer becomes advanced.

The goal of screening and early detection is to reduce morbidity and mortality from particular diseases so that people can live longer, healthier lives. The best way we know of to determine the value of a screening test is to compare a group of people who were offered screening with those who were not and compare how many people died in each group. If there were significantly fewer deaths in the group who was screened, the screening test is considered to be effective.

Some poor health habits can be found during a health interview. The clinician questions the patient regarding behaviors that put him or her at risk for disease or injury, such as high-fat diet, smoking, inactivity, high level of stress, and a high level of alcohol intake. Screening for some behaviors can also be undertaken with standardized questionnaires, rather than relying on individual clinicians to ask certain questions. Standardized screening instruments exist for alcoholism, depression, and dementia.

Screening practices are an integral part of the physical examination. Ascertaining information regarding the patient's health history and family history is a type of screening. Measurement of weight, blood pressure, vision, hearing, pulmonary function, and examination of body organs for cancer (oral cavity, breasts, abdomen, testicles, skin, pelvic exam, rectal/prostate exam) are also screening tests. Most people identify screening with laboratory tests, particularly measurement for anemia, diabetes, elevated cholesterol, HIV, electrocardiogram for heart abnormalities, tuberculosis skin or blood test, the Pap smear for cervical cancer, prostate-specific antigen (PSA) test for prostate cancer, and the stool tests for microscopic blood. Finally, screening can entail more elaborate tests, such as X-rays (e.g., mammography), colonoscopy (placing a tube in the rectum and passing it up through the colon to detect cancer), and exercise treadmill tests. The same test can serve as a screening test or a diagnostic test.

It is called a diagnostic test when performed on a person with symptoms of the illness, and called a screening test when performed on a person who has no symptoms.

Although it may seem as if the best thing would be for everyone to undergo every screening test "just to be sure," in actuality this would be poor preventive medicine for a number of reasons. Why? First, as mentioned earlier, no test is perfect. Any test has a potential to indicate that you have a certain disease or condition when you really don't (false positive), or a test might indicate that you are free of a condition when you actually have it (false negative). The chance of a test being inaccurate is increased if the health condition is rare.

Imagine that the local health department decided to screen all elders for cancer with a blood test and that the incidence of this cancer was one in a million. If the test was 99 percent accurate, this would mean that out of every 100 normal elders who were screened, one person would be told, in error, that he or she had cancer. If you screened a million elders, you might find the one elder who has cancer, but you would have to tell at least 100 elders that they might have cancer when they don't. Worse still, you might have to put those 100 elders and their families through a lot of other tests, some of them painful, dangerous, or expensive, just to be sure that they do not have cancer. Obviously, false positives can cause a lot of unnecessary worry.

Aside from being inaccurate, screening tests may cause pain and embarrassment and waste money that could be used to diagnose and treat more common health problems. Further, some tests may be very time-consuming.

How can we know which screening tests are worthwhile? Many types of studies can help us answer this question. We might do a case control study, comparing women who have had breast cancer with those who have not and asking if they had mammograms. But how will you know if it is the mammogram that was helpful? Perhaps it was just that the types of people who get mammograms (those who are educated, concerned about health, richer, insured) are less likely to get cancer in the first place.

Another type of study is to look at the cancers discovered by mammograms. For example, you may find that the cancers found by the mammogram are smaller and easier to treat than those found in other ways. That sounds convincing—of course it is better to find cancer early. But what if the mammogram is finding cancers that would never have grown and subjects these women to unnecessary procedures, surgeries, and worries? What if these findings cause someone to be depressed, suicidal, or to have psychological or financial stress paying for this unnecessary care? And none of these studies addresses the risks of the mammography—what if the procedure finds more cancers, but also causes some because of the radiation risk?

The gold standard of tests to answer the question about whether the screening tests save lives is the randomized controlled trial. This type of large-scale study randomly assigns its subjects into two groups. One group gets the intervention (for example, mammograms every year), and the other group does not. Then the study follows those subjects for many years to determine whether individuals who received the intervention are less likely to die (e.g., from breast cancer) than those who did not receive it.

Randomized controlled trials are excellent, but they are so time-consuming and expensive that few interventions have been evaluated in this way. For breast cancer, however, randomized controlled trials suggest that screening women over age 50 does save lives, and the benefits outweigh the risks for most women.

The majority of screening tests have not undergone randomized clinical trials. But even if a screening test has undergone a randomized clinical trial, it may not offer clear-cut benefits. Even fewer studies address the efficacy of screening tests for elders, so most recommendations for that group are based on studies of middle-aged adults. Thus, in most cases, screening for older people is restricted to individuals likely to live at least 10 years longer. In general, screening tests are not recommended for elders with life-threatening chronic illnesses because they are not likely to live long enough to benefit from the treatment. For example, an elder with

Whole Body Scans, or Scams?

Why not scan your entire body every few years, inside and out, "just to be sure" no illnesses are lurking? Your health is worth it, right? If something is going on inside your body, you want to know early and get it taken care of—so what if insurance doesn't cover it! Why not sign up for a total body scan? Why, a friend of mine had one, and they found a mass in his kidney—his regular doctor had missed it! They did surgery and removed it. It wasn't cancer after all, but what a close call! I'm definitely having a body scan!

A new trend in consumer health is the total body scan. A total or whole body computerized tomography scan (CT or "CAT" scan) creates images of almost the entire body, generally from the chin to below the hips. The scan creates a set of images that are akin to multiple horizontal slices of the body. A whole body scan for a healthy individual is not covered by most insurance plans, but if a problem is suspected, the subsequent evaluation and diagnosis probably are covered.

Whole body scans are touted to discover illnesses early, before symptoms are apparent. Although there are many accepted reasons for scanning parts of the body with CT scans, the U.S. Food and Drug Administration, the American College of Radiology, the American Cancer Society, and other professional groups do not recommend whole body scanning. Why would these professionals oppose a test that might save your life?

CT scans expose the body to far more radiation than a single X-ray. A CT scan of the abdomen involves 400 times the amount of radiation exposure needed for a chest X-ray; and if abnormalities are found, more scans or X-rays are needed. Radiation is dangerous to cells and may induce tumors or cancers.

Because there is no governmental oversight, the centers do not need to substantiate the claims made in their advertisements. A machine might emit far more radiation than it should or supply insufficient radiation for detailed images or have a low rate of accuracy (false positives and false negatives), and the consumer would never know.

CT scans find a lot of abnormalities that, in most cases, turn out to be no more than unimportant changes related to normal aging. However, following up on the abnormalities with more tests can be expensive, painful, or deadly. For example, initial results in a study looking at CT scans of smokers to screen for lung cancer found that the scans identified nodules in 1,049 out of 1,520 current or former smokers. A total of 2,832 nodules were discovered (3 per person!). Of these, 36 were cancerous and 2,796 were benign. That is a 98.7 rate of false positives.[3]

The CT body scan is not a substitute for other, more accurate screening tests, such as mammography, bone densitometry (X-ray screening for osteoporosis), colonoscopy, and the measuring of blood pressure, glucose, and cholesterol levels. It is best to reserve CT scans for instances when symptoms or risk factors indicate the need.

It is important for those who undergo these scans to understand the risks they are taking for "peace of mind."

end-stage heart disease who has had multiple heart attacks is likely to die of cardiovascular disease. Obtaining a mammogram and discovering the simultaneous presence of breast cancer would be counterproductive. First, the individual probably would not be healthy enough to undergo surgery, chemotherapy, and radiation treatments. Second, the diagnosis of cancer might be psychologically detrimental, reducing the quality of the few years of life remaining.

Various professional groups make recommendations regarding screening tests—who should undergo them, how frequently to be tested, and what the expected outcome is. These groups include professional organizations by medical specialty (e.g., geriatrics, family practice, urology), patient or consumer groups (e.g., the American Cancer Society), expert panels, and government agencies. These groups vary in the methods they use to make their decisions and their recommendations. Some groups convene councils of experts who use their expert medical opinion, experience, and reviews of the literature to determine recommendations. Others, such as the U.S. Preventive Services Task Force, conduct a highly structured, systematic review of the literature to determine recommendations that are later reviewed by experts.

In general, specialists tend to recommend more tests. They have seen the worst cases of an illness and feel earlier discovery just has to be better. In contrast, preventive experts often are less likely to recommend screening because they look at both the benefits and harms and the research supporting screening and long-term outcomes. For example, instead of saying, "I recommend mammograms starting at age 20 because I have seen cancers in young women and mammograms found them," preventive experts say, "There are very few breast cancers in 20-year-old women, mammography for a whole population of women would have a lot of side effects including excessive radiation and unecessary tests and worries, and there is no evidence that conducting mammograms on all women age 20 would prevent death. Therefore, we will not recommend mammograms for 20-year-old-women."

Professional groups differ in their biases. The American Cancer Society and oncologists (cancer specialists) see a lot of cancer patients and have seen firsthand the devastation that cancer can cause to the patient and family. Cancer specialists are more likely to recommend any screening that detects cancer early because they have an ever-expanding arsenal for fighting cancer and a strong belief that any cancer that was "missed" could have been treated. Often the costs (both emotional and financial) of screening are not considered. In contrast, the U.S. Preventive Services Task Force is biased toward interventions that have been proven effective, and it adopts a more population-wide approach. For example, a screening test that offers significant risk to the patient and often misses a very rare but terrible disease might not be recommended by the U.S. Preventive Services Task Force but might be recommended by experts who commonly work with that disease.

Conflicting recommendations by different professional groups can cause confusion among both the public and health care professionals and can lead to the belief that "No one knows what to do." Over a year or two in the 1990s, for example, multiple groups came out with recommendations about mammography that were quite different and caused a public outcry from patients, physicians, the public, and politicians. Sometimes there is a great deal of emotion wrapped up in recommendations, reflecting individual experience. For example, a woman who has survived a breast cancer that was detected by a mammogram may advocate mammograms for everyone. Conversely, a woman whose cancer was missed by a mammogram and who is now dying may vehemently assert that mammograms are useless.

Ideally, screening recommendations are made not because of emotionality or personal experience but by following a scientific rationale. However, the science behind recommendations—particularly the review of studies and analysis of epidemiologic concepts—is quite complicated and not easily understood by the lay public.

The controversy surrounding the value of some screening tests should not obscure the fact that there is a core set of recommendations for preventive services and screening tests that are widely agreed to have documented benefits. If everyone adhered to this core of recommendations, there would be dramatic improvements in health. Unfortunately, even when most professional groups agree on a screening recommendation, far too many professionals and laypersons do not comply. Professionals may feel they do not have enough time to devote to screening measures, they may feel they are unskilled at recommending these tests, or they may be uncertain of their benefits. And some individuals may not want to know if they have a disease, may not take the time or spend the money to find out if they do, or would not wish to follow up if something was found.

It is difficult to get individuals to comply with screening tests. By definition, screening tests are for those without symptoms. People who have no symptoms of illness are unlikely to visit a physician or go to the hospital to undergo a screening test. Further, they are not likely to want to pay for testing and counseling. And when an individual makes a visit because of a symptom, both the physician and the patient are more likely to focus on current complaints rather than devote precious time to disease prevention and early detection.

Some individuals are quite frightened of illness and ask physicians for every test to prove they are not harboring something curable. Others adopt a more fatalistic attitude: "If I'm going to get cancer, I'm going to get it, and this test isn't going to make any difference." Some find screening tests stressful and develop anxiety or depressive states while waiting for the results. Often people's biases are surprising. A chronically ill patient with a limited life expectancy might insist on routine mammograms, while a healthy elder who could benefit from such screening might refuse it. Although many people say they favor preventive efforts, few actually make appointments and act on health professionals' recommendations.

Most experts believe that before a health screening test is ordered, three questions should be considered: How many more years of life does the individual have? What is the current state of the individual's health? Will aggressive treatment affect the quality of the person's remaining years? If an elder, for example, is so frail that he or she cannot undergo surgery, then a test to detect a cancer that is only treated with surgery should not be done. Alternatively an elder with advanced dementia who can no longer speak or walk, for example, should probably not have a colonoscopy—the elder already has a severe and life-threatening illness, and the procedure and follow-up would cause discomfort, fear, confusion, and a higher risk of complications. In other words, the risks outweigh the benefits. In the frail, most times the focus of care is on quality rather than quantity of life. In addition, the frail are more likely to suffer complications from diagnosis and treatment. For those with other severe conditions, those with terminal illness, and those who desire only comfort rather than life extension, screening tests are not recommended.[4]

In the rest of this section we discuss the screening recommendations from the U.S. Preventive Services Task Force that are most relevant to the elder population. We consider major diseases and conditions for which screening tests are available (see Table 12.1), describe screening procedures, and note the pros and cons of screening.

Breast Cancer

A *mammogram* is an X-ray of the breast used to detect breast changes in women who have no signs or symptoms of breast cancer. Usually two X-rays of each breast are obtained. With a mammogram, it is possible to detect small deposits of calcium or small tumors that may indicate the presence of breast cancer. Several large-scale randomized controlled studies report a reduction in mortality (death) in women over age 50 who have had a mammography compared to those who have not. The U.S. Preventive Services Task Force strongly recommends screening mammography every two years for women between 50 and 74 years old.

Techniques are being developed to screen breasts for cancer without radiation, but none are in widespread use. It is evident that better screening devices are needed for breast cancer.

Colorectal Cancer

Cancers of the colon and rectum are common causes of death in the later years. Screening for these cancers is very effective. It finds cancers at an early stage and detects precancerous polyps that are easily removed before they become cancerous. Several tests are able to detect asymptomatic colon cancer: the fecal occult blood test, digital rectal exam, barium enema, and colonoscopy and sigmoidoscopy. These tests vary widely in cost, ease of administration, and patient comfort.

The *fecal occult blood test* can be performed at home or in the physician's office. The test involves placing smears of stool on special cards that are sent to a laboratory for analysis. The presence in the stool of occult blood (blood not visible to the eye) signals an increased risk of colon cancer and the need for further testing. A *digital rectal exam* calls for a health practitioner to insert his or

Problem Drinking

Alcoholism is a pervasive medical problem in the United States. However, even people who do not meet the criteria for alcoholism may have significant emotional, social, or medical problems related to drinking. Although the risk of alcoholism and problem drinking declines with age, elders who do drink excessively suffer detrimental effects. Screening for problem drinking should involve careful questioning about alcohol consumption, including quantity, frequency, and degree of intoxication. Clinicians may want to use standardized questionnaires designed for this purpose. All people who drink should be provided with information about the dangers of excessive drinking, including drinking while driving, and be referred to counseling when necessary.

In most cases, screening for the diseases and conditions mentioned above is initiated at the physician's office. A disadvantage of some community screening programs (for example, health fairs at malls or at senior centers) is that they are usually accomplished without the knowledge of the participant's physician. Thus, information obtained or exchanged in those settings may not be transmitted to the primary care physician for evaluation and follow-up. Ideally, these programs would have a mechanism in place to communicate with an individual's primary medical provider when abnormalities are found.

TERTIARY PREVENTION

Tertiary prevention is any intervention by the physician or by the patient who has an illness to prevent further disability, complications, or death. Tertiary prevention can include testing (e.g., monitoring blood sugar), treatments (medication, surgery, exercise, special diet), and rehabilitation (speech therapy after a stroke). This type of tertiary prevention of chronic and acute diseases and conditions is discussed in Chapters 4 through 7. A second aspect of tertiary prevention is disease-specific education directed toward individuals with a disease to improve their knowledge of their illness, warning signs of a worsening condition, and self-care strategies.

Disease-specific education, also called *patient education,* is the act of teaching an individual about his or her disease, giving him or her more control over the course of an illness. Perhaps the best-known example is the education provided to diabetics. Diabetics need to learn many things about their lifelong disease, such as what causes it, what to eat, how to exercise, complications and how to avoid them, foot care, and how to inject their own insulin and measure their own glucose levels. Many health educators focus specifically on diabetes education because of the extensive information that is passed on and the sheer number of diabetic patients. More information on diabetes education can be found at the Web site of the American Association of Diabetic Educators (www.aadenet.org). Educating individuals who have heart failure is another example of disease-specific education. Individuals are instructed about a proper diet, how to watch their weight, and learn to become aware of symptoms (such as edema or fatigue) so that their activity levels or medications can be adjusted.

There are many other examples of disease-specific education: teaching a man about prostate disease and how to insert a catheter for himself; teaching arthritis sufferers about exercises to reduce pain; teaching people with strokes how to use a walker or crutches; teaching an individual how to change a colostomy bag; discussing ways to manage breathlessness. Much of what happens during visits with health professionals involves health education, ideally tailored to an individual's background, education level, and specific situation and health problems. This education can be accomplished by a health educator who is trained in effective behavior change techniques or by another medical or health professional (doctor, nurse, physical therapist, nurse practitioner, dietician). In addition, many individuals read books and pamphlets and seek information on Internet sites in order to learn more about their medical problems.

PREVENTIVE SERVICES: UTILIZATION AND EXPENDITURES

Although most people would agree that prevention of illness and disability makes more sense than treating illnesses that have already damaged the body, care for those who are already ill dominates the health care provided in the United States. Treating advanced chronic illnesses, such as chronic obstructive pulmonary disease (COPD), cardiac disease, stroke, and cancer, consumes the majority of the health care resources in the United States, many of which are preventable.

Because there is a high prevalence of disease in older persons, the potential to prevent or decrease the severity of these diseases is great. However, prevention and health promotion programs are underutilized and underfunded. Why? The reasons are interconnected and complex.

Many individuals are unaware of the value of preventive activities and do not know when or where to access the programs. Medicare and private insurance companies too rarely reimburse for preventive services, few physicians offer them, and patients are not likely to make appointments or follow through on preventive health recommendations. It is far easier for a physician to prescribe medication for high blood pressure than to discuss weight loss, the specifics of an exercise prescription, smoking cessation, and dietary changes. Even when physicians do offer preventive services, there is not much evidence that the time spent on prevention makes an impact. It is easier for a person to take a pill every day (even that isn't easy) than to initiate and sustain a physical fitness program or to lose weight healthfully.

Some experts lament the fact that Medicare, the major payer of health services for people aged 65 and older, does not reimburse important screening activities. However, when the program was initiated, it specifically excluded preventive care. Thus, each time a preventive activity is advocated, the change is very difficult to implement because Congress must authorize it. Over the years, Medicare slowly began to reimburse immunizations and screening activities. In 2012, Medicare beneficiaries paid no deductible or copay for most preventive services if they visited a doctor or other health care provider who accepts assignment. For some preventive services, they paid nothing for the service, but had a copay for the office visit to obtain those services if the doctor did not accept assignment.

Immunizations
  Pneumonia
  Hepatitis B
  Influenza
Screening services
  Cervical cancer
  Pelvic exam
  Breast cancer
  Osteoporosis (bone mass densitrometry)
  Colon cancer
  Diabetes
  Prostate cancer
  Glaucoma
  Nutrition therapy
  "Welcome to Medicare" exam
  Cholesterol screening
  Human Immunodeficiency Virus (HIV)
  Tobacco counseling
  Abdominal aortic aneurysm screening
  Yearly wellness visit

There are some problems with Medicare reimbursement. Medicare does not cover some preventive services recommended by the U.S. Preventive Services Task Force (e.g. vision and hearing screening). But Medicare does pay for some screening that has no proven benefit and is not recommended by the task force (e.g. PSA testing for prostate cancer).

Even though Medicare pays for several types of screening, many older individuals do not take advantage of the service. There is variability among states, ethnicities, incomes, and education levels. Only half of the nation's elders receive recommended preventive health care services.

The least likely recipients are members of a minority group and are poor.

Many factors work against health promotion and disease prevention. Our health care system is geared to manage acute and chronic issues, not to prevent illness. Physician reimbursement is higher for medical procedures than for counseling and education. Patient turnover makes it hard for physicians to track the preventive services that their elder patients have received elsewhere (such as an influenza vaccine or a screening for diabetes received at a local health fair). Also, although people say they are in favor of prevention, in practice they often do not make preventive activities a priority.

The up-front costs of prevention may seem high, and the benefits may seem intangible because they occur years later. Although some preventive measures are cost-savers, others are expensive because they prolong life expectancy—deceased clients do not use health care resources. For example, smoking cessation may cost money because smokers die earlier than nonsmokers, consequently utilizing fewer health resources in their lifetimes.

HEALTH PROMOTION

Changing poor health habits has the potential to greatly reduce the development and progression of many of the chronic illnesses that are common among older people. Based on their exhaustive review of the literature, members of the U.S. Preventive Services Task Force concluded that "clinicians are more likely to help their patients prevent future disease by asking, educating, and counseling them about personal health behaviors than by performing physical examinations or tests. In other words, talking is more important than testing."[2]

Epidemiologists report that the greatest impact on chronic illness can be made through lifestyle changes rather than technological interventions such as drugs or surgery. Experts agree that the vast majority of diseases that plague Americans, including heart disease, diabetes, and stroke, are related to lifestyle. The last 20 years have shown significant declines in cardiovascular disease, largely attributed to nationwide health promotion campaigns about risk factors that encourage citizens to decrease dietary fat, stop smoking, and increase physical activity.

Increasingly, evidence points to the importance of personal health behaviors in the cause and severity of many diseases and causes of death—from lung disease to heart disease, cancer, and strokes to accidents. The most obvious example is cigarette smoking, which is responsible for one in five deaths in the United States annually from heart disease, stroke, cancer, and respiratory diseases. Two negative health behaviors, failure to use seat belts and drunk-driving, account for the majority of automobile accidents. Poor diet and physical inactivity are major contributors to heart disease, cancer, diabetes, osteoporosis, and other common diseases. Reducing these negative health behaviors is the main thrust of most health promotion efforts.

Health promotion includes a range of activities, from individual counseling and education to small-group, community, statewide, or national campaigns to improve health. In some cases, individual-based interventions are more effective than community education. For example, a health care provider can provide education, support, and medication as needed to assist an individual to quit smoking. In other situations, community-based interventions are optimal (e.g., lengthening the delay time on the street lights near a busy intersection frequented by frail elders, implementing a senior health fair, television ads). Other health promotion activities are legislative efforts to improve health (e.g., seat belt laws), community education (community forums, health fairs, billboards, television advertisements), Nationwide campaigns are also used to encourage positive health behavior change (e.g., the Great American Smokeout and the Five-a-Day campaign to increase consumption of fruits and vegetables).

In some cases, legislative options are the most effective way to improve the health of a population; legislation requiring seat belts and automatic seat belt systems has been far more effective at increasing seat belt use than individual counseling. Bans on public smoking and cigarette taxes reduce

The Health Educator's Role

Per the definition of the standard occupational classification, health educators promote, maintain, and improve individual and community health by assisting individuals and communities to adopt healthy behaviors. Health educators also collect and analyze data to identify community needs prior to planning, implementing, monitoring, and evaluating programs designed to encourage healthy lifestyles, policies, and environments. In addition, health educators may also serve as a resource to assist individuals, other professionals, or the community, and may administer fiscal resources for health education programs. Health educators may work with individuals, families, and communities in a variety of settings. They may develop educational materials such as videos, pamphlets, books, or Web sites to educate others about health. A variety of health professionals involve themselves in health promotion activities: physicians, physician assistants, nurses, dentists, nutritionists, and health educators.

Health education is a social science that draws from the biological, environmental, psychological, physical, and medical sciences to promote health and prevent disease, disability, and premature death through theory-based voluntary behavior change activities, programs, campaigns, and research. It is an essential public health service that has people practicing each of the core functions of public health: assessment, policy development, and quality assurance. By focusing on prevention, health education reduces the financial and human costs of medical treatment to individuals, employers, medical facilities, insurance companies, and the nation as a whole.

The Bureau of Labor Statistics reports that there are more than 66,000 community health educators in the United States. Many health educators specialize in health education or community health as trained or certified health education specialists. They practice in schools, colleges, workplaces, medical care settings, public health settings, community-based agencies and organizations, and other settings. Others perform selected health education functions as part of what they consider their primary responsibility (e.g., medical treatment, nursing, social work, substance abuse/HIV counseling, oral hygiene). Lay workers may learn on the job to do specific, limited educational tasks to encourage healthy behavior. Paraprofessionals and health professionals from other disciplines may offer health education services, although they may not be familiar with the specialized body of health education and behavior change knowledge, skills, theories, and research, nor is it their primary interest or professional development focus.

Being a health educator requires specialized study. Over 250 colleges and universities in the United States offer programs in health education with degrees ranging from baccalaureate to doctorate. Health education has entry-level and advanced competencies that serve as the basis for professional practice. For example, health educators can assess the need for and plan, develop, implement, manage, and evaluate health programs in collaboration with medical staff and community agencies. Nationally, a health educator may receive certification as a Certified Health Education Specialist (CHES) from the National Commission for Health Education Credentialing, Inc. The holder of CHES certification is specifically trained to effectively assess health education needs; plan, implement, and evaluate programs; build coalitions and coordinate the provision of health services; identify resources; act as an advocate for health issues; and communicate health education needs.

While health educators are traditionally associated with brochures and videos, this association only minimally suggests their capacities. Health education in practice takes an ecological approach to creating healthy communities. Health educators work at the individual, group, institutional, community, and system levels to improve health knowledge, attitudes, and skills for the purpose of changing or encouraging behaviors that relate to optimal health status.

Adapted from the Health Professions Network, www.healthpronet.org/ahp_month/07_02.html

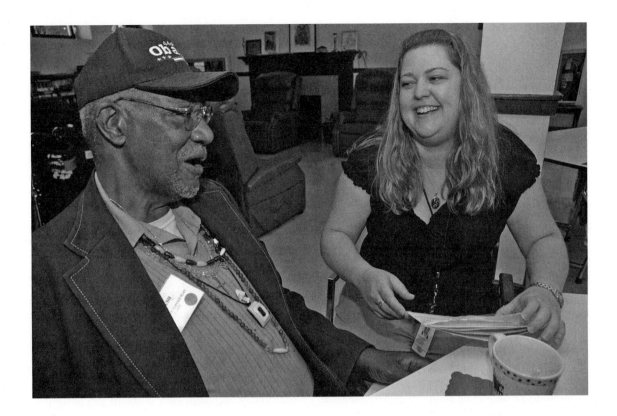

smoking more than public information campaigns. Because of the many environmental variables that affect personal health, some health professionals consider health promotion to include mobilizing individuals to become active in political change to improve health care for a far greater number of people. For instance, elders may become active in efforts to change local laws regarding smoking or to advocate more stringent nursing home regulations. In this way, professionals involved in health promotion activities can work on two fronts—not only encouraging individual health behavior change but also reducing political, social, and environmental influences that ultimately impinge on health status.

There are barriers that reduce the effectiveness of health promotion. First, there is inadequate research on which types of health promotion work best with which populations. Most people agree that people should exercise more, but there is less

agreement about the best way to get people to follow the advice of health professionals and begin an exercise program and even less agreement about what it takes to sustain or resume an exercise program. Physicians feel a lot of pressure to use their time wisely and hesitate to spend time in an activity that is not effective.

Physicians may not recognize the effectiveness of their efforts. For example, if a physician encourages smoking cessation among smoking patients and only one of 25 smokers quits, the physician may feel that the effort was in vain even though, on a population basis, the intervention was effective. In addition, physicians are not trained to provide effective counseling and education. Both physicians and patients tend to emphasize the "here and now" of patient care. Dealing with a patient's chronic disease management or acute complaint often seems more pressing than switching the topic to discuss cigarette smoking or use of seat belts.

Health promotion activities are a collaborative effort between the health care provider and the patient. Unlike many medical interventions in which the clinician initiates and controls, the patient must initiate and sustain the health behavior change. To effectively integrate prevention into medical care, the physician cannot rely on providing counseling only during checkups but must incorporate counseling into all visits. An excellent resource on integrating health promotion into medical care is *Health Promotion and Disease Prevention in Clinical Practice*.[5] The Centers for Disease Control and Prevention has extensive health promotion resources on its Web site. Go to www.cdc.gov and click on "Healthy Living."

Community-based health promotion programs have the potential to improve the health of elders. These programs may target a particular health problem (e.g., accident prevention, smoking cessation, disease screening) or include many topics as part of a comprehensive wellness program. They may be offered by health maintenance organizations or in community settings such as senior centers, assisted living facilities, and elder nutrition sites.

Changing Health Behaviors

Changing personal health behaviors (e.g., beginning an exercise program, stopping smoking, reducing fat intake) is very difficult. It usually requires a person to consciously alter long-standing patterns and often results in physical discomfort or the giving up of valued comforts. It is hypothesized that several stages are involved in the decision and follow-through. Understanding these stages helps health professionals to tailor a prevention or health promotion message to the individual.

The first and most difficult stage is acknowledging a health problem: accepting that something is not right in our lives. For example, we may decide we are gaining too much weight. Even though we admit we have a problem, we may not be willing to move to the next stage: deciding to make a change. If a goal is set (e.g., I want to lose 10 pounds), then the options for achieving that

plan are explored (e.g., cooking low-fat meals). After a plan is selected and implemented, the next stage is assessing progress toward the goal (e.g., weighing ourselves), modifying the plan as needed (e.g., I can exercise only three times a week, so I will have to lose weight slowly), and guarding against backsliding. See Box 12.1 for a 10-step guide to successfully change health behaviors.

Health Behavior Change Theories

We want our clients and ourselves to have healthier behaviors, but how can we get them to change—to eat better, to exercise more, to take their medications, to lose weight or stop smoking? People generally know what the "healthy" thing to do is. For example, smokers by and large know that smoking is unhealthy. Because of this, just educating smokers about the fact that smoking harms their health or providing them with statistics about its negative health effects is rarely effective at producing quitters. So what *is* effective and what strategies work to get people to change?

Scientists trying to understand behavioral change look at the psychological and behavioral aspects of change, such as what helps it and what slows it down. This field is called health behavioral change theory.

There are many health behavioral change theories and research looking at what works in encouraging people to make and sustain changes to be more healthy. One concept is in regard to self-efficacy, which is an individual's confidence in being successful. Another concept is risk perception—how does the individual see the risks of an action as they impact her?

Some models describing health behavior change have "stages" that people go through one after another to get to the change. One such model is the transtheoretical model, developed in the late 1970s by James O. Prochaska and colleagues at the University of Rhode Island. The transtheoretical model proposes that health promotion approaches be individualized.

B O X   1 2 . 1

How to Change Your Bad Health Habits

1. Acknowledge the need for change.
2. Believe that there is more to gain than to lose. Carefully balance the pleasures inherent in the old way of doing things (e.g., overeating, smoking, lounging) and the gains expected from the health behavioral change. If the positives outweigh the negatives, the change is more easily accomplished.
3. Feel a sense of self-worth and self-efficacy. To succeed, a person needs to feel able to accomplish the desired changes.
4. Feel a sense of ownership over the plan for change. It is important for goals to be set by the individual, not by the practitioner. If an individual is not committed to the plan for change, it is unlikely that the change will be sustained.
5. Develop realistic goals and workable plans. Often in an overzealous attempt at self-improvement, an individual will set goals that are too lofty or unattainable. For instance, a previously sedentary person should not expect to be running a marathon in three months, and a two-pack-a-day smoker may find it difficult to stop "cold turkey" tomorrow. Incremental, achievable goals are preferable.
6. Find positive reinforcement. Rewards are a well-documented way to change behaviors. Rewards can be extrinsic (I get a new

wardrobe when I lose 25 pounds) or intrinsic (a sense of satisfaction).
7. Enlist the support of others. Making health behavior changes as a family unit is often easier than making such changes on one's own. On the other hand, significant others may unwittingly sabotage health behavioral changes. For example, as one partner in a couple begins to lose weight and become more attractive, the other partner may have conflicting feelings of jealousy or fear abandonment and so may inadvertently encourage the changing partner to lose interest in the regimen.
8. Develop and implement a strategy for monitoring progress. Individuals need to frequently and continually monitor their progress toward their goal, both on their own and with the support of someone else—either a health care professional or another significant person.
9. Initiate follow-up. Even after the goals are met, follow-up is important to prevent backsliding.
10. Maintain patience and practice. It is hard to change ingrained patterns of behavior, and meaningful change takes time. Some backsliding is to be expected. It is important not to lose patience with the process and to practice new skills.

Adapted from Westberg, J., and Jason, H. 1996. Fostering healthy behavior: The process (pp. 145–162). In Woolf, S.H., Jonas, S., and Lawrence, R.S. (Eds.), Health promotion and disease prevention in clinical practice. Baltimore, MD: Williams and Wilkins. Used with permission from Lippincott Williams & Wilkins (www.lww.com).

One way of doing this is to assess the openness of each client to behavior change. Five stages through which individuals progress when making behavioral change have been identified: precontemplation, contemplation, preparation, action, and maintenance.[6]

Individuals in the *precontemplation* stage have no intention to change behavior in the foreseeable future. Many individuals in this stage are unaware of their problems. In the *contemplation* stage, people are aware that a problem exists and

are seriously thinking about overcoming it but have not yet made a commitment to take action. The *preparation* stage combines intention with previous failed attempts. Individuals in this stage are intending to take action in the next month and have unsuccessfully taken action in the past year. In the *action* stage, individuals modify their behavior, experiences, or environment in order to overcome their problems. Action involves the most overt behavioral changes and requires considerable commitment of time and energy. In the *maintenance* stage, people work to prevent relapse and consolidate the gains attained during action.

This model allows the health professional to tailor interventions for each client's stage of change. For example, in the precontemplation stage, the goal is to discuss the health hazards of a current behavior and to encourage the individual to consider changing that behavior. A smoker who refuses to acknowledge that smoking is harmful to his health and that he should stop would not be likely to benefit by setting a quit date. Instead, the goal should be to convince him about the harmful effects of smoking on his personal health and the benefits of quitting. In contrast, a smoker in the contemplation stage would not need to be told about the hazards of his harmful behavior because he is aware of them. Instead, he would need encouragement to commit to action.

Individuals in the preparation stage need encouragement, support, and assistance with strategies to carry out their plans. It would be a waste of time to discuss the negative health effects of smoking with a person who already decided to quit but is backsliding. That individual would benefit more from specific suggestions on how to avoid backsliding (e.g., using nicotine replacement) and from increased support and encouragement. Those in the action stage are expending a significant amount of energy in behavioral change, and they need support and encouragement. People in the maintenance stage need strategies to stay on track and prevent relapse.

In addition to the stages of change that are often discussed, the transtheoretical model also includes more than 20 "processes for change," decisional analysis (how people weigh the pros and cons of making a decision), and "self-efficacy." Although this model is widely discussed and seems reasonable and intuitive, in fact, multiple randomized controlled trials and reviews of the literature fail to find consistent support for it. Critics contend that people's choices aren't always as rational or as likely to fall into these specific categories, that people don't always seem to move through the stages. Nevertheless, this model is widely utilized and studied.

The Health Action Process Approach, developed by Ralf Schwarzer in Berlin, Germany, looks at *motivation to change* (thoughts, goals, and intentions) and *volition to change*.[7] Volition is the action stage—the planning, initiative, maintenance of the new behavior, and recovery from obstacles. So, for example, a smoker may have an intention to change, but not have done anything about it, or may have developed a plan including a quit date, a plan to avoid friends who smoke, and not to have cigarettes in the house, and may have thought of triggers to smoking (such as stress) and bought a book or a bag of carrots to crunch when that time comes (volition). Good intentions are more likely to be translated into action when people plan when, where, and how to perform the desired behavior.

Those who lack motivation to change can be called nonintenders. These people are not motivated to change their behavior. For these nonintenders, education about risks of the current behavior and benefits of the proposed behavior may help them at least change their mind about whether they want to consider to make a change.

Volitional phases include both those who have made these plans, but have not yet started to enact them (called intenders) as well as "actors" who are in the process of making the changes. Intenders want to change. Intenders know the risks of their current behavior and the benefits of the new behavior, but they need help getting started or in maintaining the changes. For example, intenders would benefit from assistance in planning—planning to do something (action planning) or planning on how to cope with obstacles and challenges (coping planning). Action planning gets people started (e.g., joining a gym is an action planning step), whereas coping planning keeps the behavior going. (When exactly am I going to the gym? With whom? What if my friend can't come, will I go by myself? What will I wear?)

These are just two of multiple behavioral change theories that try to explain why people behave as they do and then try to find out how to influence change behavior. It is likely that it is important to look at those who have not even decided to change (pre-intenders or precontemplative) differently from those who have decided to change but not yet acted (intenders, contemplators, or preparers) and those who have made changes, but need help keeping them going (actors, maintenance).[8]

It is abundantly clear that facilitating behavioral change requires a lot more than simply passing on information. If giving out a pamphlet or a brief admonishment were effective, nobody would smoke or overeat! The factors that keep people engaged in behaviors that are harmful to their health are complicated, as are the strategies to facilitate behavior change in others. The following strategies have been shown to be effective in patient education and counseling and are adapted from the *Guide to Clinical Preventive Services*: 2010–2011.[2]

1. Frame the teaching to match the patient's perceptions. For example, a person who asserts she is unable to exercise may be asked to reframe her definition of exercise and commit to taking the stairs whenever possible.
2. Fully inform patients of the purposes and expected effects of their behavioral change and when to expect to see these effects. For example, advice to an elder may be that muscle strength should increase over a year so that in 6 months he should be able to lift 5 pounds and in 12 months he should expect to lift 10 pounds. Advice may also emphasize that patients may experience muscle soreness over the first few weeks.
3. Suggest small changes rather than large ones. Make recommendations that you are sure the patient can accomplish, and set small goals. For example, suggest walking only 10 minutes twice a week at first. An individual who has been successful in establishing a healthy habit is more likely to be able to continue or expand that activity.
4. Be specific. It is much more helpful to suggest "a walk around the block three days a week with your dog" than to say, "You should get more exercise and drop a few pounds."
5. Adding new behaviors is sometimes easier than eliminating old ones. For example,

eating more fruits and vegetables may be easier than reducing dietary fat, and adding exercise may be more easily accomplished than stopping smoking.
6. Link new behaviors to old behaviors; help the patients see how the behavior change will fit into their usual routines. For example, people who say they have no time to exercise may agree to walk to a friend's house twice a week instead of driving, or to ask the friend to go for a walk instead of sitting and talking.
7. Use the power of the profession. Patients listen to what physicians and other health professionals tell them. Be direct about what you want the patient to do.
8. Focus on the positives, not the negatives. Reward works better than punishment, and the best rewards are intrinsic to the activity. For example, it is better to say "Exercising will give you more energy," than to say, "If you exercise, you can have a candy bar" or "If you don't exercise, you can't go to the movies."
9. Get an explicit commitment from the patient. Asking clients to describe what they plan to do helps them focus on specifics and may also reveal difficulties with the plan. Saying something aloud to another person will help clients follow through—for example, "I will walk every day after dinner, but sometimes it is dark. Well, then maybe I will ask my husband to go with me."
10. Use a variety of strategies. Combine written materials, spoken encouragement, and use of office staff or other professionals to help people change behavior.
11. Monitor progress through follow-up contact. A telephone call to assess whether changes are being made and to evaluate difficulties can be very effective.

Specific Health Promotion Interventions

A visit with a doctor or some other health professional is an ideal opportunity to discuss changes in health behavior that would enhance health and reduce the risk of disease. However, these discussions generally do not occur between elders and their health care providers. In this section we outline some health behavioral interventions that might occur individually in the physician's office or in the home, or that might occur in a group setting. The health behaviors that we focus on here have been shown to reduce rates of illness and death and increase the quality of life. As mentioned earlier, it is never too late to stop harmful health behaviors. Even the very old can benefit.

Smoking Cessation

Smoking is the most important factor contributing to premature death and disability in the United States. At least 1 of every 5 deaths are linked to smoking cigarettes. Smoking has been implicated as a causal factor in many diseases, including lung cancer, head and neck cancer, bladder cancer, pancreatic cancer, cervical cancer, heart disease, stroke, peripheral vascular disease, chronic obstructive pulmonary disease, death from fires, and pneumonia. The deleterious health effects of secondary smoke on individuals who live with a smoker also have been repeatedly documented.

About one in five Americans smokes. Almost 10 percent of older people are still smoking. Older people have a disproportionate amount of smoking-related morbidity, such as lung cancer, heart disease, and emphysema caused by a lifetime of smoking. Because of its addictive quality, smoking is a habit that can be quite difficult to change.

Although it is best never to begin to smoke, multiple studies have documented the positive effects of quitting smoking even at an advanced age. Five to ten years after a person quits smoking, cancer risks start to drop, and the risks of stroke and heart attack fall even faster. Quitting smoking also reduces the progression of and illness from lung diseases.

It is widely recommended that health professionals screen for tobacco use, frequently discuss quitting smoking with their patients, and provide tobacco cessation interventions for all who use tobacco products. Often a recommendation by a physician is enough of an inducement to quit smoking. Further, physicians should refer smokers to tobacco cessation groups, distribute written materials, ask the patient to set a specific quit date, and follow up to ensure compliance. Nicotine gum or patches may be helpful for some. It is important that clinicians strongly urge their patients to quit smoking and provide information about the health effects of tobacco and advice about how to quit. Extensive educational materials geared to help individuals stop smoking that were developed by a wide range of agencies are available at the Surgeon General's Web site (www.surgeongeneral.gov).

Physical Activity Counseling

A sedentary lifestyle is associated with multiple diseases, including heart disease, hypertension, obesity, osteoporosis, diabetes, and mental disorders. Health care professionals recommend for all age groups a regular and moderate to vigorous level of physical activity that is tailored to their capabilities. Although the benefits of exercise are clear, the value of counseling a patient to exercise is not. The USPSTF and other groups do not currently recommend that individual health care providers provide counseling and education about exercise to all their patients, not because there is a lack of good studies showing the benefits of exercise but because there is a lack of data showing that physician counseling in the office makes much difference.[2] This may be because physicians spend only a short time with patients and getting people to start exercising is a complex and challenging task. For an extensive discussion of the benefits of exercise and importance of programs to increase physical activity among older people, see Chapter 9, "Physical Activity."

Dietary Counseling

Diet plays a role in many chronic illnesses, including cardiovascular disease, cancers, hypertension, obesity, adult-onset diabetes, osteoporosis, constipation, and anemia. Although the evidence is clear that diet impacts health, the U.S. Preventive

Services Task Force (USPSTF) concluded that the evidence is insufficient to recommend for or against routine behavioral counseling to promote a healthy diet in all patients in primary care settings.[3] For individuals with elevated cholesterol or cardiovascular or other diet-related chronic disease, however, the USPSTF does recommend intensive behavioral dietary counseling by primary care clinicians or by referral to other specialists, such as nutritionists or dietitians. The USPSTF found good evidence that medium- to high-intensity counseling interventions can produce medium-to-large changes in average daily intake of core components of a healthy diet (including saturated fat, fiber, fruit, and vegetables) among adult patients at increased risk for diet-related chronic disease. Dietary counseling should include taking a dietary history; addressing potential barriers to a change in diet; offering specific guidance about food selection, preparation, and meal planning; and recommending follow-up with a counselor skilled in this area.

Motor Vehicle Injury Prevention

The elderly have a relatively low rate of motor vehicle accidents and they drive many fewer miles than younger adults. Nevertheless, motor vehicle fatalities are a significant cause of mortality among the elderly; when they are involved in motor vehicle accidents, they are more likely than younger adults to become disabled or to die. Although there is little evidence regarding whether advice provided at medical visits is effective at reducing risk factors for motor vehicle injury, all elders should be cautioned against drinking and driving, urged to use seat belts, and educated about which of their medications may impair their driving ability.

Physicians are obligated to report to the state Department of Motor Vehicles individuals with certain diagnoses (e.g., seizures) and individuals who are unable to drive safely. Although not being able to drive can be a severe blow to an elder's self-esteem, it is important for health care professionals to comply with reporting requirements to protect other drivers.

Fall Prevention

Falls are a leading cause of unintentional injury and death in the elderly. Risk factors for falls are well documented and include individual factors (e.g., sensory decrements, diminished strength, gait instability, age changes, medication use) and environmental characteristics (e.g., stairs, poor lighting, inadequate footwear). Many types of interventions have been attempted to reduce elders' risk of falls and fall-associated morbidity, including education, environmental modification, and strength, flexibility, and balance training. However, providing education about falls is not enough. The most effective programs seem to have a multipronged approach— assessing risk factors, adjusting medications, initiating exercise and education programs, and reducing the number of environmental hazards. But even the effectiveness of these programs is mixed.

At the time of the writing of the book, the updated U.S. Preventive Services Task Force recommendations regarding falls were under review. However, their extensive literature review reported strong evidence that several types of fall interventions by physicians can reduce falls among high-risk groups. The most effective interventions listed were completing a comprehensive assessment after a fall and managing the risks, prescribing exercise or physical therapy, and recommending Vitamin D supplements. More intensive intervention programs for elders show some promise and should be considered for high-risk elders: those over age 75, those using more than four prescription medications, those using antihypertensive or sedative medications, and those with impaired cognition, balance, or gait.

The Educated Health Consumer

You, the individual, can do more for your own health and well-being than any doctor, any hospital, any drug, any exotic medical device.

—Joseph A. Califano Jr.

Many people, old and young, are active consumers of health care and want to improve their health status. They seek out information about staying well, dealing with disease, and options for treatment.

Self-care is any individual effort to maintain or improve health and wellness. Self-care may include lifestyle practices that enhance health, reduce risk factors for disease, reduce the impact of disease, or prevent disease. Self-care activities are many and varied. Wearing a seat belt, meditating to reduce stress, participating in screening tests, maintaining a personal record of medications and tests that have been done, monitoring blood sugar, installing grab bars in the shower, eating a diet high in fresh fruits and vegetables, reading a book about your medical condition, attending a support group for individuals with your condition, looking up your medications on the Internet, and reading a pamphlet at the drugstore—these are all examples of self-care. Self-care allows individuals to exercise greater control over their lives and health, and it improves quality of life.

Although we recognize the importance of self-care, it is challenging to know what to set as an individual priority and how to change poor health habits. It can all seem overwhelming. The amount of health information has expanded enormously over the past few years, primarily because of the Internet. Numerous Web sites provide information about health. In addition, health newsletters, books, and articles in the popular press have become more common.

Older adults have the potential to benefit from the variety of health information available. They are at greater risk for illnesses, and they have more time to read health information. Older adults may not have as much experience with the Internet as younger adults, but studies show that they are willing and able to learn and can develop expertise quickly.

How do you separate helpful science-based health information from the flurry of "pseudo-news" and advertising claims? How do you decide what to do and what not to do with regard to your health, what health habits should be changed now and what you can leave for tomorrow? To make the best decision, you need accurate and readable information. One Web site that provides good advice about how to read health information and interpret it is www.health-insight-harvard.org This site provides tips on how to review health information and how to

make positive health changes. Information found on multiple reputable Web sites is more likely to be accurate than that found on only a few sites. Government, universities, and disease society Web sites are often well done and accurate. Remember, the URL should end in *.edu, .gov,* or *.org.*

Listed below are health education resources that elders can access directly. Offering a good overview of all health issues and problems, the most exhaustive site is Medline Plus, a search engine with extensive links to information from many organizations. It was devised by the U.S. National Library of Medicine and the National Institutes of Health. Go to www.medlineplus.gov

Those who want more technical information should access www.pubmed.gov, a search engine that can access titles and abstracts from medical journals. The site is geared to health professionals and researchers, but sophisticated consumers also find it helpful.

The following sites provide factual information suitable for the elder consumer. Several of them invite users to select large print.

AARP: www.aarp.org
National Institute on Aging: www.nia.nih.gov
Administration on Aging: www.aoa.dhhs.gov
American Society on Aging: www.asaging.org
Centers for Disease Control and Prevention: www.cdc.gov
Agency for Health Care Research and Quality: www.ahrq.gov

In addition, there are innumerable sites on particular diseases. The American Heart Association, American Cancer Society, National Cancer Institute, American Lung Association, and American Diabetes Association are just a few of the disease-specific organizations with informative Web sites.

One of the most influential preventive health organizations is the government-run Centers for Disease Control and Prevention. Founded in 1946 to control malaria, the CDC has become the last word on many issues related to health and disease prevention. The CDC operates under the U.S. Department of Health and Human Services, the cabinet-level agency in the United States government involved with protecting the health and safety of all Americans and providing essential human services, especially for those people who are least able to help themselves.

The CDC's scientists, researchers, and policy experts conduct original research and investigations and synthesize the research of others to prevent and control infectious and chronic diseases, injuries, workplace hazards, disabilities, and environmental health threats. The workforce at CDC totals more than 15,000 employees in 170 occupations with a public health focus, including physicians, statisticians, epidemiologists, laboratory experts, behavioral scientists, and health communicators. Although the agency is based in Atlanta, Georgia, CDC researchers work across the United States and internationally.

The mission of the Centers for Disease Control is to promote health and quality of life by preventing and controlling disease, injury, and disability. This is accomplished by working with partners throughout the nation and around the world to monitor health, detect and investigate health problems, conduct research to enhance prevention, develop and advocate sound public health policies, implement prevention strategies, promote healthy behaviors, and foster safe and healthful environments. For more information, see www.cdc.gov

Public Policy Change to Promote Health

Some of the most effective preventive health measures are not based on education or counseling or blood tests but instead are focused on changing public laws and policies to promote health. Perhaps the best-known example is the reduction of many previously deadly infectious diseases through the development of effective systems to provide clean water to all Americans and to have a functioning sanitation system to remove waste. Although we may like to credit the practices of our health care system and the development of antibiotics, most experts agree that these societal changes in public policies were the true catalyst behind the reduction in many deadly infectious diseases.

Legislation has had a tremendous impact on public health. Laws that mandate maximum speed limits, as well as those that mandate use of seat belts and safety features on automobiles (e.g., airbags, reinforced doors, antilock brakes), have the potential to do much more for health and reduction of injury than individual education about safe driving practices. Federal clean air legislation, often targeting certain pollutants known to cause human health problems, can have a great effect on the pulmonary health of the population. Warning labels and high taxes on cigarettes have reduced usage and increased the awareness of smokers of some of the negative aspects of their habit. States that ban public smoking note decreased smoking rates and lung cancer deaths. Laws requiring food to be labeled and packaged in a certain way, and mandating vitamin and mineral fortification of some foods, have effectively reduced many vitamin deficiency disorders. In fact, a great many of our laws—from traffic laws to pollution regulations to licensing requirements for health care professionals and facilities, to animal control to building codes—are designed at least in part to promote the health and safety of our population.

Many policy makers believe that changing public policy and issuing regulations are the most effective ways to promote changes in the health of populations and to ensure effective medical care. Regulations may specify certain aspects of care—for example, mandating that insurance companies cover mammograms. Alternatively, they may set standards by which facilities and health care are evaluated. Regulations and policies may be enacted most effectively if the government enacting these changes is also paying the bill. Thus many regulations are linked with participation in Medicare or Medicaid. Nursing homes and hospitals, for example, are governed by volumes of complex regulations pertaining to everything from their management structure, the food they provide, care coordination, and doses of particular medications, to the size and layout of rooms. All of these regulations are designed to forestall potential problems with care and to provide standards and penalties for violations of those standards.

SUMMARY

A large proportion of illness in this country is caused or aggravated by unhealthy lifestyles that can be changed. This chapter discusses many ways in which individuals can take responsibility for their own health. Three main areas of prevention are addressed. Primary prevention is initiated to prevent a disease from occurring. The most effective means of primary prevention are positive health behaviors—things we do every day to keep healthy. These include getting vaccinations, wearing seat belts, eating healthful foods, getting sufficient exercise, and not smoking, to name a few. Secondary prevention consists of screening tests that are administered to individuals who have no sign of disease in order to detect illnesses at an early, more treatable stage. Tertiary prevention includes treatments and education that help people deal with their existing illnesses and reduce the risk of further disability, complications, or death. Because there is a high prevalence of disease in older persons, the potential to prevent or decrease the severity of these diseases is great. However, prevention and health promotion programs are underutilized and underfunded.

Several health behaviors listed in this chapter are known to reduce the rate of illness and death and to increase the quality of life. However, knowledge of the right thing to do does not necessarily lead to changes in behavior. Behavior theorists have developed a model of behavior change that allows health care professionals to tailor a health education message to individual clients and patients.

Health promotion activities, including counseling and education, help people to make positive lifestyle changes and may be offered to an individual, a group, or community-wide. Health promotion efforts directed at a national audience and public education campaigns have made a significant difference in the lives of many Americans.

Public health campaigns and the efforts of public health professionals, industries, and government have resulted in positive health trends among Americans. However, health promotion is limited by inadequate funding, and insufficient research in the area of health promotion to determine what methods are effective for which populations. Nationwide efforts, such as the Healthy People Initiative, have set goals and objectives to strive to improve the health of all Americans and to reduce health disparities.

ACTIVITIES

1. Develop a health education module on a topic that is relevant for a particular elder group. Clearly specify the problem, develop measurable objectives, an outline of the topic, and choose teaching methods and materials to enhance the presentation. Use the Web site www.medlineplus.gov to help you gather information and materials.

2. Survey a group of adults of various ages regarding their knowledge of and compliance with recommended screening guidelines. Ask them why they made the decisions they have. What kinds of reasons do they put forth? Can you counter their arguments with data?

3. Develop a single-page health education campaign for a health behavior you wish to influence (e.g., smoking cessation, exercise, screening tests, seat belt use, etc.). Develop a separate flier or pamphlet for people who are intenders and a second for people who are actors. How do your approaches differ for the two population groups?

4. Ask friends and family members of various ages to recall their visits with a physician in the last year. Did the doctor ask them about their personal health behaviors? What screening tests were they offered? Was health promotion counseling offered? How many of the elders comply with any of recommendations outlined in this chapter?

5. Download the checklist for women, "Women: Stay Healthy at Any Age—Checklist for Your Next Checkup," at www.ahrq.gov/ppip/healthywom.htm or the checklist for men, "Men: Stay Healthy at Any Age—Checklist for Your Next Checkup," at www.ahrq.gov/ppip/healthymen.htm Which screening tests have you had? According to the guidelines, which ones do you need? Which immunizations have you had to prevent disease?

Are you due for any boosters? Discuss what health behaviors you might change to improve your chances of staying healthy. Make another copy of the checklist and work with a relative to complete it.

6. Choose a particular disease common to older people. Do an Internet search and see what comes up. Who is the audience for the health information? Who wrote it? How do you know it is true? Compare the information you obtain from various sites. Look up the disease on www.pubmed.gov Compare the two sites. What are the advantages and disadvantages of each? Would you use these sites again? Why or why not?

7. Review at least one major law enacted by the federal government in relation to health. Assess what prompted this legislation. How might it impact the health of older adults?

8. Find some health education and health promotion resources and examine them critically. Can you see any evidence that particular populations or stages of change are being targeted?

9. An elder comes to you and asks for help. She is interested in exercising more, but just can't seem to get started or to keep up the program for more than a week. Devise a strategy to assist her, based on health behavioral change theory.

BIBLIOGRAPHY

1. Nichols, K.L., Nordin, J., Mullooly, J. et al. 2003. Influenza vaccination and reduction in hospitalizations for cardiac disease and stroke among the elderly. *New England Journal of Medicine* 348:1322–1332.

2. U.S. Preventive Services Task Force. 2010. *Guide to Clinical Preventive Services, 2010–2011: Recommendations of the U.S. Preventive Services Task Force.* AHRQ Publication No. 10-05145, Rockville MD: Agency for Healthcare Research and Quality.

3. Swensen, S.J., Jett, J.R., Hartman, T.E., et al. 2003. Lung cancer screening with CT: Mayo Clinic experience. *Radiology* 226(3):756–761.

4. Clarfield, A.M. 2010. Screening in frail older people: An ounce of prevention or a pound of trouble? *Journal of the American Geriatric Society* 58(10): 2016–2021.

5. Woolf, S.H., Jonas, S., and Kaplan-Liss, E. 2008. *Health promotion and disease prevention in clinical practice.* Baltimore, MD: Williams and Wilkins.

6. Prochaska, J.O., and DiClemente, C.C. 2005. The transtheoretical approach. In Norcross, J.C., and Goldfried, M.R. (eds.), *Handbook of psychotherapy integration*, 2nd ed. New York: Oxford University Press, pp. 147–171.

7. Schwarzer, R. 2008. Modeling health behavior change: How to predict and modify the adoption and maintenance of health behaviors. *Applied Psychology: An International Review* 57(1):1–29.

8. Schüz, B., Sniehotta, F.F., Mallach, N., Wiedemann, A., and Schwarzer, R. 2009. Predicting transitions from pre-intentional, intentional and actional stages of change: Adherence to oral self-care recommendations. *Health Education Research* 24:64–75.

CHAPTER 13

Medical Care

America has the best doctors, the best nurses, the best hospitals, the best medical technology, the best medical breakthrough medicines in the world. There is absolutely no reason we should not have in this country the best health care in the world.

Bill Frist

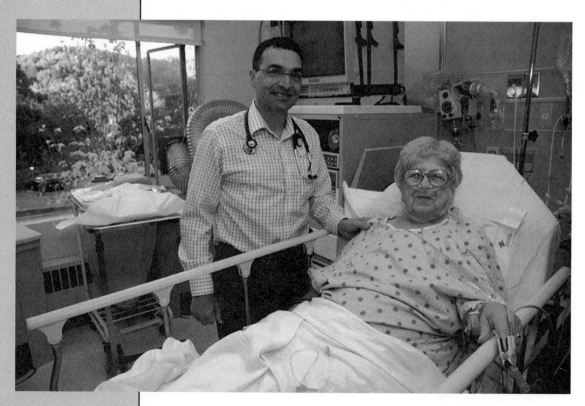

Elders use a disproportionate amount of health care services when compared to younger people. This high use is attributed to a higher rate of disability and disease, as well as more secure health care coverage to finance these visits. Elders' higher use of health care is reflected in all aspects of the health care system—they use more medications; they visit doctors more often; they are more likely to be hospitalized, and when they enter the hospital, they stay longer; and they are more likely to undergo surgery, live in nursing homes, and need medical equipment and devices. Looking at statistics, elders comprise only about 13 percent of the population, but they use about one-third of all health care resources and use services at a rate of 2–3 times those of younger populations.

Government programs are in place to cover a portion of elders' medical expenses. Many older persons also carry private health insurance to pay for a portion of their health care tab not covered by Medicare. Generally, older people still pay a significant portion of their medical expenses out of their own pockets.

Those working with older people need to know about the government programs that finance their medical care so they can better assist them in navigating a complex system of benefits and exclusions. Although learning about the workings of governmental programs may be tedious, it is an important part of becoming an effective professional in human services. A sufficient income and access to medical care is the linchpin of health in the later years.

The chapter also examines the problems of the medical system that affect the quality of care: high cost, inequalities in treatment, patient safety concerns, lack of geriatrics training, and more. We also explore the many innovations in medical care that are being implemented to increase the quality and efficiency of our medical system. Complementary and alternative medicine is becoming more accepted by both laypersons and health professionals and research in that area will be addressed.

FINANCING MEDICAL CARE

Given the preponderance of chronic disease among older people, it is no surprise that they are the highest users of physician services, hospitals, prescription drugs, and long term care. An increased use of medical care and increased number of health conditions results in increased health care costs. In this section, we discuss the major public and private sources that elders rely on to partially reimburse their health care expenses.

How do older people pay for their medical care? As you learned in Chapter 1, "Our Nation's Elders: The Facts," the median annual income of older people living alone was close to $19,167 in 2009, and one in six older people was either below or 25 percent above the poverty line.[1] If out-of-pocket health expenditures are subtracted from their incomes, it is evident that a high proportion of older people cannot afford medical care on their own.

The federal government pays a significant portion of the medical bills of individuals 65 years of age and older through the Medicare program. In addition, for those elders who are poor, Medicaid (MediCal in California) contributes all or a portion of the remainder. Military veterans may obtain medical care through the U.S. Department of Veterans Affairs, and American Indian elders access the Indian Health Service. Most elders without Medicaid, Indian Health Service, or veterans' benefits enroll in a private supplementary health insurance policy. Even with these programs, the amount that older people must pay from their own funds (out-of-pocket expenditures) is substantial and rising.

In this section we detail the major health care financing mechanisms for the 65 years and older population in the United States. The details of these programs are complex and constantly being revised. However, learning the basics of the programs is necessary for individuals planning to work with older people, to help older family members, and, sooner or later, to use the information for themselves.

Medicare

Medicare, Title XVIII of the Social Security Act, was signed into law by President Lyndon Johnson in 1965 to provide selected medical benefits for people who are 65 years of age and older who qualify for Social Security, regardless of income. In 1972 and 1973, further legislation expanded the coverage to those aged 65 and older who previously did not qualify for Social Security, as well as to certain disabled people.

Billions of dollars are paid into the Medicare fund each year, the majority from payroll taxes levied on working adults. Look at your paycheck and you can see the contribution you make every month to this program. Upon reaching age 65, elders are eligible to receive its benefits. The costs are also partially borne by the users of the service, who must pay premiums (monthly costs), deductibles (a fixed amount they must pay each year before Medicare "kicks in"), and copayments or coinsurance (an amount that is contributed by the consumer for every doctor's or hospital visit). The cost of premiums, copays, and yearly deductibles to Medicare recipients described below is accurate for 2007. Since costs increase regularly, the dollar amounts are listed to give a general idea of the cost of the program to the Medicare recipient. Yearly updates are detailed in the booklet *Medicare and You,* which can be found at local Social Security offices, ordered at 1-800-MEDICARE, or downloaded from www.medicare.gov

Medicare is divided into four parts: A, B, C, and D. To put it simply, Part A is a hospital insurance, Part B is a medical insurance, Part C is a private managed care plan, and Part D is a prescription drug insurance. Each part of Medicare has different rules, different copayments, deductibles, and different services that are covered or not covered.

Part A is supported by working adults who contribute to the fund as part of their payroll tax on their earnings. For those 65 and older who have paid into Social Security by working at least 40 quarters, there is no monthly charge (premium) for Part A. Those who did not put in 40 quarters

pay monthly premiums. Part A mainly reimburses hospital care, but it will finance limited stays in nursing homes after a hospital stay, and home health services and hospice services for the terminally ill if certain guidelines are met. A deductible is required for almost all hospital services. A deductible is the dollar amount paid by the recipient before Medicare begins payment for that particular year. Coverage ceases if hospitalization is prolonged beyond 150 days; at that point, the individual is responsible for the full amount.

In addition to hospital costs, Medicare Part A finances skilled nursing home care, but only if the skilled nursing home stay occurs after a three-day qualifying hospital stay and care is directed toward rehabilitation. Qualifying care includes skilled nursing and rehabilitation services such as care for wounds or physical therapy. These services are provided only on a short-term basis. If an elder needs to stay at the nursing home longer to continue care and supervision when the Medicare benefit is exhausted, this must be paid for in another way. For particulars, refer to Chapter 14, "Long-Term Care."

In the home setting, Medicare Part A finances some home health and hospice services. In order to receive home health care under Medicare, an older person must be homebound and under a physician's care and must require some skilled nursing care or physical, speech, or rehabilitative therapy. *Homebound* means that a person leaves home only for church and for medical appointments. Medicare does not pay for full-time nursing care or for custodial care (homemaker or personal care services). Also, Medicare does not cover home services to assist someone with activities of daily living, such as bathing, dressing, and housekeeping. In order to be reimbursed by Medicare, home health services must be prescribed by a physician and must be part of a treatment plan. Skilled nursing services in the home are covered for a maximum of 8 hours daily and for no more than 28 hours weekly.

Medicare Part A provides a variety of hospice services to aid the dying (including prescription drugs) and respite care to relieve individuals caring for a Medicare beneficiary, charging small copays for those who qualify. See Chapter 15, "Dying, Death, and Grief," for further information on the Medicare hospice benefit or refer to the current *Medicare and You* booklet at www.medicare.gov

In contrast to Part A, Medicare Part B pays for physicians, therapists, outpatient care, medical equipment, and some home health services. If an elder is hospitalized, Medicare Part A reimburses the hospital while Medicare Part B reimburses the doctors, surgeons, and physical therapists.

Parts A and B are funded differently. As mentioned earlier, Part A is funded from payroll taxes on workers, and Part B is financed through the general revenues of the federal government and the monthly premiums paid by the individuals who are enrolled. Part B can be thought of as a medical insurance plan that reimburses 80 percent of reasonable charges for medically necessary medical services after the insured person pays the yearly deductible. The monthly premium and yearly deductible for Medicare Part B increase each year. In 2011, the Part B monthly premium that beneficiaries paid was $115.40.

The government estimates that more than one-fourth of the Medicare recipients can qualify for assistance through Medicaid to pay for the entire Part B premium. Individuals who are 65 and older with an annual modified gross income of $80,000 or more, or $160,000 for a married couple (4 percent of the elder population), pay a higher monthly premium. The increased monthly premium paid by that group is projected to save Medicare almost $21 billion by 2017, significantly improving the stability of the Medicare program (www .medicare.gov).

Part C (Medicare Advantage) is a managed care plan that is approved by Medicare and administered by private companies. It might be a health maintenance organization, a preferred provider organization, or a private fee-for-service plan. Part C offers combined coverage of Part A, Part B, and most include Part D. These managed care plans are designed for individuals aged 65 and older who are willing to give up some choice in provider, physician, or hospital in exchange for increased benefits. Medicare Advantage is not available in all areas, and these plans are less common in rural areas.

Medicare Part D is a prescription drug insurance program offered by private companies to all individuals eligible for Medicare. It was initiated in January 2006. The program is thoroughly discussed in Chapter 8, "Medication Use." For the most recent updates, call 1-800-MEDICARE or visit www.medicare.gov

A big advantage of Medicare is that almost any elder can qualify. There are no exclusions for preexisting conditions, no need to stay with a certain employer, and little need to worry that the coverage will be exhausted. However, there are also many challenges with Medicare. The complexity of Medicare with its various parts and what each part covers is confusing, particularly the payment mechanisms (monthly premiums, copays, and yearly deductibles) and what is covered by the various "parts." Individuals still spend a significant amount of money on medical care because of the monthly premiums, copays, and deductibles. Medicare does not cover all needed services or reimburse fully for the services it does cover. National figures show that Medicare covers only about half the health care costs of those 65 years and older. Significant medical expenses are not covered: most nursing home care, vision screening and eyeglasses, hearing screening and hearing aids, and dental care. Unlike most private insurance plans, Medicare places no cap on what a person has to pay out-of-pocket. Many older people enroll in a private supplementary health insurance plan to help cover the cost of Medicare premiums, deductibles, and copays.

Types of Medicare Plans

Theoretically, individuals have several options for how they receive services under Medicare: the Original Medicare Plan (fee-for-service), Medicare Advantage Plans (managed care), and Other Medicare Health Plans. In some areas of the country, the Original Medicare Plan is all that is available. The Original Medicare Plan enrolls more than three-fourths of all elders, and the managed care options within Medicare enroll about 22 percent. These two options are discussed here.

The Original Medicare Plan, also called fee-for-service, lets elders visit any general physician, specialist, hospital, or pharmacy that they wish as many times as they wish, but they must pay co-payments and deductibles for both Medicare A and Medicare B. In contrast, Medicare Advantage Plans provide "managed care," which means that the primary care physician and the health plan manage (or restrict) access to services. Managed care options differ in the types and extent of services they offer and in the cost of the monthly premium, the copay per visit, and the yearly deductible, but the benefits of Medicare A, B, and commonly D are lumped together. By law, these plans must cover at least the same services that Medicare Part A and B cover.

From an administrative viewpoint, the fundamental difference between the fee-for-service and managed care plans is the way in which they finance health care services. The Original Medicare Plan (fee-for-service) reimburses physicians and hospitals for services rendered. The more often an older person visits a physician, the greater will be the amount the physician receives in fees. In contrast, a Medicare Advantage Plan (managed care) receives a fixed payment from Medicare for each individual enrolled, regardless of how many or how few services are used. This method of payment is called *capitation*. Managed care plans actually profit the most if people do not go to the doctor or are never hospitalized. This method of payment may be an incentive for a plan to institute preventive services for the plan will profit if members stay healthy and do not need hospitalization. But this method of payment can also be an incentive to reduce services, for the plan can profit if sick members can't get tests, treatments, and follow-up care.

Another difference between the Original Medicare Plan (fee-for-service) and Medicare Advantage Plans (managed care) is in who assumes the risk or the costs of an expensive patient. In fee-for-service Medicare, the government must pay more for the sickest beneficiaries. In managed care,

the health plan or physician loses money when caring for the sickest people and hopes to recoup those losses by enrolling elders who are well and will need fewer medical services. The managed care organization profits if it is able to hold costs down and limit access to expensive services. To entice healthy older people, managed care organizations offer some benefits (e.g., smaller copayments, no deductibles, lower drug costs) beyond those offered by the Original Plan. Healthier elders use fewer resources, so it is hoped that the cost of offering increased benefits to healthy elders is lower than the amount of money spent to diagnose and treat elders who have many health problems.

Managed care is provided by two types of organizations: preferred provider organizations (PPOs) and health maintenance organizations (HMOs). A PPO contracts with doctors and hospitals in an area to provide care for its enrollees at a bargain price. A doctor may contract with many different PPOs and generally has both fee-for-service and PPO patients. A person who enrolls in a PPO must see a doctor and use a hospital that has contracted with that PPO. The physicians are not hired by the plan. They sign a contract with the PPO, agreeing to see the PPO patients. Often the PPO pays them a fixed amount a month based on the number of patients assigned to them. If PPO patients see their doctor once a week or once a year, the doctor gets paid the same monthly amount. Alternatively, the payment received by some PPO physicians is based on numbers of visits, but at lower rates than they would charge their fee-for-service patients. In 2006, regional PPOs that serve one or more states became available, bringing more options to elders.

A health maintenance organization brings hospital and medical services under a single umbrella. The services can be provided in one location, or in multiple hospitals and physician offices. The administrator of an HMO receives the monthly premiums from Medicare and pays each physician a monthly amount for each patient. In some cases, called staff-model HMOs, the physicians are employed by the HMO, but more commonly, the HMO contracts with various physician groups. For the patients enrolled

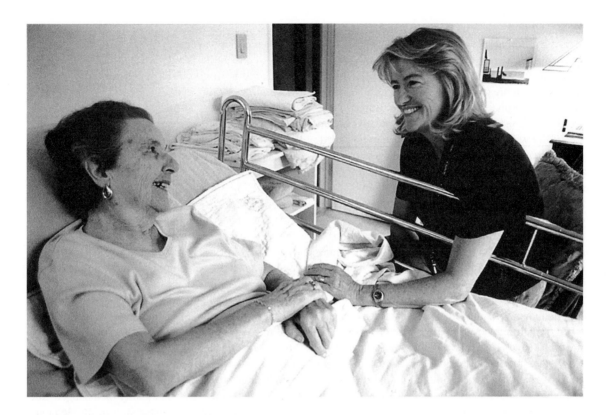

in an HMO, many services (including physician services, consultations, equipment, medication, and hospitalization) are provided by the HMO.

Both PPOs and HMOs limit patients' choices in exchange for some benefits with the goal of increasing coordination and efficiency of care. When Medicare enrollees choose a managed care option, they agree to a set of terms and conditions. In general, they sacrifice choice of physicians for expanded benefits and decreased costs.

The main benefits of joining a managed care plan are increased benefits and lower out-of-pocket costs. Depending on the organization, elders may receive more hospital benefits (for example, more hospital days or lower copayments), lower monthly premiums for Medicare Part B, a lower or no yearly deductible, a smaller copay, and a greater drug benefit. In addition, elders may receive free yearly physical examinations, free vision and hearing screening, and reduced prescription drug costs. Also, a private supplemental insurance policy is not needed because

the Medicare Advantage plans generally cover many of the same benefits that a private policy would cover—a significant savings to the elder consumer.

Ideally, managed care increases the efficiency and coordination of care. In Medicare fee-for-service plans, physicians can easily order more tests, hospitalize patients, encourage repeat visits, and refer patients to specialty care. This may result in unnecessary services and, consequently, unnecessary costs. In fee-for-service plans, care may be uncoordinated because elders can seek care from whatever providers they choose. In contrast, in Medicare managed care plans, the use of services is controlled by a single primary care physician, and the result could be greater coordination of care and an expansion of preventive services.

There are also many drawbacks to the Medicare Advantage Plans (managed care). In many areas, particularly rural areas, managed care programs are not available. In urban areas where they are available, multiple competing plans are marketing their services to elders, and comparing plans can be difficult. Plans may differ in the benefits they offer, the drugs they cover, the size of premiums, copays, and deductibles, and the coverage of "extras." Monthly premiums, deductibles, and benefits in the Original Medicare Plan (fee-for-service) are the same no matter where an elder lives, but they differ widely from region to region in managed care plans. A Commonwealth Fund survey reported that about half the elder population does not have the skills to make good decisions about which plan to enter and may not make the best health care choices.[2] The premiums and benefits of the fee-for-service Medicare program have been stable for decades. Managed care plans cannot make the same claim: Increasing premiums, decreasing benefits, high provider turnover, even withdrawing a plan from a region are not uncommon as businesses find they cannot make a profit. What happens to patients when a managed care provider folds or withdraws from a region? They need to find another PPO or HMO, and if none is available in the area, they sign up for a fee-for-service plan and purchase supplemental health insurance.[3]

Elders who choose managed care are limited in their choice of doctors to those who participate in the plan. When they select a plan, if their personal doctor is not a member of that HMO or PPO, they must switch doctors. In most managed care plans, a patient may see a specialist only if the patient's primary care physician authorizes the visit. In addition, enrollees are generally restricted to one hospital system or geographic area (except in an emergency). Before a particular medication, treatment, or specialized visit can be "covered," they may have to wait for health plan authorization. If services are denied, they must appeal. Because the system profits from reduced use of services, there is an incentive for managed care organizations to deny expensive care.

Managed care programs market their services to the healthiest elders (a process called skimming). Enrolling healthy elders enables them to make a profit. If too many sick elders sign up, costs increase and revenues decrease as the use of services rises.

As if Medicare Advantage or Medicare managed care plans weren't complicated enough, they are also a target for governmental health reform efforts and the requirements, incentives, and rules governing them are ever-changing. The government was surprised to find that Medicare managed care plans were making money at a high rate and were actually costing more than standard Medicare. It was estimated to be about 10 percent more expensive. However, the extra money didn't all go to profit; the members of the managed care programs also received extra benefits.

This made the managed care program a target for cost-cutting health reform efforts in 2010. Thus, a complex formula was developed, which targets payments based on geographic areas and gradually lowers rates of payment. In general, rural areas will get more money and urban providers will get less. These plans limit administrative costs to 15 percent and maintain quality standards that providers must meet. This is a challenging time as providers scramble to find ways to cut costs and maintain quality.

The Centers for Medicare and Medicaid Services (CMS) measures the quality of managed care organizations with a five-star system. If Medicare advantage plans can maintain a 4–5 star rating, they can actually get a 5 percent payment boost and even qualify for rebates. Stars are determined by levels of performance such as screening elders for disease with mammograms, providing checkups, high satisfaction scores, and telephone access.

Benefits and Limitations of Medicare

Unlike most government programs, Medicare is available to all those aged 65 and older regardless of their health and income status. Medicare pays a good proportion of both hospital and physician costs of a group with a high level of disease and disability who otherwise would find it difficult to purchase private insurance. By its universal availability, Medicare equally spreads the costs of health care between the sick and the healthy. Further, the Medicare fee-for-service plan offers something that private insurance policies are increasingly eliminating—free choice of providers. An elder can see any physician who accepts

Medicare as often as desired, and special permission is not needed to seek out specialists. Elders can choose to enroll in a managed care program (PPO or HMO) during the annual open-enrollment period if they are dissatisfied. Because Medicare is so big, it has the clout to initiate positive changes in health care (e.g., by means of peer review and physician reimbursement). Medicare has consistently been one of the most popular social programs ever implemented.

Despite its benefits, Medicare has been criticized on a number of counts. A major criticism is that Medicare does not reimburse some important medical needs. Although Medicare does reimburse nursing homes or home health services after hospitalization, it does not cover home or institutional custodial care for long-term chronic conditions, a much more common situation among elders. In addition, Medicare does not reimburse for dental care and dentures, routine physical examinations, vision and glasses, hearing exams and hearing aids, or routine foot care.

Some critics assert that Medicare is too complex: monthly premiums, copayments, yearly deductibles, need for supplementary insurance, and benefit restrictions. The Medicare choices can be confusing, and the best choice depends heavily on the elder's health situation, preferences, and location. And, in a way, the program discriminates against minorities. Even though they have paid into the system throughout their lives, they are less likely to live long enough to receive its benefits. Still others criticize Medicare for providing significant benefits to all elders while many poor people under age 65 are unable to afford any health insurance. Doctors and hospitals are critical of the continual decrease in reimbursements for services rendered and the increase in paperwork. In the past, Medicare reimbursements to hospitals were somewhat inflated—these monies helped build hospitals and purchase new technology. As Medicare reimbursement rates shrink, hospitals are increasingly facing financial troubles and bankruptcy.

Perhaps the biggest concern about the Medicare program is its tremendous cost. Medicare is projected to grow, primarily because of the aging of the population and increasing numbers of older people receiving Medicare benefits, and the cost of the Part D prescription drug benefit. But other factors are driving health care costs up as well. Health care costs have been rising more rapidly than the cost of living for at least the last 20 years. Spending is expected to exceed income beginning in 2012. By the year 2030, the number of people on Medicare will have almost doubled, from 40 million to 78 million, and the number of workers is projected to have declined from 4 workers per beneficiary to 2.4 workers per beneficiary. According to experts, Medicare reserves are projected to be depleted in 2029.[4]

Several proposals have been made to increase the financial stability of the Medicare program. One suggestion is to reduce costs by enrolling a greater percentage of older people in managed care plans. Other suggestions include raising copayments and deductibles, increasing the Social Security payroll taxes paid by working adults and employers, increasing the cap on taxable earnings (in 2011 Social Security tax was not paid on earnings above $106,800), privatizing Medicare, and reducing payments to hospitals or physicians. It has also been suggested that the age of eligibility for Medicare be increased to 67 years of age or even older. Another suggestion is that Medicare copayments and deductibles should be determined by a sliding scale, taking into consideration an individual's income and assets. In January 2007, a sliding scale was implemented to determine the annual Medicare Part B premiums for elder individuals with annual incomes of $80,000 a year and above and elder couples with annual incomes of $160,000 a year and above. Experts agree that more changes are needed to keep Medicare viable for future generations.

Supplemental Health Insurance

How are elders to finance the copayments and deductibles of Medicare? How do they shield themselves against the risk of huge medical bills from a catastrophic illness? The poor turn to Medicaid programs. Some elders continue in employer-sponsored health insurance plans. As more elders stay in the workplace longer, many maintain health insurance benefits from an employer, which helps finance their expenses. With employer-sponsored insurance, they can pay for benefits not covered by Medicare. While more than one-third of all Medicare beneficiaries have additional coverage from an employer, the share of employers offering retiree health benefits has declined, from 66 percent in 1988 to 28 percent in 2010.[4] Other elders without this option pay out-of-pocket. But the majority purchase supplemental health insurance policies (often called Medigap insurance) that pay many of the medical bills that are only partially covered by Medicare, such as the copays and the Part A and Part B deductibles.

The cost of Medigap insurance depends on the benefit level of the plan that elders select: the greater the coverage, the higher the cost. In the past, these insurance policies were not regulated, and there was great confusion about which policy covered what services. As a result, many elders purchased coverage they didn't need. Because of strong advocacy efforts, Congress passed legislation that requires private insurance companies to standardize and simplify their policies so elders can more easily compare benefits. All Medigap policies are now based on one of 10 model packages, ranging from basic coverage of physicians' fees and extended hospitalization coverage, to more complete policies with extended benefits such as long-term care costs and short-term in-home assistance. The policies are labeled "A" through "N" to allow consumers to easily compare prices. Four of those policy choices are now closed to new members.

A benefits package may cost from $50 to over $1,000 per month, depending on the type and extent of coverage. This monthly cost is in addition to the monthly premium an individual must pay for Medicare Part B. A person should purchase one of these policies around his or her 65th birthday (from one month before to five months after), because during that period, Medigap insurance companies cannot turn anyone down. Federal regulations require all policies to be renewable even if an elder becomes disabled.

Many elders are still working and thus may be covered by their employer for Medigap insurance. Other employers might provide a stipend to be used to purchase a Medigap plan. Usually the elder is responsible for a premium, copays, and deductibles. Some employers provide a retirement package that includes all or part payment for Medigap insurance until death.

Despite the legislation to control Medigap policies, loopholes in laws regulating the sale of private insurance policies to elders result in billions of dollars of unnecessary spending by elders on coverage they do not need. Some policies duplicate Medicare's benefits; others cover only certain illnesses. Further information is available in the booklet *Choosing a Medigap Policy,* the official government guide to health insurance for people with Medicare. To receive the brochure, call 1-800-MEDICARE or access the print version from the Medicare Web site, (www.Medicare.gov). Also, AARP and the Center for Medicare Education offer a guide on Medigap insurance (www.aarp.org).

Medicaid

Medicaid, Title XIX of the Social Security Act, was enacted at the same time as Medicare to provide protection against the high costs of extended hospital and nursing home care and physician care for the poor, blind, and disabled of all ages. Medicaid (MediCal in California) is financed jointly by the states and the federal government. The federal government provides matching grants to each state to finance several mandatory services: in- and outpatient hospital care, physician services, skilled nursing facility services, lab and X-ray diagnosis, home care nursing services, screening mammograms, and some home health services. In addition, some states provide private nursing, dental care, physical therapy, drugs, dentures, glasses, and hearing aids. The program is administered by the states, and each state has the option to offer broader coverage. In most states, physicians who agree to participate must accept the Medicaid reimbursement as full payment and cannot bill the patient for any additional expenses.

Eligibility for Medicaid is based on the individual's monthly income and total assets. Because each state administers its own program, there is much variation among states regarding which groups of people can be covered, the financial criteria for eligibility, the amount, duration, and scope of coverage, and the rate of reimbursement for services. In addition to mandated coverage for many special younger populations, states are required to provide services for older persons who fit into the following categories: (1) those who receive Supplemental Security Income (SSI) and (2) Medicare beneficiaries with incomes at or below 85 percent of the federal poverty level and resources at or below twice the standard allowed under the SSI program. A few states provide Medicaid coverage for everyone below the poverty level, but most do not. In some states, Medicaid also pays a portion of elders' health costs if their income is less than 150 percent above the poverty level.

Medicaid finances hospital care, physician visits, medications, treatments, and a wide range of both medical and personal care services in the home and nursing home. However, Medicaid reimburses hospitals and physicians far less than private insurance or Medicare, so doctors and hospitals are not eager to take Medicaid patients. Similarly, Medicaid reimburses nursing homes less than the true costs of care for full room and board, personal assistance, and skilled nursing care. Because of low reimbursement by Medicaid, many nursing homes, especially those that cater to residents in the middle- and upper-income brackets or have no trouble filling their beds, do not admit applicants who qualify for Medicaid or have few assets. Some nursing homes will accept only a small proportion of applicants who are eligible for Medicaid.

Approximately 21 percent of elders on Medicare also received Medicaid benefits in 2007. For these "dual-eligible" elders, Medicaid finances all or part of the yearly deductibles, copayments, and monthly premiums required of all Medicare recipients, depending on income and assets. Dual-eligible elders who are not in a managed care plan are enrolled in the Medicare Part D prescription drug program. Depending on their income, Medicaid pays all or part of the monthly premiums, deductibles, and copays for each of their prescriptions.

Coordination of care for those with dual eligibility for Medicare and Medicaid is complicated because these individuals represent some of the sickest and poorest older Americans. They often have multiple chronic illnesses and disabilities and have difficulty in negotiating the health care system. Because this small population uses a disproportionate amount of health care resources, attention has been focused on improving health care delivery and reducing costs for that group. Managed care has been proposed as a solution, and most states now have managed care programs for their Medicaid recipients. These individuals are often eligible for special programs (such as Pace programs, disease management programs, or other Medicare demonstration programs) that look for innovative ways to keep these elders out of nursing homes and hospitals. In addition, there is widespread concern about ensuring quality care for chronically ill, poor, and disabled beneficiaries.

Department of Veterans Affairs

The federal Department of Veterans Affairs (VA) operates the largest centrally directed hospital and medical service system in the United States. It is a tax-financed agency that delivers care directly through salaried physicians and goverment-owned facilities and relies on annual federal appropriations for its money. There is at least one Veterans Administration hospital in every state except Alaska and Hawaii.

The VA system was developed in response to the need to treat and rehabilitate veterans with service-related injuries and disabilities. Over the years, the system has helped poor veterans with medical needs unrelated to their military service. Currently, four overlapping groups of veterans are eligible to receive VA medical care: (1) veterans with service-connected disabilities, (2) recipients of VA pensions, (3) veterans age 65 and older, and (4) medically indigent veterans. Veterans with service-connected disabilities receive top priority;

however, other veterans may be cared for when resources are available. All veterans over age 65 are classified as disabled, making the VA a major health care resource for that group. Veterans Administration facilities also play an important role in medical education and research because they are staffed by medical school faculty and physicians in training. Schools of nursing, dentistry, rehabilitation medicine, and social work have also developed affiliations with the VA hospitals.

The system has undergone rapid and substantive changes in the past 15 years. The role has changed from hospital-based specialty-focused health care to outpatient primary care, including case management and preventive services that are linked with local physicians. To increase efficiency, the management of the Veterans Administration is now decentralized, and the existing medical sites are grouped into 23 Veterans Integrated Service Networks (VISNs). Their charge is to create a continuum of care by integrating VA resources with local general-practitioner groups.

The Department of Veterans Affairs provides physician services, hospitalization, home health, and long-term care services to eligible veterans. It also contracts with thousands of other services to serve veteran beneficiaries.

The major challenge currently facing the VA system is to accommodate the increased utilization of its medical services due to the aging of the veteran population and the influx of combat veterans returning from the Persian Gulf. The U.S. Census Bureau reports that in 2009 there were almost 22 million veterans in the United States, and 9 million were 65 and older.

For more information about the scope of health benefits from the Department of Veterans Affairs, refer to www.va.gov/Health_Benefits/

Indian Health Service

The Indian Health Service, an agency within the Department of Health and Human Services, was initiated in 1955 to provide community-based primary care to all American Indian and Alaskan Native peoples in cooperation with and commitment from the tribes. Currently, health services are provided to 2 million American Indians and Alaskan Natives who belong to about 565 tribes in 35 states (serving a little more than half the Indian population in the country). The Indian Health Service cooperates with tribal members to manage 49 hospitals, 247 health centers, and 339 health stations, satellite clinics, and Alaska village clinics. Other health services are purchased from private providers in the regions. Most of the clients live on or near reservations in remote poor areas of the country. Urban Indian health programs are available in 34 urban areas for about a quarter of the Indian population living in urban areas.[5]

Indian elders comprise less than 6 percent of the Indian Health Service population, but they consume a much higher proportion of its funds. Even though they are high users of the services offered, Indian elders receive fewer than half the services provided to the general elder population in our country. Older Indians tend to become disabled more often than elders in other ethnic and racial groups, and the Indian Health Service does not have appropriate resources to help them, particularly in rehabilitation and long-term care. This places a tremendous burden on family members to care for them. Although the tribes identify the need for home health and nursing home services, the Indian Health Service has never received funds to provide them. Rising health costs and increasing patient needs make it more difficult to contract for services that are not available within the Indian health system.[5]

The Indian Health Service faces many challenges as current resources cannot meet the needs of the expanding population. Federal funds allocated to the agency amount to only 60 percent of funds available to the rest of the population in the United States. Further, although health care services are available to all members of recognized tribes, the types of resources vary in each location. Even though all are eligible for health services, in reality, because of low funding, people with the greatest need get care first, and often the money runs out before the year ends, postponing care for many patients with lesser problems.[5] Interestingly, no Healthy People 2020 objectives have to do with disparities between races and ethnicities.

For further information on the Indian Health Service, see www.ihs.gov

Out-of-Pocket Expenses

Despite the huge outlay of federal dollars for medical care for older people, elders still pay a significant proportion of their medical bills out of their own pockets. And, as health care becomes increasingly expensive, the amount financed out-of-pocket continues to rise. In 2006, Medicare recipients spent an average of $4,241 from their own resources, close to 16 percent of their yearly income. The cost generally increases with advancing age and health status. The cost breakdown was as follows: for Medicare premiums alone, 39 percent; long-term care, 19 percent; medical providers and supplies, 15 percent; prescription drugs, 14 percent. Elders' out-of-pocket expenses for just the premiums for Medicare and supplemental policies increased from 5.5 percent of their median income in 1997 to 8.0 percent of their income in 2006.[4] Unfortunately, elders often have to cope with high medical expenses at a time when their income is fixed or declining.

Medicare was originally implemented decades ago because elders were paying about 15 percent of their income for health care, necessarily reducing money left for food, shelter, and other basic needs. Ironically, after all these years, elders now pay a higher proportion of their income for medical expenses than before the Medicare program was implemented. A big reason for this is that medical care costs have increased much faster than inflation. Nevertheless, with the increasing relative and absolute costs of health care services, it is obvious that Medicare, Medigap insurance, and Medicaid do substantially reduce elders' out-of-pocket costs.

MEDICAL CARE: ISSUES TO ADDRESS

The United States has the most technologically advanced medical care system in the world. Physicians have a variety of diagnostic tests, drugs, surgical treatments, and modern equipment and facilities at their disposal, and research continues to expand knowledge and treatment of many diseases. Many of the latest drugs and treatments are discovered and perfected in the United States, and we have a plethora of specialists. Some of the most respected medical centers in the world are in the United States, and individuals from other countries visit to take advantage of American medical care. Despite these advances, our medical care system has several deficiencies that affect the quality of care offered to many elders. This section highlights some of the characteristics of the medical system that affect the quality of care for older people.

The High Cost of Care

Experts agree that medical care in our country comes with a high cost. The share of gross national product spent on health care in the United States is greater than the health care share of GNP spent in any other industrialized nation. In 2009, annual health care spending in the United States was $2.5 trillion, or $8,086 for every person in the United States, comprising almost 18 percent of the gross domestic product, more than any other country.

The United States differs from other industrialized countries in the way in which medical care is financed. In other developed countries, the government is responsible for providing health care for everyone. In our country, federal and state governments help finance medical care for those 65 and older, the disabled, blind, poor, and veterans. Other people purchase private insurance, have employer-sponsored insurance, pay out of their own funds, or go without. It is estimated that 50 million people in the United States are uninsured.

There are a number of complex reasons for the high cost of medical care in our country. The expense of hospitalization, physician services, prescription medications, high-technology procedures, and diagnostic tests is significant and continues to rise faster than inflation. Furthermore, each year our country is facing increasing numbers of older people (particularly those 75 years and older) who are high users of medical services. Those aged 65 years and older are responsible for more than one-third of the nation's health expenditures, even though they account for about 13 percent of the total population. Exorbitant profits made from prescription drugs and health insurance and the high cost of fraud and waste by unscrupulous physicians and hospitals are commonly cited as areas in which medical costs might be reduced. Finally, our nation spends a higher proportion of health care dollars than any other country for administration. Hospital administration costs in the United States were approximately 31 percent of the total hospital bill in 2003, nearly twice the percentage of Canada (16.7 percent).[6] That year, the administrative costs for hospitals alone were over $163 billion, or $1,059 per person in the United States.

Hospitalization expenses are the largest single item in the national health bill—$761 billion—accounting for about 30 percent of the total tab. Hospital costs are high not only because of the administrative costs mentioned above but also because of the services provided. Further, the hospital must maintain constant readiness to provide care. For example, even if half the hospital beds are empty, the technology must be available, the mortgage needs to be paid, and staff must be on duty to respond to emergencies.

Duplication of services wastes money. Hospital services are not distributed equitably and efficiently across the nation. In some affluent communities, there are "too many" hospitals, all competing for the business of privately insured clients, while poor and rural areas have no hospitals for many miles. Duplication also extends to diagnostic tests and to specialty services offered. For example, it is not necessary that every hospital have an MRI (magnetic resonance imaging) machine or a coronary care unit. However, most hospitals in the United States have these services and are unwilling to "share" because the presence of the latest technology is important for drawing patients and physicians to a facility.

In our country, health care spending differs from almost all other types of spending: Both the provider (the physician) and the consumer (the patient) are insulated from the actual costs of the

services. Neither doctors nor patients are aware of the costs, nor are costs even considered in their decision-making process. Before making almost every other type of purchase, the consumer may shop around for the best price or even may elect not to purchase high-cost items. Not so with health care. The illusion that "My insurance is paying for it" may prompt the increased use of health care services. People commonly say that they do not have to pay for most of their health care because it is covered by insurance. However, consumers do pay, both directly by increased out-of-pocket expenses and insurance premiums, and indirectly through increased federal taxes. Most people do not realize that health care costs add to the costs of consumer goods, and that their wages might be higher if their employers were not paying high premiums for employee health insurance.

The high cost of health care affects both individuals and the nation as a whole. We all pay for health care through payroll and income taxes, insurance premiums and copayments, as well as through the increased costs of goods and services we buy. As costs increase, businesses cannot provide coverage for their employees and individuals cannot afford it; thus, more individuals "go without" health coverage. When the uninsured get sick, they are provided with emergency services that they cannot afford. Hospitals and other providers respond to this debt by increasing charges to those who are paying, and the cycle continues. The sickest individuals are the most in need of services but the most expensive to insure. The many healthy Americans who could be paying into the system often elect not to pay hundreds of dollars a month for services they feel they can do without.

Medical care costs are a significant cause of bankruptcies in the United States. A random sample of bankruptcy filers in 2007 revealed that more than three of five bankruptcies in the United States were caused by illness and medical bills.[7]

For-Profit Medical Care

Medical care in the United States is becoming a big-business industry run by large corporations for profit. Increasingly, private and nonprofit hospitals are being bought up and subsumed into larger corporations or shut down altogether. Although the for-profit chains often tout their business acumen as important in reducing waste in the system, studies show that for-profit enterprises are costlier and less efficient than public or nonprofit hospitals. They spend more on administration and less on direct patient care.[8, 9] In addition, for-profit hospitals are less likely to have unprofitable but important services such as emergency rooms and trauma care, and they are less likely to provide charity care. Most important, for-profit hospitals have higher death rates and higher payments for care than nonprofit hospitals.[10, 11]

The trend toward for-profit enterprises is extending to other health care facilities. Unfortunately, this trend is often accompanied by the same reduction in quality of care. Studies have demonstrated poorer care and outcomes in for-profit compared to not-for-profit hospices, health plans, and nursing homes.[12–14] For-profit nursing homes have lower staffing levels and worse patient outcomes among high-risk patients than the nonprofit nursing homes and had a significantly higher rate of deficiencies compared to nonprofit or publicly funded nursing homes.[14]

In a market economy, providers of goods and services compete, and market forces drive increased efficiency, service, and profit. The provision of health care, however, does not lend itself to a market economy, for a number of reasons.

First, consumers are insulated from the costs, which are assumed predominantly by insurance companies and governmental payers. Consequently, consumers are not able to compare price and quality across providers or to distinguish which provider is better than the others. Second, health care services are needed in all areas of the country and must include all types of services, even if those services or geographical areas are not profitable. For example, emergency care, charity care, high-level intensive care, and trauma care are needed in rural areas, even though they are often money-losing propositions. Health care organizations must provide care to all who arrive with a medical emergency, even individuals who cannot pay—and charity cases reduce profits. Third, health care is becoming more sophisticated and expensive at the same time that reimbursements are declining. This discrepancy makes the profit margins small in health care, and there is little opportunity to cut inefficiencies. The best way to profit in health care is to deliver fewer services and hire less staff. But that strategy often leads to reduced quality of patient care. Fourth, good health care extends life and often results in more tests (e.g., screening) and more treatments over a longer life span. Often the best care (such as routine mammograms) boosts costs for a plan because the costs of the mammogram, the biopsies, the follow-up tests, surgery, the radiation, the chemotherapy, and the follow-up care are significantly more expensive than not discovering a breast cancer until it is too late to treat.

Inequities in Treatment

Despite universal coverage under Medicare, ethnic and racial disparities in medical care are common. Researchers consistently find that blacks are less likely to use physicians and hospitals and less likely to undergo diagnostic and surgical procedures than their white counterparts, even though they have more chronic illnesses, higher disability rates, and higher death rates. The discrepancy between blacks and whites in receiving effective care has been reported for treatments of several health problems and is consistent among those with private insurance and those receiving Medicare, Medicaid, or VA benefits. Similar differences have been found for other underrepresented minorities as well as poor whites.

Multiple reasons have been put forth to explain this disparity, including financial barriers, organizational barriers, physician and patient decision making, differences in patient treatment preferences, cultural and communication barriers, hospital characteristics, differences in disease severity, and racism. Reducing racial and ethnic disparities in the delivery of health care is one of the major goals of Healthy People 2020.

Age discrimination is evident in health care policies that prevent older people from getting the care they need. An Alliance for Aging Research report describes five key dimensions of ageism that result in poor care for older people: (1) Health care professionals do not receive enough training in geriatrics to properly care for many older patients. (2) Older patients are less likely to receive preventive care routinely provided to younger groups. (3) Older people are less likely to be diagnosed or screened for life-threatening diseases. (4) Older people are less likely to be offered proven medical interventions and more likely to receive inappropriate or incomplete treatment. (5) Older people are underrepresented or excluded from clinical trials even though they are the largest users of approved drugs.[15]

The reasons for disparities in treatment are likely many and varied. Do providers offer less care to elders because they are ageist or because elders have more medical problems that make procedures difficult or risky? A lack of research on the effectiveness of diagnostic and therapeutic modalities in older people may lead to caution among physicians. It is difficult to ascertain whether elders are offered fewer tests and treatments than other age groups or whether they are more likely to decline them. It may be that elders, who often have several health problems, are steered toward a different focus of care—such as comfort rather than cure.

Patient Safety Concerns

A cardinal principle of geriatric medicine, especially when the course of a patient turns suddenly for the worse, is to ask first, "What have I done to the patient?" rather than "What has the environment done."

—William Hazzard

The same medications and diagnostic tests and procedures that save the lives of some people can impair the well-being and cause serious problems in others. When diagnostic tests, medical treatments, or the hospital environment make a person sick, the person is said to have an *iatrogenic illness.*

Iatrogenic illnesses include a wide variety of conditions, such as adverse effects from a medical procedure as well as from the negligence of a health professional. They also include drug reactions caused by the nature of a drug itself or by the medication errors of health professionals prescribing or dispensing a medication. Although aging itself is not a risk factor for iatrogenic illnesses, the accompaniments of aging—multiple diseases, high drug use, age-associated decrements, and higher rates of hospitalization—create a higher risk for them. Iatrogenic illnesses cost more than money. They result in longer hospital stays, poor health, depression, deterioration, and even death.

Iatrogenic illnesses are common in hospital settings because of the procedures that may accompany hospitalization and the presence of virulent microorganisms in the environment. Infections acquired in the nursing home or hospital are the most common iatrogenic illness and occur when bacteria and viruses are passed from one patient to the next by equipment or the hands of health care workers. Also, some treatments can create conditions that induce nosocomial infections (see Chapter 6, "Acute Illnesses and Accidents").

There is growing attention to the failure of the medical profession to protect patients from medical errors, infections, and injuries in U.S. hospitals. Studies on their prevalence differ, but the statistics quoted are alarming. In 1999, the Institute of Medicine released a landmark report, *To Err Is Human,* that estimated that from 44,000 to 98,000 Americans die each year because of medical errors including unnecessary surgery, medication errors, and infections. The report writers based their estimates on a review of medical records of hospitalized patients and estimated rates of injury and death for the country.[16] The Institute of Medicine report was a landmark study that spawned a whole new focus throughout health care about patient safety. The term "adverse event" describes harm to a patient as a result of medical care.

What are these errors? Some are blatant and well publicized: amputating the wrong leg, failing to check for appropriate blood type before a transfusion, misreading sloppy handwriting on charts and prescriptions, and administering a toxic level of a medication. Others are more complex, such as when a patient in the intensive care unit develops a urinary tract infection from antibiotic-resistant bacteria, or when the doctor prescribes a medication that interacts with another medication the patient is currently using. Some are errors of omission—for instance, failing to give aspirin therapy after a heart attack or failing to treat an elevated cholesterol level.

The term "never events" refers to a specific list of serious events that the National Quality Forum (NQF) deemed "should never occur in a health care setting." Examples of "never events" include serious falls with injury in a health care facility, cutting off the wrong limb in a surgery, development of pressure sores in a hospital, operating on the wrong person, or death (or disability) from a medication error.

How common are these adverse events? The Office of the Inspector General issued a report in 2010 in regard to adverse events in hospitals for Medicare beneficiaries. This report was mandated by the health reform bill (The Tax Relief and Health Care Act of 2006), which required analysts to deny payments for hospitalizations when these events occurred. In other words, if a hospital treated a patient for an amputation done on the wrong leg, the hospital could not bill Medicare or Medicaid for that hospitalization. Also, if an elder developed a urinary tract infection from a catheter or a bedsore, and it was determined this was preventable, then Medicare or Medicaid might not have to finance this stay and the hospital would have to absorb these costs.[17]

An estimated 13.5 percent of hospitalized Medicare beneficiaries experienced adverse events during their hospital stays. An additional 13.5 percent of Medicare beneficiaries experienced events during their hospital stays that resulted in temporary harm. Although many cases were minor, such as low blood sugar that resolved, others were more serious or occurred in those with many other problems who were already in the hospital a long time. Not only are these events too common, but it appears that almost half are preventable. Physician

reviewers determined that 44 percent of adverse and temporary harm events were "clearly or likely preventable," 51 percent were "not preventable," and 5 percent were "not known." Complications related to procedures or surgery were less likely to be classified as preventable than hospital-acquired infections. Preventable events were linked most commonly to medical errors, substandard care, and lack of patient monitoring and assessment. Physician reviewers assessed events as "not preventable" when they occurred despite proper assessment and care or when the patients were highly susceptible to the events due to health status.[17]

How much do these adverse events cost the taxpayers? Hospital care associated with adverse and temporary harm events cost Medicare an estimated $324 million in October 2008 alone, which is estimated as a 3.5 percent excess cost. To give these figures an annual context, 3.5 percent of the $137 billion Medicare inpatient expenditure for 2009 equates to $4.4 billion spent on care associated with adverse events. The increased costs are almost all related to extending hospital stays, but do not include costs required for follow-up care after hospitalization, or the nonfinancial costs of pain, physical suffering, and psychological distress.[17]

Why do doctors and nurses make so many errors, and what should we do about it? According to the Institute of Medicine report, the majority of medical errors result not from individual recklessness but from basic flaws in the way the health system is organized. The way medications are stocked in hospitals can lead to errors, as can the practice of relying on physician handwriting for orders. There are many steps involved in prescribing: from the physician's making a decision and writing an order for a prescription, to the order's being reviewed by pharmacists and nurses and delivered, stocked, and administered to the patient. In any process that has multiple steps and involves multiple people, there are many places where errors can occur.

Practitioners cannot always keep up with the rapid pace of progress in medicine with the development of new drugs and tests. Further, the health care system itself is changing so quickly that it often lacks coordination. For example, when a patient is treated by several practitioners, they often do not have complete information about the medicines already prescribed for the patient's illnesses. Medical records systems are antiquated. Patients are often unaware of their health status, physicians and nurses may be rushed or distracted, or people involved in the process may be unfamiliar with the systems. Individuals who make errors may tend to hide these errors for fear of retribution, malpractice, or negative attention. In a high-risk system such as health care delivery, redundancies and checks and balances are needed to ensure that human errors are found and corrected.

To achieve a better safety record, the Institute of Medicine report recommends a four-part plan designed to create financial and regulatory incentives that will lead to a safer health care system: (1) developing a national center for patient safety, (2) mandatory error reporting to better indicate the scope of the problem, (3) studying physician and hospital staff behavior and introducing automation or extra checks in areas where human error is likely to occur, and (4) computerizing medical records. The Agency for Healthcare Research and Quality took the lead in developing a national Patient Safety Initiative, which established safety goals and priorities. The three top priorities are (1) to identify threats to patient safety; (2) to teach, disseminate, and implement effective patient safety practices; and (3) to maintain vigilance in correcting threats to patient safety. Some interventions in place to address patient safety include laws regarding medication reconciliation at hospital discharge and regulations prohibiting the use of certain abbreviations that are often confusing. In addition, incentives have been offered for doctors and hospitals to use electronic medical records. However, these incentives have not reduced the medical error rate. More than 10 years later, a report by the Office of the Inspector General identified similar problems and proposed similar solutions. They recommended that all adverse events be tracked and counted, using a standard system of identification and reporting, and that health care facilities implement systems to examine the "root causes" of errors and to find solutions.

Rather than letting hospitals "police themselves," the report suggests that those who license and pay for the care in these hospitals (Medicare and Medicaid) enforce the best practices. In other words, hospitals with high rates of errors receive low reimbursement and face the risk of losing their license to operate. When hospitals report adverse events, licensing organizations review the event, the processes of investigation, and the plan of correction. They may fine or shut down facilities with too many errors. Those organizations working for patient safety are funding and evaluating innovative projects that many hospitals are using to reduce errors and trying to see if these can be used nationwide. With a combination of approaches, it is hoped that the financial and personal costs of health care errors can be reduced.[17] Since the release of the study by the Institute of Medicine, there have been multiple organizations dedicated to developing tools and policies to reduce errors. Most agree that errors are more the result of poor systems than they are of individuals making mistakes, and the goal is to make systems more efficient to prevent errors. Certain practices are associated with high error rates—these include understaffing, staffing with those who are fatigued, complex systems, and systems that rely on individuals checking, especially handwritten systems. Experts ponder questions such as: Should computerized physician notes and orders be required? Should legislation enforce minimum staffing levels? There is also an enhanced focus on error reporting. Individuals may be reluctant to report errors for fear of getting fired, or a lawsuit. However, the systems benefit when errors are reported, investigated, and then fixed. Experts continue to debate about what errors should be reported and to whom, who should have authority to act, and if the reporting of errors should be used against hospitals, nursing homes, or practitioners.

Inaccessible Services

Use of the medical care system in the United States depends on an individual's making a decision to go to a physician, having the energy to travel to the site of care, and having access to transportation.

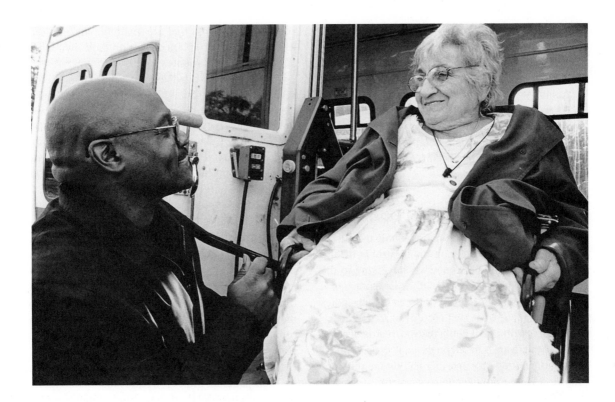

Because of mobility problems and reduced function, it is not easy for people who are very old and sick to get to the physician's office. Many older people no longer drive and must rely on friends and family members to drive them. Some older people cannot use public transportation and cannot walk easily. Further, elders usually have complex diseases that need ongoing assessment, and thus they require regular and sometimes difficult and expensive trips to the physician's office, often accompanied by a caregiver or family member. Even sitting in the physician's waiting room is more than some frail elders can manage. Some do not have the strength to leave home and, as a result, receive either crisis care or no care at all.

Another difficulty with accessibility is that many areas where elders live have few health care services available. Rural areas have fewer primary care and specialist doctors, nursing homes, hospitals, and home health agencies—they often do not have the "volume" to make these services profitable,

and health care professionals often do not live in these areas. Thus elders may have to travel for more than an hour to receive health care.

Lack of Geriatrics Training

Shifting demographics continue to increase the need for physicians with expertise in treating older adults. It is estimated that by 2030 elders will comprise half of many physicians' patient load. The majority of older people are cared for by doctors without special training in the care of older people. Experts warn that the current medical providers will not be adequately prepared because most have little or no specialized training to give optimum care to the older population. Are more geriatric specialists needed or should all primary care physicians be trained in geriatrics? Healthy People 2020 wants to increase the proportion of the health care workforce with geriatric certification by 10 percent. In 2009,

2.7 percent of physicians, 4.3 percent of psychiatrists, 1.4 percent of registered nurses, 0.20 percent of dentists, 0.30 percent of registered dieticians, and 0.6 percent of physical therapists had geriatric certifications (www.healthypeople.gov/2020). In any case, it is agreed that there are far too few physicians educated about the health needs of older persons. Professionals in nursing, social work, pharmacy, and rehabilitation with special training in gerontology will also be in demand.

Lack of Standards of Medical Practice

A vast amount of information is available to patients and health care providers on the treatment of diseases. Thus, it may be somewhat surprising to the layperson to find out how little of medical practice is based on solid evidence from well-conducted studies showing that one treatment is superior to another or that treating a disease is better than no treatment at all. Much of medicine is based on the experience, education, and intuition of a provider and on the relationship between the provider and the patient.

Many laypersons assume that a known standard of care exists and that doctors always agree on diagnosis, prognosis, and optimal treatment. Unfortunately, none of these assumptions is true. Physicians constantly debate the safety, effectiveness, and usefulness of various medical practices in their offices, at conferences, and in medical journals. Physicians' decisions on the methods to treat their patients are influenced by where and when they went to medical school, in what part of the country they trained, their personal and professional experiences, and what they have read recently.

For some diseases, best practices or evidence is available to guide treatment decisions. Unfortunately, for the overwhelming majority of diseases, standards do not exist. The Web site of the Agency for Healthcare Research and Quality provides a list of the diseases for which there are treatment standards, (www.ahrq.gov/clinic/). Various expert groups gather to review the evidence about the effectiveness of many diagnostic tests, medications, and treatments to provide guidance for physicians. Unfortunately, all too often the standards that are available are ignored as health care providers decide on their own what is best for their patients.

The trend toward evidence-based medicine seeks to improve the way in which physicians make treatment choices. *Evidence-based medicine* combines clinical judgment with the outcome of studies that are peer-reviewed, published, well designed, and placebo-controlled. In this way, physicians would be using results from large populations to make treatment decisions for an individual.[18]

The benefits of evidence-based medicine are obvious when the best available evidence is used to guide treatment decisions. However, this science is still developing, and there are many challenges to overcome. First, multiple treatment guidelines are issued by many different groups, and they may be overlapping, contradictory, or confusing. Second, there are not enough good studies in many areas to recommend one treatment over another. Third, some providers feel the evidence-based approach is too "cookbook" and not individualized enough for their patients. Many providers feel their experience is a better tool than all the studies in the world. Fourth, many providers suffer "information overload." Providers are, after all, human and can only assimilate so much information.

The challenge to those who wish to improve health care is to adapt the information from practice-based guidelines and recommendations into an up-to-date format that can be easily used by practitioners. In 1997 the Agency for Healthcare Research and Quality launched an initiative to promote evidence-based practice in everyday medical care through establishment of 12 Evidence-Based Practice Centers. These centers develop evidence reports and technology assessments on topics regarding the organization and delivery of health care that are significant for the Medicare and Medicaid populations. To look for evidence-based clinical guidelines for a specific disease, go to www.guideline.gov Literally hundreds of organizations—universities, professional societies, governmental organizations, and partnerships—are working to develop evidence-based practice guidelines.

Low Health Literacy

The ability to understand and use health information is vital to good health. Health care communication includes conversations with health care profes- sionals, reading information on medication bottles and package inserts, reading forms (patient history, insurance, informed consent), choosing a Medicare health plan, and understanding health education materials and discharge instructions. As important as it is to know how to read in order to learn about personal health care, health literacy goes beyond the ability to read. *Health literacy* is the degree to which individuals have the capacity to seek out, process, and understand basic information and services needed regarding their health.[19] Health literacy includes skills related to numbers (for example, measuring and tracking blood pressure, pulse, or blood sugar measurements, measuring medications, calculating copays or deductibles, comparing prices). Health literacy includes skills related to reading and understanding printed materials (such as reading labels or educational pamphlets and forms), and the ability to understand concepts of risk and probability (for instance, this surgery has a 75 percent success rate with a 2 percent risk of death, 4 percent risk of prolonged hospitalization, and 1 in 5 people has urinary incontinence afterwards). In addition, health literacy is the ability to learn and retain information and to understand complex words.

Health literacy encompasses abilities related to navigating health plans, completing forms, weighing choices, and locating providers and services. Those with poor health literacy skills often do not know much about the body, making it more difficult to understand and retain new information. In addition, health science is always changing; what someone learned a year ago is likely to be outdated. A person with poor health literacy may be unable to accurately complete patient health history forms, ask the right questions about his or her health concerns, understand the professional's instructions on how to get better, and read and understand the labels on prescriptions or the written materials provided at the doctor's office.

When poor health literacy is compounded by multiple chronic illnesses and short office visits, it is easy to understand why patients may not comply with treatment goals. Health literacy is affected by low educational level, language skills, vocabulary, cognitive processing speed, and motivation. Those with cognitive impairment and dementia have lower health literacy.

Health literacy is a particular problem for people who do not speak English well. Often these individuals must rely on family members—often children—to interpret for them. Their problems are compounded by low educational attainment and poor knowledge of the health care system. One study found the use of interpreters at $279 per patient per year had a significant positive effect on the amount of preventive care received, the number of office visits, and the number of prescriptions written and filled.[20]

Low health literacy is often misunderstood as a condition that affects only a specific portion of the population: the less educated and ethnic minorities. In reality, low health literacy can affect everyone regardless of background or educational level. Although ethnic minority groups are disproportionately affected, the majority of those with low literacy skills in the United States are white, native-born Americans.[21]

Poor health literacy is more common among elders than among other adult age groups. Estimates vary based on criteria, but 50 percent to more than 90 percent of older adults likely have some deficiencies in health literacy. The 2003 National Assessment of Adult Literacy, the first of its kind, sampled 19,000 individuals aged 16 and older living in the United States. Each person was given tasks related to health literacy and ranked at four performance levels: below basic, basic, intermediate, and proficient. Almost 15 percent of the entire sample scored below basic proficiency. Older adults had the lowest health literacy of all other age groups surveyed: Almost 30 percent had below basic literacy, and only 3 percent of those surveyed were considered proficient. Adults with higher educational attainment had higher health literacy, as might be expected. Adults with below basic or basic health

Tips for Communicating with Health Professionals

Before you go:

Write a list of questions in order with the most important question first, then if you run out of time, you at least asked the most important ones. If possible, submit your questions in advance through e-mail or fax or tell the nurse when you make your appointment.

While there:

- Bring a friend to the visit to help you remember.
- Bring all your medications in a list or in the actual pill bottles. If you are getting medications from different doctors, make sure you show ALL of them to EACH doctor each time. Enlist the help of the pharmacist to review the medications and help coordinate with the doctors.
- Ask what the diagnosis is.
- Ask specifically what you are being asked to do.
- Ask what the doctor has as a goal for you.
- Ask what the prognosis is—is this a life-threatening condition? Is this an annoyance only?
- If you don't understand something, don't act as if you do. Tell them, "I don't understand."

- Ask for written materials to help you understand, or you can ask the doctor to write down the instructions.
- If there are people in your family or friends that you want to be able to ask the doctor questions about you or to share information, be sure to sign a paper allowing the health practitioner to release information to them.

After your appointment:

- Look up your diagnosis on the Internet to learn more about them (try www.mayoclinic.com, for example). This helps you answer many questions on your own and saves the more difficult and personal issues for the doctor's appointment.
- Ask for and use your health plan or physician's e-mail and Web site.
- Obtain and read your medical records.
- Ask for all doctors who see you to be in contact with each other and receive copies of correspondence.
- Send lab results and test results between doctors yourself.
- Develop a relationship with the nurse.

---

literacy were less likely to get information about health issues from written sources (newspapers, magazines, books, brochures, or the Internet) and more likely to get information about health issues from radio and television. Hispanics had some of the lowest health literacy rates.[22] The health of many elders is at risk because they are not able to understand or act on health information.

The consequences of low health literacy are stark. Poor compliance with instructions leads to complications and subsequent high use of the health care system. It is estimated that these individuals average 6 percent more hospital visits and stay in the hospital an average of two days longer. A recent review of nearly 100 studies on health literacy concluded that low health literacy was consistently associated with more hospitalizations; greater use of emergency care; lower receipt of mammography screening and influenza vaccine; poorer ability to demonstrate taking medications appropriately; poorer ability to interpret labels and health messages; and, among elderly persons, poorer overall health status and higher mortality rates. Poor health literacy partially explains racial disparities in some outcomes. There were few studies about whether math skills were related to outcomes and no evidence for speaking and listening skills.[23]

How do you efficiently identify those with low health literacy quickly? Multiple tools have been developed; the simplest use just a question or two. Questions can be asked about whether elders have someone else read forms for them, how confident they are at filling out medical forms by themselves, and how they would rate their reading ability.[24]

Employing health educators or nurses to reinforce and clarify the physician's communication would be an important step in increasing adherence among older people.

Health care professionals may not realize they are not communicating effectively. Many physicians give too much information and use complicated words, speak too fast, or do not take time to find out if the patient understands their directions. Consent forms, directions on medication bottles, and communication with the physician are often in complex language beyond the average comprehension level of adults. And health professionals generally are not trained in tailoring their communication to their patients. Many do not realize that some patients are not knowledgeable about basic anatomy.

Becoming culturally sensitive, taking time to make sure patients are well informed before they leave the office, and tailoring discussion of health problems and treatment to the individual are important. A major barrier to appropriate communication between physician and patient is the time limit placed on the physician by some clinics and managed care organizations. Considering that the average office visit lasts only approximately 20 minutes (includes examination time), it is easy to understand why communication problems arise.

Health literacy skills will improve as the baby boomers age. People now entering older adulthood have more schooling than previous generations, and health knowledge in general is more sophisticated because of increased exposure in the schools and the popular media. However, an increase in the number of elder immigrants who do not speak English will continue to provide a challenge to health care workers.

The Health Resources and Services Administration has a free online course for professionals on health literacy—search for "Health Literacy Course" at www.hrsa.gov

Doctor-Patient Relationship Issues

The doctor-patient relationship is a central aspect of the provision of health care. Patients do not see themselves as seeking care from a system, but rather from an individual doctor who helps them navigate the complexities of the health care system, provides advice, and serves as an advocate on their behalf. Patients generally wish to have one doctor for their whole life and expect that the doctor maintains copies of records on their medical history (who they are and what has happened to them) and knows and cares for them personally. So, choosing a doctor can be very stressful, and those without a primary doctor they trust often delay care.

The doctor-patient relationship is based on privacy, dignity, trust, and rapport and is a two-way street. The better the relationship in terms of mutual respect, knowledge, trust, time available, shared values, and perspectives about health and disease, the better will be the amount and quality of information about the patient's disease transferred in both directions. This enhances the accuracy of any diagnosis. When their relationship is poor, the physician will not know enough to make a good decision, and the patient will be less likely to follow the recommendations.

The "old-fashioned" physician-patient relationship is one that has been called paternalistic—the physician is considered an "all-knowing" expert whose advice should be followed blindly and absolutely. Most contact occurs in the physician's office; the physician has limited and thus more valuable time; and the physician is the one with the extensive training and title. Many times the physician is called "doctor" while the patient is called by his or her first name, highlighting the differences in status. In addition, because of illness, ignorance, and fear, the patient is in a vulnerable and dependent position. For many elders and minority groups, the degree of respect for the physician is very high. Thus, patients may not share important information with the physician (for example, they may not share the information that they are not doing what was asked).

Newer concepts in the doctor-patient relationship are those of shared care and empowerment.

Plain English

Which of the following diagnoses is easier to understand?

"The cancer in your brain is not primary, but a secondary metastasis, and thus the treatment needs to focus on the primary cancer—breast cancer. We need to do palliative treatments if you develop neurologic symptoms of increased intracranial pressure."

or

"You know the cancer you had in your breast? Well, we thought we got it all when you had your breast removed. Then we did chemotherapy to try to get any cells we might have missed. But it didn't completely work. A small amount of that cancer has spread to your brain and is now growing there. I want us to try the same treatment we used to kill the breast cancer. If you start getting headaches, or you feel like throwing up, or you feel weak and dizzy, then we might have to think of other ways to kill those cells. Maybe we will have to take them out of your brain with an operation."

Plain English, also called plain language, is a way of writing or speaking that is easy to understand the first time an audience reads or hears it. It is *one* important tool for improving health literacy.

Key elements of plain English include:

- Use logical organization, putting the most important information first.
- Use everyday words and short sentences.
- Avoid technical terms and jargon.
- Be direct. Use "you" and other personal pronouns.

Know your audience: Language that is plain to one set of readers may not be plain to others.

The need to speak and write in plain language is so important that it has captured the attention of two presidents. In 1998, President Clinton issued an executive memo requiring agencies to write in plain language. Most recently, President Obama strengthened that intent with a law, the Plain Writing Act of 2010, requiring agencies to write in plain language.

www.plainlanguage.gov is a Web site to improve communication between the federal government and the public.

The physician is viewed as a consultant, one of many sources of medical information. Rapid electronic communication with physicians (such as through e-mail or Web sites), the availability of medical information from the Internet, and even "concierge doctors" kept on retainer for an individual's questions all are examples of this new trend. Although some doctors feel their position is being eroded by this new explosion of information, and others might be intimidated by the proactive medical consumer who may know more than they do about certain topics, most doctors welcome the new involvement of patients with their own health.

Strains in the relationship can occur when there are disagreements between the patient and physician about what should be done, issues of compliance, or issues of dishonesty. Areas that are difficult to talk about, such as sexuality, mental illness, prognosis (how serious is the illness and how long might I live), and end-of-life care, remain challenging and under discussed. The relationship can be developed with more face-to-face time and hindered with a hurried or rushed appearance. The standard 20-minute appointment is often inadequate to be examined and to address complex issues and account for the slowed communication of some elders, especially those of advanced age and low health literacy.

The doctor-patient relationship can be complicated at times of care transitions. Perhaps the elder has had a family doctor for years, but this person retired, and the patient now has to pick someone new in the practice—this is often a great source of stress for the elder. Perhaps the elder delays making the follow-up because of worries and fears about developing a new relationship. Another transition is related to hospitalization. Increasingly the primary doctor is not the one following the care of the elder while in the hospital—a specialist in hospital care (called a *hospitalist*) is doing so. Unfortunately, the hospitalist and primary doctor may not communicate frequently or even share medical records, leaving the patient feeling stranded and perhaps suffering adverse effects because the new doctor doesn't know his or her history. The same thing may occur with a transfer to a rehabilitation or nursing facility as the primary doctor may not provide care there. With the use of specialists, second opinions, and care transitions, it is thought ideal that the primary doctor would be the coordinator of all care, reviewing the various recommendations in light of the "whole person" and his or her care goals, other treatments, and other diagnoses. However, too often the transfer of information between doctors is poor, and elders may end up with duplicate or interacting prescriptions, unnecessary tests, and adverse effects.

Bedside manner is the terminology used to describe the way a doctor interacts with a patient. Good bedside manner makes the patient feel safe, listened to, respected, supported, and comfortable. Bad bedside manner makes the patient feel worried, scared, alone, or misunderstood. Bedside manner doesn't apply just to physicians but to all medical workers. Bedside manner is more than the words that are said; it includes the tone, the body language, and the overall feelings that are shared. One practitioner can tell a patient good news in a way that makes the patient feel bad, while another can impart catastrophic news in a manner that makes the patient feel affirmed, understood, and cared for. Spending time listening to the patient, repeating back what was heard to check for understanding, making eye contact with the patient rather than looking at the computer or chart, and sitting down to give the impression of having "enough time" have all been shown to improve bedside manner.

The Need for Comprehensive Care

A high proportion of physicians in the United States are specialists. Specialist care has many advantages for patients, especially for those with complex or severe illnesses. Older people generally have many coexisting physical conditions that need attention from more than one specialist. Whereas years ago elders may have relied on the family doctor to provide comprehensive medical care, most older people now seek care in a medical system full of "-ologists." Whether they are at home or in a hospital, elders may receive simultaneous care by two or more specialists, each ordering tests and prescribing treatments. Unfortunately when a person sees a number of specialists, it is likely that none of them is responsible for coordinating care.

Another barrier to comprehensive care for older people is a lack of connection between physicians and community resources, and among community resources themselves. Services needed by older people are varied and usually in different locations. Treatment, rehabilitation, prevention, and support services may not be coordinated. Furthermore, medical, health, and social services differ in eligibility requirements, administration, and financing mechanisms. The increase of for-profit medical and health facilities and community-based health agencies may further decrease cooperation because they compete with one another for clients. Finally, there is an insufficient range of health services for elders in many communities.

Obtaining proper care for multiple health problems and coordinating medical services and treatment are formidable tasks at any age, but the problem looms particularly large for older people. Effective use of the current health care system requires mobility, strength, competitiveness, money, and a keen awareness of ways to gain access to splintered services—characteristics not possessed by many frail elders.

Medicare managed care (also known as Medicare Advantage) has been proposed to solve the lack of coordination. With managed care, one primary care provider is responsible for the patient's medical care and must approve all specialist care. In theory, managed care promotes improved communication among the various health professionals caring for the patient. But there is no evidence that coordination is occurring.

The interdisciplinary team approach is an excellent way to ensure comprehensive care,

Team Approach to Geriatric Care

Even in locations where teams are common, teams do not function as well as they should. Teamwork takes specialized training, which is usually not part of medical training. Teamwork takes time, which is precious. Further, teams are expensive, taking practitioners away from other activities for which they could be reimbursed. Health insurance reimbursement for team meetings to plan a comprehensive plan of care is inadequate. Medicare is increasingly recognizing the importance of the team approach and is expanding reimbursement.

The use of case management services is another way to address the lack of coordination of medical and community-based services. Case managers coordinate care for elders. Case management may be provided by nurses or social workers. They may be employed by hospitals, clinics, home health agencies, HMOs, or physicians' offices. Private or nonprofit groups also offer case management services, or individuals may work on their own. Family members often serve informally as case managers. Case managers make telephone calls, maintain open communication among the patient, the family and the health care team, make sure that benefits and health insurance are in place, identify and arrange needed services (e.g., day care, nutritional programs, pharmacy), and tackle other coordinating tasks as they arise. Some managers may accompany patients to their medical appointments to ensure the patient understands the information and their questions are adequately answered.

Some case managers may play a role only when an individual is discharged to home (discharge planners in hospitals). Others have an ongoing relationship to coordinate comprehensive care of the elder to prevent the need for a nursing home. Ideally, the case manager is an advocate for the interests of the patient, but this is not always the case. Often case managers serve the interests of the organization in which they are employed and may even "ration" services.

---

especially for older people. Interdisciplinary teams are groups of two or more specialists who work together with the patient, family, and community to maximize the services for the patient. Interdisciplinary teams may include physicians, nurses, social workers, chaplains, dietitians, therapists, pharmacists, and other health care professionals. Each member contributes specialized knowledge and skills to develop a plan to meet the varying needs of the patient. The team approach is commonly used in the hospital and in home care or hospice services but is seldom seen elsewhere. Even though comprehensive medical care under one roof is uncommon, medical and allied health and social service personnel can integrate care by providing appropriate linkages to other services.

As a group, elders are somewhat less educated about health, disease, and their bodies, and they are more likely to adopt a submissive role when talking to a physician. Further, not all elders are able to act on their own behalf, especially if weakened by illness.

Patient advocates assist elders in making important health care decisions and help them to negotiate the complex medical care system. Advocates may be social workers, nurses, or trained laypersons, but most are members of a patient's family. An important role of an advocate is to accompany a patient to the medical appointment and ensure that the patient understands the information presented and asks any questions he or she may have. The main disadvantage of advocates is that their presence can interfere with the doctor-patient relationship. Members of the health care team may address their questions to the advocate, not to the patient. Advocates need to be certain not to assume an antagonistic posture toward physicians and to separate their own ideas of "what is in the best interest of the patient" from the patient's actual wishes. Elders may be less likely to bring up sensitive issues such as sexuality, death, or mental illness when an advocate is present. Because of cultural differences, the relationship that elders may desire and expect with their doctors might be different from the relationship that younger people would prefer (e.g., relying more on the doctor for decision making). Advocates need to respect the elder's wishes. Family members in particular need to separate their own agenda from that of the patient. The National Institute on Aging recently revised *Working with Your Older Patient: A Clinician's Handbook* to assist medical professionals working with older people. The free handbook is available online, and a hard copy can be ordered from www.nia.nih.gov/HealthInformation/Publications/ClinicianHB/

ADVANCES IN MEDICAL CARE

What can be done to improve medical care for older people and for everyone else? Improvements are possible at many levels. Where should the efforts begin? With the providers of care? With insurance companies? With the government or private entities? With individuals themselves? Should improvement of care be focused on prevention of illness, management of disease for the chronically ill, better end-of-life care, or improved intensive care? Should we provide more care at home and less in the hospital? What is the role of technology in improving health care? The answers to these questions will lead us to the future of health care—a future in which you will play a role. In this section we review several diverse strategies to improve the quality and efficiency of health care.

Reducing Hospital Readmissions

There is increasing concern that people are being discharged from the hospital too sick and without adequate resources to maintain health, prompting readmission into a hospital. It is clear that hospital stays have reduced in length from a decade ago, and there is an increasing push to reduce hospitalization duration in order to decrease costs. This trend not only saves money, but often saves lives—hospitals can be dangerous places for elders. Separated from

their families, homes, and routines, and sometimes kept in restraints, elders may become confused, delirious, or lose the will to live. In addition, hospitals are breeding grounds of multiple-drug-resistant infections, and they have a high rate of errors and adverse events.

Nearly one in five Medicare patients discharged from the hospital is readmitted in 30 days. The highest rates of readmissions are among those with heart failure, lung disease, psychosis, or intestinal problems and those who have had surgery (heart surgery, joint replacement, or surgery to lose weight). Those on six or more medications, those who have depression or poor cognitive function, racial minorities, those without private insurance, and those who have had another hospitalization in the previous six months are also at a higher risk. In addition when discharges occur on weekends or holidays, the risk of readmission is higher.

Hospital readmissions may occur because many "sicknesses" cannot fully be cured, or they lead to other illnesses. Some readmissions are not preventable. However, experts estimate that nearly 10 percent are preventable. There are a number of factors that prompt readmission—perhaps the patient was not able to get a follow-up appointment; lab results were not checked prior to discharge and so a problem wasn't identified; the patient was not able to get his or her prescriptions, or there was confusion about medications. Elders may be tired, confused, and unable to really understand information provided to them as they leave the hospital. Staff may be hurried and so might skip extensive education and simply provide computer-generated, generic patient information sheets for the elder to read. Discharge instructions may be unclear or conflicting with the elder's normal routine. The hospital staff often doesn't fully understand the elder's home situation, transportation needs, and level of health literacy. There can be poor communication with the primary doctor, who is supposed to resume care without an understanding of what happened in the hospital.

Another reason for hospital readmission is that the patient is declining and perhaps is in the last months of his or her life. In these cases, elders are discharged while they are still very weak and instead of recovering, they continue to decline and come back to the hospital again and again. When this type of readmission pattern is recognized and addressed with the patient and family, many times the patient and family make a choice to reduce the intensity of care and to seek services such as hospice care (discussed in Chapter 15).

Elders need to be informed about the medications they need to take upon leaving the hospital. Otherwise, they may end up back in the hospital. In the hospital setting, elders are placed on a lot of new medications, many times without their knowledge. These may be tapered, ended, discontinued, or continued after hospitalization, and they may overlap with or conflict with the medications the patient normally takes or may not be covered by their insurance. Sorting through the medications can be difficult. It is important to address questions like: What are you taking now and why? What should you be taking? Do you have them? Do you know how to take them? Are they covered by your insurance? If not, can you afford them? Are you planning to take them? Although hospitals are required to do a process of "medication reconciliation" at discharge, this is often done poorly or in a hurry and can be confusing to elders.

Interventions to address and improve hospital readmissions include the following:

1. Develop a discharge plan with clear plans tailored to the needs of patients and their families, clinicians, case managers, and payers.
2. Discuss advance directives and prognosis with each patient not only at the beginning of hospitalization, but at the end—many elders, if asked, wish to make a choice to stay out of the hospital, but they are never given the information to make this decision.
3. Improve coordination with the primary care doctor by completing and faxing summaries of the hospitalization and medications, and helping the elder make appointments and travel arrangements prior to discharge.
4. Develop a medication reconciliation plan that includes all prescription and over-the-counter medications used at home and those used in

the hospital, what each medicine is used for and dosages and how to take them, and what medications need to be discontinued or changed.

House Calls

It is difficult for some older people to get to the doctor's office or clinic for a variety of reasons. The alternative, bringing medical services to an older person's home, is a good solution. This can be accomplished through house calls when the practitioner travels to the elder's home to observe, educate, examine, and prescribe, or through electronic means when the health care worker and elder can communicate remotely. Although house calls are expensive in terms of gas, travel time, and a low reimbursement rate, these visits can be incredibly valuable. When you actually see where and how someone lives, you can better understand the elder and his or her needs, and assess which interventions will work and which will not. Recognizing the value of the home visit, Medicare and Medicaid do reimburse it, but the rate is insufficient to cover the real costs of this type of care. Home visits can be accomplished by physicians, nurses, dieticians, or health care technicians.

Advances in technology allow physicians to take their tools into a patient's home. Spirometers to measure lung function are the size of a laptop, and electrocardiographs, blood glucose monitors, and even X-ray machines are portable. In addition, electronic tools such as smartphone applications, video conferencing, digital photography, video, fax, e-mail, and texting can facilitate rapid transfer of information remotely, allowing the practitioner to diagnose, educate, and treat in her office while the patient never has to leave the comfort of his home!

One model to extend primary care for frail elders into their homes is called the Medical House Call Program.[25] It facilitates the connection between the home and hospital, provides support for family members or frail elders, and provides the health and social services needed in the community.

The Home Visit: One Physician's View

Rebecca Ferrini, MD

Mrs. Garcia was a 98-year-old Spanish-speaking woman who had been relatively healthy and active until about a month ago when she had a stroke. After the stroke, she was unable to walk or even get out of bed, her appetite lessened, and she spent more time asleep. About three weeks later, she suffered another stroke and completely lost the ability to speak. Her family physician agreed with the family's desire to keep her home and comfortable and referred her to hospice services. While with hospice, she received visits a few times a week from a nurse, and a social worker assisted the family in coping and provided referrals for low-cost burial. A home health aide assisted her granddaughter with bathing her and taught her to move and turn her in bed to prevent bedsores. However, one morning Mrs. Garcia became completely unable to swallow, and the granddaughter could no longer give her medications to her.

The nurse noted Mrs. Garcia was restless and moaning.

Mrs. Garcia had expressed a wish to never go back to the hospital and was unable to get to my office, so a house call was arranged later that morning. I drove to her tiny apartment, which was in a very poor neighborhood with bars on the windows and doors. I was led into a dim house, overflowing with belongings but scrupulously clean. Mrs. Garcia, a tiny lady of not more than 70 pounds, lay curled in a hospital bed in the living room, surrounded by medications, diapers, and religious artifacts. I was shown multiple medications and was able to tell her which were useful and which should be discarded. The granddaughter took careful notes. I gave Mrs. Garcia a small amount of morphine under her tongue, and she seemed to relax. In a 15-minute visit, I learned more about Mrs. Garcia and her family than I knew about patients for whom I had cared for years. Mrs. Garcia died peacefully about two days later in her home—comfortable and surrounded by those she loved.

Medicare Demonstration Projects

The Centers for Medicare and Medicaid Services (CMS) work with private and governmental organizations to test possible improvements in Medicare coverage, costs, and quality of care. These projects are usually geared to individuals with a specific disease (e.g., lung disease, end-stage renal disease, complicated diabetes, or heart failure). Special benefits (such as prescription drugs, case management/care coordination, home visits, different technologies) are offered in exchange for enrolling. Many of these programs have grown from pilot studies into full-fledged programs that are an integral part of the Medicare benefit; others have been less successful or less widely disseminated. Those interested can read about current programs at www.cms.gov and search for "demonstration projects."

Disease Management Programs

Medicare statistics reveal that care for people with chronic lung diseases, diabetes, and heart failure is very expensive. These individuals use a lot of medications, see the physician frequently, commonly suffer complications, and require high-cost hospital stays. It has been suggested that better management of these diseases in the community setting would reduce disease complications, lower hospitalization rates, and consequently reduce costs. Several disease management programs have been initiated across the country, many of them as Medicare demonstration projects.

The patient and caregivers are educated about the disease, are taught to monitor the disease with various instruments, and are given help in managing the disease. For instance, patients with lung disease have portable spirometers to evaluate their

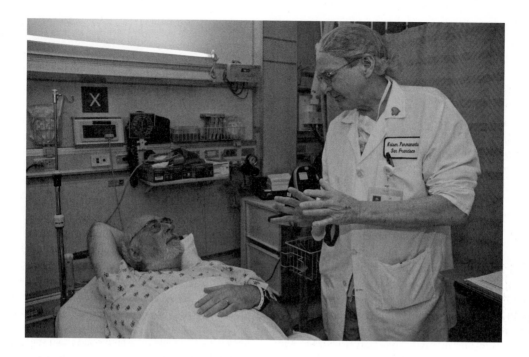

lung function, those with diabetes can measure their blood sugar, and those with heart disease can monitor their weight and symptoms. The patients are also regularly tracked and monitored. These programs are appealing: They use patient advocates, health educators, and home visits to teach patients about their illnesses and how to monitor them. They may use technology, such as a glucose monitor that sends the glucose measurements directly to a physician's office, or Internet-based interventions. They often include education of medical professionals to ensure they are providing uniform and high-quality care to these patients. The hope is that people can learn about their own illness, prevent adverse events, and discern when to seek the care of a doctor or go to the hospital.

Disease management programs improve health outcomes, but they don't seem to save as much money as was hoped. The diabetes disease management program is a good example. An analysis of several published studies revealed that the program improved blood sugar control in diabetics, reduced diabetic complications, improved the care that patients received, and reduced death rates.[26]

The program was well liked and improved enrollees' quality of life but was expensive. It was hoped that the costs of such programs would be offset by their benefits. For example, if the program reduced hospitalization, the result would be a cost savings. So far, these programs have been shown to reduce illness, but there is not enough evidence to conclude that they save health care dollars.

Patient-Centered Medical Home

In the "good old days," the family doctor took care of individuals and families from "cradle to grave." The doctor could be called at all hours and would come to the person's home to provide medical care and comfort. Fast forward to today when the medical care options are dizzying: One person sees many specialists; it is common to change doctors when insurance policies change; one household may see several different doctors, and none of them makes house calls. Even the most savvy customer can have difficulty navigating the system. To address this difficulty, a concept called "medical home" or "patient-centered medical home" has been developed.

The concept is based on the ideal that every person should have a place to go when he or she is ill or in need of health care services: a place that is relevant, coordinated, accessible, and focused on the whole person, and that includes a focus on prevention as well as treatment of illnesses. This place (whether real or partially virtual) is considered the medical home. Under this concept, the primary care physician becomes the hub of the home, with doctors taking responsibility for patients and their families and coordinating their care. This includes maintaining electronic personal health records as well as being accessible in person, through e-mail, or over the phone on short notice, even in the evenings or on weekends if necessary. The concept asserts that physicians should plan and conduct regular appointments to perform checkups and advise their patients on new health information, preventive care measures, and healthy lifestyle decisions based on their genetic and environmental risk factors. If specialist care should be needed, the primary care physician should coordinate it, approving relevant, necessary, and efficient procedures in the patient's best interest and according to his or her care goals.

In 2007, the American Academy of Family Physicians, the American Academy of Pediatrics, the American College of Physicians, and the American Osteopathic Association released the Joint Principles of the Patient-Centered Medical Home (see www.acponline.org). The principles listed were:

- **Personal physician:** "Each patient has an ongoing relationship with a personal physician trained to provide first contact, continuous and comprehensive care."
- **Physician-directed medical practice:** "The personal physician leads a team of individuals at the practice level who collectively take responsibility for the ongoing care of patients."
- **Whole person orientation:** "The personal physician is responsible for providing for all the patient's health care needs or taking responsibility for appropriately arranging care with other qualified professionals."

- **Care is coordinated and/or integrated,** for example, across specialists, hospitals, home health agencies, and nursing homes.
- **Quality and safety** are assured by a care planning process, evidence-based medicine, clinical decision-support tools, performance measurement, active participation of patients in decision making, information technology, a voluntary recognition process, quality improvement activities, and other measures.
- **Enhanced access to care** is available (e.g., via "open scheduling, expanded hours, and new options for communication").
- **Payment** must "appropriately recognize the added value provided to patients who have a patient-centered medical home." For instance, payment should reflect the value of "work that falls outside of the face-to-face visit," should "support adoption and use of health information technology for quality improvement," and should "recognize case mix differences in the patient population being treated within the practice."

Here is how patient-centered medical home might look:

Mildred and her husband Bob know Dr. Smith is there for them. They have a phone number for Dr. Smith on the refrigerator and they know they can call with any concern. They can call the office day or night and get a receptionist who can direct them to their next step. Dr. Smith knows Mildred has diabetes and heart failure, and if she misses an appointment, she is called and another one is set up. If she misses that, a nurse comes to her home to do a checkup. A dietician works closely with Dr. Smith and sees Mildred monthly to go over her weight and diet. Mildred and Bob need appointments together and their daughter has to drive them, but luckily Dr. Smith has appointments available on Wednesday evenings and Saturday morning. When Bob went to the oncologist to discuss options regarding his recently discovered prostate cancer, Dr. Smith made sure to call the oncologist before and after the visit to provide Bob's background and get a summary of the visit, so that he was ready to explain the options to Bob at his next appointment. Both Mildred and Bob are called every year to get flu shots at the office, and Mildred is reminded every two years about her mammogram. If she forgets to get one, she is reminded again until she either goes or makes a decision to refuse it. Dr. Smith has discussed emergency medical plans with Mildred and Bob, and a social worker has helped them make advance directives and fill out the correct forms so that their daughter can make decisions for them if they cannot.

Ambulatory Surgical Centers

Ambulatory surgical centers are mainly operating room facilities to which patients are referred by their physicians. Generally surgical patients stay in the facility for no more than 24 hours. More people are choosing ambulatory surgical centers over hospitals for a wide variety of procedures: cataract surgery, cosmetic procedures, colonoscopies, dental surgery, orthopedic surgery, to name a few. Some centers offer only one type of procedure, such as laser eye surgery; others offer many types of procedures. In 2006, almost 15 million surgeries were conducted at freestanding ambulatory surgery centers and almost 20 million occurred in hospitals. The top two procedures were colonoscopies and cataract surgery. Between 1996 and 2006, the number of surgeries conducted at ambulatory surgical centers increased three-fold while the number in hospitals remained steady. The big advantage of the ambulatory surgery center is that it significantly reduces time in preparation, surgery, and recovery.[27] The vast majority of ambulatory surgical centers are licensed both by the state and the Joint Commission on Accreditation of Hospitals, and the majority accept Medicare reimbursement.

Patients who elect to have surgery at an ambulatory center arrive shortly before they undergo the necessary procedure and go home soon after. The complex hospital admission procedure is absent at the center. Patients and providers both like ambulatory surgical centers. They are modern and clean and often have patient-friendly features such as on-time scheduling, improved customer service, and family-friendly waiting areas. They are often run by the physicians who work there, so the doctors have more control.

Ambulatory surgical centers tend to operate in urban areas, offering more choice to urban populations. These centers are rarely available in rural areas, where doctors are relatively scarce. The centers need to be close to a major hospital for emergency care, in case there are serious complications. Because they tend to focus on lower-risk patients, they have high success rates. They are generally (though not always) less expensive than hospital care.

Innovative Use of Personnel

One way to save money in the delivery of health care is to match the level of personnel skill to the level of care to ensure that professional time is used efficiently. For instance, instead of relying on physicians to see patients, diagnose illnesses, and prescribe treatment, other medical professionals who are less expensive are employed. Mid-level practitioners include nurse practitioners, nurse midwives, nurse anesthetists, clinical nurse specialists with special training in a particular area (such as cancer), and physician assistants. States have varying requirements for mid-level practitioners, but most permit them in some form. Many large HMOs or nursing homes are using mid-level practitioners to provide care. These individuals are less expensive, they may be able to spend more time with the patient, and often they become experts in one or more areas of practice. Further, they can handle most common ailments and may be preferred over physicians by patients for many health needs (e.g., physical exams, urgent care visits, women's health exams). Another benefit is that mid-level practitioners enable physicians to perform more complex tasks. A disadvantage is that these professionals are less trained than physicians and may miss some important findings.

Another new trend in the United States is to use *hospitalists*—physician specialists who work only in the hospital. Traditionally, when people goes to the hospital, they are cared for by their primary care physician. In some hospitals, they are cared for by a hospitalist. Hospitalists are hired by the hospital or may work in a group practice and take care of patients only while they are in the hospital. An advantage of hospitalists is that they know the hospital systems well, they are at the hospital all day so they can respond readily to emergencies, and they can stay current on the latest developments in efficient and high-quality care. A disadvantage is that they often do not know the patient as well as the primary care physician does: It may be stressful to the patient to have to meet a new face during the stress of hospitalization.

Patient Privacy

Over the past decade, concern about the privacy of health information has been increasing. Some fear that personal health information will be released to employers or insurance carriers and result in discrimination. Others are concerned about losing their insurance when they switch jobs. These concerns resulted in a federal law—the Health Insurance Portability and Accountability Act of 1996 (HIPAA)—that has had a far-ranging impact on medical care for both the provider and the patient.

This federal law raises standards for the privacy of personal health information by requiring standards to be developed for security and privacy for billing, eligibility, payment and benefit coordination claims, and all health information systems. This increased security is designed to keep health information safe from unauthorized uses and to ensure that people who receive such information receive only what they need to know and no more. The law also sets high standards for privacy regarding the release of medical information. Signed waivers are required before personal health information can be released to anyone—including the patient's family, friends, or insurance companies. The law also requires health insurance to be more portable. Provisions of the law enable individuals who lose their jobs to keep their health insurance while looking for work if they pay a monthly premium.

Electronic Medical Records

Patients may believe that there is a unified, comprehensive medical record that follows them from physician to physician, to the hospital and back, and includes all their diagnoses and treatments and test results. Providers know the truth: There is no such document. In its place is a haphazard collection of data: handwritten and often cryptic notes, incomplete lists of medications, missing lab reports, and few notes from past or concurrent providers of care. Physicians often lack the information they need to make decisions. When they refer a patient to a specialist, they may never see the results of the tests and examinations from the specialists. Doctors in nursing homes rarely see hospital records, and doctors in the hospital too often have little information about what the primary care provider has been doing. The lack of coordination can cost billions of dollars in lost productivity (hunting down the results) and redoing tests, and it can result in errors and misdiagnosis. In the worst case, failure to provide accurate information to physicians who need it can result in worsened health or even death.

In response to these concerns, in 2004, President George W. Bush requested that a comprehensive and unified electronic medical record for each patient be developed and implemented. This record would allow laboratories, hospitals, X-ray companies, pharmacies, patients, physicians, and nursing homes to input and access information. Creating these records is an enormous task. The U.S. Department of Health and Human Services is coordinating the effort with public and private agencies to develop a common language and framework. The Institute of Medicine is developing a free prototype record to be shared among all health care providers. The government offers financial incentives and penalties in order to encourage health care institutions to develop and implement a system of electronic records. Problems are arising, however, in regard to security and confidentiality, imperfectly designed systems, and educating workers on how to use the new system, leading to low rates of successful implementation, very high costs, and inability to share data across health care systems. There is still no universal template for health care facilities to use, but there are many ongoing initiatives.

Cybermedicine

Cybermedicine is a new medical practice where patients and physicians communicate through electronic mail.

Telemedicine is the use of technology—phone call, fax, e-mail, or audio-video links—to connect health care practitioners with patients or with other health personnel who are in different locations. Telemedicine allows a rural doctor to contact a specialist at a university-based medical center to discuss the treatment of an unusual cancer or even to send photos of a skin condition. Telemedicine allows patients and their doctors to communicate readily. Telemedicine is cost-efficient in rural areas because it reduces the cost of time and fuel. It also improves patient access to specialists and increases communication among health care professionals. To improve access to specialists in rural areas and to reduce transportation costs, at least 18 states currently permit Medicaid reimbursement for telemedicine services. Telemedicine can be used in intensive care units, in rural areas, or at night. One physician can actually monitor care in multiple remote ICU settings with video cameras. Telemedicine is increasingly reimbursed through insurance plans, the connections are generally secure, and there are a limited number of users involved. The American Telemedicine Association (www.atmeda.org) can provide more information.

Cybermedicine is an exciting and rapidly changing field where the technology of the Internet is used to enhance health care. It is global, anonymous, free-form, and less secure than telemedicine. It includes consumer education on diseases and disorders and support for those with certain conditions. Cybermedicine can include Web-based personal health records so patients can access their records, physician notes, and test results over the Internet. This can be through a primary care system (e.g., Kaiser has such an interface) or can even be anonymous. Cybermedicine includes the vast quantity of

health information on the Web today—you can get personalized advice, enter your symptoms and get a list of what it might be, order tests on your own, blog with a community of thousands who have your same condition, and find scientific and not-so-scientific information all for free and in the privacy of your own home.

It is not only patients but also doctors who are increasingly embracing the Web both seek information, to ask questions in online communities of physicians, and to communicate with patients. The Web, of course, is filled with good and bad information, and the consumer must be aware of which is which.

Cybermedicine is entering new frontiers. Smart devices can send GPS information to others (e.g., tracking) and may even be able to detect falls (when the person doesn't move from one position or there is a change in altitude). Microchips in devices or within the body can track health-related indices and transmit information about blood chemistry or sugar or weight directly to a health care provider to review. Applications for smartphones are increasingly focusing on health, providing another source of information and assistance. Cybermedicine is changing quickly, and there will always be something new to learn.

National Health Care Reform

In 2010, Congress passed the Affordable Care Act, a health care reform package designed to address issues of costs, health insurance availability, and quality. This bill was introduced to address the escalating costs of health insurance, the growing number of those without insurance—by choice or because of the costs of preexisting conditions. A key component is all Americans are required to purchase health insurance or pay a tax that would defray the costs of their illness if they had an emergency and went to the hospital without insurance. Medicaid, the program for the poor was expanded to cover individuals who make up to 133% of the poverty level. Insurance companies are required to standardize benefits packages, offer mental health insurance and provide insurance to everyone, even those with pre-existing conditions. Health insurance companies are not permitted to spend more than 20% on administrative costs. Elder health care may be affected because of the reduced reimbursement for Medicare Advantage plans, which were more profitable than expected. Equalizing payments for mental health and physical health services, promoting increased payments to primary care practitioners, and assuring coverage for preventive services are also provisions impacting the health of elders. The bill was controversial and was implemented step-wise with various components starting earlier and others not beginning until years later. It is being challenged politically in Congress as well as in the courts.

The Future of Health Care

The future of health care is uncertain in the United States—Medicare and Medicaid are extraordinarily costly entitlement programs, with costs increasing as the baby boomers retire and move into their later years. With a large federal budget deficit and worldwide economic woes in developing countries, it is almost certain there will be more changes in federal entitlement programs. What will change depends on the political process. Universal health care programs (for example, the United States National Health Care Act, formerly called the "Medicare for All" Act), pending in Congress, have predicted cost savings associated with elimination of insurance company overhead costs and universal preventive care. Although universal health care is generally provided in most developed countries, it seems unlikely to pass in the United States.

The future will likely bring more initiatives to link payment to quality and need. So, for example, doctors will be paid more if they work in places that are rural, underserved, and need doctors more. Medical specialists may be paid less while primary care doctors will get more. Doctors who order fewer treatments and save money may get rewarded with higher pay. Hospitals will be paid less if they have high rates of errors or hospital readmissions and will be paid more if they score high on quality measures (for example, low surgical complication rates). Doctors or hospitals who adopt evidence-based practices, encourage their patients to get flu shots or mammograms, whose patients have low rates of diabetic complications, and whose patients are at normal weight may received extra payment as an incentive.

A new concept in care coordination, called "bundling," has the potential to radically change the way that physicians and health care facilities are paid through Medicare and Medicaid. Currently both are paid "fee for service"—they are reimbursed for services provided. The current system, for example, pays more for and therefore encourages medical interventions such as surgeries and prescribed medicines (all of which carry some risk for the patient but increase revenues for the medical care industry). In fact, those hospitals with higher readmission rates actually get paid more as they can bill the second time or third time the patient returns, while those with lower admission rates might have empty beds because their patients are at home and are healthy! In addition, the current reimbursement mechanism does not pay for activities that are more time consuming like smoking cessation, dietary, and exercise counseling. Bundling means that local doctors and hospitals will not be paid on a fee-for-service basis, but will share a pool of money based on the outcome for the patient with those groups that can deliver the best outcome being paid more. Currently there are demonstration projects looking at how this might work in the "real world."

Complementary and Alternative Medicine

The type of medicine conventionally practiced in the United States is *allopathic* medicine. Allopathic medicine—more commonly known as "conventional medicine"—divides the body into different systems (respiratory, digestive, etc.), studies the biology of these systems and health conditions associated with each system, and relies on the scientific method to test hypotheses using repeated experiments and observations. Because most of us grew up with this type of medicine, we think that it is the only way to treat illness. However, there are many other approaches to healing—some of them thousands of years old, others relatively new.

Complementary and alternative medicine (CAM) is a group of medical, health care, and healing systems other than those included in mainstream health care in the United States. Whereas *complementary* medicine is used *with* conventional medicine, *alternative* medicine is used *in place of* conventional medicine.

Throughout the world, innumerable strategies to treat illness, reduce pain and suffering, and restore health have coexisted for centuries. Scientific evidence is mounting that some of these alternative or complementary medicines are effective. Many alternative healing strategies are becoming more accepted by the public and the medical community. The National Center for Complementary and Alternative Medicine (NCCAM) is the lead agency of the federal government engaging in scientific research on complementary and alternative medicine. The center conducts scientific studies regarding complementary and alternative healing practices, trains CAM researchers, and informs the public and health professionals about the study results.

The NCCAM divides complementary medicine into five categories: (1) whole medical systems (Chinese medicine, ayurveda, homeopathy, native healing practices, naturopathy), (2) manipulative and body-based practices (chiropractic, osteopathy, massage), (3) biologically based practices (dietary supplements, herbal products), (4) mind-body medicine (biofeedback, imagery, meditation, prayer, yoga), and (5) energy medicine (Qui Gong, Reiki, therapeutic touch). An in-depth description and analysis of each of these complementary medicine practices is beyond the scope of this book. For such information, refer to the NCCAM Web site (www.nccam.nih.gov). The book *Complementary and Alternative Medicine in the United States,* by the Board on Health Promotion and Disease Prevention (National Academies Press), is another excellent source and can be read online at www.nap.edu

Results from the 2007 National Health Interview Survey of American adults and children revealed that almost 40 percent of adults surveyed had used at least one form of complementary or alternative medicine in the past 12 months. According to the survey, those who use CAM tend to be highly educated, well-off, with many health conditions and many visits to the doctor. American Indians or Alaska natives were the most likely to use CAM (50 percent of the sample); rates for whites were almost as high (43 percent); and Hispanic adults were the least likely to use CAM (24 percent). Common CAM therapies were natural products like omega-3 oil, glucosamine, and echinacea (37 percent), deep breathing exercises (13 percent), meditation (9 percent), chiropractic or osteopathic care (9 percent), massage (8 percent), and yoga (6 percent). Adults were found to be most likely to use CAM therapy for a variety of musculoskeletal problems, particularly back pain (17 percent). The second highest use was for head and chest colds (9 percent).[28]

A national sample of almost 1,500 older people reported that 88 percent of the respondents aged 65 and older used some form of complementary and alternative medicine. Most commonly used were dietary supplements (65 percent) and chiropractic services (43 percent). In general, older women were higher users than older men, and blacks and Hispanics used fewer supplements and less chiropractic but reported more personal practices (deep breathing, meditation) than whites.[29] Unfortunately, many individuals using a form of CAM therapy are not likely to tell their physicians, or pharmacists, and not much is known about interactions between CAM and other therapies, about adverse effects, or even about how they work.

Even if no scientific benefits are reproducible in randomized controlled trials, CAM therapies may be beneficial. The time and attention spent with a practitioner of alternative medicine may have positive effects on health and sense of well-being. Often these practitioners focus on the whole body and encourage alteration of diet, increased exercise, and stress reduction. Alternative medicine practitioners may spend more time with their patients and empower them to improve their health. Through a gentler focus on healing the self, many, but not all, alternative healing strategies are far less toxic and invasive than conventional drugs or surgery. In addition, alternative medical treatments generally cost less than conventional medical treatments. Even if they do no good, at least they usually do no harm. Probably the most harmful consequence of CAM therapies is when they are used instead of known effective treatments. Further, some practices also waste money that could be better spent elsewhere.

Increasingly, the lines between conventional and alternative medicine are becoming blurred. Due to consumer advocacy and the demonstrated efficiency of some CAM therapies, many health insurance companies now offer coverage for some CAM therapies. At present, Medicare covers only chiropractic and osteopathic services. In addition, some medical schools have developed courses on the subject. As research supports some alternative medicine practices, they are being integrated into conventional medicine. Ideally, medicine would become truly integrative, encompassing the best of all worlds with an emphasis on personalized care, empowering patients to heal themselves, diet and exercise, and other behavioral changes and evidence-based interventions when needed.

Summary

B ecause of their higher rates of chronic illness, elders utilize physician and hospital services more than any other age group. A large proportion of the medical expenses of those over age 65 in the United States is financed through Medicare—a complex federal program with deductibles, copayments, and monthly premiums, Parts A, B, C, and D, and dizzying choices for elders. Private Medigap insurance is available for elders to reduce their out-of-pocket costs not covered by Medicare. The nation's poorest elders may qualify for Medicaid, the federal/state program that supplements what Medicare does not reimburse. The Veterans Administration provides health services to elders who have been in the armed forces, and the Indian Health Service offers medical care to American Indian elders.

The medical care system of the United States is technologically advanced, offering highly skilled medical practitioners and a myriad of diagnostic tests, drugs, surgical treatments, modern equipment, and facilities unparalleled elsewhere in the world. Nevertheless, our health care system is not working for everyone. There are multiple barriers to providing and coordinating health care services for elders. The high cost of medical care, inequities in treatment, medical errors, and lack of coordination of care are just a few of the factors that are discussed that reduce the quality of care for older people. The medical system is constantly evolving to improve the quality and efficiency of health care by such means as electronic medical records, improved safety initiatives, Medicare demonstration projects, improved use of technology, and complementary and alternative medicine, and more.

Activities

1. Read the portion of the *Medicare and You* booklet at www.medicare.gov that describes the Original Medicare Plan and the Medicare Advantage Plan. If you just turned 65, which plan would you sign up for and why? What factors might make you change your plan?

2. Informally survey several physicians in your community by telephone to determine if they accept Medicare and Medicaid patients. What percentage accepts each? Do those who accept Medicare or Medicaid set a limit on how many patients they will take?

3. Debate the pros and cons of the statement "Medical care is the right of all individuals in the United States, regardless of ability to pay."

4. Find out whether your community offers the following health services to elders: free or reduced-rate medical care, mass screening

programs, health promotion programs, medical outreach into elders' homes or neighborhood sites, and transportation to medical care.

5. Many hospitals reach out to serve the special needs of elders. Find out what special services are offered to elders by the hospitals in your community. Find out whether your community has an ambulatory surgery center. If it does, call or visit one to find out what services it offers.

6. Participate in a class discussion in which you share your views of how the health care system might be improved without increasing the cost of health care.

7. Research current legislation pending in your state regarding medical care. What problem is being addressed? Which constituents are actively influencing the debate and in which manner? Write a letter to your representative outlining the reasons why you believe the proposal should or should not be passed.

8. Collect advertisements and articles on particular alternative healing techniques from both lay sources (e.g., magazines, health food stores) and medical literature. What claims are made?

9. Contact a seller of Medigap insurance and listen to the presentation on policies for either yourself or an elderly friend or relative. What are the pros and cons? What did you like about the presentation? What questions do you still have? Do you understand what is being offered and the price? Would you purchase any of those policies?

10. Using the Web site of the National Center for Complementary and Alternative Medicine (www.nccam.nih.gov), research one complementary therapy. Then go to www.pubmed.gov to find the most recent research on that therapy. Write a brief report.

11. Look in your local phone book to see what types of complementary and alternative therapies are available in your community. Choose one practitioner to interview and write up your results. What did you learn about the therapy? Did your interview change your opinion about the therapy? Would you consider getting such therapy? Why or why not? What might be the special risks and benefits of this treatment for the elderly?

12. Gather information about a Medicare demonstration project and summarize it. When did the project begin? What geographical areas are involved? What are the expected outcomes, and what has been observed so far? How is the project funded?

13. Find a cybermedicine site on the Web, and report on how it works, how much it costs to use, and what services are offered.

BIBLIOGRAPHY

1. Administration on Aging. 2011. *A profile of older Americans: 2010.* Washington, DC: Administration on Aging. Department of Health and Human Services.

2. Institute of Medicine. 2004. *Health literacy: A prescription to end confusion.* Washington, DC: National Academies Press.

3. Biles, B., Dallek, G., and Nicholas, L.H. 2004, Jul–Dec. Déjà vu all over again? *Health Affairs* Suppl Web Exclusives: W4-586–597.

4. Henry J. Kaiser Family Foundation. 2010. *Medicare chartbook.* Menlo Park, CA: Henry J. Kaiser Family Foundation.

5. Indian Health Service. 2005, January. *Health and heritage brochure.* Washington, DC: Indian Health Service and U.S. Department of Health and Human Services.

6. Woolhandler, S., Campbell, T., and Himmelstein, D.U. 2003. Costs of health care administration in the United States and Canada. *New England Journal of Medicine* 349:768–775.

7. Himmelstein, D.U., Warren, E., Thorne, D., and Woolhandler, S. 2005, Jan–Jun. Illness and injury as contributors to bankruptcy. *Health Affairs* (Millwood) Suppl Web Exclusives: W5-63–W5-73.

8. Woolhandler, S., and Himmelstein, D.U. 2004. The high costs of for-profit care. *Canadian Medical Association Journal* 170(2):1814–1815.

9. Woolhandler, S., and Himmelstein, D.U. 1997. Costs of care and administration at for-profit and other hospitals in the United States. *New England Journal of Medicine* 336:769–774.

10. Devereaux, P.J., Choi, P.T., Lacchetti, C., et al. 2002. A systematic review and meta-analysis of studies comparing mortality rates of private for-profit and private not-for-profit hospitals. *Canadian Medical Association Journal* 166(11):1399–1406.

11. Yuan, Z., Cooper, G.S., Einstadter, D., Cebul, R.D., and Rimm, A.A. 2000. The association between hospital type and mortality and length of stay: A study of 16.9 million hospitalized Medicare beneficiaries. *Medical Care* 38(2):231–245.

12. Carlson, M.D., Gallo, W.T., and Bradley, E.H. 2004. Ownership status and patterns of care in hospice: Results from the National Home and Hospice Care Survey. *Medical Care* 42(5): 432–438.

13. Schneider, E., Zaslavsky, A.M, and Epstein, A.M. 2005. Quality of care in for-profit and not-for-profit health plans enrolling Medicare beneficiaries. *American Journal of Medicine* 118: 1392–1140.

14. Harrington, C.L., Woolhandler, S., Mullan, J., Carillo, H., and Himmelstein, D.U. 2002. Does investor ownership of nursing homes compromise the quality of care? *International Journal of Health Services* 32(2):315–325.

15. Alliance for Aging Research. 2003. *Ageism: How healthcare fails the elderly*. Washington, DC: Alliance for Aging Research.

16. Kohn, L.T., Corrigan, J.M. and Donaldson, M.S. (Eds.). 1999. *To err is human: Building a safer health care system.* Washington, DC: Committee on Quality of Health Care in America, Institute of Medicine.

17. Office of the Inspector General. 2010. Adverse events in hospitals: National incidence among Medicare beneficiaries. Washington DC: Department of Health and Human Services.

18. Sackett, D.L., Rosenberg, W.M.C., Gray, J.A.M., Haynes, R.B., and Richardson, W.S. 1996. Evidence based medicine: What it is and what it isn't. *British Medical Journal* 312:71–72.

19. Institute of Medicine. 2004. *Health literacy: A prescription to end confusion.* Washington DC: National Academies Press.

20. Jacobs, E.A., Shepard, D.S., Suaya, J.A., and Stone, E.L. 2004. Overcoming language barriers in health care: Costs and benefits of interpreter services. *American Journal of Public Health* 94(5):866–869.

21. Parker, R.M., Ratzan, S.C., and Lurie, N. 2003. Health literacy: A policy challenge for advancing high quality health care. *Health Affairs* (Millwood) 22(4):147–153.

22. Kutner, M., Greenberg, D., Jin, Y., and Paulsen, C. 2006. The health literacy of America's adults: Results from the 2003 National Assessment of Adult Literacy. U.S. Department of Education. Washington, DC: National Center for Education Statistics.

23. Berkman, N.D, Sheridan, S.L., Donahue, K.E., Halpern, D.J., and Crotty, K. 2011. Low health literacy and health outcomes: An updated systematic review. *Annals of Internal Medicine* 155(2):97–107.

24. Powers, B.J., Trinh, J.V., and Bosworth, H.B. 2010. Can this patient read and understand written health information? *Journal of the American Medical Association* 304(1):76–84.

25. Gammel, J.D. 2005. Medical House Call Program: Extending frail elderly medical care into the home. *Journal of Oncology Management* 14(2):39–46.

26. Knight, K., Badamgarav, E., Henning, J.M., et al. 2005. A systematic review of diabetes management programs. *American Journal of Managed Care* 11(4):242–250.

27. Cullen KA, Hall MJ, Golosinskiy A. 2009. Ambulatory Surgery in the United States, 2006. National health statistics reports; no 11. Revised. Hyattsville, MD: National Center for Health Statistics.

28. Barnes, P.M., Bloom, B., and Nahin, R.L. 2008. Complementary and alternative medicine use among adults and children: United States, 2007. *Health Statistics Report* 12:1–23.

29. Ness, J., Cirillo, D.J., Weir, D.R., Nisly, N.L., and Wallace, R.B. 2005. Use of complementary medicine in older Americans: Results from the Health and Retirement Study. *The Gerontologist* 45(4):516–524.

CHAPTER 14

Long-Term Care

Everyone who is born holds dual citizenship, in the kingdom of the well and in the kingdom of the sick. Although we all prefer to use only the good passport, sooner or later each of us is obliged, at least for a spell, to identify ourselves as citizens of that other place.

Susan Sontag

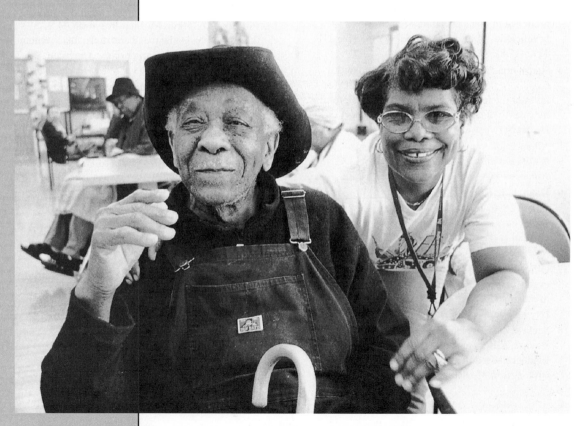

Most of us hope to maintain a high level of health and vigor until our final days. Unfortunately, many older people are not able to do so. Long-term care includes a wide range of medical, social, and personal care services designed to assist individuals to live as independently as possible by maximizing their level of physical and psychological functioning. Long-term care services may be formal or informal and may be provided at home, in the community, or in an institutional setting. Individuals needing long-term care often have a variety of physical and mental disabilities and require several types of services. The most common type of care needed is personal assistance—help with shopping, cooking, driving, bathing, dressing—rather than medical or nursing care. Various long-term services help millions of Americans who are physically or mentally disabled from birth defects, accidents, or chronic diseases and who otherwise could not manage. Some individuals need long-term care services for a short period of time while they recuperate from an illness, an accident, or an operation. Others need them for the remainder of their lives. The need for long-term care continues to expand with the aging of the population and the growing numbers of elders who are living to be very old and require daily assistance.

In this chapter, we describe the range of living situations and services that enable elders to remain as independent as possible for as long as possible, whether they reside at home, in sheltered living arrangements, or in institutions. A important factor that determines whether health and support services are used by the individuals who need them is cost. This chapter will continue the discussion of federal and state financing that assist elders to pay for the health and supportive services they need, whether they be offered in the community or at home. The cost and benefit of long-term care insurance will also be addressed. Select community-based services, including sheltered living arrangements, are discussed. The characteristics, needs and concerns of family caregivers and services to assist them are described. Elder abuse, a serious problem both in the home and in institutional settings, is explored.

Special attention is given to skilled nursing home care, including characteristics of the residents, the nature of institutional living, the many regulations governing their operation, and new alternatives. Several variables affecting the quality of care are addressed and tools to help individuals choose a quality nursing home are described.

THE NEED FOR LONG-TERM CARE

When people have physical or mental impairment that affects their ability to take care of themselves on their own, long term care is needed. They may need help in dressing, eating, or maintaining personal hygiene. They may require help to communicate, or to manage their life affairs such as shopping, cleaning, working, or managing their finances. They may need medical or nursing care such as management of feeding tubes or urinary catheters, care for wounds, or physical or speech therapy. Some may just need supervision—someone to watch and make sure they are safe, to remind them of what to do, to help them take their medications. All these are under the umbrella of long-term care. Long-term care providers or caregivers provide basic care, supervision, coordination, and assist with decisions for those who are unable to do these things for themselves. Long-term care includes a wide range of services, each with a different payment mechanism.

Who needs long-term care? Long-term care services are needed for individuals of any age who have with physical and/or cognitive impairments. For those who cannot walk, use the bathroom by themselves, or feed themselves, the need for caregivers is obvious. However, those who need supervision to make sure they do not harm themselves, those who can do things like go the bathroom and get dressed, but who would forget if they were not reminded, those who might leave the stove on, or drop a cigarette on the floor, or fall and not be able to get help—these individuals also need long-term care. Long-term care is used by individuals of all ages, but elders who have conditions that increase dependence on others for their daily routine are the most likely to need it, particularly those with dementia, those who are the oldest-old, and those who lack family members to assist them.

Need for long-term care services often begins with a question: "Does she need help with her ADLs?" ADLs, or "activities of daily living," include the ability to function independently in the following areas: eating, bathing, dressing, getting to and using the bathroom, getting in and out of a bed or chair, and mobility. Inability to complete these tasks without assistance can be life threatening and is usually the reason an individual must move from home into a sheltered living situation. Adding to the ADLs are "Instrumental ADLs," which are other skills necessary to live independently. To live an independent life, it is also necessary to get around town, keep track of money or bills, prepare meals, do light housework, use the telephone, and take medicine.

Whether individuals require formal long-term care services depends not only on what they can and cannot do, but who is willing and available to help them. If no relative or friend is available to assist the frail person to perform necessary activities,

formal services are needed. Imagine two women who both need help with bathing and shopping and cooking. One has a daughter who lives next door and is willing to check on Mom daily, shop for her, and help her with bathing and cooking. The other has no children or her children live far away. The second woman would be more likely to need services.

Changes in living patterns in our country are causing a shift from family-oriented care toward a greater need for formal services. The number of older people living alone is increasing. In 1950, fewer than 15 percent of elders lived alone; today that figure has more than doubled. Those with more money have more choices, and they often choose to live alone rather than move in with family members. The increased proportion of women in the labor force reduces the number of wives and daughters available at home to care for frail family members. In addition, the trend toward children moving away from parents, higher divorce rates, and having few or no children leaves some elders without the option of family caregivers.

Frailty

Trudy is tiny, thin, and weak. Walking slowly from her room to the kitchen table takes ten minutes, and afterwards she is exhausted. She returns to bed to rest after each meal and eats little. She spends much of the time sleeping, bruises readily, and looks as if a big wind might blow her away. Trudy can be described as "frail." Frailty has been a difficult term to categorize, although "you know it when you see it." Frailty is associated with the need for long-term care, nursing home placement, and a high death rate. Frailty has been called "the dwindles," and when someone appears to die of "old age," it is often due to frailty. Frailty is associated with low appetite, poor nutrition, and poor physical strength, endurance, and exercise tolerance. One definition of frailty is the presence of at least three of the following characteristics: The person unintentionally

lost more than 10 pounds in the past year, feels exhausted, ranks in the bottom fifth of his or her age group in grip strength and walking speed, and engages in very low levels of physical activity.[1] Frailty also implies both physical and psychological declines, decreased physical capability (through either illness or lack of use), and slowed cognitive processes. Older people who are frail often have several diseases that affect many body systems: heart disease, diabetes, vision loss, and arthritis. But frailty is more than a list of diseases. Frailty implies that individuals have little or no reserves—it is hard for them to fight off infections, to get up if they fall, to tolerate changes in weather or diet or environment. Nutritional support and exercise have been shown to reverse frailty, although the majority of those who are frail die.

The need for long-term care is increasing in our country primarily because of the rapid increase in the older population. A large proportion of this increase in the next few years will be due to the baby boomers, who become 65 years of age between 2010 and 2030. The demand for long-term care services is also attributed to the increased longevity of the population: A higher proportion is living beyond 85 and constitutes the group with the greatest need for long-term care. Another reason for the increased need for long-term care is that medical advancements are keeping the very sick and very old alive longer. Consequently, more long-term care services are needed to care for frail elders who are spending those extra years in a disabled state. A particular challenge is the increasing numbers of elders with dementia, particularly Alzheimer's disease.

FUNDING SOURCES FOR LONG-TERM CARE

There is no doubt about it: Care needed for a frail person is expensive and someone has to pay for it. Depending on the geographic location and care needed, nursing home costs range from $90 to $500 a day, and full-time 24 × 7 care at home is nearly as expensive with hourly rates estimated at $13–$28 per hour for home aides. Even part-time help can be costly. Although we may think of long-term care as medical care and assume that it is covered by insurance, in fact, very little of it is financed by either private insurance or Medicare.

Elders pay the majority of the costs for custodial home care, assisted living situations, and custodial nursing home care from their own incomes. Only when an elder becomes impoverished does the government (through Medicaid) begin to assume the costs of long-term care. Because such care is expensive and most elders do not have sufficient income or financial reserves, impoverishment comes relatively quickly. In this section we briefly review the major sources of governmental support and the government's contribution to long-term care expenses. For an overview of Medicare and Medicaid, see Chapter 13, "Medical Care."

Medicare

Medicare pays for a proportion of some services needed for long-term care but has strict eligibility requirements, and time-limited benefits. All individuals 65 years of age and older are eligible to receive federally funded health care benefits through Medicare, regardless of income. However, Medicare pays primarily physicians and hospitals and has limited funding for long-term care in nursing homes, for hospice care, or for home care. All Medicare-funded long-term care services are designed to reduce the costs of hospitalization. Home care services are designed to allow people to leave the hospital earlier to go home. Nursing home services are financed to rehabilitate and treat an elder after a major illness or hospitalization so that the person is able to return home. When the elder fails to improve fast enough or lacks skilled needs, or benefits run out, then Medicare no longer pays the bill. Hospice services are designed to reduce costly end-of-life care in the hospital and replace it with care and eventual death in a homelike setting.

To receive home health care under Medicare, elders must be homebound and under a physician's care, and they must require part-time or intermittent skilled nursing care or rehabilitative therapies. Caring for a wound, physical therapy to assist with function after a stroke, and administering intravenous medication are examples of situations calling for skilled care. Medicare does not pay for full-time nursing care or for custodial care. Also, Medicare does not cover services to assist with activities of daily living such as bathing, dressing, and housekeeping, even though such assistance might permit individuals to remain in their own homes. To be covered by Medicare, a service must be prescribed by a physician and be part of a treatment plan. Skilled nursing services are covered a maximum of 8 hours daily and no more than 28 hours weekly. Few individuals need skilled nursing care more than a few hours a day.

Medicare Part A finances a limited stay in a skilled nursing home for rehabilitation from a particular illness or injury, but *only if the nursing home stay directly follows at least a three-day hospitalization*. Further, a physician must order specialized nursing care every day *for the same condition that caused the hospitalization*. If the elder's condition stabilizes or the person needs only custodial care, then Medicare Part A coverage stops. Only a small proportion of nursing home care meets the strict requirements of Medicare Part A.

Medicare coverage for skilled nursing homes depends on the length of stay. Up to 100 days per benefit period are financed. A benefit period starts upon nursing home admission and ends when an individual has not used any nursing home or hospital care for at least 60 days. There is no limit to the number of benefit periods an individual can have. In 2012, Medicare Part A fully paid the first 20 days in a skilled nursing home. Then, for the next 80 days, the individual paid $144.50/day of the total bill. After 100 days, the individual was responsible for all charges. Consult the *Medicare and You* booklet at www.Medicare.gov for any changes in Medicare benefits and restrictions.

Let's look at an example of how Medicare funding works for skilled nursing home care. If an elder is in the hospital after a hip fracture for at least three days and is too incapacitated to return home, she may go to a nursing home for nursing care and receive physical therapy for a week or so. However, if she does not make steady progress (perhaps she becomes weaker) or she has fewer medical and nursing needs, Medicare will stop paying for the nursing home. When Medicare stops paying for her care, either she can go home or she can stay at the facility. If she stays, she can start paying the bill with her own funds, she can activate her long-term care insurance (uncommon), or, if she is poor enough, Medicaid will pay the bill. Even if she elects to pay with her own funds, she is likely to deplete them within months (average yearly skilled nursing home cost is $90,000 for a private room[2]), after which time she becomes eligible for Medicaid.

Medicare pays for hospice services to aid the dying and for respite care to relieve individuals caring for a Medicare beneficiary. However, Medicare does not pay for room and board care for a terminally ill patient in a nursing home. Hospice will pay for short-term hospital stays and for inpatient respite care (short-term care up to five days for the terminally ill patient, usually in a nursing home, to give the family caregiver a rest). Refer to Chapter 15, "Dying, Death, and Grief," for a detailed discussion of hospice services.

Medicaid

The largest public funding source for long-term care is Medicaid (MediCal in California), funded jointly by the federal and state governments. Currently, Medicaid is responsible for paying the bills of the majority of the nation's nursing home residents. For those poor enough to qualify, Medicaid is the payer of last resort, paying nursing home and home health care bills not covered by Medicare and private insurance. Unlike Medicare, Medicaid does pay for unlimited custodial nursing home care and does not require previous hospitalization.

In order to qualify for Medicaid benefits, an elder must prove that she or he has few or no assets. A person who cannot afford to pay out-of-pocket for home or institutional care but is above the cutoff for Medicaid must "spend down" his or her assets in order to qualify. The spouse of a Medicaid-eligible elder may keep their house and some income and assets. The amount varies by state.

Medicaid provides medical and rehabilitation services to the disabled, blind, and poor of all ages. By law, Medicaid must provide skilled nursing home services and home health care for persons eligible for skilled nursing services. Some states receive federal matching funds to provide other long-term care services: rehabilitation and physical therapy services and home and community-based care to certain persons with chronic impairments. Some states offer more home care services than others. Medicaid also covers the skilled nursing home expenses of those formerly middle-income older people who have exhausted their financial resources by paying for nursing home expenses. Medicaid pays for medical and personal services in a nursing home, as long as the services are authorized by a physician and are part of a treatment plan.

Medicaid reimburses nursing homes less than the full costs of care. Because of this low level of reimbursement, many nursing homes do not accept Medicaid. Nursing homes sometimes decline Medicaid patients who are "expensive" to care for—for example, individuals who require intravenous therapy, extensive wound care, or artificial feeding. Some nursing homes allow only a small proportion of their residents to be Medicaid-eligible. They make a profit on the cash-paying and Medicare-funded patients and use it to cover their losses on the Medicaid patients.

Although some states passed laws earlier, the federal Omnibus Budget Reconciliation Act of 1993 requires every state to try to recover the money the Medicaid program spent on long-term care by claiming assets left behind by deceased Medicaid recipients. However, states cannot make claims against an estate if there is a surviving spouse or a child who is disabled, blind, or under 18 years of age. Recovery programs are in effect in almost every state, and several states hire private contractors to collect at least a portion of what Medicaid spent. Detailed information on Medicaid is available at the Centers for Medicare and Medicaid Services Web site, www.cms.hhs.gov

A new legal industry has evolved to help middle-class and wealthy seniors protect their assets for their children yet still qualify for Medicaid. Elders who transfer their assets to their relatives may protect themselves from some losses. "Asset shifting" allows many people who could afford to pay for nursing home care with their own funds to use Medicaid. In an attempt to slow down asset shifting, a federal law was passed that requires any transfer of assets (except to a disabled child or spouse) to occur at least three years before nursing home admission and for trusts to be set up at least five years prior to nursing home admission. Subsequently, in 1997 another federal law was passed to make asset-shifting a criminal offense, with up to a $10,000 fine, one year in jail, or both.

Private Insurance

Medicare supplemental insurance, commonly called Medigap insurance, is voluntary, private insurance that gives elders a choice of policies with many benefit levels—the more coverage, the higher the premiums. Medigap insurance is designed to supplement Medicare coverage by paying the deductibles and copays. Depending on the plan chosen, Medigap policies may cover copayments for skilled nursing home care (days 21 to 100) and provide some coverage for short-term in-home assistance.

Long-term care insurance is a voluntary, private health insurance that is intended to supplement the reimbursement by Medicare for nursing home and home care services. There are many types of policies, and the cost of the monthly premiums depends on the age of the individual purchasing the insurance and the level of benefits. In addition to nursing home care, other long-term care services may be included: nursing care in the home, physical therapy, personal care, and homemaker services. The government offers tax incentives for individuals because long-term care insurance saves the government from expensive Medicaid outlays. Nevertheless, few people choose to buy it.

There are many reasons why an individual might not wish to purchase long-term care insurance. First, the plans are confusing, and it is difficult to anticipate what type of policy a person might need 30 or 40 years into the future. Many policies do not offer protection against inflation, and premiums may increase without notice. Also, there are few protections for the policyholder if the insurer goes out of business or if the policyholder can no longer pay the monthly premium. The older the person is when the policy is initiated, the higher is the monthly rate. Depending on the policy, long-term care insurance can cost thousands of dollars a year for life.

In addition to the high cost, long-term care policies often have exclusions and limitations. Preexisting conditions may be excluded, particularly disabling diseases, such as Alzheimer's disease. Long-term care policies also restrict the type and length of care covered. Further, they usually place an upper limit on payment to the policyholder. Policies may have other restrictions.

Potential buyers of these policies should contact their local Area Agency on Aging for advice before making a decision to purchase.

Other Sources of Funding

In 1965, the Older Americans Act was passed with the goal of improving the lives of all people 60 and older by funding a broad range of health and social services and supporting education and research in gerontology. This legislation established the federal Administration on Aging, which drafts regulations and provides funds for health and social services for anyone age 60 and older. Each state has a Department of Aging that receives funds and direction from the Administration on Aging, then disperses those funds to the network of Area Agencies on Aging that reach every area of that state. Each Area Agency on Aging plans and coordinates services to benefit elders in its region, then contracts out the services needed in its area to other public or nonprofit providers. The majority of the funds are used for the following services: information and referral, in-home support, nutrition, transportation, and legal services. In addition, each Area Agency on Aging is mandated to offer ombudsman services to protect the rights of persons in nursing homes and assisted living facilities in its area. Many of the services are based on a sliding scale, dependent on income.

Title XX of the Social Security Act, implemented in 1975, significantly expanded the availability of home health care services to the poor and disabled of all ages. Under Title XX, the federal government matches the state's contribution to fund selected social services. Each state must determine income criteria, the populations to be served, and how the federal government funds will be allocated. Ten percent of Title XX funds is spent on in-home services, mainly homemaker and home health services. Eligibility and available funds vary from state to state.

The Department of Veterans Affairs provides institutional care for veterans. The VA has 133 Community Living Centers (formerly called nursing homes), the majority of which are on or near the VA medical centers. They also contract with community nursing homes and other long term care services so that veterans can receive care near their homes and families. and contracts with thousands of other agencies to provide long-term care services for veteran beneficiaries. The department also pays for home health assistance to disabled veterans with service-connected disabilities. Several VA hospitals have established their own programs to deliver home health care services.

HOME CARE

Where would you want to be if you were sick and disabled: living in your own home, living with your relatives, or living in an institution? Most people, young and old alike, want to remain in their own homes for as long as possible. Staying at home gives a person control over when, how, and what type of personal care is received, unlike the care in a nursing home. Also, there is pressure to keep elders at home as long as possible to avoid, or at least delay, the high costs of a nursing home.

Elders may remain in their own home because they have only a few disabilities and can manage on their own, or they may stay at home with severe disabilities and capable caregivers. Some elders choose to stay at home even when those who love and care for them feel the situation is unsafe; many refuse help and services offered. Only about one-third of frail elders needing services use them. And, among elders with severe limitations, more than half use no formal services. The location of a person's home, the presence of loved ones and money to provide care, the physical arrangement of the home, the degree of the elder's physical and cognitive impairment, and the elder's preferences play

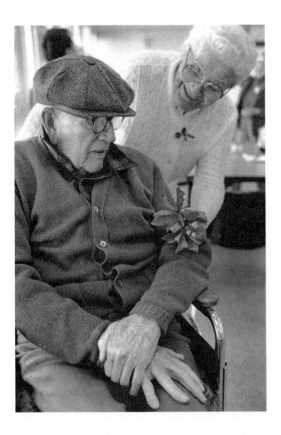

an important role in determining whether an elder is cared for at home.

Family Providers of Home Care

Graciella works full-time as an office manager in a small manufacturing company. Every day at lunchtime, she visits her elderly father in his home to be sure he takes his medications and eats something. She returns after work to make dinner and tidy up. She does his shopping and spends one weekend day each week "helping out."

Agnes and her sister Myrna alternate visits with their 90-year-old mother in her apartment in an assisted living complex. Agnes calls to remind her mother to take her medications and accompanies her to her many physician visits. Myrna takes her grocery shopping and to Sunday church services.

Bill and Anna found it easier to move their elderly aunt with Alzheimer's disease into their suburban home, where they can get up with her if she needs to use the bathroom at night and provide her meals and supervision.

Pearl, who is 80 years old, diligently cares for her husband, Frank, who is 86 and has advanced Parkinson's disease. She has chronic bronchitis and arthritis but is still able to manage on her own. A member of her church comes to visit with Frank once a week for a couple of hours so that Pearl can shop for groceries and do other errands.

What do all those people have in common? They are all caregivers for a family member, and the help that they provide enables their relatives to stay in their own homes. Unpaid family caregivers provide the majority of home care to frail elders. Almost 44 million people (family, friends, and neighbors) provide care to individuals 50 years and older who need help with daily activities. The single most important consideration in determining whether a frail elder can remain at home is whether there is a close family member or friend willing and able to perform the physically and emotionally taxing role of the caregiver.

What is the profile of a person who cares for an elderly family member? Women are more likely to be caregivers than men. And, when duties are compared, women spend more time and are more likely to handle personal tasks (bathing, toileting, and dressing) while men are more likely to handle finances and arrange for care.[3] The average age of an individual caring for an older person is 69.[3] Many caregivers of older persons are also in the workforce, often having to change work schedules, reduce hours, or take unpaid leaves to be able to care for their kin.[3]

How taxing is the caregiving role? The average family caregiver for adults works 20 hours a week, but if the caregiver also lives in the home, the average caregiving time spent is 39 hours/week.[3] The number of hours per week spent in caregiving tasks has been shown to increase with the age of the caregiver.[4] Further, the amount of time spent caregiving increases with the degree of cognitive impairment of the older person, commonly reaching more than 40 hours a week for those with severe dementia.[5] The length of caregiving might last from weeks or months to decades.

Cultural differences make a difference in the extent of care given by family members and friends. Even though ethnic elders have higher rates of disability and poorer health than whites, yet they use a smaller proportion of long-term care services (nursing homes, community services, home health care). It has been suggested that ethnic elders are more likely to be cared for at home because of stronger intergenerational family networks and cultural values to care for their kin. Some groups, particularly Asians and those from the Middle East, have long traditions of honoring the elderly, and family members are expected to care for elderly members in their own homes. There may also be differences in expectations between different cultural groups. If ethnic minorities tend toward larger families and the children are less likely to move away from the parents, there are more available caregivers than in populations where the children leave the city, state, or country. Higher rates of unemployment also can leave more adults available to care for frail elders. Some ethnic minorities distrust formal health care services, are not located near them, or may be unaware of them.

Caregiver effectiveness depends on a number of factors: the frail elder's degree of disability and dependence, the caregiver's own health and mobility, and the availability of emotional support. Generally, if a spouse is available, he or she gradually takes on more responsibility for the home and for the partner's personal care. If the spouse is unable or unwilling, or if the individual lives alone, the caregiving role usually goes to an adult child or his or her spouse. The caregiver's other roles and responsibilities in the family and community and the degree to which the caregiver can obtain relief can also affect the ability to serve a frail elder. The caregiver may have to move or make room for the elder to move into her or his home. The caregiver may have to juggle paid work and caring for a relative.

Caregiving encompasses a wide variety of behaviors and commitments to a frail relative, from visiting or running errands for a couple of hours a week to living with the relative and being responsible for round-the-clock care. Such care commonly includes the following: medically related care, personal care, household maintenance, transportation, supervision, paying bills, and shopping. Caregivers may make medical appointments, accompany elders to the doctor, pick up their prescriptions, negotiate their benefits, help with their medical bills, and keep their checkbooks balanced. They may do shopping, house cleaning, yard maintenance, and small repairs. Perhaps a caregiver calls a few times a day and drops by multiple times a day or week. In some situations, an elder needs to be taken to a day care program, or a caregiver with paid employment hires a companion to care for the elder during working hours. Caregivers may need to bathe, feed, and toilet a frail relative. They may need to move into the elder's home or move the elder into their home. Just like parenting a small child, the task of caregiving can be a 24-hour commitment with minimal support and no reimbursement.

The demands of caring for a frail elder can be physically, financially, and emotionally draining. It is often hard physical work, particularly if the patient needs to be moved, requires constant supervision, or is violent. It can be constant work to care for someone who fights caregivers, wanders, does not believe he or she needs care, or no longer recognizes loved ones. Disruption of sleep during the night is common. Caregivers often need to quit their jobs or reduce their hours to provide care to a family member, often at great financial expense. Watching the physical and mental deterioration of someone you love can be very sad. Furthermore, juggling the demands of a disabled parent with the needs of a spouse and children, with career responsibilities, and with their own health needs can be overwhelming. Caregivers who are old themselves may have to deal with their own disabilities, failing health, and declining energy. Studies show that caregiving places a physical and psychological burden on the caregiver.

Why do they do it? The most common reason is love for a family member and a sense of duty. Children care for parents who cared for them. Many spouses see caregiving as a part of the marriage vows, "in sickness and in health, until death do us part." Sometimes family members provide care because they see no other option. They have limited financial resources, they cannot afford outside help, or they want to protect their inheritance. Many individuals and their families see nursing home placement as a last resort and strive to do what they can to prevent it. Often the family member who lives the closest assumes the lion's share of caregiving responsibilities, particularly daughters.

When parents care for a child, there is a progression toward independence. Within a few years, the job of caregiving eases as the child becomes increasingly responsible, eventually leaving the home. Caring for a parent or a spouse is more difficult because the road is less predictable, and the difficulty increases with time as the elder becomes more and more dependent. Caregiving can impact family relationships, creating or worsening conflicts among relatives about who provides what care and how much. Another common consequence of caring for another person is the accompanying confinement within the home and restriction of outside activities: Many caregivers become as housebound as the family member they serve. Caregiving activities demand increasing time and energy, often without relief. Isolation from friends and from other family members, and even alienation from the frail elder, may occur. Caregivers may feel guilty because they sometimes wish the frail elder would die.

Formal Support for Caregivers

Given the multiple stresses placed on those caring for an invalid at home, it is not surprising that many families find coping difficult. The stress of caregiving can create or aggravate emotional and physical health problems. Because of this, it is important that caregivers obtain help, either formally or informally. The services outlined here are available in many areas to provide support to caregivers.

Education programs can increase caregivers' skills and feelings of competence in dealing with

Life of a Caregiver

"At first, although he couldn't remember what day it was or what he had for breakfast, his memory of long-ago events was still sharp. So we'd talk a lot about our wonderful years together and the great times we'd shared.

But soon, those memories left him too. Now they're fading for me as well. Because the person who sits across from me staring blankly into space is *not* the same person from those memories. He no longer even knows who I am.

The dreams we had for our "golden years"? *Forgotten.* The money we saved to make those dreams come true? *Gone.* Used up for medical expenses and supplies. Even though our little house is paid for, I can barely pay the taxes on it. Our friends are enjoying retirement, always making travel plans. *I have to make plans just to take a walk!*

The worst part is, I look at my husband and sometimes find myself hating him. Then I hate myself for feeling that way. But I can't help it. At least when someone dies, the grief eventually ends—you accept the loss, pick up the pieces of your life, and go on. With Alzheimer's, *the grief doesn't end because death doesn't come even though you find yourself praying it will!*"

Letter to the Alzheimer's Family Relief Program, 15825 Shady Grove Road, Suite 140, Rockville, MD 20850.

the medical needs of a frail relative. Such education might include information about the patient's illness or disability, how to deal with crises as they arise, use of special equipment, transport techniques, rehabilitation strategies, and how to administer medications. Caregivers also can learn about available community services and their eligibility standards.

Support groups provide emotional and practical support to caregivers, providing them with an opportunity to share experiences, develop coping strategies, enhance knowledge about disease and treatment, and gain access to community resources. Support programs also can assist caregivers in making the difficult decision to continue home care or place their frail relative in a nursing home. Support groups encourage members to air feelings of resentment, anger, and hopelessness. Some support groups may also become politically active in advocating for frail elders. For example, they may initiate changes in laws or develop a respite care program in the community. A professional facilitator may or may not be present. Some group membership is specific to the illness of the frail elder (e.g., Alzheimer's disease). Support groups may be offered by the local Area Agency on Aging, nonprofit health associations such as the American Cancer Society, the American Lung Association, and the American Heart Association, and the county mental health department. There are also Internet support groups for caregivers.

Financial support to caregivers can make a significant difference in the availability and quality of caregiving. As part of the Medicaid program in some states, reimbursement may be provided to family members to care for a disabled relative for up to 24 hours per week as an in-home support service aide (IHSS). In some states, caregivers qualify for medical benefits.

Often caregivers need *legal support and assistance*. Legal experts can help deal with questions that can arise: Who determines when Mom can no longer make her own medical or financial decisions? How can we access the appropriate resources to care for Uncle Jim? Who can help create a durable power of attorney, draw up

wills or trusts, and help with estate planning? One resource is the National Academy of Elder Law Attorneys, at www.naela.org

Case management services can assist family members, particularly those who need to access and supervise services from a distance. These are discussed more fully later in the chapter.

One opportunity to "get a break" from caregiving is respite care. *Respite care* is a service that offers temporary, infrequent care or supervision of frail and disabled adults to provide relief for caregivers from the stress of constant care. Let's say you are caring for your husband with Parkinson's disease and you need to have knee surgery. Respite care allows you to place him in a nursing home or special wing of the hospital temporarily while you get on your feet. Or, if you need something on a smaller scale, a trained individual can come into the home and temporarily care for the frail elder for an hour or two so that you can leave the home for errands, a short trip, or a visit with friends. Adult day care facilities and homemaker and home health aides may also provide respite care. Respite care can prevent institutionalization by temporarily relieving the intolerable level of stress experienced by the caregiver. Medicaid and Medicare both provide some funding for limited respite services.

The Administration on Aging, through an amendment to the Older Americans Act, established a program specifically for caregivers called the National Family Caregiver Support Program. The funds allocated to the program are distributed to the states, which are mandated to work with local Area Agencies on Aging and other community agencies to offer direct services to caregivers in their areas. The services include the following:

Information to caregivers about available services
Help for caregivers to access support services
Individual counseling, support groups, and caregiver training
Respite care
Supplemental services to enhance the work of the caregiver

The local Area Agency on Aging provides information and linkages to a variety of local programs. In addition the Administration on Aging sponsors a Web site, The Eldercare Locator (www.eldercare.gov) that connects caregivers with sources of information on local senior services. Other important sites for family caregivers include the National Alliance for Caregiving (www. caregiving.org), the Family Caregiver Alliance (www.caregiver.org), and the National Family Caregivers Association (www.nfcacares.org). The National Respite Locator Service helps caregivers to find respite services in their local area (www.respitelocator.org).

Domestic Elder Abuse

As older persons become frail and dependent on others, they become more vulnerable to abuse by their caregivers. Elder abuse occurs when an elder suffers harm or loss from one or more behaviors, including physical abuse, psychological abuse, sexual abuse, financial exploitation, and neglect. Variable definitions of what constitutes abuse and neglect result in conflicting data on its prevalence. For example, everyone agrees that kicking, hitting, or biting an elder is abuse, but some situations are subject to interpretation. Can an elderly woman with dementia consent to a sexual relationship, or is that abuse? Can an elderly man who has cognitive impairment give all his money to his children when they ask for it, or has he been abused? Can a 98-year-old woman live in her own home when it is infested with vermin and she cannot properly care for herself, even if she refuses to leave? What about an older person who refuses to eat—is this neglect? As you can see, often the identification of abuse is not simple. It is obvious that the consequences of abuse can be devastating and include the loss of independence, homes, life savings, health, dignity, and security.

Estimates of the extent of elder abuse in our country vary from 2 percent to 10 percent of the elder population, depending on the definition of abuse, the survey methodology, and sampling technique. It is generally agreed that data on elder abuse in our country are sparse, and the figures on

Two Examples of Elder Abuse

Glenda, age 83, was admitted to the hospital with a ruptured left eye due to untreated glaucoma. Her hair was matted and her clothes were soiled. She had sores on her legs. Her toenails were so long that they curved around her toes. Glenda lived with a daughter who had a history of mental illness. Their home was infested with roaches and cluttered with trash, both inside and out.

Harry, age 72, was hospitalized in order to amputate his leg. He signed over power of attorney to his son, John. John did not have a job nor did his wife. Harry had an estate of $400,000, plenty of money to support all of them. The son and his wife moved in and took over, remodeling the house and spending significant amounts of money on luxury items. They said they remodeled a bathroom for Harry, but the bathroom was not wheelchair accessible, and no ramps were built to enable Harry to enter and exit the house. Harry was very mentally capable but was told whom he could see and was never included in making decisions about how his money was to be spent. Kept hostage in his own home, he never telephoned anyone because his son and daughter-in-law would listen in on the conversations and then yell at him. Other family members were told that they could not visit Harry unless they made prior arrangements with John, who summarily denied all of them contact.

Source: National Center on Elder Abuse. 2003. *A response to the abuse of vulnerable adults: The 2000 survey of state Adult Protective Services.* National Center on Elder Abuse, 1201 15th Street, N.W., Suite 350, Washington, DC 20005;202-898-2586.

abuse differ. Some experts say that 500,000 elders have been abused, others say the number is 1 or 2 million, and some put the number at 5 million. In this section we discuss domestic elder abuse, or abuse outside the institutional setting, usually in the individual's own home.

Probably the most important study on elder abuse in the home is the survey of state Adult Protective Services conducted by the National Center on Elder Abuse. Using data gathered from local Adult Protective Services across the country, the study revealed that more than 550,000 persons aged 60 and older experienced abuse and neglect in domestic settings.[6]

The most frequent forms of elder abuse were self-neglect (37 percent), caregiver neglect (20 percent), emotional/psychological abuse (15 percent), financial/ material exploitation (15 percent), and physical abuse (11 percent). (Some individuals experienced more than one type of elder abuse.) Two-thirds of the elder victims of all types of abuse were women, and about two in five victims were 80 years and older. In two-thirds of the incidents, the perpetrator was a family member, and two-thirds of the perpetrators were adult children or spouses. Adult children were the largest perpetrators of elder abuse (33 percent), followed by other family members (22 percent), and spouses or partners (11 percent).[6]

It is estimated that there are far more cases of elder abuse than are reported. Why? The abused might not report the problem because of confusion, shame, fear of retaliation, or loyalty to the abuser. Often the abused are part of a family where abuse has been long-standing and may even seem "normal." Frail elders may also fear that they will have to be moved to an institution. When confronted, they may deny they have been abused or may internalize the blame and believe they caused or deserved the abuse.

Experts once believed that the stress of caring for a disabled elder was the major contributor to elder abuse. However, we now know that most caregivers are stressed but do not abuse their loved ones. In fact, abuse generally occurs because of long-standing personality problems of the caregiver and a history of using abusive methods to solve problems. For instance, adult children who are financially dependent on an elder relative are more likely to be abusive than children who are financially independent. Relatives with mental illness or substance abuse problems and a history of violent or antisocial behavior are also at higher risk for being abusers. The abusers are often part of a cycle of violence. They may have been abused as children, or they themselves may have been child abusers or wife abusers. Many suffer from drug or alcohol abuse, or mental illness.

All states have enacted elder abuse laws that require health care providers to report any type of suspected elder abuse to Adult Protective Services, part of the county Department of Social Services. If you suspect elder abuse or are concerned about the well-being or safety of an older person, report it immediately. Each state has an elder abuse hotline that can be accessed at www.elderabusecenter.org If there is an emergency, call 911.

Prevention of elder abuse may include programs to assist caregivers in dealing with the stresses of caring for a dependent adult and to teach anger management and other skills. Programs for professionals who work with older people to identify signs and symptoms of abuse can help. Multidisciplinary teams are by far the best way to address the problem of elder abuse—its prevention, identification, and resolution. The National Committee for the Prevention of Elder Abuse, funded by the U.S. Administration on Aging, is a gateway to resources on elder abuse. Go to www.preventelderabuse.org

Self-Neglect

One of the most challenging situations for health care professionals and family members arises when a person behaves in a way that threatens his or her personal health and safety. Among older people, these behaviors include the refusal or failure to provide themselves with adequate food,

Box 14.1

Signs of Self-Neglect

- Failure to keep the home free of vermin
- Failure to take care of trash
- Hoarding
- Failure to take needed medicines
- Refusal to seek medical treatment for serious illness
- Malnourishment

- Lack of food, or spoiled food, in the home
- Poor hygiene
- Not wearing suitable clothing for the weather
- Confusion
- Inability to prepare adequate meals
- Dehydration
- Pets not cared for

water, clothing, shelter, safety, personal hygiene, and needed medication. This behavior is called "self-neglect." Box 14.1 lists common signs of self-neglect. In some cases, it begins in old age and is often associated with dementia. For example, an elder who was normally fastidious may stop caring for herself and her home. In other cases, such behaviors have been ongoing for years but worsen with age. Most self-neglecting older people have difficulty caring for themselves, and most have confusion. The following is an example of self-neglect.

Ruth W. has lived like a miser her entire life, watching every penny and refusing to throw anything away. Her home is unbelievably cluttered with her life's treasures, which others would call junk or trash. There is spoiled food in her refrigerator. She refuses to wash herself or flush the toilet in order to save water. As she ages, she becomes increasingly eccentric and isolated as she refuses to let anyone in for fear that someone will steal her things or remove her from her home.

In cases of self-neglect, there is a fine line between elders' right to live as they please and society's obligations to ensure individual health and safety and sanitary conditions. These issues are often very complex and are best solved by an interdisciplinary team, generally consisting of medical personnel, mental health professionals, law enforcement,

family members, and, at times, an attorney. Many elders who exhibit self-neglect are capable of making their own decisions and have chosen their lifestyle. They generally are not violating any laws and, although one might question their judgment, are competent to make their own decisions. When this is the case, there is little that can be done, and it is best to develop a relationship with the elder so that the situation can be monitored, improved little by little, and action can be taken if it worsens significantly.

If an elder is unable to manage his or her own affairs due to physical, mental, or cognitive difficulties, a conservatorship may be sought by the family or by a health or social service professional who has become aware of the problem. A *conservator ,* also called guardian, is an individual employed by a public agency, or a friend or relative of the elder, who is appointed by the court to make decisions on behalf of an individual who cannot make decisions for him- or herself. These decisions might be financial (such as probate conservatorships established to protect the assets or money of frail or disabled elders) or, rarely, LPS conservatorships, which are designed specifically for the mentally ill (see Chapter 7).

There are many types of conservatorships, and rules governing each type are complex and vary among states. All are characterized by the loss of rights. Some arrangements are permanent;

others are temporary and are renewed periodically. Many times, conservatorships result in institutionalization.

Placing an individual under a conservatorship to protect his or her health and assets can be complex, expensive, and emotionally draining. It is important to remember that a conservatorship is a removal of rights and is a very serious act. Many times health professionals and families are unhappy with the decisions made by their clients or loved ones and consider conservatorship. However, individuals generally have the right to make poor or unpopular decisions about their health and body as long as they fully understand the risks and benefits of those decisions.

In-Home Services

Formal care enables frail elders to remain as independent as possible in their own homes and includes a range of services. Skilled services include medical services (physician services, nursing services) and rehabilitation services (physical, speech, and occupational therapy). Personal care services are provided by nursing assistants and homemaker aides and include bathing, toileting, dressing, and meal preparation. These services are discussed in the following pages. Home care may be provided by one individual who lives in the elder's house or by several individuals (generally under the auspices of one agency) who go into the home. The primary consumers of home-based services are individuals recuperating from hospitalization, the chronically ill who need rehabilitation or help with daily living activities, the acutely ill who can be managed at home with help, and the dying. Companies that offer home medical equipment (e.g., hospital beds, respiration devices, medical and surgical supplies, and home infusion therapy) are also expanding in response to an increased demand.

The availability of home care services may postpone, or even eliminate, the need for a nursing home. When the elder is able to remain at home, the network of family and friends remains intact. Furthermore, the individual and family can select particular services that meet their needs without financing unnecessary care. However, many frail elders choose institutional care because they do not want to be a burden to their family, they lack a caregiver, or they cannot coordinate or find services that would enable them to live at home.

If round-the-clock care is not needed, home care is less expensive than institutionalization. Live-in care can be less expensive than care provided by those working in shifts. Costs for 24-hour care in one's home are generally close to the expenses of a nursing home. However, they do not include food, utilities, rent, and supplies. Even if costs are similar, home care provides one-on-one contact with a caregiver, unlike institutionalization, where one caregiver's time is spread out among multiple patients.

For the elder poor who qualify, Medicaid finances some home health and homemaker services, although not 24-hour custodial care. Elders who do not qualify as poor must bear the costs of home care from their own assets. Thus, whether or not an elder is eligible for governmental financial support is often a significant factor in deciding between home care and institutionalization.

Home care does have limitations. Home care quality is uneven and depends greatly on who is providing the care. There are few quality or training standards for caregivers. This is especially true in cases where a caregiver is hired privately, not through an agency. Although most states license or regulate some or all home care organizations, few have licensure requirements for workers in the home care industry. All states must maintain a registry for nursing home aides according to federal law, but most states do not register or require background checks for home care workers.

In theory, home-based care is comprehensive and accessible, but in practice, the services may

What Will I Do with Mom?

Mom has fallen three times in the last two weeks. She looks bruised, but says she is fine. Last time she fell on her back porch, and it took two hours before a neighbor heard her cry for help. This scared me—I do not want to go to her house and find her dead alone.

She wants to stay in her own home with her friends and go to her church, and she promises to be more careful. When she last went to the doctor, it appeared she was not taking her medications correctly and she had lost weight. She cannot really keep the house clean anymore and food I leave for her is often untouched in the containers in her refrigerator.

So, they ask me what I am going to do? It sounds as if living alone just isn't working out for her. Should I try to keep her in her own house—hire a caregiver to come in 24/7 or maybe just during the day? Maybe get a companion who can rent a room in her house and watch out for her? What about that nursing home down the street where her friend lives—maybe it is best if she goes there? It's so expensive! She'll have to sell her house, and that means she can't come back. Maybe assisted living—I saw an ad about a place that offers a place to sleep, meals, and supervision, and the price was cheaper than the nursing home. My sister said she can help in the

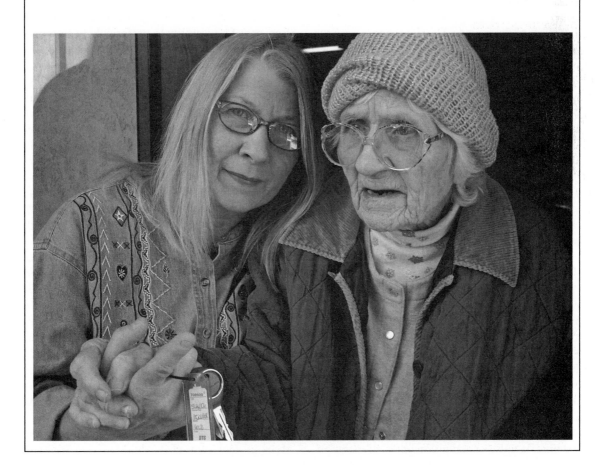

What Will I Do with Mom?

summers, but she lives out of state and wants Mom to fly to her house. Can Mom fly alone? I could bring her to live with me, but there is no one there in the daytime, and the room I have available is upstairs. I'm not so sure she can handle the stairs, and my husband isn't too excited about your Mom mom living with us. Maybe I can get her one of those alarms—at least she could call me if she needed help, but my boss is already making remarks about how much time I have been taking off work to help her shop or remind her of things or check on her during the workday.

And what does she think? Will she go along with my plan or will she fight me and insist on staying in her home by herself? If she insists on staying at home—can I make her leave? Should I get some kind of power of attorney so I can help her manage her money and help her make decisions?

Welcome to the world of caregiving.

---

fall short of these goals. Despite the rapid growth in home health care, most small communities have only a few types of services. Services can be underdeveloped and fragmented, focusing on a specific health need or professional specialization. When many different services are utilized, none has full responsibility. This fragmentation makes it difficult for elders, especially those with multiple disabilities and language difficulties, to coordinate their home care services to meet their needs. Even when all needed services are available, older people may be unaware of them and may not know whether they might qualify for reduced or free services. Case managers, social workers, and hospital discharge planners can assist in piecing together services.

Home Health Services

Home health services are the most common and most important services to enable an individual to stay as independent as possible in a comfortable and familiar environment and to postpone or prevent institutionalization. Services include personal care, homemaking, nutrition, and health care. *Homemaker aides* perform a full range of homemaking activities, including light housekeeping, laundry, shopping, and meal preparation.

Because elders' ability to perform daily activities is often limited, these individuals can be instrumental in avoiding institutionalization. *Home health aides* provide personal care, such as assisting with bathing, grooming, toileting, supervising medication use, and exercise. In many cases, one worker performs a variety of housekeeping and personal care activities. In many cases, the frail elder relies on family members for this type of assistance.

Home health care is available through public health departments, hospitals, and home health care agencies. Medicare reimburses home health services but not homemaker services. For individuals poor enough to qualify, both homemaker and home health aide services are funded through local departments of social services (funded by Title XX). Sometimes, a family member will be paid for caregiving services through Medicaid's in-home support services (IHSS) program. For individuals who do not qualify for those programs, some agencies funded by the Older Americans Act offer services and charge a variable fee based on income and assets.

To find and compare the home health services in your area, go to the Medicare Web site (www.medicare.gov) and click on Resource Locator to find Home Health Compare.

Skilled Nursing Services

Nurses commonly visit sick individuals at home to evaluate their condition and determine the type of nursing care required to carry out the prescribed medical treatment plan. They provide direct patient care, monitor treatment, and refer the client to other social and medical services as needed. Care provided by registered or licensed vocational nurses is skilled and includes care for wounds, catheters, and IV lines, and assessing and monitoring patients. Nurses provide health education and instruct the patient and family on basic home care techniques such as changing sterile dressings, catheter care, and insulin injections.

Nursing services are commonly provided by registered nurses or licensed vocational nurses from visiting nurse associations, public health departments, or home health agencies. Nurses working under the auspices of health departments provide free services, mainly to poor inner-city elders. Other agencies adjust fees based on the client's income.

Physician Services

Physician services to the home-bound elders may be provided by a primary care doctor or a doctor who works through the home health agency. These physicians may work with a nurse practitioner or physician assistant. In some cases, a physician assistant or nurse practitioner makes home visits to assess the patient and develop a treatment or rehabilitation plan under the direction of a physician. In general, the family or home health agency staff implements the plan and periodically informs the physician about the patient's health status. Agency physicians or their representatives may be involved in short-term home care after hospitalization as well as maintenance care for those with chronic illnesses. More information on house calls is found in Chapter 13, "Medical Care."

Physical, Speech, and Occupational Therapists

Rehabilitation therapists help patients who have suffered a debilitating illness or injury to improve their ability to care for themselves. A physical therapist is needed to improve patients' use of limbs or muscles. A speech therapist helps patients whose speech has been affected to relearn and maintain this skill and can also treat memory and cognition, and swallowing skills. An occupational therapist helps patients to improve their ability to perform routine functions with their hands such as daily activities (dressing, sewing, teeth brushing, use of a computer, cooking, driving) and community reintegration. Activities and devices (such as walkers) are also introduced to maintain or restore skills needed to function independently. Elders who suffer a stroke or hip fracture are the most likely to need these rehabilitation services.

After assessing the client, the therapist develops a treatment schedule and may routinely visit the home, or the client may go to the office until therapy is no longer needed. A therapist may also instruct the patient and family on rehabilitation activities that can be accomplished between visits.

Emergency Response Services

Elders living alone may use an emergency response system to decrease their isolation and reduce the fear that they won't be able to summon help in a medical crisis. These services vary in the way they monitor a frail elder. Monitoring services may be personal or electronic.

An example of a personal emergency response service is when a volunteer makes a phone call at a prearranged time every day to a home-bound elder to check on his or her physical status. If the caller receives no answer after several calls within an hour, a friend, neighbor, police officer, or nurse is dispatched to the home to check if the elder has had an accident or needs help.

Electronic devices are worn 24/7 allowing an injured elder to get help whenever needed. When the button is pushed, a device attached to a standard telephone automatically dials a central office, and a trained professional dispatches help. The dispatcher then calls the elder to determine the problem. If there is no answer, the dispatcher contacts a relative or neighbor who has previously agreed to be called to check on the person, or an ambulance is sent to the home. In many assisted-living facilities, call buttons are commonly placed in the bathroom and bedroom. Electronic technology using pagers and cell phones, GPS tracking, webcams, and motion/position sensors provide new options for monitoring and summoning help.

Telephone and Visiting Programs

Friendly visitor programs send volunteers, who are usually old themselves, to the homes of isolated or homebound elders once or twice a week. The visitors are trained to recognize health problems and environmental dangers, and they serve as an information and referral source for local services. Some communities have friendly visitor services that, in addition to visiting, help the elder with errands, writing letters, or other activities. Some programs contact elders by phone instead of visiting their homes. In some communities, mail carriers are trained to check up on homebound elders on their routes.

Home-Delivered Meals

Home-delivered meal programs—Meals on Wheels—provide homebound elders one hot meal a day, five days a week. The programs prepare meals for those with special dietary restrictions. Sometimes the service provides an additional meal to be refrigerated for the evening. The services are usually provided by voluntary organizations, and costs vary widely. Often, the program is funded through city government, the United Way, or senior organizations. The demand far exceeds the service capability in many communities, and often there is a long waiting list.

For those needing tube feeding, home health agencies may provide this service in the home. This program is reimbursed by Medicare.

Hospice Care

Hospice care was developed as a humane alternative to dying in a hospital. In order to qualify, the individual must have a physician's prognosis that he or she has six months or less to live. A team of medical and social service personnel and trained volunteers coordinate physical and psychological care to the dying person and family. Hospice services may be provided in hospitals and skilled nursing facilities but are most commonly provided in the home. For elders with terminal illnesses, hospice services offer the advantage of skilled nursing, social work, home health, and homemaker services in the home. Medicare reimburses these services without the stringent requirements imposed on home health services. Hospice services are discussed in more detail in the next chapter.

Community-Based Services

Some programs provide services in the elder's home, but they are often expensive and time-consuming. Other programs service a greater number of elders by having the elders come to them. The following sections describe services available in the community that support elders' desire to live in their own homes with assistance. Also described are sheltered living arrangements that permit those who can no longer live without assistance but do not yet need the level of medical care provided in nursing homes.

Congregate Meals

What can be better than sharing a warm, balanced meal, prepared in accordance with your special dietary needs, with a group of friends? For those who can leave the house, congregate meal programs serve a hot lunch and offer an opportunity to socialize at selected community sites. Transportation to and from the site is included. Additionally, the sites often provide education, outreach, health screening, and social activities.

Funding for congregate meals comes primarily from federal funds that the Administration on Aging passes on to the local Area Agencies on Aging, which then contract with local providers. Although this service is free to everyone, donations are encouraged. This service is discussed more fully in Chapter 10, "Nutrition."

Adult Day Care Centers and Adult Day Health Centers

Just as day care services are provided to children while their parents are employed, adult day care centers provide supervised social, recreational, and health-related activities in a group setting to elders who are too frail to be left alone during the day. Several have special programming for those with Alzheimer's disease. Meals and transportation to and from the site are usually included. For elders with more complex medical needs, some centers offer more health care services. Adult day health centers, in addition to services mentioned above, offer nursing and rehabilitation services. Sometimes adult day health centers or day hospitals are located in a wing of a nursing home or hospital.

Both adult day care centers and adult day health centers are especially valuable for working families who care for a dependent adult. For many families, if a day care center were not available, the frail relative would have to be placed in a nursing home. Even for caregivers who do not work, the program provides a welcome respite. Adult day health centers are more likely to have a high proportion of elders who have dementia and psychiatric disorders compared to other elderly in the community. Medicaid covers the cost of adult day health care, and for those who do not qualify, many centers adjust cost according to income. Unfortunately, many communities do not yet have adult day centers, and those that do often have long waiting lists or strict eligibility requirements.

Multipurpose Senior Centers

Multipurpose senior centers were designed to be the community focal point for older adults—a place to come together to receive services and participate in activities that increase their involvement in the community and support their independence. Two basic types of programming are available: recreation/education and service provision. The recreation/education component is generally seen as the central component of the senior center. Ideally, the program reflects the needs of the elders in the area and should be developed in cooperation with elders who participate in the center. The activities can be as varied as the interests of the center participants and as resources permit.

The service component is also important to the success of the center. The services offered depend on the facility, the local community resources, and the defined needs of elders in the area and of the center participants. The services might be provided directly by center staff, or outside agencies might come to the center on a rotating basis. The services with the highest number of participants are congregate meals, information and referral, and recreational activities. The success of the senior center can be measured by the variety of services and activities provided and the degree of volunteer participation. Depending on the survey, between 10 and 20 percent of the older population utilizes senior centers. The challenge is to find ways to recruit more older people to participate.

Transportation Services

In our society, the ability to drive is a sign of independence, providing ready access to visit friends, go to the doctor, attend social functions, and shop for life's necessities. In the later years, many people reduce their driving miles and some give up driving altogether. In order to freely move within the community, those who do not drive must rely on their family or friends, utilize public transportation, or walk to their destination. Provision of transportation to enable individuals who cannot drive to get to social and cultural events is a high priority for elders.

Transportation services are sometimes part of other community-based services. Many nutrition programs and adult day care programs include transportation services (usually a wheelchair-accessible van). Many assisted living facilities also offer transportation services for residents for medical appointments, shopping, and selected social events. Some communities have implemented a senior taxi service that responds to calls, taking elders wherever they need to go for a low fee. Others have a wheelchair-accessible minivan service that responds to elders' calls. Many times the cost of transportation services is subsidized by federal funds through the local Area Agency on Aging.

Case Management Services

The delivery of long-term services to older people has become complicated, mainly due to the varying qualification criteria and payment mechanisms among the services offered. Case managers, sometimes called care coordinators, assist the client and family to design the optimal package to meet an elder's special medical and social needs: arranging for and coordinating the appropriate services, monitoring the effectiveness of services, and reassessing them as needed.

Hospitals and some local Area Agencies on Aging offer case management services, as do private companies. Fees can be a flat rate or range from about $40 to $120 an hour. These programs enable elders who would otherwise be institutionalized to remain in the community. Case management services are especially helpful for children of frail elders who live some distance away. These services enable the relative to work with a case manager by phone to ensure the elder is receiving appropriate care. Although these services are not inexpensive, the case manager is more skilled in accessing local health and social services than a frail elder or an out-of-town relative.

A good case manager not only can coordinate many services to enable the older person to remain at home but also can facilitate the move to an appropriate sheltered setting when needed. Even if the individual is placed in an assisted living facility or a nursing home, periodic visits by a case manager to communicate with the elder and the health care providers can facilitate continued appropriate care. The National Association of Professional Geriatric Case Managers (www.caremanager.org) has more information.

Coordinating long-term care services can be difficult, particularly in metropolitan areas, because there are so many different services, funding mechanisms, and eligibility criteria. San Diego's Aging and Independence Services (formerly San Diego County's Area Agency on Aging) has implemented an innovative program that simplifies access to the many and varied long-term care services needed by older people and their family members. Called Network of Care, the program provides a single access point for older people and others to locate a variety of long-term care services and to determine their eligibility. Older persons residing in the county can call the Network's Call Center toll-free for information on needed services and be assessed for eligibility for long-term care programs offered by Aging and Independence Services. Callers are referred to other appropriate local programs as needed. The Call Center combines information and referral, case management, program intake, and the elder abuse reporting function. Another way to access information regarding long-term care services is through the Network Web site (www.sandiego.networkofcare.org). The Web site won an award for innovation and quality from the American Society on Aging.

Comprehensive Community-Based Care

The Balanced Budget Act of 1997 authorized an integrated system of comprehensive community-based care for elders who are "dual eligible," that is, eligible for both Medicare and Medicaid funding. The comprehensive option is called Program of All-Inclusive Care of the Elderly (PACE). The program was designed for frail elders who are certified by the state to be eligible for nursing home placement to instead enter an inclusive long-term care program that enables them to remain at home. Services offered include medical care, medications, home care, adult day health center, and social and transportation services. If necessary, the program also pays for hospital and nursing home care.

The On Lok Senior Services in San Francisco, which served as the PACE model (*on lok* means "peaceful happy abode" in Chinese), was created in 1971 to serve the Asian community in San Francisco. The program began with a day care center that also offered health and supportive services to a group of frail elders. In the evening, elders were returned to their families. In 1983, On Lok obtained Medicare and Medicaid funding and other waivers to allow them to experiment with providing both acute care (medical care and hospitalization services) and long-term care services.

The PACE centers combine dollars from Medicare and Medicaid and other sources to enable personalized delivery of individualized social and health services that enhance the participants' health and well-being. The uniqueness of the program is that the providers of the program deliver all medical and social services to participants according to need rather than dealing with the paperwork and restrictions of the traditional Medicare and Medicaid reimbursements. The services have a simple financing mechanism. Instead of each elder participant negotiating complex payment schemes and seeking out various health care providers, PACE receives a monthly fee for each person cared for from Medicare and Medicaid and uses it to provide any services the interdisciplinary team thinks are needed. One limitation is that the elder participants in PACE cannot receive care outside the comprehensive care center.

Upon entry into the PACE program, an extensive evaluation is conducted by a multidisciplinary team to identify an elder's social and medical needs and resources. The team, in collaboration with the elder and his or her family, develops a care plan and delivers all services, including hospital and nursing home services when necessary. The social and medical services are usually provided within an adult day health center, and sometimes in the home, depending on individual need. Periodically, the team reevaluates the client and care plan to modify services. Thus, PACE integrates care between the primary care doctor and the specialist and the hospital, as well as all the community services (day care, transportation, meal programs, etc.) and home care, hospital, and nursing home services—all the while making the

integration seamless to the elder. PACE programs put the health care providers at risk for the costs of care. At the risk of oversimplifying, it works like this—if the health care team can link together services to keep enrollees out of the nursing home or hospital, they can make money, but if the elder requires nursing home placement, the PACE program will lose money. For more information, refer to the Web site of the National Pace Association (www.npaonline.org).

Community-Based Sheltered Living

Community-based living alternatives to nursing homes serve elders who need daily assistance but do not need the 24-hour nursing care and supervision mandated in nursing homes. There are varying levels of care; some provide only room and board and others provide comprehensive services. Standards of care vary among states.

Single-room-occupancy hotels and *boarding houses* provide room, board, and some supervision to physically and mentally disabled adults who are fairly independent but need some protection. Some places might also offer other services, such as personal care, transportation, laundry, and housekeeping, but medical care is not provided. In some areas, there are board and care homes or other licensed entities that provide meals, board,

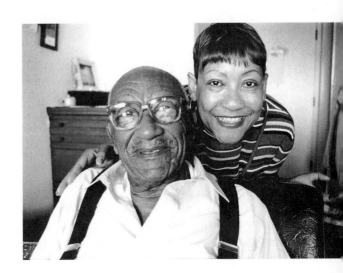

and some supervision. These homes are often licensed and can be large or small within a community or a personal home. The group homes differ widely in size, atmosphere, and amount of supervision and care. Many residents rely on public funding (Supplemental Security Income) to pay for room and board. If that is not sufficient, most states will supplement the SSI income to make up some of the difference between the monthly board and care fee and residents' income, allotting the resident a small allowance for personal needs. These homes are the primary repository for the chronically mentally ill, and they house many other groups of people who need sheltered living, such as those with developmental disabilities.

Ideally, board and care homes provide for supervision and social needs in a safe, secure, homelike living environment. Some board and care homes are family homes in neighborhoods where residents live for years, enjoying home-cooked meals and a sense of belonging. Other board and care homes are run-down and dirty, with inadequate food, isolation of the residents, and little supervision or care. States differ widely in licensing requirements. In some states, only facilities with three or more residents must be licensed. About half the board and care homes in the United States are not licensed.

Adult foster care is geared to an adult population who is unable to live independently. Adult foster care is a type of sheltered living arrangement in which a substitute family provides care and protection for one to four older people in a homelike setting. Usually, the programs are administered by local social service departments and have strict income requirements. Customarily the clients served are developmentally delayed or mentally ill. The family is paid a monthly fee for caring for one or more older persons in their home. A limitation of this program is that it is difficult to recruit foster families so the demand is higher than the available homes.

When elders need more care than they can get at home but do not need the level of care offered in a nursing home, *assisted living* is a good solution. The Assisted Living Federation of America defines an assisted living residence as a special combination of housing, personalized supportive services, and health care designed to meet the needs—both scheduled and unscheduled—of those who need help with activities of daily living. Assisted living is a relatively new type of supportive housing that enables older people to maintain their independence and privacy with their own living space, without having to deal with housecleaning, grocery shopping, and meal preparation. In addition, staff is available to assist with personal care if needed. Many individuals choose assisted living because it is a safe, secure environment and help is available 24 hours a day. Assisted living may be less expensive, is often unlicensed, and may look appealing and offer a little more privacy than board and care or nursing homes. Assisted living residences usually include the following services:

- Three meals a day served in a common dining area (sometimes meals in the room when ill)
- Housekeeping and laundry services
- Transportation
- Assistance with activities of daily living, such as eating, bathing, dressing, toileting, and walking
- 24-hour security and staff availability
- Emergency call systems
- Medication management
- Social and recreational activities

It is important to note that services and assistance offered vary enormously from facility to facility. Some places give almost as much care as a nursing home while others do not offer much more than a room and meals. Ownership of the facility may be church sponsored or government subsidized, but most facilities are private for-profit endeavors.

The costs and quality of assisted living facilities vary greatly. A national study conducted in 2009 report that the average monthly rate for a private room in an assisted living facility is $3,300.[2] The rates also depend on the size of living area, services provided, type of assistance needed, and location of the facility. Some state and local governments offer subsidies for rent or services for low-income elders. Others may provide subsidies in the form of an additional payment for those who receive Supplemental Security Income (SSI) or Medicaid. For instance, if an elder is to be placed in a facility that costs a bit more than his or her SSI payment, the government may provide a little extra money to finance that living situation, to pay for rent or to cover the cost of incidentals. Some states also utilize Medicaid waiver programs to help pay for assisted living services.

In assisted living, residents often live in their own room or apartment within a building or group of buildings and take their meals in a common dining room. Residents usually pay a monthly rent and then pay additional fees for extra personal services. See the Assisted Living Federation of America Web site (www.alfa.org) for an online directory of assisted living residences and tips for consumers on what to look for when choosing a facility.

Assisted living residences must comply with local building codes and fire safety regulations. Although several federal agencies have jurisdiction over consumer protection and quality of care in assisted living facilities, states have the primary responsibility for developing standards and monitoring the care. Licensing regulations vary from state to state. Some states regulate facilities under board and care standards, others developed new standards specific to assisted living, and still others are in the process of developing standards. There is a tension between those who want more oversight and regulation over assisted-living residences, and those who feel that increased regulation will increase costs and decrease access and flexibility. Because of this, it is important for consumers to fully investigate a facility before entering into a contract.

Continuing care retirement communities offer a range of living accommodations from independent living facilities to skilled nursing home care in one location. Continuing care retirement communities allow individuals to "age in place" by enabling an older person to move into the community while independent and providing higher levels of health and supportive care in the same living environment as the person's health needs dictate. The services provided usually include a room or apartment, meals, 24-hour emergency call service, laundry and housekeeping service, recreational facilities, transportation, support services, and guaranteed health coverage for life. Continuing care offers several advantages. Relationships formed in the community may be easily maintained. The stresses of relocation are reduced because moving from one level of care to another is easily accomplished. This type of care eliminates the problem of finding an appropriate level of care in the community with short notice. It also eliminates the problem of financing the high cost of skilled nursing care and gives elders a sense of security.

The cost to move into a continuing care retirement community varies but is high. The American Association of Retired Persons reports that entrance fees range from $100,000 to $1 million and monthly charges can range from $3,000 to $5,000, but may increase as needs change. These fees are dependent on a variety of factors including the health of the resident, the type of housing chosen and the type of service contract, among others. Additional fees may be incurred for housekeeping, meal service, transportation and social activities. A resident who decides to leave the multilevel care home may lose the initial fee. In most cases, the entry fee is lost upon death, but sometimes the family may inherit the apartment. Some of these facilities have gone bankrupt, losing the life savings of elders who lived there. Membership in one of these communities is a major investment decision and should not be undertaken without a great deal of thought and review of the solvency of the organization.

NURSING HOMES

Nursing homes are designed for individuals who need 24-hour care and supervision by a health professional. They provide short-term care for individuals who are recuperating from acute health problems, such as a heart attack, hip fracture, or stroke, to ready them to return home. Nursing homes also serve as "home" for people with chronic physical and mental problems and disabilities. Nursing home placement is sometimes called "institutionalization."

Nursing homes in the United States have a bad reputation. Many people envision frail, drugged, hopeless individuals who are either slumped in wheelchairs or shuffling aimlessly down dimly lit halls that smell of urine, all waiting for death. Media attention on the deplorable quality of care in a few homes with stories of neglect and abuse serve to tarnish the image of the rest. Because of the negative press, most families are hesitant to place a family member in a nursing home. Despite their tarnished image, nursing homes are an important component of long-term care since they are the only alternative when care at home or other living arrangements are not suitable or available.

In fact, nursing homes are more like hospitals these days. Residents live in single or double rooms and bring some of their belongings with them, but space is limited. If they are able, they decorate their corner and walls with familiar objects. They sleep in a hospital bed and most use a wheelchair, walker, or lounge chair/recliner to spend the majority of their days. There are group rooms where people gather during the day and watch TV or play cards, lobbies where people can watch the world pass by, and dining rooms for those who can eat socially. Nursing homes offer recreational activities, and there is a posted schedule of activities (for instance, reading of the newspaper, pet interaction, bingo, Bible study, card games, singing activities, chair exercises, and crafts). Some residents receive physical or occupational therapy. Others participate in programs that keep their joints moving or keep them able to walk short distances.

There is tremendous variability in the physical structure, the quality of care, the price, and the atmosphere of nursing homes. Some homes provide excellent personalized care in a homelike setting, while others provide impersonal, uneven, or even substandard care. They may house only a few residents, or be extremely large. Elders may have private rooms or share with others. Some nursing homes specialize in rehabilitation while others primarily take individuals with chronic health problems. Some nursing homes offer special dementia units with increased security and locked doors to prevent confused residents from wandering from the facility. A few hospitals operate nursing homes inside their walls or nearby. Called hospital-based, transitional or distinct part units, they specialize in treating elders with complex medical problems, such as those who are on a ventilator, and those who need intravenous medication or artificial feeding.

Nursing assistants comprise the majority of staff in nursing homes, and they perform the majority of the hands-on care for residents (e.g., bathing, dressing, toileting, changing diapers, moving them from bed to chair, exercising arms and legs, and more). Nursing assistants can be certified, but the job requires only brief training and does not pay well. Licensed nurses, including LPNs (LVNs in some states) and registered nurses, are available to pass out medications, monitor and assess patients, change wound dressings, run tube-feeding machines, provide IV therapy, and contact the physician when needed. Other staff members may include a dietitian, social worker, therapists, and an activity director. Physicians or their representatives—nurse practitioners or physician assistants—are mandated to visit each nursing home resident at least once a month.

Ownership of nursing homes varies. They may be owned by individuals, hospitals, for-profit chains, nonprofit chains, managed care organizations, religious organizations, or governmental entities. The National Nursing Home Survey is an ongoing series of national surveys of nursing home personnel to gather information on a variety of demographic characteristics of nursing homes and their residents. It began in 1963 and continues to the present. The latest survey reveals that the number of beds is 1.7 million, with the average number of beds per facility at 107. There is also a trend for nursing homes to be for-profit instead of nonprofit and government-sponsored facilities. The survey reported that 61 percent operated for profit, 31 percent were nonprofit, and 8 percent were operated by the government.[7]

Although for-profit large chains may have some economy of scale, there is concern that for-profit chains must necessarily place profit above the quality of care. A national study, using inspection data from almost all nursing homes in the United States, compared deficiency citations and nurse staffing ratios between investor-owned, nonprofit, and government-supported nursing homes. Investor-owned nursing homes had significantly more citations from the licensing agency for substandard care and a markedly lower staff ratio than the nonprofit and government-supported homes.[8] Several studies have reported significant differences in care between for-profit and nonprofit nursing homes. For-profit nursing homes also have worse patient outcomes among high-risk patients than the not-for-profit nursing homes.[9]

The Nursing Home Population

The latest National Nursing Home Survey indicates that 1.5 million people are housed in nursing homes, with close to 90 percent of them aged 65 years and older. The proportion of elders in nursing homes increases with advanced age.[7] While less than 1 percent of those aged 65 to 74 are in nursing homes, 14 percent of those aged 85 and older are institutionalized. However, the proportion of elders residing in nursing homes is lower than most people think: Less than 4 percent of the nation's elder population resides in nursing homes at any one point in time.

Almost three-fourths of nursing home residents are women of all races and ethnicities, and the majority of residents are widowed.[7] These figures are reasonable since men are less likely to need nursing home care because they generally marry younger women who are likely to care for them until death whereas women generally outlive their spouses. Those residents who were married had the shortest length of stay, and those who were single or never married had the longest[7] Childlessness increases the risk that an elder will enter a nursing home, and those who lack a spouse or children often have a longer duration of stay. The average length of time individuals remain in nursing homes is more than two years. About one-fourth of individuals who are admitted to a nursing home die there. Some are discharged to a hospital (30 percent), likely because of an acute illness or worsening of a medical condition. However, many individuals spend a short period in the nursing home for rehabilitation, such as after surgery, an accident, or acute illness, and are then discharged back home.[7]

The most common diagnosis for admission to a nursing home is cardiovascular problems, the second is mental disorders, and the third is nervous and sensory system disorders. Almost half the residents had nine or more medications the day before the survey was taken. Eleven percent had pressure ulcers, most of which were stage two or higher.[7]

Those admitted into a nursing home generally have multiple chronic illnesses, and cannot perform many of the tasks of daily living.[7] More than half needed assistance in four activities of daily living: bathing, dressing, toileting, transferring.[7] Comparisons of impairments between white and black nursing home populations showed a higher proportion of blacks had impaired mobility and were more likely to need help toileting and eating.[7] Check the National Center for Health Statistics Web site for the latest survey information at www.cdc.gov.nchs

As mentioned earlier, ethnic groups are underrepresented in nursing home populations even though they are reported to have higher levels of disability. Researchers offer many hypotheses for this disparity. One hypothesis is that black populations are congregated in the South, where few elders of any ethnicity are institutionalized. Another hypothesis is that ethnic groups may have more extensive kinship networks, which minimize the need for institutionalization. Black elders and their families may not trust the medical profession and care system. They may have a strong cultural bias against institutionalization, or there may not be nursing homes close to their families. Economic strife may result in more adult children living with elderly parents and thus available for caregiving.

Furthermore, black American, Hispanic American, and Native American elders have a shorter life expectancy, and fewer survive to need a nursing home. A lower risk of hip fracture among non-white elders may also explain some of the differences as hip fracture is a common cause of institutionalization among white women. Finally, racial discrimination is a likely barrier that keeps many from receiving such care. It may be that members of this population wait until they are sicker than their white counterparts before they enter a nursing home, possibly for one or more of the reasons mentioned above.

The aging of the population, especially the unprecedented numbers of individuals who are over 85 years old, will likely result in an increased need for nursing homes, whether for temporary care (for example, after a hip fracture) or for permanent care due to physical or mental disability. Further, the greater proportion of older people without children and the greater geographical distance separating children and parents increase the likelihood that older people will face institutionalization.

Nursing Home Costs

Nursing home care is expensive, and the price tag continues to increase, causing a substantial drain on both federal and state budgets and on personal finances. A national survey on nursing home costs in 2010 reported that the average daily rate for a private room in a nursing home was $247 or $90,155/year.[2] Payment for the services of the nursing home usually originates from one or more of the following sources: Medicaid, Medicare, private insurance, managed care programs (PACE), and the residents' personal savings. Upon admission, more than a third of those entering a nursing home use Medicare as their primary source of payment, but many of these become Medicaid patients within two years after exhausting their personal funds. Individuals may qualify for Medicaid when their personal resources are almost depleted. Currently 60 percent of nursing home residents rely on Medicaid to finance long-term care.[7]

Skilled nursing facilities are not required to admit Medicaid recipients but most do. Because of the limited reimbursement available through Medicaid, facilities that rely on a large number of Medicaid recipients can be expected to have less staff and fewer amenities and services than facilities that rely on Medicare or private-pay services. Medicaid pays less per day than it costs to provide care, so a facility often loses money on Medicaid patients. The only way to recoup these losses is by charging private-pay and Medicare patients a little more. Some facilities deny admission to Medicaid recipients who are viewed as medically challenging because Medicaid pays a flat fee for residents no matter how much care they need. Many times the skilled nursing facility accepts a frail elder who is covered by Medicare; then when Medicare runs out or the elder can no longer pay, Medicaid kicks in to enable the elder to stay in the facility.

Nursing Home Regulations

Nursing homes are increasingly subject to extensive regulations intended to ensure that residents are treated appropriately and their rights are respected. Federal and state regulations affect every detail of nursing home care. The particulars of these regulations are beyond the scope of this text. However, an understanding of them is important for everyone caring for older people who are now receiving or may eventually need nursing home care.

The federal government issues and enforces regulations through multiple sources: through the Centers for Medicare and Medicaid Services (which administers Medicare and Medicaid), through Congress and its laws, through the Office of the Inspector General, and through the Health Care Financing Administration, a division of the Department of Health and Human Services. Nursing facility reform regulations, spelled out in the 1987 Omnibus Budget Reconciliation Act (OBRA '87), were the first major revisions of federal nursing home requirements in almost two decades. For the first time specific expectations for nursing home care were required, revolutionizing the standard of care in nursing homes. The regulations were again updated in 1990.

Nursing home regulations are now part of the Code of Federal Regulations (CFR) and the Federal Register. These guidelines have been revised many times as new areas are identified as problematic and new laws and regulations are added. Recent additions to the regulations include an expanded role and responsibility for the nursing home medical director, new guidelines for prevention and management of pressure ulcers, new guidelines on incontinence, and new requirements for pharmacists to review the medications for residents in nursing homes. Regulations also specify the training of facility staff and staff responsibilities from those of the nursing assistant to the administrator, director of nursing, and medical director. In addition, the federal regulations are being changed to strengthen the way in which nursing homes are inspected and the quality of care is monitored. Up-to-date summary information on federal nursing home regulations can be found at the National Long Term Care Ombudsman Resource Center Web site www.ltcombudsman.org: click "Library," then click OBRA.

The goal of the federal regulations is to ensure that the care provided in nursing home facilities meets the highest practical level of physical, medical, and psychological well-being of every resident. The regulations are intended to focus on actual performance in meeting residents' needs rather than on the capacity or potential to provide such care. A facility cannot be licensed and cannot receive payment from Medicare or Medicaid unless it agrees to comply with these regulations and to undergo annual surveys and drop-in inspections to ensure it is doing so. CMS has the authority to apply a wide array of sanctions for noncompliance. Some states have adopted these or similar requirements for all nursing facilities, even those that are not reimbursed by Medicare or Medicaid.

Many states have more restrictive regulations than those required by the federal government regarding the operation of skilled nursing facilities.

For example, California authorities issue licenses for the operation of those facilities, but the county offices of the Department of Health Services are responsible to conduct the surveys and issue deficiencies and citations and, when necessary, revoke licenses. In addition to abiding by federal and state regulations and undergoing surveys, nursing homes are subject to an annual safety inspection by the local fire marshall to ensure compliance with building and safety codes.

The federal government ensures compliance with the regulation in many ways. Currently, facilities are inspected at least once a year at irregular intervals to introduce an element of surprise. In addition, surveyors enter the facility when there is a complaint of abuse or when the facility reports an unusual incident or when a patient or family member or the ombudsman makes a complaint about the facility. The Health Care Financing Commission trains inspectors to oversee nursing homes and ensure compliance with all regulations. Currently, the inspectors must interview a sample of residents and observe their daily routine, meet with the home's residence council, inspect kitchen and dining facilities, review medical records, observe the administration of medications and treatments, and interview the ombudsman assigned to the facility and a sample of family members.

Almost inevitably the review team notes one or more performance deficiencies, areas that need improvement, and the inspector files a report. The inspector issues deficiencies and links the deficiencies to certain aspects of the regulation (e.g., quality of care, quality of life, resident assessment). The facility has to respond to the deficiency or citation with a written plan of correction to ensure that the problems identified have been corrected, that other residents who may be affected by the problems have been assessed, and that there are ongoing activities and review to ensure the problems do not recur.

Deficiencies are classified as to severity. If any deficiency leads to a serious negative outcome, a citation is given to the facility. Facilities can still operate with deficiencies and citations. In rare cases, when a facility is very substandard, the state may send inspectors to monitor the progress of correction for a time or, in the worst-case scenario, may shut the facility down. Deficiency reports are available to the public in a book located inside each nursing facility, at the local Social Security office, at the state health department, and on the Internet at the Nursing Home Compare Web site (www.medicare.gov/NHcompare/).

The effect of so many regulations on the nursing home environment and on patient care can be good or bad, depending on who is asked. From the nursing home administrators' perspective, excessive regulations and demands for documentation prevent staff from caring for the patients. From the inspectors' perspective, inspectors who don't find any performance deficiencies are not doing their job. Inspectors perceive their role as helping the nursing home when they find deficiencies that can be improved. From the perspective of the residents, their families, and the public, any deviation from the high standard of care they expect is unacceptable and the more regulation the better. Ample statistics document that the magnitude of serious deficiencies in nursing homes is unacceptably high.

The Federal Government Accounting Office collects statistics on topics ranging from nursing home ownership, quality, survey and deficiency results, to indicators of care in nursing homes such as the use of atypical antipsychotic drugs among demented elderly. Current and past reports can be found on the Web. In 2009, the Government Accounting Office documented over 50,000 complaints against nursing homes, but found wide regional differences in rate and severity. They reported that large, for-profit chains some of which are private investors, are becoming more common, and it is not always clear who is the nursing facility owner. These chains account for a higher proportion of the homes that provide poor-quality care.

The Minimum Data Set (MDS)

One of the federally mandated aspects of nursing home care is the implementation of regular comprehensive interdisciplinary assessments of every resident, and the results, called the Minimum Data Set (MDS), are reported to the federal government. Nurses and other staff who work closely with each older person complete the assessment. Regulations require that the MDS assessment be performed at admission, quarterly, annually, and whenever a resident experiences a significant change in status. For residents in a Medicare Part A stay, the MDS also is used to determine the Medicare reimbursement rate. These assessments are performed on the 5th, 14th, 30th, 60th, and 90th days of admission.

The assessment includes information on the resident's health, physical functioning, mental status, and general well-being. The document is extensive: demographics, likes, dislikes, behaviors, amount of assistance in activities of daily living, medical and psychiatric diagnoses, treatments received, medications, continence or incontinence, cognitive status, indicators of delirium, physical restraints, disabilities, and abilities. The data are entered on a computerized form by the facility staff and transmitted to the federal Centers of Medicare and Medicaid Services (CMS), where they are compiled and reviewed. CMS provides a monthly report to the facility listing each resident and the "problems" in his or her care that must be addressed—physical restraints, weight loss, loss of ability to do activities of daily living, depression, incontinence, and so on. The facility reviews and corrects the data that CMS has compiled based on the MDS assessment. The facility ensures that the data are accurate (for instance, does Mr. Smith still have an indwelling catheter?) and that each resident has an appropriate care plan that addresses the issues raised in the assessment.

Individual Care Plans

The doctors, nursing activity specialists, social workers, and therapists in the nursing home assess each patient's needs and goals of care. These assessments, combined with the assessment done through the MDS, provide the information needed for care plans. A new concept in care

Case Study: The First Week in the Nursing Home

Ms. Alvez entered the nursing home on the afternoon of August 5. She was exhausted from a long day in the hospital and had been told she was going to the nursing home because she couldn't care for herself at home anymore. She arrived by ambulance at the nursing home and had a sheaf of papers to sign. She was tired and did not understand all the paperwork but felt she could show it to her daughter later on. She was put in a hospital bed in a room with another woman who didn't talk to her. Her bed was by the doorway. A steady stream of people came in and asked her questions, did a physical examination, and asked more questions. They completed more paperwork and appeared hurried, and Ms. Alvez knew she would never remember all their names.

She had dinner in her room that night. The facility quieted down in the evening, and she rested and felt a bit better in the morning. She began physical therapy to assist her in moving from the bed to a chair, and the nurse's aide gave her a shower in a large tiled shower room. A commode was placed by her bed. Because of her stroke, she slipped and fell when trying to use it on her own. The nurse's aide reminded her to use the call bell to ask for help before she moved. Once she pushed the bell, but nobody came and she wet herself. The nurse's aide

apologized and said she had been helping another resident.

In about a week, Ms. Alvez and her daughter met with the nursing home staff. At the meeting, Ms. Alvez's medications, her diagnoses, her diet, her likes and dislikes, and her plan for therapy were discussed. The staff told Ms. Alvez that they were working on her plan of care. They summarized her diagnoses, listed her medications, enumerated the tasks in which she needed assistance, reported their assessment of her ability to think clearly and her mood, and told her she was "at high risk for falls" and was to be put on a bladder program so that she would be taken to the toilet on a schedule. Although the staff were pleasant, they seemed rushed. Ms. Alvez wanted to go home, but her daughter said that she needed too much help and would have to stay at the nursing home for a while until she got stronger.

DISCUSSION QUESTIONS

What went well? What needed improvement? What are some differences among the resident, family, and staff perspectives? What services could be put in place for Ms. Alvez so that she could go home? Who decides where she lives?

planning is the "I" care plan, which presents the resident's story and goals. (See Box 14.2 for three examples.) The individualized plan of care is a federal mandate intended to serve as the cornerstone of care in the nursing home. The doctor makes various diagnoses—both medical and psychiatric—and writes orders for medications and treatments, the social worker identifies psychosocial issues and needs, the dietitian evaluates dietary needs and deficiencies, and the recreational therapist identifies suitable activities. Nurses assess safety risks, fall risk, and pressure ulcer risk and identify nursing needs. Then, in an ideal situation, the interdisciplinary team, the

resident, and the resident's family meet and discuss the resident's problems, concerns, strengths, and resources; identify measurable goals; and set timetables to achieve them. The members of the interdisciplinary team work together to meet these goals through selected interventions. For instance, Mrs. Smith has diabetes. One goal is to maintain her blood sugar in the normal range, and the goal is to be accomplished through a special diet (dietitian), a mild exercise program (recreational therapist), frequent checking of blood sugar and administering insulin (nurse), and checking the person's feet for diabetic ulcers (nurse's aide).

BOX 14.2

Three Individual Care Plans

Mrs. Patricia Smith, age 80
Likes to be called Mrs. Smith

PROBLEM:	Impaired blood sugar control
DUE TO:	Diabetes
GOALS:	To maintain blood sugar in the range of 80–120 for 90 days
	To minimize complications related to type II diabetes for 90 days
INTERVENTIONS/ APPROACHES:	Blood glucose measurement before meals with a fingerstick (RN)
	Administer insulin on sliding scale per MD order (RN)
	Check blood sugar if resident has signs or symptoms of hypoglycemia (low blood sugar), such as sweating, confusion, or decreased response (RN)
	Diet low in concentrated sweets (Dietition)
	Instruct patient and family to avoid highly sweetened foods (All)
	Light daily exercise program as designed by physical therapist (Nurse's Aide)
	Encourage participation in Tai Chi program MWF 10–11 AM (Nurse's Aide)
	Check feet daily for skin breakdown (Nurse's Aide)

Fred Williamson, age 86
Likes to be called "Buddy"

PROBLEM:	Impaired decision-making capability
DUE TO:	Alzheimer's disease, advanced behavioral disturbances related to dementia
GOAL:	Patient will make as many decisions in activities of daily living as able for 90 days
INTERVENTIONS/ APPROACHES:	Approach resident quietly and respectfully (All)
	Offer simple choices, such as "Do you want to wear the red shirt or the blue shirt?" (Nurse's Aide)
	If patient begins to scream, tell him you will come back when he is done, then leave the room and return in five minutes (All)
	If patient becomes very agitated, call his daughter and have patient talk with her on the phone (All)
	Monitor for side effects of Ativan (RN)
I CARE PLAN	A new concept in care planning is the "I" care plan, which presents the resident's story and goals in a more understandable format.
	I am Mildred and I am 78 years old. I am very independent and do not want to be here. I never ever wanted to go to a nursing home, but when I broke my hip, I could not live alone. I want to get better to go back home as soon as I can, but sometimes I am afraid I will never get better. I have pain mainly in the morning, and I tend to not want to get up—I think I am a bit depressed. Please come in quietly and encourage me to get up slowly. Help me move from the bed to the wheelchair. I can pivot on my good left leg if you hold me. I like a blanket placed over my legs. Once I brush my teeth, I often feel better, but if I want to go back to bed or skip therapy, remind me of my goal to go home and see my dog Claire. I can be forgetful about my glasses—please check to make sure I have them around my neck.

When the resident has a new problem or need, the care plan must be updated. The individual care plan must be followed by all nursing home staff. Staff is expected to aggressively prevent deterioration of the resident's medical and functional condition and to justify any invasive procedure, such as a catheter or feeding tube. In addition, special attention must be paid to issues identified as problematic by the MDS assessment, such as pressure ulcers, physical restraints, pain, antipsychotic medication, and incontinence. For example, if Mr. Smith is taking an antipsychotic medication, needs to be physically restrained, and has a urinary tract infection, his care plan needs to be revised. The new plan would aim to reduce his medications by managing his behavior and thereby reduce his need for physical restraint, and it would get Mr. Smith into a bladder training program.

The care plan is only one of many requirements within the complex web of federal and state regulations that govern nursing home care. OBRA regulations cover many aspects of nursing home care—from environmental issues such as the size of the rooms, to staffing of nursing homes, to details about the kinds of care and even the dosages of medications to be prescribed for nursing home residents. Regular medical visits are required—every 30 days for the first three months of care, then every 90 days for Medicaid recipients and every 60 days for Medicare beneficiaries. A physician or a nurse practitioner or a physician's assistant under the physician's direction must review each resident's treatment plan and medications at every visit. In addition, more patients' rights are recognized. Nursing homes are required to survey residents to determine how to increase their quality of life.

Five-Star Rating of Nursing Homes

Just as hotels and restaurants are rated by stars, so CMS developed a five-star rating system for skilled nursing facilities. Nursing homes are given stars for the results of their health inspections, the level of staff they have available to take care of residents, and the results of the data on quality of care. Health inspections occur about every year and examine whether nursing homes are following the state and federal regulations. Generally facilities are inspected by state health departments and all surveys are unannounced. When surveys find many deficiencies or deficiencies that are more severe and more widespread, they get a lower number of stars. Nursing facilities submit the numbers of staff they have available each day to care for the residents to the Centers for Medicare and Medicaid Services (CMS). The numbers include those who are registered nurses as well as lower level caregivers. Staffing data are reported by the nursing home once a year over a two-week time period. Staffing is reported in hours per patient day—how many staff work how many hours divided by the number of residents under their care. Numbers can range from about one hour per patient day to more than seven hours per patient day. Staffing data includes number of staff, but does not include the quality of the staff, the qualifications of staff, staff satisfaction, and staff turnover, all of which can affect the experience the individual resident will have.

Quality measures are also reported by the nursing home. Nursing home staff perform comprehensive assessments of their residents on admission, with transfer to the hospital and return, with change of condition, quarterly and annually. All data are submitted electronically to CMS. CMS uses that data to determine the quality of care the nursing home is providing--is the nursing home immunizing their residents? Do they use restraints? Are their residents losing weight or developing pressure ulcers? Each facility can be readily compared to others in their county, state or the United States. From 2011–2012 quality measures were not reported as the system was moving to a new assessment instrument.

The five-star quality rating system enables the viewer to compare one nursing home to another, but this single measure is not sufficient to make a decision. The five-star rating is not designed to be used alone, but in combination with visits to the nursing home, interviews with staff, and visiting

Advancing Excellence in America's Nursing Homes

A national quality improvement campaign called Advancing Excellence in America's Nursing Homes is under way. The mission of the campaign is to help nursing homes achieve excellence in quality of care and quality of life for nursing home residents across the nation. In order to achieve this, they work with long-term care providers and their associations, consumers, and advocates; nursing home practitioners including nurses, health care professionals, medical directors, nursing home administrators, and certified nursing assistants (CNAs); caregivers and other frontline support staff; government agencies, quality improvement organizations, foundations, and private organizations supporting nursing home education and person-centered care. The eight goals of the campaign include reducing staff turnover, increasing consistent assignment, restricting the use of restraints, appropriately treating pressure ulcers, minimizing pain, discussing preferences and goals for care including advance care planning, increasing resident/family satisfaction, and maximizing staff satisfaction. The campaign provides educational sessions and other resources to help facilities achieve these goals including implementation guides. Each guide includes the campaign goal, flow diagrams, process framework, process review tools, and resources. These guides are designed to assist all nursing homes in meeting their selected campaign goals. More information can be found at their Web site: www.nhqualitycampaign.org

the home to see if there is a good fit. Many individuals prefer to go to a nursing home near their friends and family, or one that shares their religions affiliation or other reasons that are more important to them than the number of stars a facility has received.

Selected Areas of Concern

Several indicators point to problems of concern both to the public and to health professionals: physical restraints, chemical restraint (overuse of sedatives or antipsychotic drugs), pressure ulcers, falls, unnecessary medications, use of catheters to treat incontinence, and abuse of residents. These problems result in lawsuits and bad outcomes for patients, and staff work to minimize them. State and federal regulations use a regulatory approach to solving these problems. Detailed regulations govern care in these homes. Six areas of prime concern are discussed below: physical restraints, chemical restraint/antipsychotic medications, pressure ulcers, staffing levels, hospital readmissions, and elder abuse.

Physical Restraints

Physical restraint devices—belts, vests, pelvic ties, specialized chairs, bed side rails—have been used for years to manage the care of forgetful or unsteady patients to keep them safe. It makes sense, doesn't it? Mrs. E. can't stand well, but she forgets and keeps trying and falls. Why not put a waist belt on her that is attached to the wheelchair? Mr. P. keeps getting out of bed, but he needs help and keeps injuring himself. Why not pull up long side rails on his bed to make it like a crib and keep him in there so he can be safe? Unfortunately, although restraints have been used to increase safety, there is no evidence that they do so and ample evidence that they cause serious problems, including worsened agitation, increased debilitation, pressure sores, incontinence, and even death by strangulation. Further, each resident has the right to be free from any physical or chemical restraints used for discipline or caretaker convenience, unless it is done to treat a medical problem.

A *physical restraint* is "any manual method or physical or mechanical device, material or equipment attached or adjacent to the resident's body

Bed Rails

*Y*ou visit Ms. Smith in her hospital room. She is
lying in a hospital bed and is frail, confused, and
weak. As you leave, you carefully pull up the bed side
rails to keep her safe. You don't want her to roll out
of bed and break a hip.

Bed side rails have been a source of confusion
and ongoing discussion in the physical restraint debate. Hospital beds have rails. They are for safety,
right? Doesn't it make sense to pull up the rails to
keep people from falling out of bed? In fact, evidence
is accumulating that bed rails do not promote safety
for many patients. They serve as an impediment to
getting out of bed, but a confused elder will still try
and may topple over the rails, become entangled in
them, or otherwise sustain an injury by trapping an
arm or a leg between the rail and the mattress. In
1995, the U.S. Food and Drug Administration issued
a Safety Alert regarding the dangers of injury and
death due to entrapment in bed side rails.

This is not to say that bed side rails should never
be used. Bed side rails can help some patients who
are not confused to move and adjust their position in
bed. OBRA regulations permit bed side rails for
mobility purposes. However, if the bed side rails are
used to keep a person in bed, they are considered a
restraint and are subject to the same assessment, informed consent, and attempt to find alternatives as
other restraints.

What are the alternatives to bed side rails? New
hospital beds are able to be kept very low to the
ground. They are raised up to the waist height of the
caregiver but then lowered nearly to the floor. That
way, an elder who falls out of bed falls only a short
distance. Often these newer beds have very short rails
for mobility. Mattresses can be designed with a little
lip on the edge to help an ill elder know "where the
edge is." Mats or pads can be placed on the floor
beside the bed to cushion a fall.

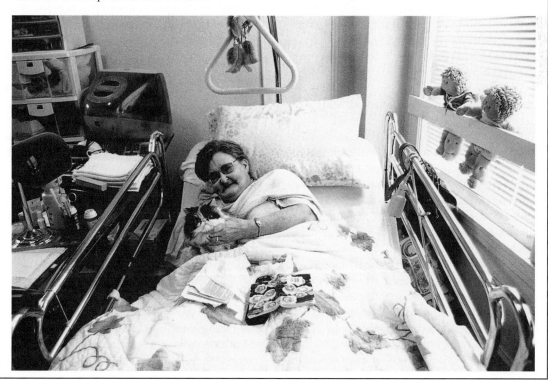

that the individual cannot remove easily which restricts freedom of movement or normal access to one's body."

OBRA did not prohibit restraints. It required a thoughtful process before a restraint could be used, and when a restraint was used, OBRA called for careful monitoring of the restraint and documentation of efforts made to discontinue its use and to find alternative methods. Alternatives include closer resident monitoring, placing residents in low beds with mats alongside, bladder programs (many people try to stand or move because they need to use the bathroom), strengthening and rehabilitation programs, use of assistive devices (e.g., hearing aids, walkers), use of bed and chair alarms to alert staff when a resident needs help, and making the environment safer.

Prior to the implementation of OBRA, an estimated 40 percent of nursing home residents were physically restrained. After the regulation was enacted, this number was cut in half and continues to decline, but levels are variable, differing between facilities and even differing by state. Many facilities in the United States and abroad are able to reduce rates below 5 percent or even to go "restraint free."

Some nursing homes are "restraint-free." When the regulations were enacted, staff were concerned that fewer physical restraints would result in an increase in antipsychotic medications to keep patients from moving. However, this did not occur. In fact, antipsychotic drug use was also reduced when OBRA was enacted.

Restraint use also occurs at home and in the hospital. Use of restraints in the hospital is now regulated, but use of restraints by family members in the home is not.

Families may desire that a family member be restrained. A nursing home or a hospital cannot apply a restraint even if the family insists unless there is a medical diagnosis that supports its use. An assessment needs to precede the application to use a restraint: Why is the patient falling? Is there pain? Infection? Does the patient need to use the bathroom? Are there particular times when the elder is especially agitated? If a restraint is ordered, the patient or family must give informed consent, indicating their understanding of the risks and benefits of the restraint and the alternatives.

Decreased reliance on physical restraints can be accomplished in nursing homes without an increase in staffing. Transition to limited restraint use requires an organized, planned effort to change the attitudes, beliefs, practices, and policies of a facility.

Chemical Restraint

In response to concerns in the 1980s that nursing home patients were being tied down and drugged up, OBRA initiated regulations for the use of psychoactive medication. The use of psychoactive drugs for the purpose of sedating persons or changing their behavior so that they do not place themselves or others at risk is called *chemical restraint*.

The most commonly used psychoactive drugs for chemical restraint are sedatives and antipsychotics. These drugs do have medical purposes and can be used for mental and physical diagnoses. For instance, benzodiazepines can be used for seizures, muscles spasms, or severe anxiety. Antipsychotics can be used for nausea, hallucinations, or delusions. However, when these medications are prescribed to keep elders from getting out of their chair, talking incessantly, or wandering (by putting them to sleep), they are referred to as chemical restraints.

Experts are concerned that too often these drugs are being prescribed as chemical restraints, especially when used in elders with behavioral problems related to dementia. The behavioral problems observed are often things that medications just can't fix (like repeating the same comments over and over again, being restless, or resisting care they don't understand). In these cases, the drugs sedate these elders, sometimes increasing confusion and disorientation. In addition, they can cause urinary retention, constipation, increased risk of falls, diabetes, abnormal movements, and even sudden death.

In response to the overuse of these medications, stringent federal regulations have been put in place. Antipsychotics contain a large warning that they are seriously risky in elders with dementia. In nursing homes, the use of these medications is controlled by dose, diagnosis, and indication. There are mandated drug reductions, meaning the medications must be reduced every few months as a trial, unless there is a medical justification for their use. The nursing home must monitor the patient and carefully document medication side effects as well as have informed consent from the resident or his or her family to continue these medications. Nondrug alternatives such as activities, distraction, redirection, and consistent staffing are preferred ways to deal with the difficult behaviors of dementia.

These regulations have resulted in some reductions in the use of antipsychotics, but they are still prescribed. The federal Office of the Attorney General released a report based on medical records review of claims in 2007. This report noted that half of the Medicare claims for atypical antipsychotic drugs for elderly nursing home residents were questionable, amounting to $116 million. The report revealed that one of six elderly nursing home residents had been prescribed psychotic drugs, primarily for dementia.

Why are these drugs being prescribed so often for elders with dementia, even though they have been shown to be ineffective and have significant side effects? The behavioral symptoms for those with dementia can be very disturbing, and there are no medications available that are approved to treat aggression or the behavioral challenges of dementia. The drugs are effective for some elders with psychosis who experience delusions and hallucinations and for those with long-term mental illness as well as dementia. Although it is likely that these drugs are overused in many cases, in some individuals they reduce symptoms and increase quality of life. Some professionals and caregivers are willing to accept an increased risk of serious side effects for a reduction of symptoms. However, other ways to manage unacceptable behaviors should be tried first.

Pressure Ulcers

One of the most common reasons for lawsuits against nursing homes arises when a frail elder develops a pressure ulcer, also called a bedsore. The latest National Nursing Home Survey reports that eleven percent of nursing home residents have pressure ulcers.[7] Regulations regarding the prevention and treatment of pressure ulcers are comprehensive. To ensure that a facility is providing the best care, inspectors often focus on patients who have developed pressure sores. Nursing homes must maintain a high degree of vigilance to prevent these sores from occurring. The residents of nursing homes are at high risk: They are often immobile and incontinent and have poor nutritional status.

The most effective way to prevent pressure ulcers begins with a comprehensive assessment of risk factors and the implementation of strategies to reduce those risks. For example, Mildred is painfully thin, with bony hips. She has diabetes. She experiences numbness in her feet, she is occasionally incontinent, and she eats like a bird. Mildred is a high-risk patient. Her care plan would address these issues: She might have a special cushion on her wheelchair and a special mattress on her bed. She would be turned in her bed every two hours (even when she is sleeping), and her skin would be checked daily for redness or signs of breakdown. She might have creams applied to reduce friction against the bed sheets or to protect her skin from the irritating effects of urine. Her arms and legs would be moved frequently so she does not develop stiffened joints or contractures. The dietitian might give her nutritional supplements and tempt her with her favorite foods. The podiatrist would examine her feet regularly, and she would have special diabetic shoes fitted. If she does develop a pressure ulcer, the facility is mandated to investigate why it occurred and initiate a plan to treat it and continue to work to prevent others.

Many pressure ulcers are preventable with good interdisciplinary care. Pressure ulcers are discussed in detail in Chapter 6, "Acute Illnesses and Accidents."

Unnecessary Emergency Room Use and Hospital Readmissions

Transitions from one facility to another can be problematic and are associated with higher risk of errors and poor outcomes. When an elder is home, she might receive care from her doctor. When she develops a fever and confusion, she goes to the emergency room and is admitted to the hospital—however, her care there may be managed by a hospitalist physician or perhaps by her regular doctor or someone who works in the same practice. At the time of discharge, she is ready to go to a skilled nursing facility and have a different doctor (hers doesn't practice at that nursing home). Each provider knows the patient at least somewhat, but these various providers rarely talk with one another and share what they know about the patient. The medical record is rarely shared among the providers. Medications can be started or stopped, diagnostic tests can be done and then repeated, and medical records almost never contain all the information really needed to care for the patient well.

Poor-care transitions can be expensive—both in money costs and also in risk. Errors can happen with changes in care—medications are not continued that should be, while other medications are started that may not be safe. Tests are done, but the new site of care doesn't check the results. Every time an elder moves from one site to another, there is a chance of poor communication. What happens too often is missing diagnoses, failing to make and keep follow-up appointments, not knowing what the elder's "baseline" status is, and not transmitting critical information like allergies, diagnoses, advance directives, preferences, and who is involved within the family. Much effort is being expended to look at these care transitions and see how they might be improved. Efforts focus on improving communication among health care providers—for example, through telephone conversations, shared medical records, and easy-to-read summaries. Informing the family about the patient's status and needs helps make a smooth transition. And it is important that one of the health professionals talk frankly about prognosis and end-of-life concerns and whether elders want to go back and forth to hospitals. Policies need to be developed and implemented regarding transition from one facility to another and staff need to be aware of the policy and play a role in transition planning for each patient. Best practices include a process of "teach back" in which staff not only tell elders and their families what has happened and what has to be done, but take the time to listen to what the elder and family understand and have heard. Another best practice is to examine practical barriers (such as transportation, financial) that might hinder the elder from getting the recommended follow-up care, medications, or equipment.

Staffing Levels

Overall, the more staff a nursing home has, the better the care is going to be. Of course, the quality of the staff matters—their training, commitment, attitude, and actions—but at very low staffing levels, even with high-quality care, supervision and care suffers. An area of controversy is the appropriate level of staffing for nursing homes. How many residents can one person care for during the workday? On one hand, the families and patients want even more staff to attend to them, and on the other hand, those who are responsible to pay the bill (or in charge of making a profit for the shareholder) want to be efficient by hiring no more staff than necessary.

Federal regulations are not specific about staffing levels, only that staff be sufficient and that there be a licensed nurse on each shift (and that the director of nursing cannot count as the one nurse if there are 60 or more beds). However, states have filled in the gap with a myriad of different regulations on required staffing hours and ratios. These patchwork regulations cover issues such as how many staff should always be available, which kinds of staff "count" under the regulations, and under what circumstances ratios can be increased or reduced. Some state regulations even specify the hours of the day when various staffing levels are required or what has to happen during break or lunchtimes to make sure there is coverage. At the time of this writing, California and Vermont had the most stringent staff requirements: three hours of licensed staff per patient per day.

Three hours of patient care per day—what does this mean? This means that in every 24-hour shift, a resident of a nursing home will receive 3 hours of some kind of attention from a staff member and 21 hours without direct attention. The attention might be changing their briefs, feeding them, bathing them, helping them to the bathroom or to a chair, giving them medications, or applying cream to their skin. When people think of "24-hour care," they often do not realize that in most facilities, a resident receives very few hours of direct care each day.

Usually, more staff work during the day, when the patient's needs are greater for meals, bathing, morning care, and medications; fewer staff work in the evening, and even fewer at the night shift. It is not uncommon for one certified nursing assistant to have 10 or even 30 or more patients to care for during an 8-hour shift.

Institutional Elder Abuse

All states have enacted elder abuse laws that *require* health care providers to report any type of suspected elder abuse. Mandatory reporting means that every employee in a health care facility caring for elders or dependent adults must immediately report any suspected abuse (financial, physical, emotional, sexual, or neglect) to the state Department of Health Services, which licenses the nursing home, and to the long-term care ombudsman or the local law enforcement. A staff member who fails to make a report could be found guilty of a misdemeanor.

The reported cases are investigated. If abuse is substantiated, the facility may be sanctioned with a deficiency or citation. A health professional who

abuses a patient may lose her or his license. In addition, each state is required to maintain a registry—a list of names of staff accused of abuse. The list is available for review to ensure that these individuals do not go from facility to facility.

One way to reduce the chance of elder abuse in a facility is through careful screening of the staff. A significant proportion of elder abuse in nursing homes is perpetrated by individuals with a criminal record. In 2009, the office of the Attorney General investigated a national sample of 260 nursing home workers' FBI records to determine the extent of their criminal backgrounds. Their investigation revealed that 92 percent of nursing facilities had at least one employee with at least one criminal conviction, although the type of conviction was not identified. A total of 5 percent of nursing home employees of those nursing homes investigated had criminal backgrounds—more employees in laundry, housekeeping, maintenance, and security had convictions than those involved in direct care.[8]

In 2010, President Obama signed the Patient Protection and Affordable Care Act into law. Part of that law requires states to conduct national and statewide criminal background checks on all employees.

One way to stimulate patients, decrease maltreatment, and increase the quality of care is to make sure nursing homes have frequent and many visitors (community "sentinels"). Members of the community may act individually or as an organized group to improve nursing home care in their locale. Some individuals, especially the relatives of residents, can facilitate better care for family members by making unannounced visits to nursing homes to ensure conformity to the Residents' Bill of Rights. It is important to speak out with concerns and report any suspected abuse, neglect, or mistreatment to the ombudsman assigned to the facility. Case managers can be hired to check up on elders, review medical records, and arrange other services as needed.

A recent phenomenon is legal action to sue nursing homes for poor-quality care. Elder abuse has also become lucrative for personal injury attorneys. Many sizable damage awards, including punitive damages, have been granted. Among nursing home employees, fears are increasing that an accusation of abuse could result in the loss of license and livelihood. Agencies in charge of investigating elder abuse, however, are often understaffed and unable to effectively investigate every complaint.

Benefits and Limitations of Nursing Home Care

Nursing home care has significant advantages. The resident has access to 24-hour a day medical supervision, and most of the services needed are at the site. The ability of the staff to collect information on the resident's behavior enhances the opportunity to make effective treatment decisions. Coordination of care is facilitated because many services are located under one roof. Furthermore, the group-living environment provides elders with opportunities for social interaction. Nursing homes must follow multiple governmental regulations that promote optimal care. Finally, nursing homes provide a safe, secure environment for frail elders when nobody is available to adequately care for them at home or when their condition requires medical supervision.

Nursing homes are an important and necessary component in the continuum of long-term care, but they have their limitations. Although the full implementation of the Nursing Home Reform Act goes a long way to improve these homes, many problems are still unresolved. We explore several of them in the remainder of this section.

A major complaint about nursing homes is the difficulty in recruiting, training, and retaining qualified, sensitive staff. Nursing home work is demanding, sometimes depressing, and does not pay well. In many facilities, staff turnover is more than 100 percent a year. High turnover increases training costs as waves of employees come and go and few get to know the facility or its residents well. Registered nurses who work in nursing homes generally perform administrative duties rather than direct patient care, leaving poorly trained and poorly paid nurse's aides to provide one-to-one patient contact. For less than $10 an hour, nurse's aides do some of the most backbreaking work

there is—changing diapers, moving heavy patients, feeding, and cleaning—and may be assigned 16 patients or more. Because they are overworked, nurse's aides are often more concerned with finishing the necessary "bed and body work" than spending time to encourage independence in their patients and offering emotional support. Because of the hard work and low pay, many nurse's aides positions are vacant at any one time, compromising the quality of care.

The atmosphere of nursing homes often feels more like a hospital or institution than like a home, and this environment may not be the best to maximize the function and quality of life of the residents. The buildings are often old and were designed for staff efficiency, not for the residents' comfort. The unvarying appearance of rooms and corridors can cause orientation problems. Glare, caused by enameled walls, waxed floors, and fluorescent lights, reduces vision. Background noise, such as piped-in music, overhead paging, call lights, and institutional clatter, can make hearing even more difficult for the hearing-impaired. The monotony of the days may reduce the type and amount of sensory input. Further, many nursing home residents have uncorrected vision and hearing problems, which exacerbate already serious problems of sensory deprivation.

Although too much care sounds like an oxymoron in an institution caring for the very frail, it can undermine the residents' ability and confidence to care for themselves, causing further dependence and disability. In an environment where there is a lot of help, some people stop doing things for themselves. For instance, aides may insist on feeding elders or using wheelchairs to transport them because it is quicker and easier than allowing patients to feed themselves or use their walkers. It is easier for staff to allow patients to urinate in diapers, or even to insert a catheter, than to help patients get up every two hours to use the bathroom.

Institutional life, no matter what its type or quality, creates an impersonal and depersonalizing environment. The prominent sociologist Erving Goffman asserted in his book *Asylums* that many types of total institutions (e.g., prisons, mental

care in nursing homes, assisted living, and board and care facilities. Each long-term facility in the United States is assigned an ombudsman—a volunteer who is trained and certified by the state to investigate and respond to specific complaints made by, or on behalf of, residents in long-term care facilities. Ombudsmen serve as advocates to improve the quality of care in their assigned facilities and to facilitate a constructive working relationship among administration, staff, patients, and their family members.

In addition to dealing with complaints, the ombudsman can provide general information to potential residents and their families about how to select a nursing home or residential care facility. To contact a local ombudsman, or to become one yourself, contact your local Area Agency on Aging. To find the Area Agency on Aging serving your area, go to www.eldercare.gov

Resident councils provide another way to ensure that the residents of long-term care facilities are satisfied with their care. Resident councils allow a forum for residents to air their concerns and have them addressed. In an ideal situation, a self-governing board of elected residents leads a council that is empowered to make decisions affecting the lives of residents. Unfortunately, these councils may be inclined to make only small decisions (e.g., what movies to see) instead of tackling the larger issues of patient care and patient rights. Generally, an ombudsman is invited to attend meetings of the resident council. Some institutions also have grievance boards to enable patients, family, staff, and administrators to air their differences and arrive at workable compromises without outside intervention.

Assessing Nursing Home Quality

The goal of federal laws for nursing homes is to provide a high quality of care to each resident. But how is quality measured? A quality nursing home might be one that has few residents who have to be physically restrained, or one in which residents have their pain managed or do not get pressure ulcers. The federal government measures quality by using the MDS (described in an earlier section) gathered by the staff from each resident in the

nursing home that is sent to the Centers for Medicare and Medicaid Services. CMS combines the information on several quality measures for each facility and calculates the percentage to determine the performance of each nursing home on the quality measures listed in Box 14.4. The percentages are posted on the CMS Web site to enable consumers to compare the performance level among various nursing homes in their area.

The Nursing Home Compare site is very valuable for potential residents and family members who need to find a good nursing home, for the quality measures from several facilities can be directly compared to one another on the Web site. State and national averages for each measure are also included in the display. A facility that appears better or worse than average either provides lower-quality care or serves a special population. For instance, a facility may have a high number of pressure ulcers because it is a specialized care center for pressure ulcers and attracts patients from other facilities on account of its care, or because it has a high percentage of patients at high risk for ulcers, or because it delivers substandard care and pressure sores develop.

Another measure of the quality of care in nursing homes is staffing ratios: the number of residents assigned to a specific staff member. As mentioned earlier, staffing can also be measured as "hours per patient day"— the number of hours of direct, face-to-face nursing care a patient will average in a day. Hours per patient day and resident-to-staff ratios are important because these ratios are correlated with quality of care. It is intuitively obvious that if one certified nursing assistant is assigned 16 residents to change, feed, and interact with, those residents will get far less attention than if the nursing assistant has only 6 residents to serve. Likewise, a licensed vocational nurse who has to pass medications to 32 residents and assess each of them for pain, infection, or worsened illness is less effective than she would be if she had only 12 patients.

Nursing and patient advocacy groups have introduced legislation in many states to mandate certain minimum levels of nursing staffing, but the overwhelming majority of these bills are defeated.

BOX 14.4

Quality Measures for Nursing Homes

SHORT-STAY QUALITY MEASURES

- Percent of residents on a scheduled pain medication regimen on admission who report a decrease in pain intensity or frequency
- Percent of residents who self-report moderate to severe pain
- Percent of residents with pressure ulcers that are new or worsened
- Percent of residents assessed and given, appropriately, the seasonal influenza vaccine
- Percent of residents assessed and given, appropriately, the pneumococcal vaccine

LONG-STAY QUALITY MEASURES

- Percent of residents experiencing one or more falls with major injury
- Percent of residents who self-report moderate to severe pain

- Percent of high-risk residents with pressure ulcers
- Percent of long-stay residents assessed and given, appropriately, the seasonal influenza vaccine
- Percent of long-stay residents assessed and given, appropriately, the pneumococcal vaccine
- Percent of long-stay residents with a urinary tract infection
- Percent of low-risk residents who lose control of their bowels or bladder
- Percent of residents who have/had a catheter inserted and left in their bladder
- Percent of residents who were physically restrained
- Percent of residents whose need for help with daily activities has increased
- Percent of long-stay residents who lose too much weight
- Percent of residents who have depressive symptoms

Why? More staff costs more money, and nursing home reimbursement is low. Higher staffing costs would be passed to consumers and to the government through Medicare and Medicaid. If required to provide more staff, many facilities could no longer stay open. Because of the importance of staffing ratios in assessing quality, facilities are required to post them on each unit. For each facility, the average ratios of three types of staff (nurses, licensed vocational nurses, and nurse's aides) are posted on the Nursing Home Compare Web site for public review. Just like the other measures, staff ratios can be compared from facility to facility on that site.

A third measure of quality is the number of health deficiencies and citations a facility has received. Various federal, state, and county inspectors periodically inspect all nursing homes and issue reports. These reports are available to the public in a book inside each nursing facility, at the local Social Security office, the state health department, and on the Nursing Home Compare

Web site. A report may contain citations, health deficiencies, and the inspector's comments about other shortcomings. The challenge for the consumer is to determine the seriousness of the violations: To the layperson, all seem serious.

Health deficiencies are classified under broad categories such as "resident rights," "resident safety," and "quality of nursing services" and sound ominous at times. Indicators of the seriousness of health deficiencies are the severity of the outcomes (e.g., did a resident suffer injury or death?) and the pattern and extent of the deficiencies (was the problem identified in only one resident or throughout the facility?). Each deficiency is categorized as (1) has the potential for minimum harm, (2) caused minimal harm or has the potential for actual harm, (3) caused actual harm, and (4) resident is in immediate jeopardy. If a major deficiency is found, a plan of correction is required, which is also available for public review.

Keep in mind that all these measures of quality—staffing ratios, quality measures, and health deficiencies and citations—are available on the Web site Nursing Home Compare (www.medicare.gov/nhcompare/) and are updated at least quarterly. The Web site lists each deficiency and classifies it by level of harm, when it was corrected, and how many individuals were affected.

PLANNING FOR LONG-TERM CARE

All elders, regardless of their current health and ability, should consider their eventual long-term care needs. Elders who do not currently need such services may plan for their future by surveying programs and institutions in the community and discussing their preferences with family and friends. In addition, they must consider how to pay for long-term care. For example, they may determine whether they wish to purchase long-term care insurance or pay out-of-pocket, or whether they are likely to qualify for Medicaid. Reverse mortgages are another possibility for those who have little savings but own their own homes. In this case, the bank agrees to pay the owner a specified amount each month in return for the bank recovering the property upon the owner's death.

Ideally, planning for long-term care is accomplished before the need arises. Too often the recognition that long-term care is needed occurs when an elder is hospitalized from an accident, an acute illness, or a crisis in a chronic illness and is too weak to be sent home without additional help. Many times the need is not recognized until the home situation fails (e.g., an elder falls and is not discovered for some time). When this occurs, hospital nurses and physicians assess the elder's current level of function and potential to be rehabilitated, and they recommend an increased level of care or surveillance. Social workers, case managers, or hospital discharge planners are responsible for discussing long-term care options and financial issues with elders and their families. They can also make appropriate referrals and arrange for home care services or institutional placement. Many times, these plans must be made on short notice because hospitals are under pressure to discharge patients rapidly.

When individuals need 24-hour care or can no longer live independently, families must make the difficult decision between home and nursing home care. When given a choice, most individuals prefer to remain at home as long as possible. Often, family members promise an older relative that "We will never put you in a nursing home." However, home is not always the best choice. Spouses and working children often cannot provide the care needed and cannot afford to pay for further help. If an individual needs more care than the family or community can provide, institutionalization may be the only option. Further, elders might dislike their current living situation and prefer to move to a safe, sheltered environment. Some elders would rather move into an institution than move in with grown children. Finally, caring for frail elders who have severe and debilitating illnesses, such as severe dementia, is often best accomplished in an institutional setting where patients are less isolated and can consistently receive the extent of personal and medical care they require.

When choosing a nursing home, families are often given a list of nearby facilities and are instructed to visit them. Each Area Agency on Aging has a list of nursing homes in its region and a record of violations. Generally, the time frame in which families must select a home is short. The federal government has an excellent Web site to help with deciding which home is best (www.medicare.gov/nursing/overview.asp). Among other information, the site provides a *Nursing Home Checklist* and *Nursing Home Compare,* a listing of a variety of indicators on the past performance of every certified nursing home in the country.

The best place to start is to visit all potential nursing homes in the area. Call in advance for an appointment. Ask the director of nursing or the nursing home administrator to provide you with a tour, an interview, and any descriptive materials. Schedule your visit during a meal. Talk with the residents, their family members, and staff to inquire about their satisfaction with the home. A return visit should be unannounced. If a return visit is not permitted, choose another home. Use a nursing home checklist to ensure that all areas of concern are addressed. Examples can be found on the Medicare site (www.medicare.gov), the National Citizen's Coalition for Nursing Home Reform site (www.nccnhr.org), and the American Association for Retired Persons site (www.aarp.org).

SUMMARY

Long-term care includes a wide variety of health and social services and living arrangements for frail elders in the home, the community, and nursing homes. The need for long-term care services and facilities in this country is increasing drastically as the population ages. Federal and state funds finance much of long-term care, but a significant out-of-pocket expenditure must be made by the elder or family members.

In-home and community-based services include a wide variety of programs provided in the home or community to frail elders to delay or avert institutionalization. Despite the availability of these services, family members still provide the lion's share of home care for their loved ones, often at great emotional cost. Many support programs and respite care services are available in some communities for caregivers to reduce their stress. Also, there are many supportive living environments in the community for individuals who can no longer remain in their own homes.

Nursing homes may be utilized for short stays after a hospitalization, illness, or hip fracture, or they may be a longer-term option. Nursing homes are subject to extensive regulations that spell out the care to be provided, that require every nursing home to publicly report on the characteristics of its patients, and that safeguard residents' rights. Individualized plans of care govern treatment of nursing home residents. Ombudsmen assigned to each nursing home advocate for residents when needed.

There are many advantages and disadvantages to institutionalization. However, to the public, the disadvantages are often more evident. New directions in nursing home care may result in places that feel like home. Planning for long-term care involves knowing what resources are available in the community and understanding funding mechanisms, as well as personal preferences and the availability of family or other support.

ACTIVITIES

1. If you were preparing to enter a nursing home, what five personal items would you consider most important for your comfort and well-being? Contact a local nursing home and ask about the types of personal belongings permitted in the facility.

2. Tour a local nursing home as if you were planning to place a loved one there. Inquire about the following: daily costs, admission requirements, personal items permitted, how roommates are matched, available interaction between residents and the outside community, activities offered within the home, and nutrition services. Observe the activity of the residents. Are services available for residents' families? Use a checklist to gather additional information. Alternatively, two students could go to the same facility, assess it separately, then discuss what differences they reported.

3. Compile a list of home care services for elders in your community. Check with the local Area Agency on Aging. What services discussed in this chapter are not available?

4. Do you think you would prefer home or institutional care? Why? What health problems would convince you that your own institutionalization was necessary?

5. Using material from this chapter and other information about the health needs of elders, design a topic outline for nurse's aide training in a nursing home.

6. If you were given unlimited funds to build a nursing home, what would it be like? Describe the physical environment, staffing, food service, rehabilitation, social, and educational activities, admission procedures, residents' rights, services for families, how residents would participate in

decision making, and interaction with the community. Remember that most residents have moderate to severe disabilities.

7. You have just been hired as a nursing home administrator. List five policies or procedures you want to implement to enhance the residents' quality of care. What arguments will you use to convince the board of directors of the cost-effectiveness or benefit to residents?

8. Do you, your parents, or grandparents have long-term care insurance? Why or why not? Contact a broker who sells this type of policy and inquire about its purchase. Compare rates and benefits among various policies.

9. Interview a case manager or discharge planner from a local hospital regarding his or her opinions about local home care programs and nursing homes. How much time do families typically have to arrange for placement? What options does the case manager recommend? How is the determination between institutional and home care made? What happens if elders refuse to follow recommendations for institutionalization or long-term care?

10. Find out the costs of a nursing home and costs of the same services provided at home to a frail elder and compare the out-of-pocket costs of the two alternatives. How does eligibility for Medicaid affect this financial analysis? Attend a support group meeting for caregivers. Who is there? What issues are addressed? Who is facilitating the group? What did you learn?

11. Identify three local nursing homes and compare data on each from the Nursing Home Compare Web site. Visit each home and review the data on its licensing surveys and deficiencies, which should be posted in an accessible location. Which nursing home would you select for yourself or a family member? Why? What information did you find most important in making this choice?

12. Identify three local home health agencies, and make the same comparisons as in item 11. Which agency would you select and why?

13. Question your parents and grandparents regarding their use of community services. Which services were used? Ask them to discuss their benefits and drawbacks.

BIBLIOGRAPHY

1. Fried, L.P., Tangen, C.M., Walston, J., et al. 2001. Frailty in older adults: Evidence for a phenotype. *Journal of Gerontology: Medical Science* 56:M146–M157.

2. Univita. 2011. National cost of long term care survey. June 2010. www.univitahealth.com

3. National Alliance for Caregiving and AARP. 2009. *Caregiving in the U.S.* Bethesda, MD: National Alliance for Caregiving, and Washington, DC: AARP.

4. Partnership for Solutions. 2002. *Chronic conditions: Making the case for ongoing care.* Baltimore, MD: Johns Hopkins University.

5. Langa, K.M., Chernew, M., Kabeto, M., et al. 2001. National estimates of the quantity and cost of informal caregiving for the elderly with dementia. *Journal of General Internal Medicine* 16:770–778.

6. National Center on Elder Abuse. 2006. Fact Sheet. Abuse of adults age 60+:2004 survey of state Adult Protective Services. www.elderabusecenter.org/pdf/2-14-06%2060FACT%20SHEET.pdf

7. Jones, A.L., Dwyer, L.L., Bercovitz, A.R., and Strahan, G.W. 2009. National Nursing Home Survey: 2004 Overview. *NCHS Vital Health Statistics* 13(167):1–164.

8. Office of the Inspector General. 2011. Nursing facilities' employment of individuals with criminal convictions. Department of Health and Human Services, OEI-07-09-0011.

9. Goffman, E. 1961. *Asylums.* New York: Doubleday.

10. Hamilton, N., and Tesh, A.S. 2002. The North Carolina Eden Coalition: Facilitating environmental transformation. *Journal of Gerontological Nursing* 28(3):35–40.

CHAPTER 15

Dying, Death, and Grief

Life is pleasant. Death is peaceful. It's the transition that's troublesome.

Isaac Asimov

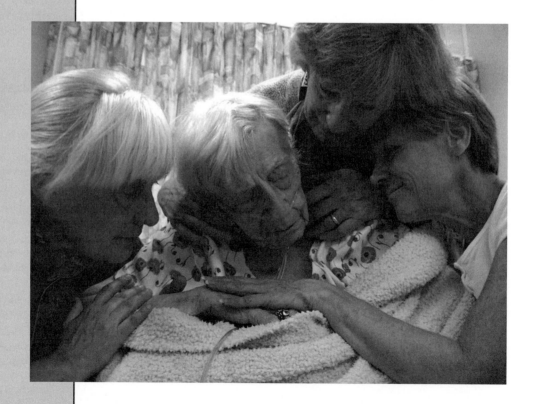

Atext on health and aging is not complete without a discussion of dying, death, and grief since death occurs more frequently among elders than among other age groups. Although that statement seems self-evident, it has not always been true. In 1900, those aged 65 and older comprised only 17 percent of all deaths. Now, about three-fourths of those who die are 65 and older. Reductions in infectious disease, infant mortality, and deaths from childbirth have contributed to this changing pattern. Not only are deaths more common among older people, but also older people more often experience the deaths of family and friends than younger groups.

Professionals working directly with elders, especially those in the health and social services field, inevitably confront death, whether they work with people who die while in their service or deal with others' grief. To be effective, professionals have to face their own attitudes toward death and dying. In this chapter we address issues commonly faced by the dying, the bereaved, and those who work with them.

DEATH DEFINED

The moment of death used to be easy to determine: A person was pronounced dead when the heart stopped beating. Now, the availability of new technology blurs the distinction between life and death. Sophisticated medical equipment can keep the body functioning whether or not the individual is capable of thinking, eating, or breathing. Machines can ventilate the lungs, feed a patient through a tube or a vein, and remove waste products from the bloodstream through dialysis.

The federal Uniform Determination of Death Act in 1981 mandated that each state define death as the loss of all brain function. The brain cells involved in higher thought and voluntary action are the most sensitive when trauma, heart attack, or stroke robs the brain of oxygen. Some believe these cells are irreversibly damaged after less than six minutes without oxygen. If an individual is revived after the brain has been deprived of oxygen for more than a few minutes, the lower brain—less sensitive to oxygen deprivation—can be revived, and heartbeat and respiration will continue. However, these individuals show no evidence of higher brain function as measured by an electroencephalogram (EEG) and are considered "brain dead." In practice, an EEG is rarely done to determine death. Instead, the absence of spontaneous heartbeat and breathing and the loss of pupil response to light are used as indicators.

There are many levels of near death states that are referred to as coma. Individuals may be unconscious and unable to be awakened, but not dead. In a deep coma, a person cannot be awakened, even with pain, light, or sound. The person lacks the normal sleep-wake cycle and does not generally move in a directed way or react to the outside environment. A person in a coma is said to be comatose. However, in general use, the word *coma* refers only to the deepest state of unconsciousness, but other "lighter" states can also be thought of as coma. One of the most common ways to measure coma is the Glasgow coma scale. This scale evaluates whether individuals open their eyes on their own, or respond to loud noise, pain, or not at all; whether they can speak at all and whether the words make sense; whether they can obey a command or withdraw from pain; and whether they have begun to develop the abnormal body positioning that occurs when the brain is injured. Coma is serious and the prognosis depends on what caused it. Strokes, overdoses, low oxygen, low blood sugar trauma, and hypothermia can all cause coma. Sometimes comas are reversible and a person returns to nearly the state he or she was before, but other times, even if the individual wakes up, functioning will remain impaired. Individuals who have suffered extensive brain damage may pass into a chronic state of unconsciousness and have no self-awareness. They may spontaneously open their eyes, make unintelligible sounds, or make facial movements; however, they cannot speak coherently, comprehend speech, or make any voluntary movement. When the condition lasts for more than a few weeks, it is called a persistent vegetative state.

A *persistent vegetative state* is permanent and irreversible unconsciousness in which there is no voluntary movement or behavior or thinking or reaction, and the individual cannot communicate or interact with the environment. A persistent vegetative state exists when a person is awake but not aware. The person may sleep and awaken or may always appear to be awake. Some automatic behaviors such as smiling, grunting, moaning, puckering the lips, or crying tears may occur, but there is not a consistent stimulus that brings on these behaviors. Most health professionals feel that individuals who are truly in a persistent vegetative state never recover; some reports of people recovering are usually thought to be due to an initial misdiagnosis.

One important consideration for those with dementia is their capacity to make decisions for themselves. In the United States, there is a legal presumption of competence for adults—that is to say, all adults are presumed to be competent to make their own decisions unless proven otherwise by a court of law. When a court proves someone is no longer competent, the court orders a conservatorship or guardianship—someone to make decisions for that person. Some elders, especially those with severe mental illness or developmental delay/mental retardation, may have guardianships or conservatorships. However, the majority of elders with cognitive decline do not. For most elders with dementia, a family member helps them make decisions when they can no longer do it themselves. Some elders have considered in advance whom they wished to make decisions for them if they could not do it themselves and have created an advance directive. If they have not, some states have hierarchies (for example, the spouse would be the first asked, and if he or she cannot, the oldest child, etc.), while others state that the person who is the closest and showing the most interest and concern should be the one making the decision.

How do we know when elders cannot make their own decisions? First, decision making is not all or none. For example, an elder who is impaired may be able to decide what to wear and who can visit, but not be able to make the informed consent decision to have a surgical procedure. However, if there is no conflict—for example, the health care team, the individual, and the family all agree what is the best course of action—then there is usually no difficulty. The difficulty arises when there is conflict—either the health care professional wants to do something that the patient or family refuses, or perhaps the elder refuses something, but the family wants him or her to have it. When conflict occurs, one of the first steps is to determine whether the elder has the capacity to make his or her own decisions on this issue.

In most cases, a clinical capacity determination is made—the person is asked questions, and the answers determine the person's ability to make decisions. To make a clinical capacity declaration, individuals are assessed as to whether they understand the decision to be made and its risks and benefits, whether they can communicate a choice, and whether they can provide a reason or explanation for their decision. For example, the doctor recommends an amputation of the leg. If an elder can state, "You want to cut off my leg because the wound is so bad you don't think it will ever heal. The surgery has a small risk of death, but without the surgery the risk is greater, and I may not even live a month. I choose to keep my leg—I am ready to die anyway, and I want to die with my leg," then this demonstrates that the elder can make his or her own decision. On the other hand, if the elder only says "No, no, no, go away" and cannot understand, reason, or communicate his or her decision, then a surrogate may be appointed.

When a surrogate makes an important decision for an impaired individual, the surrogate is supposed to act under an ethical concept called *substituted judgment,* which means the surrogate makes the decision the elder would have made if not impaired. So, in the example above of the elder who cannot make the decision and just says "no," his wife would be asked, "If he could tell us what he wanted, what do you think he would have chosen?" If the wife said, "He always hated doctors and didn't want anything extending his life," this would be substituted judgment, and the health care team would likely honor this as his decision. If the wife had no idea what he would have wanted, then she can use another ethical construct called *best interests*. In this case, she would be asked to make the decision in his best interests—maybe this would be to get the life-saving surgery, but maybe, if he had a lot of other problems, had been suffering, and had a low quality of life, her assessment of his best interest would be to allow a natural death.

It can be difficult to be a surrogate—a surrogate is often emotionally involved with the patient and has to make a complex "life and death" decision while very sad, fatigued, or overwhelmed. Sometimes there is conflict in the family about what is the best course of action. For example, what if the wife stated that the surgery should not be done, but an out-of-town daughter called and insisted the surgery be done right away? Some surrogates may themselves have dementia or another mental illness. Many people are worried about doing the wrong thing. Perhaps they tell the health care team, "Do everything you can," or ask for advice. For very complex cases, ethics committees can help. There can be cultural differences, which add stress or complexity to the process. Surrogates can feel guilty about participating in this kind of decision.

Individuals can make things easier for their loved ones by completing advance directives (discussed later in this chapter). As part of the advance directives, individuals should choose a surrogate or surrogates to make their decisions if they are unable and should discuss their values and preferences in advance so that those who have to make these tough decisions have a better understanding of what the individual wants.

WHO SHOULD DECIDE?

Most of us would like a quiet, dignified death. Anyone who works in a hospital knows that this reasonable wish is almost never fulfilled and most of us now die in hospitals. The last rites of respirators, dialysis machines, nasogastric tubes and gastrostomy tubes along with cardiopulmonary resuscitation and the nth round of chemotherapy are wonderful when prolonging useful life but have changed death into a mechanized spectacle in which no sane person would like to be the main actor.

—C.M. Kjellstrand[1]

The advances of technology have created many complicated ethical dilemmas. Most people will agree that maintaining life at any cost is not necessarily better than death. However, there is a controversy surrounding the role of individual choice in dying and who should decide—the patient, the family members, the physician, or the law. Although most people support the right of conscious, mentally stable adults to refuse medical treatment even if it means death, who decides when very frail individuals are not able to decide for themselves? Should life be artificially prolonged if there is only a minute chance of recovery? If not, then who should decide when a life is no longer of worth and death should be allowed? Should a relative, friend, or physician be permitted to assist a terminally ill patient to die more quickly? Although it is generally accepted that life-sustaining measures, such as feeding tubes and ventilators, may be refused, who should decide whether they are to be removed once they are in place? If a person suffers a heart attack, who should decide whether resuscitation should be initiated or not? Should family members be permitted to request that everything be done to keep the patient alive, even if the chance of recovery is minimal, the treatment causes pain for the patient, and the cost of the treatment is exorbitant and borne not by the individual but by the taxpayers? When does the cost of care become a part of the decision?

Whether or not measures are implemented to maintain life depend on the patient's age, the patient's income, the preferences of the patient and family, the type and severity of illness, and

What Is Your Opinion?
The Case of Terri Schiavo

Theresa Marie "Terri" Schiavo captured the attention of the country in 2005 when the conflict and legal wranglings between her husband and family became the main topic of conversation in many homes about the "right to die." Ms. Schiavo suffered sudden and unexpected cardiac arrest and collapsed in her home in early 1990. Due to lack of oxygen, she suffered massive brain damage and remained in a coma for more than two months. When she regained consciousness, she was found to have little reaction to her environment, and within three years she was diagnosed to be in a persistent vegetative state. Despite intensive attempts to rehabilitate her, she remained in this condition.

Beginning in 1998, eight years after Terri's collapse, Michael Schiavo, her husband and guardian, petitioned the courts to remove the feeding tube that was keeping his wife alive. He stated that she had expressed to him that she would not want to live in this way. The courts agreed to his petition. However, Terri's parents, Robert and Mary Schindler, did not want the feeding tube removed and submitted appeal after appeal against their daughter's husband. By March 2005, the legal history around the Schiavo case included 14 appeals and innumerable motions, petitions, and hearings in the Florida courts; five suits in federal District Court; and four denials from the United States Supreme Court. The governor of Florida, the U.S. Congress, and the president of the United States used extraordinary measures to support Terri's parents in their desire to not remove her feeding tube.

In October 2003, when the family lost their "last" court battle, the Florida legislature passed "Terri's Law," giving Governor Jeb Bush the authority to intervene in the case. Bush immediately ordered the feeding tube to be reinserted. Later, Terri's Law was found unconstitutional and when it was overturned, the Republicans in the U.S. Senate took action. They decided to subpoena both Michael and Terri Schiavo to testify at a congressional hearing. This maneuver was intended to provide protection to Terri by threatening her husband with legal action if he interfered with her role as a "witness." However, Congress did not enforce the subpoenas. Then, the Senate tried something else. On March 20, 2005, the Senate, with only three members present, and the House passed a law that transferred the case into federal courts. The bill passed the House on March 21 at 12:41 a.m. EST. President George W. Bush interrupted his vacation in Texas to travel to Washington, D.C., in order to sign the bill into law a half hour later, at 1:11 a.m. EST.

All these interventions from politicians did not change the outcome. All of the Schindlers' federal petitions and appeals were denied, as they had been in the state courts. The United States Supreme Court supported the decisions of the lower court that Terri Schiavo was in a persistent vegetative state with no hope for recovery and would want to end life support. Her feeding tube was removed a third and final time on March 18, 2005. She died at the hospice on March 31, 2005, at the chronological age of 41.

The case and the legal wrangling and political grandstanding were all over the papers. Politicians, physicians, religious figures, "right to life" advocates, and supporters of the "right to die" made their opinions known.

DISCUSSION QUESTIONS

Who was in the best position to decide what was right for Terri, given the fact that an advance directive wasn't completed? The doctors, the husband, the parents, the politicians, the courts, the president? Defend your answer.

If you had a strong belief that something was morally wrong and that a political or legal decision was going to result in a needless death, what would you do?

Would you make a different decision if Terri was 70 years old? 90 years old?

Was letting Terri die a humane act, or was it an invalidation of the worth of the disabled?

What is your opinion regarding the withholding of artificial nutrition?

What would you have done if you were Terri's husband and had to make this decision?

What would you want done if this happened to you?

Source: Information gathered primarily from http://en.wikipedia.org/wiki/Terri_Schiavo

the prognosis. For example, an elderly person with widespread cancer who finally succumbs to pneumonia will generally not be resuscitated, tube-fed, or put on a ventilator. But a young college student involved in a serious motor vehicle accident would probably be aggressively treated even if his or her chance for recovery was minimal. Even in the face of an extremely poor prognosis, some patients or their families are adamant that "everything should be done," including treatments that may be medically futile. In other cases, people with a good chance of partial recovery may refuse life-extending treatment, perhaps motivated by fear of prolonged suffering.

Ethical issues surrounding care at the end of life become more complex when the cost of treatment is considered. Although patients themselves are somewhat insulated from the actual costs, it is true that money allocated to health care is limited. It is commonly believed that the aging of the population, combined with newer, more expensive technology to prolong life, has markedly increased the costs associated with care for the dying. Actually, the proportion of Medicare funds for medical care during the last year of life has remained fairly stable over the past 20 years—about one-fourth of the Medicare budget. Interestingly, the older one is at death (especially those 85 and older), the fewer Medicare resources are spent during the last year of life, largely because the aggressiveness of

medical care in the last year of life decreases with increasing age.[2]

What proportion of the nation's health care dollars should be spent on the terminally ill, especially those who are very old? There is an ongoing debate about the best use of scarce health care resources. On the one hand, utilizing health care dollars (provided by the government or insurance companies) to support a dying patient results in fewer resources for other patients, many of whom have a better prognosis. On the other hand, it is difficult to place more value on one person's life than on another's. The dilemma takes on a different focus when the dying individual is you or your loved one.

ADVANCE DIRECTIVES

Advance directives are legal documents that enable individuals to convey their desires about life-prolonging medical treatment when they are no longer able to make their wishes known. Ideally, advance directives are completed *before* the person is ill, to provide information to help health professionals and families make difficult medical decisions. Although the directives are completed when individuals are mentally competent, they are not enforced until individuals can no longer decide for themselves. Without advance directives, medical care teams may do everything possible to keep

---

Ethicist Callahan: 'Set Limits' On Health Care
By Beth Baker

For decades, Daniel Callahan has argued that expensive medical care be parceled out carefully–essentially rationed–for elderly patients. Now, at 79, his quest to stem late-in-life spending is coming face to face with his own mortality.

Twenty-two years ago, the co-founder and president emeritus of the Hastings Center, a nonpartisan

bioethics research institute in New York, wrote the highly controversial book, "Setting Limits—Medical Goals in an Aging Society." It made the case for limitations on care based on age–a topic that recently provoked intense, if sometimes hyperbolic arguments during the health care debate—and against the provision of extraordinary,

Continued

Continued

Ethicist Callahan: 'Set Limits' On Health Care
By Beth Baker

expensive medical procedures for people who have already lived a full life. But recently Callahan himself underwent $80,000 worth of treatment for a heart condition.

That drew a rebuke from blogger James Pinkerton, a fellow at the New America Foundation. He called Callahan a hypocrite for having the expensive heart procedure.

Callahan laughs off the criticism, but notes that his experience is indicative of the difficulty in trying to contain medical costs. After a period of dizzy spells, he fainted last summer, and his cardiologist insisted he go straight to the hospital. The doctors diagnosed a ventricular tachycardia, or rapid and irregular heartbeat that starts in the ventricles, and performed a seven-hour ablation procedure that burns off tissue causing the problem. Before he knew it, Callahan had received $80,000 worth of treatment.

When he asked, his physician didn't even know the price tag. That's why, he says, decisions can't be left to individuals and their doctors.

"I want Medicare to determine what benefits it will make available, based on costs and other considerations, and then simply not pay for those that don't pass their tests," he says. That doesn't sound especially incendiary–except that Medicare isn't supposed to consider cost and the health overhaul bills in Congress bar the program from using the results of comparative-effectiveness studies to decide what to cover.

His new book, "Taming the Beloved Beast–How Medical Technology Costs Are Destroying Our Health Care System," critiques costly pharmaceuticals and medical devices that Callahan says drive costs ever upward. "Our whole health care system is based on a witch's brew of sacrosanct doctor-patient autonomy, a fear of threats to innovation, corporate and (sometimes) physician profit-making, and a belief that, because life is of infinite value, it is morally obnoxious to put a price tag on it," he writes.

He has written or edited 41 books and amassed a host of professional honors, but Callahan also has plenty of critics. Dr. Kenneth Prager, professor of Clinical Medicine at Columbia University Medical Center and director of clinical ethics for the hospital, said he considers efforts to limit who gets treatment "unethical and arrogant."

"I have patients that I'm sure would be considered to have an awful quality of life who are taken care of and loved by their families and to whom every day is of inestimable value," Prager said.

Callahan, however, continues to believe that after people have lived a reasonably full life of, say, 70 to 80 years, they should be offered high quality long-term care, home care, rehabilitation and income support, but not extraordinary and expensive medical procedures. He rejects the effort to find a medical remedy to every condition. (Of erectile dysfunction, he says, "You get old. That's the way it goes, guys.")

He has little faith that political leaders will set limits he deems necessary. Calls to cut waste and inefficiency have been made for decades, he says, to no effect. "Liberals believe in progress and are heirs to the enlightenment," he says, "and conservatives want individual choice." Neither address the heart of the problem.

QUESTIONS TO PONDER

We are developing new and expensive technologies to keep people alive and Medicare funds are limited. Limits need to be put in place.

But who should set those limits-the marketplace? state or federal your own physician?

Is it better to cover treatments that benefit the young rather than those who only provide small benefits to those who are already aged and disabled?

This article was excerpted from kaiserhealthnews.org with permission from the Henry J. Kaiser Family Foundation. Kaiser Health News, an editorially independent news service, is a program of the Kaiser Family Foundation, a nonpartisan health care policy research organization unaffiliated with Kaiser Permanente. Beth Baker is author of "Old Age in a New Age—The Promise of Transformative Nursing Homes" someone alive or may have to rely on decisions made by family members who do not know what an individual would really want. It is suggested that all adults complete an advance directive and discuss personal choices with family members. Because older people are at higher risk of becoming ill or dying than other age groups, they are encouraged to prepare advance directives and sign legally binding documents regarding medical treatments while still mentally capable.

The two most common advance directives are the living will and durable power of attorney for health care. A *living will* outlines specific medical treatments to be withheld or withdrawn in certain situations. Living wills are usually generic and focus on choices of specific interventions, such as cardiopulmonary resuscitation (CPR), artificial feeding, or use of a ventilator machine. *Proxy,* or *durable power of attorney for health care,* specifies the name of a family member or friend to assist in medical decision making for the individual who is no longer physically or mentally competent. A durable power of attorney for health care is more flexible because the individual appoints a trusted person (also called a proxy or surrogate) who ideally makes decisions based on the individual's wishes and in the individual's best interest.

Each state has its own specific requirements regarding advance directives. In general, these documents must be signed and witnessed when a person is mentally capable. A witness should not be a blood relative or beneficiary of property. Completed copies of the document should be kept in the home or car and given to physicians and family members and a copy should accompany the individual to the hospital or nursing home to be included in medical records.

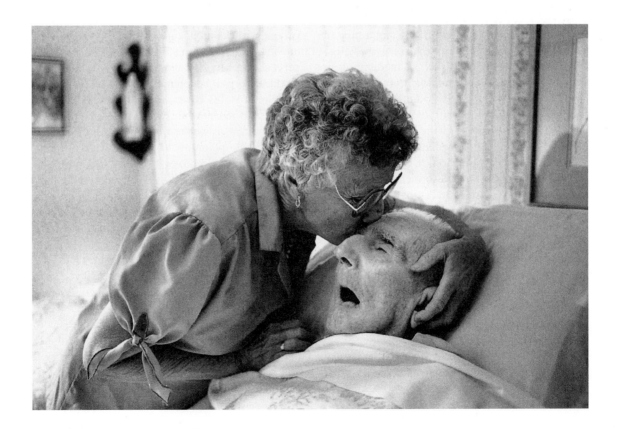

Federal law, the Patient Self-Determination Act of 1990, gives certain rights to individuals who are in hospitals, nursing homes, and other institutions that receive Medicare or Medicaid funds: (1) the right to participate in and direct their own health care decisions, (2) the right to accept or refuse medical or surgical treatment, and (3) the right to prepare an advance directive. The law further requires all health care institutions to provide written information regarding advanced care directives to all patients and residents on admission. For those who do not have the mental capacity, the information must be given to the family or surrogate. The act also prohibits institutions from discriminating against patients who do not have an advance directive. Finally, the law requires institutions to document patient information and provide ongoing community education on advance directives.

The DNR order (do not resuscitate) is an advance directive particular to cardiopulmonary resuscitation (CPR) procedures used when the heart stops or the person stops breathing: artificial respiration and intubation (placing a tube in the airways), chest compressions or use of electrical stimulation to the heart, or medication to support or restore heart function. If an individual (or the surrogate) does not want to be resuscitated, a conversation is initiated with the physician, who then writes up the DNR order and places it in the person's medical records (usually at the hospital or nursing home). Only physicians can write DNR orders. Unless such orders are on file, CPR is provided to every patient who has cardiac or respiratory arrest in a hospital or nursing home.

If a person is dying at home and does not want to be resuscitated, the physician may need to write, and have the individual or surrogate sign, a prehospital DNR order to be kept in the home to show emergency personnel. More than half the states have prehospital DNR programs. Some states also utilize DNR bracelets or medallions similar to the Medic Alert bracelets.

If an individual has an advance directive, such as a living will or durable power of attorney for health care, this document should be available in the home. Not all states honor prehospital DNR orders or advance directives when emergency medical personnel are called to a home. Even if a state accepts such documents, if they cannot be found, emergency medical personnel called to the home are required to start CPR procedures. On the other hand, the DNR order can be revoked by destroying the document or telling the paramedics to disregard the order.

When death is anticipated, the family needs to resist calling 911 for emergency medical assistance. Physicians and hospice workers need to be able to reassure families that they can support their loved ones in privacy and comfort at home with nonparamedic resources (e.g., a hospice nurse) when death is imminent.

A new paradigm is gaining popularity in many U.S. states in regard to advance planning. The Physician Orders for Life-Sustaining Treatment (POLST) program is designed to improve the quality of care people receive at the end of their lives. It is based on effective communication of patient wishes and documentation of these wishes and medical orders on a brightly colored form that serves as a physician order, like a promise by health care professionals to honor these wishes.

Some states have individually developed a form that is meant to serve as a physician note and order for care, as well as a record of a discussion on advance care planning. These forms are different from advance directives because they are completed with and signed by a physician and are honored as a physician order in hospitals, nursing homes, by emergency medical personnel, and in the home. These forms prompt certain discussions: If you developed pneumonia and needed a tube to breathe, would you want that to happen? If your hearts and lungs stopped suddenly, would you want CPR? Do you want to have a tube placed for feeding if necessary?

Many individuals elect less formal means to convey their preferences regarding end-of-life care. Perhaps as a reaction to the living will and other directives that state what treatments individuals do *not* want, a *life-prolonging procedures declaration* requests the use of all medical

Physician Orders for Life-Sustaining Treatment

Physician Orders for Life-Sustaining Treatment (POLST) is a new program being implemented state by state to find out what people want for end-of-life care and to document it in a way that is quick and easy to understand and that will be honored across the health systems.[3] The POLST program began in Oregon in the early 1990s. By the beginning of 2010, at least 12 states had adopted the POLST paradigm, and proponents in most other states were developing programs. The idea for POLST is different from advance directives in that POLST involves a structured conversation between a health care worker and a patient. The patient's preferences are stated on a form that is standardized, recognized as a physician's order, and can travel with the individual. It is actionable—that means if the patient is unconscious and the paramedics come in and see a POLST that says do not resuscitate, they are protected if they do not try CPR. States have used differing terminology for the POLST program, including POST (Physician Orders for Scope of Treatment), MOLST (Medical Orders for Life-Sustaining Treatment), MOST (Medical Orders for Scope of Treatment), and COLST (Clinician Orders for Life-Sustaining Treatment). Two states (Oregon and Minnesota) used clinical consensus rather than

legislation to establish POLST, while 10 states used legislation of varying nature and complexity. In all cases, the POLST form can be signed by a doctor; however, in some states a nurse practitioner or physician assistant are also allowed to sign it. POLSTs are not mandatory and are designed for those with significant illnesses for whom death is a possibility in the next few months or years.

Problems identified include the following:

- How do you tell if the person who is signing it is able to make that kind of decision for him- or herself and is not being coerced?

- Who can sign it if the patient cannot?

- How can this form be integrated into various medical records systems and electronic records?

- How do we make sure physicians have these conversations with patients and those who care for them?

Various states have slightly different forms and policies and rates of implementation and success. The Web site of the Oregon Health Sciences University is a good place to seek information on the policies of each state (www.ohsu.edu) and type POLS in the search bar, then click on In Your State.

procedures that would extend life without regard to the cost or chance of recovery. *Organ/tissue donation* is another type of advance directive for individuals who want someone else to benefit from their tissues or organs after their death. Many states include an organ/tissue donation card as part of the driver license registration. Contact 1-800-DONOR or www.organdonor.gov for more information.

The simplest advance directive is talking to a health provider or family member about preferences and decisions regarding end-of-life care. Whether or not individuals complete a formal advance directive, it is important for them to discuss their preferences with the people who may be

called on in the future to make decisions on their behalf.

Advance directives are theorized to provide proof of the patient's wishes when the patient is no longer able to make decisions, but studies show they are not widely used in decision making for care of the dying. Studies show that advance directives are becoming more common, but are underutilized in nursing homes and among elders living at home. In 2004, 28 percent of elders receiving home care had advance directives, nearly 70 percent of nursing home patients did, and nearly all hospice patients did. The most common advance directives were "do not resuscitate" orders or living wills.[4]

Research indicates that the preference for having an advance directive can be influenced by individual attitudes, cultural beliefs, health conditions, and trust in health care professionals. Those with more education and whites are more likely to complete an advance directive than those of other ethnic backgrounds and educational level. Blacks may distrust health professionals and the health care system and worry that a do-not-resuscitate order will be an excuse to "do nothing" for them or their loved ones. Those with illnesses that are more likely terminal, such as cancer, may be more likely to complete an advance directive than those with diseases like cardiac or pulmonary chronic disease who are less sure when the end of their life is near. An important factor is the comfort the health care professional has in discussing the prognosis and advance directives. If physicians, nurses, or social workers never discuss these issues with patients, they are less likely to complete an advance directive. Decisions on end-of-life care will fall to the physician, family, or a court-appointed guardian.

Why are advance directives not more widely used? Healthy people may not complete a living will because their death seems so far off. Others may not want to think or talk about their death, and still others know nothing about end-of-life planning. People may mistakenly believe that completing an advance directive gives away the opportunity to make their own decisions. Or they may not know which family member or friend would be the best choice. Individuals rarely discuss their end-of-life wishes with their physicians, and copies of advance directives (from home or nursing home) too often do not make it to the hospital to influence decision making there. Further, advance directives may be completed without full knowledge of all the potential issues that may arise in the future.

It is common for people to change their minds over time about what type of life-prolonging technology they would desire and under what circumstances. For instance, an individual may believe that if she became dependent on a ventilator she would not wish to live. However, if this situation actually happened, she might change her mind.

Individuals with multiple disabilities often have a high quality of life if they have appropriate supports and care.

It is difficult to predict the situations that might come up and to write a directive detailed enough to handle all contingencies. There are hundreds of possible scenarios, and it is impossible to micromanage one's own dying before one becomes ill. For instance, a person may refuse chemotherapy for one type of cancer because of its poor success rate but choose to undergo this treatment for another type of cancer. A person may not desire artificial feeding in one situation but be willing in other circumstances.

The average citizen knows precious little about the realm of therapeutic possibilities that differ substantively from one diagnosis to another. Without knowing the benefits and risks of each type of life-extending procedure for one's personal situation, how can anyone make a good choice regarding cardiopulmonary resuscitation, artificial feeding, intravenous fluids, intensive care, chemotherapy, or surgery? Because so few patients understand advance directives, it is questionable whether advance directives truly represent the patient's wishes.

It can be challenging to imagine situations in which you cannot speak for yourself. News stories in 2005 about Terri Schiavo brought at least one condition, the persistent vegetative state, to the awareness of more Americans. Box 15.1 describes a possible scenario in which you would be unable to make a life and death medical decision for yourself. Notice how your decisions change with different circumstances. The exercise is a reminder that, not matter what your age, it is important that such life and death decisions be discussed with your loved ones so that they might better relay your wishes when they are asked to make that decision for you.

Finally, it is often difficult for the patient and family to admit, or for the physician to determine, that the patient is dying and that it is time to implement the provisions of the living will. Studies show that physicians often wait to write do-not-resuscitate orders until patients are very near death. Because "a little more" treatment is almost

Box 15.1

What Is Your Opinion?
Will you choose to live or die?

Can you imagine a more difficult decision to make than whether you want to discontinue treatments that may be keeping you alive? Now imagine this—someone else is making that decision for you.

That someone is usually a wife, husband, daughter, son, parent, or friend who cares about you. Unfortunately, that someone is also scared, grieving, and uncertain of the future. They are asked not to make the decision THEY would make for themselves, but instead to think what you would have wanted. If they have talked to you about the topic, they are better able to make the best decision for you, and will be left with less worry about doing the "wrong thing."

But how can you have these conversations? Nobody wants to imagine the dire situations we might encounter and it is even harder to determine what our response would be in every case. Many considerations influence such decisions—health status, religion, culture, personality, values, support from family and close friends, even the physician—to name a few.

The following vignette illustrates a life or death scenario in which a decision has to be made about your living or dying by someone you love without your input.

You have just been seriously injured in a car crash and have been brought to the intensive care unit of your local hospital. You cannot talk or communicate with the outside world and are not aware of what is happening around you. The doctors tell your family that you might get a little better, but to keep you alive now you need to be placed on a breathing machine and a tube must be inserted in your stomach for nutrients. If you were conscious, what would you choose?

THE DECISION

Do you want the tube to breathe placed?
Do you want the tube to eat placed?
Do you want to be resuscitated?

WOULD YOUR DECISION CHANGE ANY UNDER THE FOLLOWING CIRCUMSTANCES?

You are 20 years old.
You are 60 years old.
You are 88 years old.
You have two small children.

The doctors recommend that life support be discontinued and say, "That's what I would do if it were my family member."
The doctors say you are "brain dead" and may never regain consciousness, but you can be kept alive with life support machines.
Your condition stabilized so you don't need to remain in intensive care, but you still cannot talk, move, or interact with others and now you are going to a nursing home to live.
You already have cancer and so didn't expect to live more than a few months anyway.
The physician said there is no chance of getting better, but you may be able to breathe on your own or be fed small amounts by mouth.
Your family has to make financial sacrifices to keep you alive.

We cannot plan for every circumstance and we certainly cannot know all the ramifications of the outcome. Nevertheless, giving your loved ones a guide to follow will make it more likely that your intentions are followed. So think about this and talk to you loved ones. Complete an advance directive where YOU decide who is to make decisions for you in the event you cannot and tell your loved ones about it. And, think of people for whom YOU might be the one to decide—talk to them about what they would want. Knowing what the person would have wanted makes a difficult decision/situation just a little bit easier.

always possible and patients with terminal illnesses may live a long time, it is often difficult to decide when certain therapies are "heroic" or "ill advised" and should be avoided or terminated. Doctors may not communicate their own opinions to the patient about his or her poor prognosis, leaving the patient to believe that treatments may be helpful. Ideally, treatment alternatives should be communicated to the patient with specifics about the risks and benefits. Unfortunately, many of the treatments have not been rigorously tested. Even if an advance directive is signed and given to the physician, there is no guarantee that the patient's wishes will be honored.[5]

Although advance directives may not influence the nuts and bolts of medical treatment, they may serve to initiate conversations with family and friends regarding desires and preferences. Despite attempts to improve communication between patients and their physicians and to improve the implementation of advance directives, many physicians remain unaware of their patients' wishes and provide overly aggressive care at the end of life, resulting in poor outcomes for both patients and their families.

Some of the problems with advance directives can be minimized by a durable power of attorney: The patient appoints a relative or friend to make medical decisions when he or she is no longer mentally capable. Without an advance directive, decisions about care are generally made quietly between family members and the health care team. In rare cases when the family and the health care team disagree, the court will intervene.

Each state has its own advance directive laws and unique procedures to enable a dying person's wishes to be carried out. Documents for each state may be downloaded from Caring Connections (www.caringinfo.org). Click on Are you planning ahead then click on State-specific advance directives for free download. The site also operates a national crisis and information hotline dealing with end-of-life issues. Aging with Dignity (www.agingwithdignity.org) offers a simple advance directive for a small fee. Called "Five Wishes," it is easy to use and is legally valid in 34 states. The five wishes are (1) Whom do I want to make care decisions for me when I can't? (2) What kind of medical treatment do I want toward the end? (3) What would help me feel comfortable while I am dying? (4) How do I want people to treat me? (5) What do I want my loved ones to know about me and my feelings after I'm gone?

EUTHANASIA AND ASSISTED SUICIDE

A topic that continues to engage heated public debate is *euthanasia,* the painless putting to death of a person suffering from an incurable condition. *Passive* euthanasia is withholding treatment that otherwise would prolong life, allowing death to occur naturally. If a person with severe lung disease is not put on a ventilator or given antibiotics to prolong life, this is *passive* euthanasia. In contrast, *active* euthanasia occurs when someone takes an active step to deliberately end another's life, such as giving an overdose of medication. Active euthanasia is considered murder in our country. The differences between active and passive euthanasia are not always clear-cut. For instance, "pulling the plug" on a ventilator is sometimes considered passive because it allows the death to progress naturally, but it is active in that it is an intentional, conscious act to end life.

Assisted suicide is the procedure in which a physician helps a seriously ill individual to comfortably end his or her life, generally by prescribing a lethal dose of a drug. In recent years, the most publicized advocate of assisted suicide was Dr. Jack Kevorkian, a retired Michigan pathologist. He facilitated the suicides of 130 terminally ill patients. However, in 1998, he did more than provide the drug. He actively administered the injection to a man suffering from ALS. The videotape of the incident was subsequently aired on *60 Minutes.* A jury in Michigan found him guilty of second degree murder in 1999; he was released in 2007 with the condition that he not offer suicide advice. He died in 2011.

Assisted suicide is a very controversial issue. Depending on the survey, from one-half to two-thirds of the American public think it should be legal for physicians to help terminally ill patients end their lives painlessly. Most respondents are also aware of the need for safeguards to protect the vulnerable. Proponents of assisted suicide argue that people have the right to decide when to die in order to prevent prolonged suffering from an incurable or terminal illness. Opponents argue that assisted suicide is the first step on the "slippery slope" of devaluing human life and suggest that the pain and depression that kindle a desire to end one's life can often be effectively alleviated. Some opponents fear that patients might choose euthanasia for the wrong reason, such as saving families the burden of paying for nursing home care.

On the one hand, allowing very sick people the option of dying can be a humane act. On the other hand, it can be an excuse to provide inferior medical care. In some cases, those who desire to end their life are clinically depressed. Medications, support, and therapy can reduce symptoms and increase the will to live. In some ways it is easier and less costly to end someone's life than to secure the social and medical supports necessary for the patient to live the remainder of life more fully. Although many illnesses are incurable, modern medicine, if used appropriately, can make the last days more comfortable. Most pain and suffering can be managed by specialists in palliative medicine.

Most physicians support a terminally ill patient's right to die, and some would practice assisted suicide if it were legal. Through high court decisions, legislation, and voter initiatives, states are clarifying the limits of active and passive euthanasia and assisted suicide. In many states, voter initiatives have been put on the ballot, sometimes to permit physician-assisted suicide, other times to prohibit it.

In 1994, a physician-assisted suicide initiative, called the Death with Dignity Act, was successful in Oregon. However, state and federal court battles delayed implementation until 1998. In 2009, the state of Washington passed a similar law. Both Oregon and Washington complete annual reports in regard to the numbers of prescriptions written for lethal purposes and the number of completed deaths and who chooses this. In general, most have cancer, are white and educated, and have insurance

through Medicare or Medicaid. There is often a delay from getting the prescription to using it, and some people do not choose to use it. In general, fewer than 100 people a year obtain the medication, and even fewer use it to end their lives. Most cited the following reasons for their actions: concern about loss of autonomy, loss of dignity, and losing the ability to participate in activities that made life enjoyable. For further details, see the annual reports from the Oregon and Washington Departments of Public Health on the Internet in regard to their "death with dignity acts."

At this writing, no other state has passed a similar law although voters in several states have defeated the measure on the ballot. "Right to die" groups in those states challenged the initiatives, asserting that individuals have a constitutional right to physician-assisted suicide. Several cases went through the higher courts. Finally, in 1997, the United States Supreme Court unanimously ruled that physician-assisted suicide was not a constitutional right, allowing state laws permitting or outlawing assisted suicide to stand.

CHOOSING TO DIE/SUICIDE

Choosing to take one's own life is the ultimate human decision. What are the circumstances in which it is justified? And when is it condemned? Suicide may range from an irrational act committed by a mentally unstable individual to a premeditated, rational decision to end a life of physical or mental anguish.

What opinions do those who are closest to death, the terminally ill, have regarding physician-assisted suicide? One study interviewed over 900 terminally ill patients to determine their attitudes. More than half of the terminally ill patients reported that euthanasia or physician-assisted suicide should be an available option, but only about 10 percent reported that they were seriously considering those options for themselves. Those who seriously considered them were more likely to be depressed, to be in pain, and to have a substantial need for care. Interestingly, less than half had talked to a physician or hoarded medications.

Those who were black, who were over age 65, or who "felt appreciated" were less likely to consider hastening their death. When researchers questioned the individuals again from two to six months after the original interviews, they found that half of the responders had changed their minds. Those who were depressed or had difficulty breathing were more likely to change their minds toward hastening their own death. Of the 256 terminally ill patients who died during the study, only a very small minority actually took concrete action to hasten death: One individual died by euthanasia or physician-assisted suicide, one attempted suicide, and one repeatedly requested that her life be ended but the family and physician refused.[5]

The study mentioned above has several implications: Very few individuals take advantage of the opportunity for euthanasia or assisted suicide. Psychological symptoms such as depression and feeling appreciated play a large part in individuals' attitudes. Many individuals who are terminally ill waver between choosing life and choosing death. A waiting period can be a safeguard. Many more people obtain the prescription than use it.

There is yet another option to deal with the physical and mental anguish of those who are dying. In 1997, during their deliberations regarding physician-assisted suicide, the Supreme Court justices became sensitized to the need of the terminally ill to be free of pain and suffering while dying. They requested experts in the field, such as members of hospice groups and the American Medical Association, to make a statement about controlling pain during the dying process. The group assured the justices that pain can be controlled for most patients without heavy sedation, but for a few, sedation to a sleeplike state may be necessary in the last days or weeks of life to prevent the patient from experiencing severe pain.

A part of the Supreme Court ruling that was not as well publicized as the decision on assisted suicide is the decision that individuals have the right to adequate palliative care (care to alleviate pain and other suffering). The Supreme Court prohibited any state law or regulation from obstructing the provision of adequate care to alleviate pain and other physical symptoms of people facing death. This ruling invalidated several states' regulations that unduly restricted the prescribing of opiates for pain relief and also eliminated the power of state regulatory boards to discipline physicians who prescribe high doses of opioids to their patients. Although physicians may not intentionally hasten death with drugs (except in Oregon), that ruling permits them to use a drug to hasten death if the drug is intended for other purposes, such as pain relief. This is a significant departure from the past.

Because of that ruling, a physician may now prescribe high doses of opioid drugs to relieve extreme suffering of those who are dying if there is no other way to remove suffering. This is called *terminal sedation*. In general, it is thought that it is acceptable to provide pain relief that may result in quicker death, if the goal is not to kill but to relieve pain. However, patients, their families, and their health care providers need to work together to ensure that the patient's wishes are being followed and that the risks and benefits of each treatment are explored and understood.

A small proportion of terminally ill individuals whose suffering becomes intolerable hasten their own death by voluntarily refusing food and fluids. Some believe this behavior is a form of suicide; others believe patients have a right to refuse treatment. The advantage of choosing this way to die is that the method does not depend on the physician or legislation but rests on the desire and action of the individual. The time it takes to die ranges from less than a week to several weeks.

Contrary to popular belief, it is unlikely that fasting is painful. A study of hospice nurses reported that one in four had witnessed the death of at least one patient who chose to refuse food or drink as a means to end his or her life. When asked about the overall quality of death of those who refused food and drink on a scale of 0 to 9 (0 was very bad; 9 was very good), three-fourths of the nurses' ratings were 7 or above. In the majority of cases (85 percent), death occurred within 15 days. Most nurses also described their patients' suffering

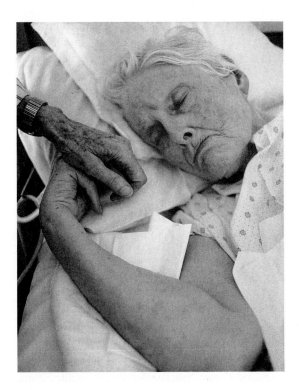

as minimal and the dying process as peaceful.[6] Since a reduced appetite and refusal of food and fluids are a natural part of the dying process, it is hard to differentiate "self-induced starving" from a natural death, especially for the onlooker. Although the study is not definitive and relied on recollection, it raises awareness of fasting as an option to accelerate the dying process.

Recognizing that terminal sedation and refusal of food and fluids are viable choices of last resort for some terminally ill individuals, the End of Life Care Consensus Panel of the American College of Physicians–American Society of Internal Medicine published guidelines for physicians to consider these last resorts in response to patients' requests to die. The panel also discussed the moral and legal dimensions of those choices.[7]

In 1980, the founders of the Hemlock Society began to advocate for dying persons to be able to choose from a full range of end-of-life options. Its proponents argue that the right to take one's own life is as important as the right to life, that death with dignity is preferable to prolonged life with a terminal illness, and that the quality of life, not its duration, is most important. As part of that movement, Derek Humphrys authored a book, *Final Exit: The Practicalities of Self-Deliverance and Assisted Suicide for the Dying* (1981), on methods that may be used by the terminally ill to hasten death. The Hemlock Society has since changed its name to Compassion and Choices (www .compassionandchoices.org).

ATTITUDES TOWARD DYING AND DEATH

Because death is universal (we all will die) and mystifying (we can never understand it), it is reasonable that death anxiety is a part of everyone's life. It is known that the young think about their own deaths less frequently than the old, possibly because they believe that death is something that happens to old people. With advancing age, however, the inevitability of death becomes clear, and the number of years left to live becomes finite: Time no longer stretches out endlessly as it did in adolescence and young adulthood.

Studies consistently report that death anxiety is higher among young adults than among old adults. Why might this be so? Older persons generally have more experience with the death of friends and family than do younger groups. Further, the urgency of staying alive diminishes when individuals no longer have dependent children. The young may see death as missing out on what life has to offer, whereas the old may be satisfied with their life experiences. Older people who are institutionalized or those who are chronically ill or depressed may welcome death as a release from continued disability and pain. Many have lost much of their autonomy, have started to withdraw from family and friends, and have been separated from some of the pleasures in life that made it meaningful. Finally, death looms closer and is expected in the later years, so older persons are likely to be more prepared and resigned to it.

OPTIONS ON WHERE TO DIE

A century ago, most dying people were cared for at home. New, institutions have taken more responsibility for the dying: Most Americans die in hospitals (almost 60 percent), about 20 percent die in nursing homes, and about 20 percent die at home.[8] It is assumed that most people prefer to die at home, but some studies show that is not the case. Some people prefer to be home with their families, but others are fearful of pain or suffering, do not want to burden their families with caregiving or "bad memories," and feel more comfortable in a medical setting. Difficulties arise when there is disagreement—for example, an elder may wish to die at home, but her elderly spouse is uncomfortable with that option. One researcher questioned more than 400 adult patients hospitalized with end stage cancer and other end-stage conditions and their family caregivers regarding preferred location for the patient to die. About half the patients questioned reported a preference for a home death as did the family caregiver group. However, in half the cases, the patient and caregiver dyad disagreed regarding preference for home or hospital. It is evident that conversations between the patient and caregiver need to occur before death is imminent so that both the patient and caregiver are clear on patient's choice of place of death.[9]

The transfer of responsibility from the family to the institution has altered the motives for care of the dying. Families are motivated to care for their dying kin largely because of emotional ties, whereas institutions are motivated by economic gain. Because hospitals focus on controlling physical problems, care is less personal and seldom meets the emotional or social needs of the patient. Advanced medical technology and prescription medications have extended the length of life, but they also have prolonged the dying interval, isolated the terminally ill, and placed an added strain on the family. With the advent of cost-cutting measures in hospitals by promoting recovery at home, the trend toward dying in hospitals may be reversed in the future.

The place of death may be determined by many factors, such as the health condition of the person, the amount of care needed, the availability of a willing caretaker, and available in-home services. Elders who live alone are more likely to go to an institution or hospital to die than those who live with family. Married men are more likely to die at home than married women because wives are more likely to be alive to care for dying spouses than vice versa. Personal preference also plays a role. Most elders prefer the familiar surroundings and personalized care at home, but some do not want to burden their families and prefer hospitalization. The older the individual is, the more likely it is that he or she will die in a nursing home.

Hospitals are the most common place of death, but some experts believe that they may not be the most appropriate place. Physicians generally subscribe to the view that death is pathological, not natural, so they value cure more than easing of symptoms. Their training is geared toward saving lives and controlling death rather than alleviating symptoms and meeting the psychosocial needs of the dying. Many doctors are fearful of using the high doses of opioid medications required to alleviate pain or are uneducated about the proper use of medications for symptom relief. Doctors and nurses in the hospital setting must meet the acute medical needs of patients and have less time to provide a restful, supportive, and comfortable patient- and family-centered environment. Furthermore, the bureaucratic nature of hospital policies and procedures (for example, frequent blood draws) can deplete the scarce energy resources and depersonalize the dying person.

Home care services can provide an alternative for dying persons and their families. Such services include everything from homemaking services to around-the-clock nursing care (see Chapter 14, "Long-Term Care"). Frail elders who cannot be cared for at home by family or hired help generally live in skilled nursing facilities. Although some individuals die in these facilities after being there for an extended period, others are transferred to a hospital for their final days or hours. Despite the fact that many individuals in skilled nursing facilities die, generally staff are not trained to deal with the multiple medical, social, and psychological needs of the dying resident and are not provided with education and support in their work with dying patients.

Hospice

Hospice provides compassionate care for the terminally ill. The emphasis of hospice care is on making the patient as comfortable as possible by managing symptoms while providing psychological and spiritual support to the individual and family during the dying process. No curative, life-prolonging treatment is provided. This type of care is called *palliative care.*

The first hospice inpatient facility was set up in London in 1967 as a reaction against the disease- centered hospital care of the dying. In the United States, hospice services may be provided in a variety of settings. Most commonly, hospice workers go into the home, but hospice care can be delivered in hospitals, special facilities, and nursing homes. However, some communities offer hospice facilities where palliative care is given. Hospice programs use multi-disciplinary teams composed of physicians, nurses, social workers, counselors, clergy, and trained volunteers who offer medical services, personal care, and emotional and spiritual support for the dying, and respite care and grief counseling for bereaved family members. Some teams also include physical and occupational therapists and nutritionists.

Members of the hospice team are available 24 hours a day, 7 days a week to provide support for the dying person and the family members. The goals of the hospice staff are to relieve pain and suffering, to provide education, case management, and support to the caregivers, to facilitate interactions with the physician, to arrange for and provide services, and to provide a dignified death for the dying person. It should be noted that hospice does not provide 24-hour *care* to the dying individual at home or in the nursing home; instead, hospice provides around-the-clock *support* to the ill person and the caregivers. Medical equipment and supplies and drugs for symptom control and coordination of pain relief are included.

The use of hospice care is increasing dramatically. According to the National Hospice and Palliative Care Organization, in 2009 there were about 5,000 hospice programs in the country serving about 1.56 million patients. About 41 percent of those who died that year had been cared for by hospice workers. Eighty-three percent of patients who used hospice care were over 65, and more than 80 percent were white. Close to half the patients using hospice had cancer; some had other diagnoses, such as end-stage cardiac or pulmonary disease and dementia. The median stay for individuals was 26 days. Because of the type of care given, hospice patients are more likely to die at home than those without hospice even though they may be admitted to inpatient facilities for their final days or to reduce symptoms. Even if they move to hospitals or nursing homes, they still receive hospice services.

Hospice care differs from conventional medical treatment in that patients are not admitted to the program unless the individual and physician believe further treatment and cure are no longer possible. In order for a sick individual to receive hospice care, a physician must certify that the person has six months or less to live. Many physicians wait too long to prescribe the services. Many referrals are made too late in the course of illness for patients and families to fully benefit from the services available from hospice.

Many more seriously ill individuals could benefit from hospice. However, requesting hospice care is an acceptance that death is inevitable, and many physicians, dying individuals, and their family members continue to search for new treatments even when death is near. Many endure pain and suffering in a hospital or nursing home, then seek hospice care when they have only a few days to live, reducing the benefits of pain-reducing medications and social services. Experts assert that physicians and terminally ill patients and their families should consider enrollment in hospice as early as patients can qualify to improve the quality of their remaining days by receiving pain-relieving medicine and support services not covered by a hospital.

Medicare offers a hospice benefit for those who are 65 and older that covers almost all aspects of care with little out-of-pocket cost to the patient or family. In addition, most private health plans and Medicaid in most states cover hospice services. To be eligible, both the patient's physician and the hospice director must certify that the patient is terminally ill and has six months or less to live. The patient or designated family member must sign a statement to choose hospice care rather than the standard medical benefits. Again, it should be stressed that hospice does not provide or pay for day-to-day care of the patient at home or in an institution but supports and aids the providers of such care. In addition, Medicare provides respite care to the caregiver by providing short-term hospital or nursing home stays to patients. For information on hospice services and referral to the nearest hospice, call the National Hospice and Palliative Care Organization, at 1-800-658-8898, or go to the Web site, www.nhpco.org

THE DYING TRAJECTORY

The dying trajectory is the period of time from the individual's first awareness of impending death until death occurs. Up to the early twentieth century, the common dying trajectory was a short but dramatic struggle against infection or injury. The individual either "pulled through" or died within a few days, even hours. There were few drugs and medical procedures to delay the outcome. Now, people who are dying are more likely to live for an extended period, moving from chronic-progressive to terminally ill, with unclear boundaries between the periods. The major killers of adults are chronic diseases, and individuals can live for months, even years, in a debilitated state through medical intervention.

Those dying of a chronic illness generally follow one of these trajectories: (1) a short period of obvious decline at the end, (2) long-term disability with a period of worsening health and unpredictable timing of death, or (3) inability to care for oneself and a slowly dwindling course to death, usually the result of frailty or dementia.[10] The first trajectory is the most familiar one and is common among those dying of cancer. The significant decline (inability to perform activities of daily living and extensive weight loss) occurs in the last two months. The second trajectory is common among those dying of multiple organ failure (heart failure, obstructive lung disease, cirrhosis of the liver). These patients are seriously ill for many months, even years, with occasional dramatic medical events. However, dwindling physical reserves and worsening of the condition eventually cause death. The timing of death with long-term disability is less certain than for those with cancer. The number of individuals following the third trajectory, progressive disability, is increasing. This group includes those coping with stroke, dementia, and the frailty of old age.

Physicians recognize the third type of death trajectory as the "dwindles" or "geriatric failure to thrive." It is common for those who are very old to eventually undergo a decline in abilities, become increasingly apathetic, and lose the desire to eat and drink. This behavior ends in death, even in the absence of terminal disease. Failure to thrive seems to be a downhill spiral in which poor nutrition affects cognitive function, which in turn leads to worsening nutrition, which increases susceptibility to disease and decreases the will to live as well as the ability to respond to the stressors of illness. Failure to thrive carries a high rate of morbidity (e.g., poor recovery from surgery, pressure ulcers, repeated hospitalizations) and mortality. Some professionals have suggested that among the very old (individuals in their 90s and 100s), the "dwindles" may be what is meant by dying of "old age." The case study of Mrs. Y. exemplifies this natural process (see Box 15.2).

Even though the third trajectory, dying of the dwindles, is probably the most natural way to die, physicians often make medical efforts to reverse the natural decline, partly because it is difficult to differentiate the dwindles from reversible and treatable conditions (e.g., a urinary tract infection). Patients and family members are more comfortable

BOX 15.2

A Case of the Dwindles

Mrs. Y. is a 94-year-old widow who was hospitalized three times in three months for dehydration, urinary tract infection, and stool impaction. Despite treatment for her illnesses and a trial of an antidepressant, she continued to lose weight and functional ability until she was bed-bound. She denied having sleep disturbances or problems with appetite, although she ate little. She had previously been married to a man with high rank in the military and still maintained a close-knit group of other widowed socialites. She missed her husband very much but thought her life was "all right." Medically there was nothing found that could be treated to explain her decline. She developed a decubitus ulcer (bedsore) from lying in bed. She remained cheery, even when talking about death, but maintained she was "tired of living" and "ready whenever the good Lord wants to take me." She was very polite with caregivers and friends who attempted to motivate her to become more active, and she vowed to "get on the ball after her birthday." She died peacefully of unknown causes after a brief decline only days before her 95th birthday.

with a diagnosis of "the dwindles" after other conditions have been ruled out.

No matter if the dying trajectory is brief or lengthy, the status of the dying person changes. Someone who used to be a contributing member of the community withdraws from social activities as it becomes obvious that time is running out. Former friends may be uncomfortable around the sick individual. Alternatively, family members may travel great distances to visit, become more open about their feelings toward each other, or renew estranged relationships. As weakness progresses, even conversation may be difficult; the sick person may no longer desire to interact with more than a handful of friends and family members. As a result, the social sphere of the sick person becomes very small. Many former activities and broader interests disappear as the sick person becomes more focused on the tasks of dying and on activities directly related to day-to-day comfort and survival. Although many people face their own death fully awake or die suddenly while sleeping, often the process of dying involves days, weeks, or months, characterized by a withdrawal from communication, diminished appetite, increased sleepiness, disorientation, and a dulling of consciousness.

It is commonly thought that the end of life is fraught with existential concerns, anguish, or spiritual rebirth. In actuality, the concerns of the dying more often are focused on coping with symptoms, dealing with pain, loss of control and dignity, and being a burden to their families.

One of the most significant fears of dying is the uncontrollable pain that is often associated with it. The fear of pain is well founded. Although estimates vary widely, between one-third and three-quarters of cancer patients report uncontrolled pain near the end of life. How should this pain be handled?

There is overwhelming theoretical agreement that pain at the end of life should be treated with appropriate medications. However, achieving this objective is problematic. Elders may not report pain, or they may not be asked about their pain. Consequently, members of the health care team may mistakenly believe pain medications are not needed. Patients may have had bad experiences with pain medication or fear the pain medication and are reluctant to take it. Even if pain medications are prescribed, the dosages may not be effective. They might be too strong, leading to drowsiness and other side effects, or too weak to have any effect on the pain. If either the physician or the patient is not comfortable with pain medications, one or both might give up before appropriate medications and dosages are found.

There are drawbacks to pain medication that may make physicians and patients resistant to their use. First, opiates (medications that contain opium or its derivatives, such as morphine) dispersed to a frail person may induce confusion or even unconsciousness that is unacceptable to someone who wants to be alert. Second, and more important, the drug may ease the pain, but it could suppress breathing, induce unconsciousness, and even cause death. Despite the drawbacks, proper dosages of opiates are the most effective drugs available to keep people comfortable in their final hours. Medical school curricula are giving increased attention to the importance of pain relief for those who are dying, both to medical students and in continuing education for practicing physicians.

Those who are dying experience significant psychological changes. The first professional to propose a psychological process that individuals undergo in order to cope with their impending death was Elisabeth Kübler-Ross, a Swiss-born psychiatrist who worked with the terminally ill. She described five distinct stages through which many terminally ill patients pass, each stage a defense mechanism to cope with impending death.[11] Dr. Kübler-Ross observed that the stages were not absolutes. The time spent in each stage and the sequence varied among individuals, and many stages overlapped. Superimposed on each stage was hope, which remains possible in all five stages. The five stages are as follows:

Denial: When first learning that he or she is terminally ill, the patient registers shock and disbelief. The individual rejects the diagnosis, thinking that the lab reports must be mistaken or that the physician made a wrong diagnosis. This stage is generally short unless the family also continues to deny the illness.

Anger: The diagnosed terminally ill patient laments, "Why me?" The patient may become resentful that others are healthy while he or she must die. The individual may express anger at family members, at health professionals, or at him- or herself, or the anger may be unfocused. Irritability and complaining are common.

Bargaining: During this stage, death becomes a reality, but the individual attempts to postpone the time of death by bargaining. Most deals are struck with God, even if the person has never talked with God before. Most deals are secret. During this period, the dying individual may seek out alternative treatments, such as faith healers, unusual drugs, or vitamin supplements, to postpone death.

Depression: When it becomes obvious that a bargain cannot be struck, depression occurs. Death is recognized as inevitable, and feelings of loss become overwhelming. Whereas before the individual may have been talkative, crying, agitated, or seeking sympathy, during this stage the individual often withdraws from visitors and mourns silently. Mourning for loss of capability and lost relationships allows an individual to prepare for death and to attempt to make sense of life and death.

Acceptance: Individuals at this stage are often devoid of emotion and disengaged from the outside world. Many limit contact to one or two people who are very close. The dying are often tired and weak and spend their days sleeping, resting, and reminiscing.

Dr. Kübler-Ross' work was revolutionary in that it sensitized the public and the medical profession to the range of emotions that dying people experience. However, her research has been criticized on a number of counts. For one, there are no clear, observable behavior patterns for each stage; differentiation among stages relied on her subjective interpretation of patients' emotions or motivations. Critics question her findings because they believe her subjects' emotions were probably highly vulnerable to suggestion and manipulation and may have been influenced by medications, since this variable was not controlled in her study. Another problem with the Kübler-Ross model is that, even though she did not envision these stages as a "correct" way to die, many health professionals erroneously interpret the stages as a prescription all must follow for a "good death." In some instances, this expectation leads to labeling patients and attempting to move them to different stages rather than helping them deal with their feelings and accepting their individuality. Finally, her findings were not confirmed by other studies.

Other research has revealed that there are many emotions associated with the dying process other than those Dr. Kübler-Ross described. Many experts agree with psychologist Edwin Schneidman's description of the dying process:

> Rather than the five definite stages . . . my experience has led me to posit a hive of affect, in which there is a constant coming and going. The emotional stages seem to include a constant interplay between disbelief and hope and, against these as background, a waxing and waning of anguish, terror, acquiescence and surrender, rage and envy, disinterest and ennui, pretense, taunting and daring and even yearning for death—all these in the context of bewilderment and pain.[12]

The general consensus is that the way someone copes with the dying process varies with the individual. One expert's analysis of Kübler-Ross' work suggests that the most valuable lessons for families and professionals are (1) to assist the dying in resolving unfinished needs, (2) to actively listen to those who are dying, and (3) to help them identify their own needs.[13]

A prominent gerontologist, Dr. Richard Kalish, speaks for many when he expresses his views on his own dying process: "For some people and under some circumstances, acceptance of death is certainly the way to an appropriate death. For others, it is not. Perhaps anger, even fury, is the most appropriate way to die: what a mockery death is; how destructive it is; how

absurd it is—there is nothing good about death, at least about my death and I have no intention of being peaceful or submissive or accepting!"[14] Kalish echoes the words of Dylan Thomas' famous poem:

> Do not go gentle into that good night,
> Old age should burn and rave at close of day;
> Rage, rage against the dying of the light.

Rights of the Dying

Dying people are very vulnerable. The process of dying takes a lot of physical and psychic energy. Sedatives, painkillers, and some medical treatments can further reduce energy and cause disorientation and diminishing capabilities. As strength decreases, dying individuals are progressively less able to carry out daily activities. Because those who are dying are generally in a weakened state, family members and professionals are responsible to ensure that their rights are not violated. Following is a description of these rights.

Right to Open Communication about Death

Most Americans believe that individuals have the right to know about their impending death and would want to be told if they were dying. Because individuals commonly deny that they are dying in the early stages, it is generally most sensitive to inform them first that their condition is serious and allow them to ask questions. Knowledge of impending death allows dying persons to complete certain tasks before dying and to close their life in accordance with personal wishes. Additionally, full awareness of impending death allows an individual to make responsible decisions, such as where to die and what treatments to allow. However, individuals from some cultures do not believe that dying relatives should be informed of the severity of their illness.

What Is Your Opinion?
How Do You Want to Die?

Harold M. hadn't felt well for the past three days and had actually been on his way to the doctor when he experienced sudden chest pressure. He decided to drive directly to the hospital emergency room. He was found dead in the driver's seat from a heart attack and fatal arrythmia in the parking lot of the hospital. His wife of thirty-seven years was shocked to learn of his death—he had been so healthy (except for a little high blood pressure and cholesterol) and had not yet retired. They had plans to travel the country in an RV upon his retirement later that year. She regretted they had not had a chance to say goodbye and knew little about the family finances. Their children, arriving for the funeral, thought it may have been better to die quickly, with a minimum of pain and suffering and worry about death. Their dad had been so independent and proud, they reasoned, he wouldn't have tolerated the indignities of a slow death.

Margaret S. had lost some weight over the past six months and had a nagging stomach ache, and her over-the-counter antacids were not working anymore. When her stomach cancer was diagnosed, it had already spread to most of her liver, and the doctors said there was little they could do. She underwent chemotherapy but felt ill, and the tumor's growth was not slowed, so she elected to stop treatment. As she became weaker, her children were able to visit her and say goodbye, and she resolved a long-standing dispute with her eldest daughter. Her husband became overwhelmed with caregiving and hired a live-in helper (despite his concerns about spending their savings). He had promised never to put her in a nursing home. She had some pain, and this was treated with morphine. She spent the last two weeks of her life in a coma and died in her sleep with her husband in the bed next to her.

DISCUSSION QUESTIONS

What are some of the advantages and disadvantages of a sudden death? A more prolonged dying? Which would you prefer for yourself or your loved ones?

What have been your personal experiences with death and dying?

What are your biggest fears about dying? Your greatest hopes?

Do you think people have any control over the kind of death they have?

If you have six months to live, what would you want to accomplish in that time? What if you were very weak and unable to travel?

What issues do you think people must resolve before they die?

Right to as Painless a Death as Possible

A common fear among elders is that their death will be painful. However, severe pain when one is near death is not common, and most patients can become pain-free with proper medication. Painkillers, including strong addictive drugs (those containing opium and morphine) should be given freely to dying persons who are in severe pain. Other symptoms causing discomfort (e.g., nausea, difficulty breathing) should also be controlled.

Right to the Presence of Concerned Others

Elders are more likely to die in lonely, isolated conditions than younger people. In fact, one of elders' greatest fears is dying alone. A high proportion of elders may spend their dying interval without a concerned person to help make medical decisions or advocate adequate medical treatment. If a family member or friend is not present, it is imperative that those who are dying alone be assigned a nurse or volunteer.

Right to as Much Control over the Environment as Possible

Because dying people often experience loss of control over their environment and declining health, it is imperative that health professionals and family allow the dying person as much control as possible. Allowing some choice over meals, frequency of nursing interruptions, visiting hours, roommates, and medical treatments can greatly enhance feelings of autonomy.

Right to Have All Treatments Fully Explained and to Refuse Treatment

The dying, like other patients, have the right to have all medical treatments fully explained, including a description of the prognosis, methods of treatment, and potential risks, benefits, and side effects. For instance, chemotherapy, a common cancer treatment, has a variable success rate and is accompanied by many uncomfortable side effects, including hair loss and nausea. Because of this, many patients refuse the therapy, opting for a more comfortable though perhaps shorter life. As discussed earlier, patients have the right to refuse all heroic, artificial efforts to sustain life. On the other hand, it should not be assumed that all elders are ready to die and would refuse life-sustaining measures. Elders should have the right to all the technologically advanced equipment and treatments available to younger groups to prolong life and should be allowed to seek out alternative treatments, even those not condoned by the medical profession.

Tasks of the Dying

Individuals who are dying must cope with significant challenges that threaten all aspects of life—body, mind, and spirit. Individuals who know they are dying often feel compelled to complete a number of tasks before they die. The importance of each task and the time spent on each vary with the degree of disability, the nature of the illness, the time left to live, the personality of the individual, and the environment. The tasks generally center around the following themes.[14,15]

Completing Unfinished Business

Individuals vary in the types of activities they wish to complete before death. The unfinished business may include reuniting with a distant family member, completing a photo album, or sharing intimate feelings with their family. It is important to let the dying person decide what tasks to accomplish and the ways in which the family and the health professional can help.

Dealing with Medical Care Needs

The dying need to understand their diagnosis and prognosis, learn of alternative treatments and pain control methods, and decide on life-sustaining treatments. Furthermore, they need to tell others what measures should be taken if their condition worsens to a point where they are no longer in control. They may complete a living will or direct a family member to make medical decisions. The dying individual also needs to be involved in the decision of whether to die in a hospital, in a nursing home, or at home.

Allocating Time and Energy Resources

We all have thought of what we would do if we knew we had five or six months to live. The usual answers—such as traveling or accomplishing a significant project—generally include tasks that require more mental and physical energy than most dying persons possess. How much time and energy a dying individual can allocate depends on the nature of the illness and its progression. As the disease progresses, individuals generally become weaker and must be selective about which tasks can be accomplished before death and which must be left behind. Additionally, dying persons must choose whom to spend time with during their last days.

Arranging for Death

Another important task for the dying is to arrange what will happen after death. The dying person may need to make a will and distribute valued possessions to loved ones before death. Many make decisions on cremation, burial, or donation of body organs. Some plan the details of their funeral. Others arrange for people to take care of finances and insurance policies and their pets.

Life Review

The dying often spend time reminiscing about their life and its meaning. Some contemplate on what it means to die and their belief in an afterlife. Many individuals turn to religion during this time to give them hope or justification for their suffering.

CARING FOR THE DYING

What does the dying person need or want in order to experience a good death? In the 1990s, concerns about the experience of dying in America prompted increased research on the care and needs of individuals with terminal illness. One of the most prominent studies of the dying, the Study to Understand Prognosis and Preferences for Outcomes and Risks of Treatments (SUPPORT), set out to answer that question by interviewing dying patients, their loved ones, and the physicians and nurses who cared for them during the end of life.[16]

The initial findings of the SUPPORT study documented that many individuals had prolonged and painful deaths. Some experienced unwanted, expensive, and invasive care at the end of life. Interviews revealed that patients and families have several needs: symptom management, preparation for death, involvement in decision making, achieving a "sense of completion," and "being treated as a whole person." Terminally ill patients also reported other needs during their last days: to be mentally aware, to not be a burden on their families, to help others, and to have peace with God. Interestingly, they ranked freedom from pain as most important and dying at home as least important at the end of life.

One of the important findings of the SUPPORT study was the lack of awareness of health professionals regarding their patients' wishes.

In fact, the study reported that health professionals' estimation of the wishes of their patients was about as good as chance. Health professionals, although they often had good intentions, fell far short in meeting the expectations of dying patients and their families.[16] These studies and others have helped to identify the discrepancy between the kind of care patients want and the kind they receive, documenting the need for better communication with dying patients.

Within the last few years, there has been an effort on several fronts to enhance the quality of end-of-life care: recommendations from the medical community, education of health professionals, and legislative endeavors. The American Medical Association issued a statement, "Elements of Quality Care for Patients in the Last Phase of Life," available at www.ama-assn.org, that lists eight elements of care that every person should expect from physicians and health care institutions. Another medical organization, the Institute of Medicine, issued a lengthy report, *Approaching Death: Improving Care at the End of Life,* outlining the problems with end-of-life care and proposing solutions. On another front, a medical specialty in hospice and palliative medicine has been initiated to train physicians to effectively care for the dying person.

Federal and state legislation has addressed the quality of care at the end of life. Some states have legislated physician training in pain and symptom management and end-of-life care as a condition of ongoing physician licensure. Federal regulations mandate discussion of end-of-life preferences and

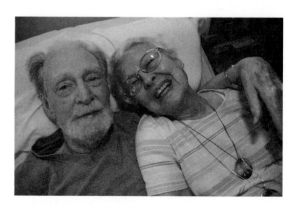

advance directives with all patients admitted to hospitals. All these efforts focus on achieving a comfortable and dignified death in accordance with the patient's wishes. However, attempting to make incremental changes in the way heath care is provided is very difficult.

The Family

Family members, not formal services, provide the vast majority of the care for the terminally ill. The presence of a family member to care for a terminally ill person can mean the difference between dying at home or in an institution.

Since one of the greatest fears of the dying is dying alone, perhaps the most important aspect of caring for the dying is to reduce this fear by being a trustworthy companion. Open communication with the terminally ill about their illnesses and treatments and day-to-day concerns, and frank discussions of death and the past, can reduce feelings of isolation and bolster their feelings of control over their last days or weeks. The family is often intensely involved. The family may have to struggle with decisions about when to come and help, trying to predict the moment of death to be present, coordinating work and child care with caring for a loved one and making end-of-life

---

What Does Dying Look Like?

When you are called to the deathbed of a close friend or family member, it is a time of great emotion, uncertainty, fear, and often extended waiting. It is common to wonder, "What is going on?" "How long will it take?" "Is he suffering?" "What should I do?" When extended families lived together and life expectancy was shorter, everyone had more experience with birth, illness, dying and death. Now with families flung far and wide, the advent of hospitals and nursing homes and longer life expectancies, many individuals have never seen somebody die. The symptoms listed below are evidence that the body systems are shutting down and death is near. Any one of the symptoms may be present, all may be present, or none may be present.

- The skin often becomes cooler, especially in the arms and legs, and may even become mottled-looking from low circulation.
- Secretions and congestion may build up in the lungs and breathing may sound raspy or uncomfortable. There may be periods of not breathing (apnea) or unusual breathing patterns.
- People are no longer interested in eating or drinking—they may wet their lips or take a sip, but they no longer desire food.
- Dying persons may withdraw from even their closest family members and friends.

- The person may become restless, moving in bed and perhaps appearing uncomfortable—this may or may not be due to pain.
- People make less urine and are usually incontinent.
- The person spends more and more time asleep and less and less time awake.
- They may be confused when awake or say things you cannot understand. Contrary to popular belief, few people have meaningful last words before death.
- They may maintain awareness, even when they appear to be sleeping.
- Many times those who are dying have an awareness that it is "their time" and might tell you if you ask.
- They may or may not be in pain in their final hours.

Many families believe that their loved one would want to die with them so they want to stay by the bedside for the last breaths. However, there are many stories of individuals who passed away only when their loved ones left the room. Dying is defined as taking the last breath and many times it is the silence that is noted. After death, the eyes are often open, the body slowly cools down, and over the next few hours becomes rigid.

Grandpa Pat

Wendy Gabrielle Evans, medical student, University of California at San Diego, School of Medicine

Until Grandpa Pat died in the summer of 1995, I hadn't had much close experience with death and dying. He was diagnosed with prostate cancer about ten years before he died. The radiation treatment he underwent soon after his diagnosis did little to slow the course of his disease, and during the spring of my junior year in college, we learned that the cancer had metastasized to his bones and Grandpa Pat started to plan for his death. All his life, he had been a difficult man to get along with, reluctant to show his feelings and too proud to apologize to anyone or say he was wrong. While his stubbornness brought him great success as a leader in the longshoreman's union in San Francisco and later as a lobbyist in Washington, it left significant battle scars on his relationships. Coming closer to his end mellowed him, though, and he made many reconciliations. He had been estranged from his son Dan since Dan's teens, and my mother and I feared that Grandpa Pat would die without talking to his son. But Dan and Grandpa Pat proved us wrong. During that last year, Dan took care of my grandfather. He was there every day fixing his medication schedule, getting his food, taking him to the doctor.

My relationship with Grandpa Pat was different from his relationship with other members of our family in that it was not wrought with as many conflicts and hard feelings. He was infinitely proud of me, thought I was the smartest, most beautiful girl in the world. His pride in me was so unconditional and he talked about it so often that being around him always made me feel special. As his condition declined, we talked more and more on the telephone. He developed a real interest in his disease; I guess he wanted to figure out why he was dying. I tried to explain cancer to him in simple terms, translating from what I was learning in college biology, and went to the medical library and copied articles about prostate cancer for him. He said his doctors never explained his cancer to him in common terms, and it seemed to mean a lot to him to understand his illness.

The week my grandpa died was in late August. I was in Berkeley on vacation when my mom called to tell me that Grandpa Pat had been admitted to the hospital because he was acting strangely and seemed paranoid to Dan. We thought he was having trouble with the dosing of his hormone treatments and narcotics, but it turned out that tumors were encroaching on the drainage from his kidneys, so it wouldn't be long. His nitrogenous wastes would build up in his bloodstream, he would slip into a peaceful coma, and die. Though my family told me that I didn't need to stay, I wanted to because I felt my presence would mean a lot to my grandfather. Staying with my family during that last week was one of the most wonderful experiences in my life. Working together to take care of Grandpa Pat, I felt closer to my family than I ever have before and that closeness stayed with us after he died.

I had always assumed that dying of cancer was not painful because drugs relieved the pain. I'm glad I was able to watch someone close to me suffer through his last week so that I will know what it is like for my patients. The narcotics, it is true, relieved the pain, but mentally made him feel awful. He became confused and agitated, so he was given another drug which made him groggy and sedated. We finally moved him home, where we cared for him—with much help from hospice, for the second half of the week. The hardest thing for us was determining when he needed more pain medication, especially when he could not communicate well through the drugs and uremia. Even when he could articulate how he was feeling, he didn't want to take the drugs because they took him away from us, but then his pain would become terrible and he would have to take more, but then he would become more groggy. It was an unending cycle.

For all of that, though, I have to say—and I know this sounds strange—that the last week of my grandfather's life was a fun and joyful time. Once he was home, my mom and I and my uncles took shifts staying with him. Once, when my mom and I tried to change his sheets, he resisted and resisted and kept whining "Wait, Wait" and we waited and finally he

Grandpa Pat

said okay he was ready and as soon as we started to lift him he started wailing "Wait, Wait" again. It turned out that he was embarrassed for us to see him naked, so when we closed our eyes and rolled it was okay. He laughed the whole time, though, becoming a comedian, and I think he loved having everyone there to pay attention to him and baby him.

Finally, I had to fly back to school and my mother back to work. Grandpa Pat could no longer speak, and could barely squeeze a hand. I think many people would wonder whether he knew at all what was going on around him. Before we left from our second to last day in San Francisco, I went to his room and sat with him and held his hand and explained that my mom and I were leaving the next day and that we were sorry we couldn't stay with him. I also told him that he should not be afraid, that he didn't need to hang on any longer and that he could just let go and leave us. He died three hours later.

Though we did mourn for my grandpa after his death, much of our grieving took place that week as we slowly said good-bye while watching him fade from a robust, overbearing man to a skinny, paralyzed vestige of what he once was. I also think that his week with us was what allowed him to die peacefully and happily. He was cremated, and we had a memorial for him a month later. There was more laughter than crying at the memorial. People told their stories about him and reminisced and we all heard some very funny stories. Afterwards, we scattered his ashes in the Pacific Ocean off San Francisco, so that he would always be near the city which symbolized his life and his work to him. The whole family gathered around my mother as she opened the bag that contained what was left of Grandpa Pat. The ashes were a beautiful purple color and glinted when the sun shone on them as they fell to the water, swirled around, and were gone.

decisions. When the task becomes overwhelming or the sick person needs specialized care, institutionalization usually occurs. Placement in an institution can release families from the need to do all daily body care, leaving them energy to provide companionship, advocacy, and presence.

Caregiving can be an enormous commitment: It impacts the physical, emotional, and social life of the individual or individuals giving care. Caring for a dying relative may bring about profound changes within the family. A parent, once the caregiver for his or her children, now must depend on them for physical care and emotional support. Children may have to toilet or clean or lift their parents, and this can be physically exhausting, awkward, or embarrassing. Caregivers must cope with feelings of loss and grief while dealing with the physical, emotional, and financial needs of a dying loved one. The care of a very sick older person usually requires tremendous personal commitment, physical strength, and financial resources. Family members may become overwhelmed with

responsibility, and they may resent the dying relative, even sometimes wishing the sick person would die. Finally, the cost of care may be substantial, even with Medicare, and may cause stress.

Health Professionals

Most people who work in health and social services have to deal with death and dying at one time or another. Health and social services professionals, like the rest of the population, do not like to be confronted with death. Health care workers who see their role as restoring an individual to health and productivity may have intense feelings of failure and emotional conflict as they watch a patient deteriorate and die. Health professionals may have different cultural beliefs about death. They may fear providing treatments that they believe may promote dying. They often find it uncomfortable to communicate with the dying and their families or to talk about dying. They may be uncertain of their abilities to predict death and may feel there is nothing they can do.

Some professionals might respond by detachment, others by avoidance, and others may get overinvolved and sad, having difficulty separating themselves from the grief experienced by the family. Some health care professionals, in an effort to be positive, may offer false hope while others, in an attempt to be realistic, may speak too harshly. The situation becomes more complicated when there are different cultural beliefs between the health care professionals on the team and the family. A person frankly talking about death can be very discomforting to some cultures. Professionals who work closely with dying patients need to have deep compassion for the terminally ill and their families, while preserving a distance from the death that keeps them from falling into depression every time a patient dies. It is important that health professionals who work with dying people receive training and support in their work.

As discussed earlier, a likely contributor to ineffective end-of-life care is inadequate training in end-of-life care. An important part of education for physicians, nurses, and social workers is to learn about the beliefs, customs, and rituals regarding death, grief, and bereavement among ethnic and racial subgroups. Such knowledge can enable the professional to better understand members of these groups and offer help.

No matter what the level of professional training, burnout (emotional and physical exhaustion) is common among those who work with the dying.

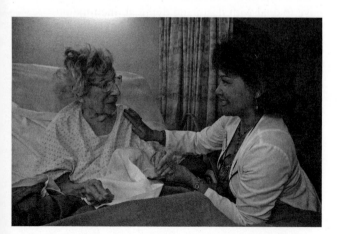

Burnout is characterized by job dissatisfaction, cynicism, withdrawal from the dying and their families, and, in some cases, termination of employment. Burnout can affect job satisfaction, performance, and home life. Those professionals who work in the home with the terminally ill, such as home health aides and visiting nurses, need special support.

Hospital and nursing home administrators can support those who work with dying patients by providing training on the psychological, physiological, and social needs of the dying and how to communicate with the dying and their families. Institutions may also offer both formal and informal support to staff, allowing them to vent their frustrations and concerns. Supervisors can also help employees to work through the complex emotions associated with caring for the dying. Supervisors may serve as role models for new professionals who are learning to give good care without burning out. However, supervisors need to be aware that not all employees are qualified to work with the terminally ill, and some staff may need to be transferred. Furthermore, supervisors need to recognize that even the most competent staff needs a break from working with the dying.

BEREAVEMENT AND GRIEF

Bereavement is a natural, even necessary, response to the death of a loved one and is generally manifested as an acute feeling of despair. The process of grieving is very complex, involving a host of physiological, psychological, and social reactions. The grief response is highly individual and dependent on the personality of the aggrieved, whether death was expected or unexpected, and the intensity of the previous relationship. Additionally, the number of past losses, the number of other love relationships, and the available social supports of the grief-stricken influence the extent of mourning.

The Grieving Process

The loss of a loved one is one of life's most traumatic events. *Bereavement* is the experience of being deprived of another's presence by death.

During bereavement, intense emotional suffering caused by a loss occurs. *Grief* is the outward expression of the loss. It is a natural, even necessary, response to the death of a loved one. Healthy grieving can be a slow and difficult process that lasts for months, even years. Most survivors eventually accept the loss and carry on with meaningful lives even though the deceased is not far from their thoughts.

Similar to the earlier discussion of the dying process, it should not be assumed that everyone who is grieving should experience grief in an orderly, stereotypical way. There is an extraordinarily wide range of healthy responses to the death of a loved one. Grieving may invoke multiple, contradictory emotions: denial, despair, anger, confusion, numbness, sadness, relief, and guilt. Emotional reactions, such as anxiety attacks, chronic fatigue, depression, obsession with the deceased, and thoughts of suicide, are not unusual. The varied feelings are common reactions to loss. Further, the emotions may change quickly, and it is common to doubt one's mental stability. Physical symptoms that commonly accompany grief are stomach pain, loss of appetite, intestinal upsets, sleep disturbance, and loss of energy. Existing chronic illnesses may worsen and new ones may appear. Over time, the impact of the loss is absorbed and the pain eases, but missing the presence of the lost loved one lingers.

The state of recovery or resolution following loss, thought to be the goal of grieving, is also being reconsidered. It seems that feelings of meaninglessness, painful memories, and anxiety persist for years after the loss in many people. Some degree of physiological disturbance is common among the bereaved: Sleeplessness, appetite loss, and lack of energy are common. Other symptoms include a hollow feeling in the stomach, heart palpitations, dizziness, tightness in the chest and throat, breathlessness, and muscle weakness. Furthermore, after a loved one dies, a survivor is more likely to become ill or die than others the survivor's age who have not experienced a recent loss. Experts think that grief may impair immune system function. Persistent elevated levels of stress hormones can reduce immunity, raise blood pressure and cholesterol, and induce abnormal heart rhythms. Survivors, especially widowers, commonly experience insomnia, changes in appetite and weight, increased consumption of alcohol and other drugs, and increased physician visits and hospital admissions.

My Wife Seems Gone Already

I sit vigil over the body in the bed, chin up, eyes at half-mast, breathing, rattling.

It won't be long, they tell me, until she is at peace.

She doesn't squeeze my hand, doesn't notice when I come and go.

She looks like my wife, she sometimes responds to my wife's name,

But my wife seems gone already.

I sit and remember our first kiss, when Jesse broke her arm, that big fight, our anniversary in Hawaii, how she looked putting on her stockings.

"You know how it is," she always said. "you win some, you lose some."

I know her, she'd tell a joke about now— about how long this is taking and whether we're getting our money's worth from those doctors and how young they all look.

I chuckle thinking of it, lean over to share it with her,

But she is silent.

I see her clothes in the closet, her shoes lined up, her make-up, and her jewelry.

I smell her smell.

Hang on, I want to say, I want to tell you something.

Wait, I want to cry, what will I do without you?

Stop! I want to scream. I am not ready!

Tears streaming down, I climb in next to her cool skin and sleep.

It is difficult to distinguish normal symptoms of grief from true clinical depression that should be treated. Some experts assert that early intervention for major depressive disorders should occur whether the person is grieving or not. Others advocate that treatment be instituted if symptoms persist beyond six months after the loss. Cultural background affects the interpretation of grief symptoms. What might be excessive grief in one subculture might be normal in another. If and when treatment is initiated, it may include psychotherapy alone or in combination with antidepressant medication.

It is commonly believed that an important part of the grieving process is the importance of emotional expression (e.g., crying and writing about the deceased). But recent research is calling this belief into question. It seems that "getting the feelings out" may not be helpful to everyone. Two studies on widows and widowers suggest that people who have difficulty sharing their feelings should not be pressured to do so because neither talking nor writing about the loss reduced distress of those widowed who were followed for a period of years.[17]

Assisting the Bereaved

Methods to assist the bereaved in coping with the death of a loved one vary depending on the situation and personality of both the helper and the bereaved. It is not uncommon for those approaching a newly bereaved person to be unsure how to act. Even though visits to the bereaved may be uncomfortable, friends should not avoid the bereaved or avoid discussion of the loss because of not knowing what to say. However, well-intentioned but thoughtless comments from friends and family may exacerbate the grief. In contrast, giving of your time to help, being a good listener, and sharing fond memories are more helpful (see Box 15.3).

Some physicians prescribe drugs to help individuals deal with grief, but others believe this practice may not be in the best interest of the mourner. Mild sedation when used shortly after the death of a loved one can relieve exhaustion and insomnia. However, some fear that sedatives can cause a grieving person to "miss out on" the support and rituals that surround the process after the death when family and friends offer intensive

---

B O X   1 5 . 3

Showing That You Care

If someone you care about has lost a loved one, there are many ways in which you can help:

- Be there. Your presence alone will serve to support the grieving person. Sit quietly when appropriate.
- Listen. Allow, even encourage, the grieving person to express feelings of loss and to share memories of the deceased.
- Express your sorrow. Don't be afraid to say the word *death* or to discuss the cause.
- Talk about special qualities of the deceased; relate a memorable anecdote about how the deceased impacted your life.
- Don't offer false comfort. "Don't question God's will," "Your wife is at peace," and "I know how you feel" are usually not helpful.

- Remind the bereaved of his or her strengths—resilience, patience, religious faith, optimism—that can help in coping with loss.
- Make yourself useful. Rather than asking, "How can I help?" make specific offers of assistance and follow through: Run errands, bring in food, and do yard work.
- Offer to take the person out of the house: Go out to eat, or take a walk.
- Stay in touch. Grief can last months or years, and often assistance offered later is more needed.
- Encourage professional help when it looks as though the individual is not coping.

support. These medications do not "cure" the emotion, but rather postpone it.

Resources are available for the bereaved but vary significantly among communities. Though seldom used by older people, psychotherapy can help the bereaved deal with their feelings and reminisce, and it can orient them to the future. Group therapy may be especially appropriate for widows and widowers, enabling them to deal with their grief and the problems of living alone while facilitating social interaction. Perhaps the most inexpensive, accessible programs for the bereaved that offer both social and psychological support are widowhood programs.

Most newly widowed persons have lost their most important social support base. A circle of supportive family and friends buffers the effects of losing a spouse. Self-help/support groups can supplement those natural networks. Some utilize volunteers who are also widowed to contact a recently bereaved person (from obituaries or funeral home referral) to provide psychological support. Other programs utilize social gatherings or discussion groups of widows or widowers led by a professional or a trained layperson. Many hospice programs offer bereavement programs.

Several types of resources for people who are dealing with the grief and the loss of a loved one are available on the Web. GriefNet.org lists almost 50 e-mail support groups. The AARP Web site www.AARP.org/griefandloss/ provides educational materials and online support on grief and loss. It also has a toll free grief support line (1-888-797-2277). MedlinePlus, www.nlm.nih.gov/medlineplus/bereavement.html, provides educational materials and Web links on bereavement.

SUMMARY

It is important to learn about dying, death, and grief when studying aging and health because death occurs more frequently among individuals who are aged 65 and older than among any other age group. Furthermore, elders are more likely than younger persons to have to confront the deaths of friends and loved ones. Modern technology allows the prolongation of life, but many ethical questions about euthanasia and the right to die accompany it.

The dying can choose to die in a hospital, at home, or in a nursing facility. The dying have certain rights, such as the right to full knowledge of their condition and treatment, and the right to the presence of supportive others. Furthermore, dying individuals have certain tasks to complete, such as finishing projects, planning funeral arrangements, and deciding on medical treatment.

Caring for the dying is physically and emotionally draining. Family and professional caretakers must cope with their own feelings while meeting the needs of the dying. Grief reactions are inevitable following the death of a loved one. Support groups and professional assistance are often available for those who need help in the grieving process.

ACTIVITIES

1. Download and fill out the advance directive forms for your state at www.caringinfo.org Who would you appoint as the proxy to make decisions on your behalf? Share this activity with your family members.

2. Have you signed an organ donor card and placed in your wallet? If not, would you be willing to be an organ donor? If you would like to sign an organ donor card, go to www.organdonor.gov Talk with your classmates and family members about your decision.

3. Would you be more likely to sign a living will to refuse treatment or to ask for heroic efforts? Give reasons for your choice. Discuss this issue with your family and friends.

4. Make a will stipulating what should be done with your body and your personal possessions after your death. Discuss this plan with your family and close friends.

5. Write your own funeral ceremony. Include poems, essays, religious scripture, and music. Would you prefer to be buried or cremated? Will the ceremony be public or private? Will you have pallbearers? If so, who? Whom would you want to attend your funeral?

6. Question your parents and friends to determine who has completed advance directives. Discuss with them the advantages of doing so.

7. If you were given six months to live and you knew your health would be failing considerably toward the end, what tasks would you wish to complete? What significant others would you like near you? Would you prefer to die in a hospital or at home? Why?

8. What services or programs in your community help bereaved elders (churches, senior organizations, funeral homes, hospitals)? How are the programs or services publicized? What is the cost?

9. Design an administrative policy for a hospital or nursing home on care for the dying. Outline goals, policies, and procedures to meet the social, psychological, and medical needs of the dying and their families.

10. Visit a local nursing home or hospital and question staff on their policies regarding the dying. Is there a special section for the terminally ill? Are patients told they are dying? Are there professionals or volunteers available who are trained to work specifically with the dying? How do other residents react to the death of an elder? What is the organization's policy on advance directives? How is a death in the facility handled?

11. Are there any circumstances in which assisted suicide would be a solution for you? Discuss them with the rest of the class.

12. Debate: Assisted suicide should be legalized in your state. Utilize the Web sites www.longwood.edu/ library/suiweb.htm and www.religioustolerance.org/ euthanas.htm

13. Visit a funeral home and crematorium. What are the costs ranges for various types of services? What kinds of strategies are used in the process of selling these items? What are the options in your community for someone who dies without any funds to pay for burial or cremation?

14. Find a form on the Internet for Physicians Orders for Life Sustaining Therapies. Review the form and how it is completed. Attempt to complete one for yourself or with a loved one. What did you find out about the process of discussing these issues with someone or thinking about them yourself?

BIBLIOGRAPHY

1. Kjellstrand, C.M. 1992. Who should decide about your death? *Journal of the American Medical Association* 267:103–104.

2. Levinsky, N.G., Yu, W., Ash, A., et al. 2001. Influence of age on Medicare expenditures and medical care in the last year of life. *Journal of the American Medical Association* 286(11):1349–1355.

3. Sabatino, C., and Kemp, N. 2011. Improving advanced illness care: The evolution of state POLST programs. Washington, DC: AARP Public Policy Institute. www.aarp.org/ppi

4. Jones, A.L., Moss, A.J., and Harris-Kojetin, L.D. 2011. Use of advance directives in long-term care populations. *NCHS Data Brief* 54, January 2011.

5. Emanuel, E.J., Fairclough, D.D., and Emanuel, L.L. 2001. Attitudes and desires related to euthanasia and physician-assisted suicide among terminally ill patients and their caregivers. *Journal of the American Medical Association* 284(19):2460–2468.

6. Ganzini, L., Goy, E.R., Miller, L.L., et al. 2003. Nurses' experiences with hospice patients who refuse food and fluids to hasten death. *New England Journal of Medicine* 349(4):325–326.

7. Quill, T.E., and Bock, I.R. 2000. Responding to intractable terminal suffering:: The role of terminal sedation and voluntary refusal of food and fluids. ACP-ASIM End of Life Care Consensus Panel. American College of Physicians-American Society of Internal Medicine. *Annals of Internal Medicine* 132(5):408–414.

8. Weitzen, S., Teno, J.M., Fennell, M., and Mor, V. 2003. Factors associated with site of death: A national study of where people die. *Medical Care* 41(2):323–335.

9. Stajduhar, K.I., Allan, D.E., Cohen, S.R., and Heyland, D.K. 2008. Preferences for location of death of seriously ill hospitalized patients: Perspectives from Canadian patients and their family caregivers. *Palliative Medicine* 22(1):85–88.

10. Lynn, J., Schuster, J., and Kabcenell, A. for the Center to Improve Care of the Dying and the Institute for Healthcare Improvement. 2000. *Improving care for the end of life: A sourcebook for clinicians and managers* New York: Oxford University Press.

11. Kübler-Ross, E. 1969. *On death and dying.* New York: Macmillan.

12. Schneidman, E. 1973. *Deaths of man.* New York: Quadrangle/New York Times, p. 7.

13. Corr, C.A. 1993. Coping with dying: Lessons that we should and should not learn from the work of Kübler-Ross. *Death Studies* 17:170–176.

14. Kalish, R.A. 1985. *Death, grief and caring relationships.* Monterey, CA: Brooks/Cole.

15. Butler, R.N., and Lewis, M.J. 1982. *Aging and mental health.* St. Louis: C.V. Mosby.

16. Covinsky, K.E., Fuller, J.D., Yaffe, K., Johnston, C.B., Hamel, M.B., Lynn, J., Teno, J.M., and Phillips, R.S. 2000. Communication and decision-making in seriously ill patients: Findings of the SUPPORT project. The Study to Understand Prognoses and Preferences for Outcomes and Risks of Treatments. *Journal of the American Geriatrics Society* 48(5 Suppl):S187–193.

17. Stroebe, M., Stroebe, W., Schut, H., Zech, E., and van den Bout, J. 2002. Does disclosure of emotions facilitate recovery from bereavement? Evidence from two prospective studies. *Journal of Consulting and Clinical Psychology* 70(1):169–178.

INDEX